An Instructor's Guided Tour of

Fit & Well

Core Concepts and Labs in Physical Fitness and Wellness

SECOND EDITION

by Thomas D. Fahey, Paul M. Insel, and Walton T. Roth

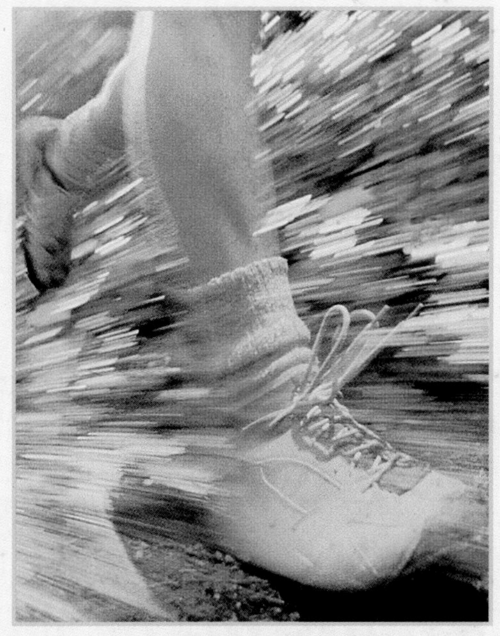

Please take a few minutes for this guided tour of the second edition of *Fit and Well*. You'll find examples of the book's outstanding features, writing, and pedagogy, as well as information about the comprehensive teaching package that accompanies the book.

Building on the success of the first edition, this edition continues to provide students with the knowledge, tools, and motivation they need to take charge of their wellness-related behavior. New features and refinements make *Fit and Well* an excellent choice for any fitness or wellness course. For a complete description of changes, see the annotated table of contents on pages ix–xix.

You already know that a lifestyle based on good choices and healthy behaviors maximizes quality of life. Let *Fit and Well* help you share that message with your students.

Fit . . .

Fit and Well provides accurate, up-to-date coverage of key concepts in physical fitness, including cardiorespiratory endurance, muscular strength and endurance, flexibility, and body composition. It also gives students the practical tools they need to create successful, individualized exercise programs. Author Thomas D. Fahey is an exercise physiologist, teacher, and author of numerous exercise science texts.

Illustrated Exercise Sections

To ensure that students exercise safely and effectively, *Fit and Well* includes full-color photographs showing proper technique for exercises and stretches that develop muscular strength and endurance, flexibility, and low-back health. This example from Chapter 4 illustrates how to perform back extensions on a weight machine.

EXERCISE 8

Low-Back Machine (Back Extensions)

Muscles developed: Erector spinae, quadratus lumborum

Instructions: **(a)** Sit on the seat with your upper legs under the thigh-support pads, your back on the back roller pad, and your feet on the platform. **(b)** Extend backward until your back is straight. Return to the starting position. Try to keep your spine rigid during the exercise.

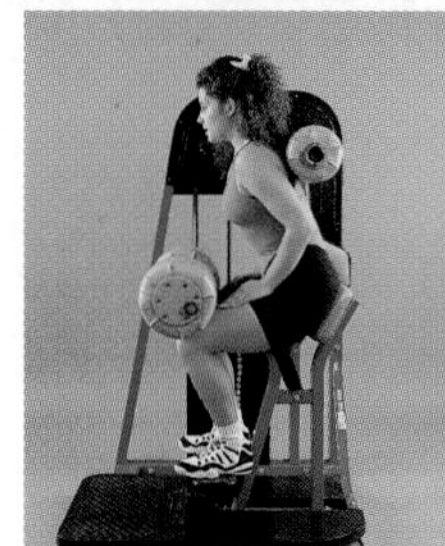

(a)

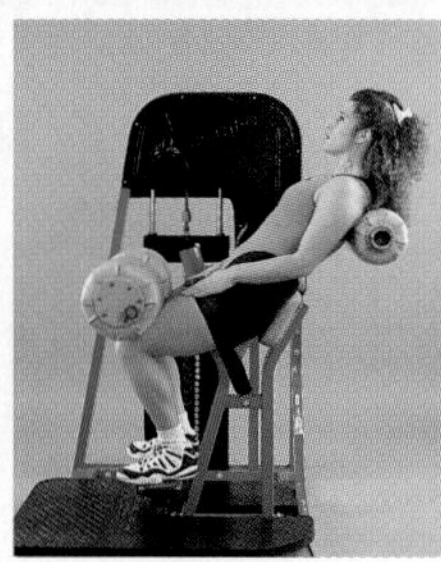

(b)

Sample Fitness Programs

To help students get started on a lifetime of regular exercise, Chapter 7 includes six complete sample programs built around popular cardiorespiratory endurance activities: walking/jogging/running, bicycling, and swimming. This page from the beginning walking program explains how to start a walking program and how to adjust intensity, duration, and frequency as fitness improves.

TABLE 7-2 Calorie Costs for Walking/Jogging/Running

This table gives the calorie costs of walking, jogging, and running for slow, moderate, and fast paces. Calculations for calorie costs are approximate and assume a level terrain. A hilly terrain would result in higher calorie cost. To get an estimate of the number of calories you burn, multiply your weight by the calories per minute per pound for the speed at which you're doing the activity (listed in the right-hand column), then multiply that by the number of minutes you exercise.

	Speed		
Activity	*Miles per Hour*	*Minutes: Seconds per Mile*	**Calories per Minute per Pound**
Walking			
Slow	2.0	30:00	.020
	2.5	24:00	.023
Moderate	3.0	20:00	.026
	3.5	17:08	.029
Fast	4.0	15:00	.037
	4.5	13:20	.048
Jogging			
Slow	5.0	12:00	.060
	5.5	11:00	.074
Moderate	6.0	10:00	.081
	6.5	9:00	.088
Fast	7.0	8:35	.092
	7.5	8:00	.099
Running			
Slow	8.5	7:00	.111
Moderate	9.0	6:40	.116
Fast	10.0	6:00	.129
	11.0	5:30	.141

Source: Kusinitz, I., and M. Fine. 1995. *Your Guide to Getting Fit*, 3d ed. Mountain View, Calif.: Mayfield.

your program. To select the variation that's best for you at your current fitness level, consult Table 7-3, p. 164.

VARIATION 1: Walking (Starting)

Intensity, duration, and frequency: Walk at first for 15 minutes at a pace that keeps your heart rate below your target zone. Gradually increase to 30-minute sessions. The distance you travel will probably be 1–2 miles. At the beginning, walk every other day. You can gradually increase to daily walking if you want to burn more calories (helpful if you want to change body composition).

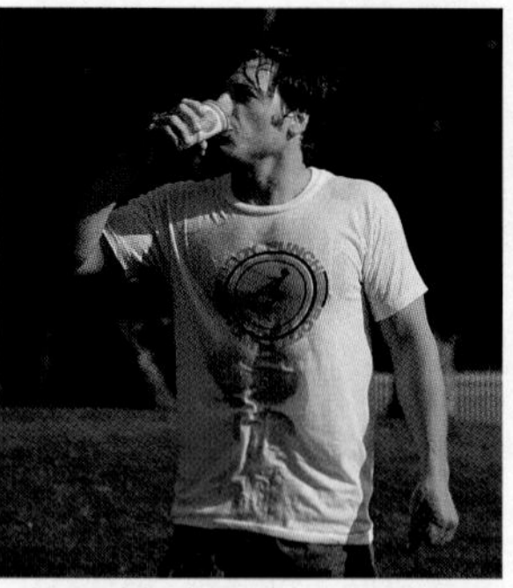

Drinking water before, during, and after exercise helps prevent dehydration from the loss of body fluids through perspiration. About 8 ounces of water or other fluid should be consumed for every 30 minutes of heavy exercise.

Calorie cost: Work up to using 90–135 calories in each session (see Table 7-2). To increase calorie costs to the target level, walk for a longer time or for a longer distance rather than sharply increasing speed.

At the beginning: Start at whatever level is most comfortable. Maintain a normal easy pace, and stop to rest as often as you need to. Never prolong a walk past the point of comfort. When walking with a friend (a good motivation), let a comfortable conversation be your guide to pace.

As you progress: Once your muscles have become adjusted to the exercise program, increase the duration of your sessions—but by no more than 10% each week. Increase your intensity only enough to keep your heart rate just below your target. When you're able to walk 1.5 miles in 30 minutes, using 90–135 calories per session, you should consider moving on to Variation 2 or 3. Don't be discouraged by lack of immediate progress, and don't try to speed things up by overdoing. Remember that pace and heart rate can vary with the terrain, the weather, and other factors.

Walking/Jogging/Running Sample Program 161

and Well

Fit and Well balances its coverage of physical fitness with a comprehensive, current discussion of other critical parts of a wellness lifestyle. Leading personal health textbook authors Paul M. Insel and Walton T. Roth provide students with the information they need to choose a nutritious diet; maintain a healthy body weight; manage stress effectively; avoid tobacco and other harmful drugs; and protect themselves from disease and injury.

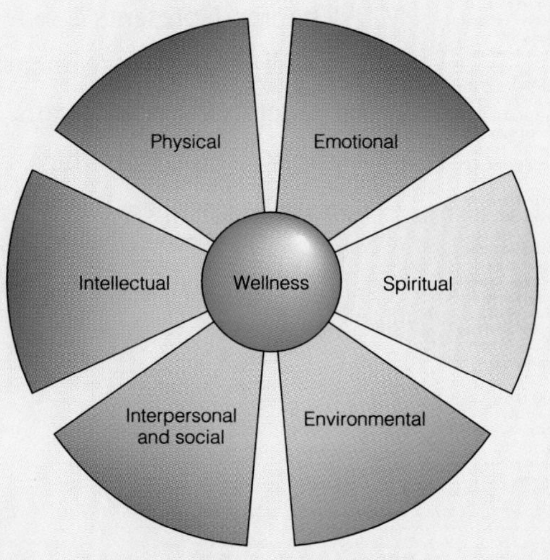

Balanced Coverage of Wellness

Fit and Well emphasizes wellness as a multidimensional concept. It explains to students that total wellness involves the balanced development of physical, emotional, intellectual, spiritual, interpersonal and social, and environmental wellness.

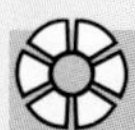

WELLNESS CONNECTION

Exercise, Mood, and Mental State

Many people report that exercise puts them in a better mood, but studies have also shown that exercise is an effective treatment for mild to moderate cases of depression. Researchers have found that exercise can be as effective as psychotherapy in treating depression, and even more effective when used in conjunction with conventional therapies. This is an important finding because major depression is a common condition among Americans; the estimated lifetime prevalence is about 5% for men and 10% for women. Although depression is a highly treatable condition, only about one-third of affected individuals seek professional help.

The ties among exercise and physical, emotional, and social wellness become clear when one looks at the variety of theories that have been proposed to explain exercise's antidepressant effects:

- Exercise provides a distraction from stressful stimuli.
- Exercise provides a way for people to gain mastery or control over their bodies and lives and enhance their self-esteem.
- Psychological benefits accompany the positive social interaction that can occur during exercise.
- Exercise causes an increase in the activity of certain brain chemicals, including dopamine, serotonin, and norepinephrine (low levels of these substances are linked to depression).

What type of exercise is most effective for treating depression? Cardiorespiratory endurance exercise seems to work the best. In a study of moderately depressed individuals, those involved in endurance training experienced a significant improvement in their condition, compared with individuals involved in a stretching program that did not include endurance exercise. Exercise recommendations for depressed people are similar to those given to the general population: a program of regular, moderate endurance exercise that is fun, convenient, and includes lots of opportunities for positive feedback.

How does exercise affect mood and depression levels in the rest of the population, those not suffering from clinical depression? Research indicates that exercise elevates mood in nondepressed people who feel fine or who feel a little bit "down." Physical fitness also seems to have a protective effect. National surveys suggest that sedentary adults have a much higher risk of feeling fatigue and depression than those who are physically active. A study of college students found that among those who were exposed to high levels of life stresses, the students who had low cardiorespiratory fitness subsequently developed more health problems and scored higher on tests measuring depression than those who were more fit.

The bottom line is that exercise is important for your emotional wellness—now and in the future. A program of regular exercise will enhance self-esteem and increase your feelings of well-being and vigor; it will decrease depression, anxiety, and the impact of stressful life events. Exercise is essential for the development of all aspects of wellness.

Sources: Nicoloff, G., and T. L. Schwenk. 1995. Using exercise to ward off depression. *Physician and Sportsmedicine* 23(9):44–58. Nieman, D. 1995. Physical activity and psychological health, in *Fitness and Sports Medicine: A Health-Related Approach.* Menlo Park, Calif.: Bull Publishing.

NEW! Wellness Connection Boxes

These boxes highlight important links among the different dimensions of wellness. They show how developing one dimension leads to changes in other dimensions. The Wellness Connection box from Chapter 3 shown here describes how exercise, in addition to developing physical wellness, can also improve emotional and social wellness.

Positive Choices

A Step-by-Step Guide to Behavior Change

Chapter 1 presents a six-step lifestyle management model that students can apply to behaviors they want to change.

TABLE 1-2 *Selected* Healthy People 2000 *Objectives*

Objective	Estimate of Current Status	Goal
Increase years of healthy life.	64 years	65 years
Increase the proportion of people age 6 and over who engage regularly, preferably daily, in light to moderate physical activity for at least 30 minutes per day.	24% (5 times/week) 17% (7 times/week)	30%
Increase the proportion of people age 18 and over wh... vigorous physical activity that promotes the developr... maintenance of cardiorespiratory fitness 3 or more d... for 20 or more minutes per occasion.	14%	20%
Increase the proportion of people age 6 and over wh... perform physical activities that enhance and maintair... strength, endurance, and flexibility.		
Reduce dietary fat intake.		
Increase the consumption of fruits and vegetables.		
Reduce the prevalence of overweight among people a...		
Reduce the proportion of people age 18 and over wh... adverse health effects from stress each year.		
Reduce deaths from coronary heart disease.		
Reverse the rise in cancer deaths to achieve a lower d...		
Reduce the prevalence of cigarette smoking among p... and over.		
Reduce the proportion of college students engaging i... occasions of heavy drinking of alcoholic beverages.		
Increase the proportion of sexually active, unmarried... used a condom at last sexual intercourse.		
Reduce the average amount of solid waste (garbage) ... each person each day.		
Increase the proportion of people who have a specific... ongoing primary care for coordination of their health...		
Increase the use of helmets by bicyclists.		

Sources: U.S. Department of Health and Human Services. 1... *Objectives.* Washington, D.C.: U.S. Government Printing Of... *Healthy People 2000 Review,* 1994. Hyattsville, Md.: Public H...

lives. Once you have the knowledge, motivatio... commitment, behavioral self-management techn... will give you the means to change your behavior.

Putting Together a Behavioral Self-Management Program

What follows is a self-management model that yo... apply to behaviors you want to change. The key t... cess in this six-step approach is to be both consiste... persistent. Don't skip steps or rush through. Yo...

1. *Monitor your behavior, and gather data.* Begin by isolating a **target behavior** that you wish to change. Concentrate on one behavior at a time; making even a few small changes in your life requires energy and effort. Once you've identified this behavior, keep track of when it occurs and the circumstances surrounding it. Keep your records in a health journal, a small notebook in which you record your observations and comments. Note exactly what the behavior was, when and where it happened, what you were doing, and what your thoughts and feelings were at the time.
   This record helps you identify and get information about the factors in your environment and in yourself that support your target behavior or make it difficult to resist. If your target behavior is eating too many candy bars, for example, you might note that the presence of candy in your home is a factor outside yourself—an environmental factor—that encourages you to indulge. Hunger or anxiety might be a factor within yourself—an internal factor—that also supports this behavior. (Examples of other behaviors a person might wish to change are smoking cigarettes, consuming too much caffeine or alcohol, and not wearing a seat belt or a bicycle helmet.)
   Keep your records for a week or two to get some solid information about the behavior you want to change. You can also use this period to gain information relating to your target behavior: How many calories are there in a candy bar? How much sugar, and how much fat? How does it compare nutritionally with other snacks? And how does it fit into a healthy diet?
2. *Examine the data, and identify patterns.* Now examine your records to discover patterns. When are you most likely to eat a candy bar? What events seem to trigger your desire for candy? What are you doing? Whom are you with? Note any connections between your feelings and environmental factors, such as time of day, location, and the actions of others around you.
3. *Set specific goals.* Whatever your ultimate goal, it's a good idea to break it down into a few small steps. Your plan will seem more manageable, increasing the likelihood that you will stick with it. Breaking it down into pieces will also give you milestones by which to measure your progress and opportunities to reward yourself for the progress you make. For example, if you want to eliminate candy from your diet, plan to work on one part of the day at a time. If you want to lower the fat in your diet by 15%, plan to lower it by 5% at a time. Take the easier steps first and work up to the harder ones.
4. *Make a personal contract.* Once you have set your goals, prepare a personal contract. A serious personal contract clearly states your objective and your commitment to reach it. You may include details of your plan, such as the date you'll begin and the date you expect to reach your final goal; the interim goals and the rewards you've established for reaching them; and the time and resources you've committed to the plan. It often helps to have another person witness the contract, especially someone whose help you're enlisting in the plan. A sample contract is included in Lab 1-2.
5. *Devise a plan of action, and put it into effect.* When you filled in your health journal, you gathered quite a lot of information about your target behavior. Now you can probably trace the chain of events that led to the behavior; you can probably also see points in the chain where other choices are possible. Begin to break this chain by making other choices. For example, if you buy candy bars when you take breaks while studying at the library, try studying in your room for a while. That may be enough to break the habit. For more ideas on interrupting habits, refer to the box "Breaking Behavior Chains."
6. *Keep track of your progress, and revise your plan if necessary.* Use your health journal to keep track of your progress. Record your daily activities and any relevant details. If you don't seem to be making progress, analyze your plan to see what might be causing the problem. Be ready to revise your plan if

TERMS

target behavior An isolated behavior selected as the basis for a behavior change program.

10 Chapter 1 Introduction to Fitness, Wellness, and Lifestyle Manage...

Laboratory Activities

To help students apply the principles of fitness, wellness, and behavior change to their own lives, *Fit and Well* includes 29 laboratory activities. These hands-on activities give students the opportunity to assess their current level of wellness, to create plans for changing their behavior to reach wellness, and to monitor their progress. The labs have a user-friendly format and are located on perforated pages at the ends of the chapters. In this sample lab from Chapter 7, students complete a contract for starting an exercise program.

Name ______________ **Section** ______________ **Date** ______________

LAB 7-1 *A Personal Fitness Program Plan and Contract*

A. I, ______________ (name), am contracting with myself to follow a physical fitness program to work toward the following goals:

1. ______________
2. ______________
3. ______________
4. ______________
5. ______________

B. My program plan is as follows:

Activities	Components (Check ✓) CRE	MS	ME	F	BC	Intensity*	Duration	Frequency (Check ✓) M	Tu	W	Th	F	Sa	Su

*You should conduct activities for achieving CRE goals at your target heart rate or RPE value.

C. My program will begin on ______________ (date). My program includes the following schedule of minigoals. For each step in my program, I will give myself the reward listed.

______________ (minigoal 1) ______________ (date) ______________ (reward)

______________ (minigoal 2) ______________ (date) ______________ (reward)

______________ (minigoal 3) ______________ (date) ______________ (reward)

______________ (minigoal 4) ______________ (date) ______________ (reward)

______________ (minigoal 5) ______________ (date) ______________ (reward)

LABORATORY ACTIVITIES

Lab 7-1 A Personal Fitness Program Plan and Contract 175

Positive Changes

NEW! Behavior Change Activities

These activities give students the opportunity to work through each step in a behavior change program in detail and to develop strategies for overcoming common obstacles to behavior change. This Behavior Change Activity from Chapter 10 helps students manage their time more effectively by showing them how to plan and set priorities.

BEHAVIOR CHANGE ACTIVITY

Managing Your Time Successfully

"Too little time" is a common excuse for not exercising or engaging in other healthy behaviors. Learning to manage your time successfully is crucial if you are to maintain a wellness lifestyle. The first step is to examine how you are currently spending your time. Use your health journal to track your current activities; use a grid broken into 15-, 20-, or 30-minute blocks. Next, list each category of activity and the total time you engaged in it on a given day on the chart below (for example, sleeping, 7 hours; eating, 1.5 hours; studying, 3 hours; working, 3 hours; and so on).

Take a close look at your list of activities. Successful time management is based on prioritization. Rank each of your activities according to how important it is to you: essential (A), somewhat important (B), or not important (C). Based on these priority rankings, make changes in your schedule by adding and subtracting hours from different categories of activities. Add your new activities to the list, and assign a priority and time period to each.

Activity	Current Total Duration	Priority	Goal Total Duration

Prioritizing in this manner will involve tradeoffs. For example, you may choose to reduce the amount of time you spend watching television, listening to music, and chatting on the telephone while you increase the amount of time you spend sleeping, studying, and exercising. Don't feel that you have to miss out on anything you enjoy. You can get more from less time by focusing on what you are doing. Strategies for managing time more productively and creatively include the following:

- *Schedule tasks for peak efficiency.* You've probably noticed that you're more productive at certain times of the day (or night). Schedule as many of your tasks for those hours as you can.
- *Avoid unnecessary distractions and interruptions.* Find a pleasant setting where you can focus on your current activity.
- *Listen actively and effectively.* Good communication can prevent misunderstandings and save time in the long run.
- *Set realistic goals.* Attainable goals will spur you on. Impossible goals, by definition, generate frustration and failure. Write down your goals, then fully commit yourself to achieving them.
- *Budget enough time.* For each project you undertake, calculate how long it will take to complete. Then add another 10–15% as a buffer against mistakes or unanticipated problems. If you wind up with extra free time, use it to do something you particularly enjoy.
- *Divide long-term goals into short-term ones.* Instead of waiting for or relying on large blocks of time, use short time periods to start a project or keep one going. For example, suppose you have a 50-page report due and are about to panic. Divide the assignment into three tasks: research, outlining, and writing. Then budget enough half-hour or hour-long time slots to complete each task. Steady progress will keep you encouraged and committed.
- *Visualize the achievement of your goals.* By mentally rehearsing your performance of a task, you can reach your goal more smoothly.

(continued)

NEW! STUDENT SUPPLEMENT
Daily Fitness Log

This easy-to-use booklet is available from Mayfield in a special shrinkwrapped package with the book at no additional cost to students. The *Daily Fitness Log* allows students to plan and track the progress of their fitness program for up to 40 weeks. The sample log shown here is for weight training exercises.

Weight Training Logs

Exercise/Date								
	Wt							
	Sets							
	Reps							
	Wt							
	Sets							
	Reps							
	Wt							
	Sets							
	Reps							
	Wt							
	Sets							
	Reps							
	Wt							
	Sets							
	Reps							
	Wt							
	Sets							
	Reps							
	Wt							
	Sets							
	Reps							
	Wt							
	Sets							
	Reps							
	Wt							
	Sets							
	Reps							
	Wt							
	Sets							
	Reps							
	Wt							
	Sets							
	Reps							
	Wt							
	Sets							
	Reps							

Weight Training Log

Complete lists of all Behavior Change Activities and Laboratory Activities can be found on pages xviii–xix in the table of contents. For instructors who want to make more extensive use of Laboratory Activities, an additional 42 labs, formatted for easy duplication, are included in the teaching package.

Building Lifelong Skills

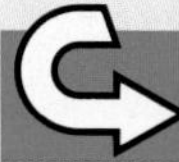

TACTICS AND TIPS

Keeping Your Fitness Program on Track

- Set realistic goals. Unrealistically high goals will only discourage you.
- Sign a contract, keep records of your activities, and track your progress.
- Start slowly, and increase intensity and duration gradually. Overzealous exercising can result in discouraging discomforts and injuries. Your program is meant to last a lifetime. The important first step is to break your established pattern of inactivity.
- Make your program fun. Participate in a variety of different activities that you enjoy. Vary the routes you take walking, running, or biking.
- Exercise with a friend. The social side of exercise is an important factor for many regular exercisers.
- Focus on the improvements you obtain from your program, how good you feel during and after exercise.
- If your program turns out to be unrealistic, revise it. Expect to make many adjustments in your program along the way.
- Expect fluctuation. On some days, your progress will be excellent, while on others, you'll barely be able to drag yourself through your scheduled activities.
- Expect lapses. Don't let them discourage you or make you feel guilty. Instead, feel a renewed commitment for your exercise program.
- Reward yourself often for sticking with your program.
- If you notice you're slacking off, try to list the negative thoughts and behaviors that are causing noncompliance. Devise a strategy to decrease the frequency of negative thoughts and behaviors. Make changes in your program plan and reward system to help renew your enthusiasm and commitment to your program.
- Review your goals. Visualize what it will be like to reach them, and keep these pictures in your mind as an incentive to stick to your program.

CRITICAL CONSUMER

Using Food Labels to Make Dietary Choices

Food labels are designed to help consumers make food choices based on the nutrients that are most important to good health. A food label states how much fat, saturated fat, cholesterol, protein, dietary fiber, and sodium the food contains. In addition to listing nutrient content by weight, the label puts the information in the context of a daily diet of 2000 calories that includes no more than 65 grams of fat (approximately 30% of total calories). For example, if a serving of a particular product has 13 grams of fat, the label will show that the serving represents 20% of the daily fat allowance. If your daily diet contains fewer or more than 2000 calories, you need to adjust these calculations accordingly. Refer to p. 184 for instructions on setting an appropriate limit on your fat intake.

Food labels contain uniform serving sizes. This means that if you look at different brands of salad dressing, for example, you can compare calories and fat content based on the serving amount. Regulations also require that foods meet strict definitions if their packaging includes the terms "light," "low-fat," or "high-fiber." Health claims such as "good source of dietary fiber" or "low in saturated fat" on packages are signals that those products can wisely be included in your diet. Overall, the food label is an important tool to help you choose a diet that conforms to the Food Guide Pyramid and the Dietary Guidelines.

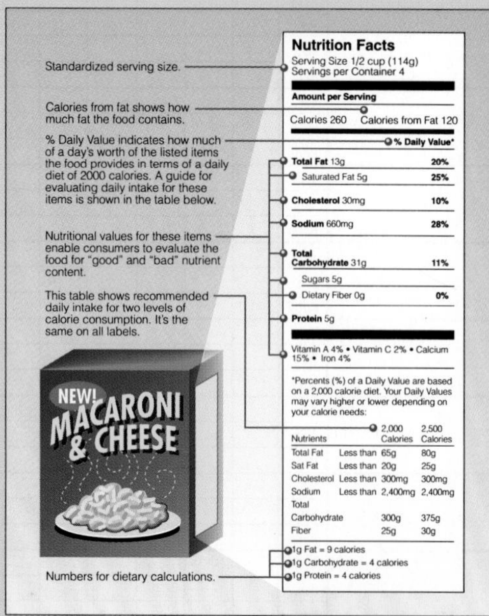

Standardized serving size.
Calories from fat shows how much fat the food contains.
% Daily Value indicates how much of a day's worth of the listed items the food provides in terms of a daily diet of 2000 calories. A guide for evaluating daily intake for these items is shown in the table below.
Nutritional values for these items enable consumers to evaluate the food for "good" and "bad" nutrient content.
This table shows recommended daily intake for two levels of calorie consumption. It's the same on all labels.
Numbers for dietary calculations.
NEW! MACARONI & CHEESE
Nutrition Facts
Serving Size 1/2 cup (114g)
Servings per Container 4
Amount per Serving
Calories 260 Calories from Fat 120
% Daily Value*
Total Fat 13g 20%
Saturated Fat 5g 25%
Cholesterol 30mg 10%
Sodium 660mg 28%
Total Carbohydrate 31g 11%
Sugars 5g
Dietary Fiber 0g 0%
Protein 5g
Vitamin A 4% • Vitamin C 2% • Calcium 15% • Iron 4%
*Percents (%) of a Daily Value are based on a 2,000 calorie diet. Your Daily Values may vary higher or lower depending on your calorie needs:
Nutrients 2,000 Calories 2,500 Calories
Total Fat Less than 65g 80g
Sat Fat Less than 20g 25g
Cholesterol Less than 300mg 300mg
Sodium Less than 2,400mg 2,400mg
Total Carbohydrate 300g 375g
Fiber 25g 30g
1g Fat = 9 calories
1g Carbohydrate = 4 calories
1g Protein = 4 calories

Tactics and Tips Boxes

These boxes present the practical advice students need to apply information from the text to their own lives. This example from Chapter 7 offers strategies for beginning and maintaining a successful fitness program.

NEW! Critical Consumer Boxes

These boxes are designed to help students develop and apply critical thinking skills, so they can make sound choices related to wellness. The Critical Consumer box from Chapter 8 shown here helps students learn to use food labels to make healthy dietary choices.

Assessments/Laboratory Activities

Many of the laboratory activities contain assessments that help students evaluate their current level of fitness and wellness. The lab activities also help students pinpoint lifestyle behaviors that they could change. In this lab from Chapter 5, students assess their level of flexibility in important joints.

Name ______________ **Section** ______________ **Date** ______________

LAB 5-1 *Assessing Your Current Level of Flexibility*

LABORATORY ACTIVITIES

Part 1. Sit-and-Reach Test

Equipment

A flexibility box or measuring device (see photograph). If you make your own measuring device, use two pieces of wood 12 inches high attached at right angles to each other. Use a ruler or yardstick to measure the extent of reach. Set the footline at 6 inches.

Preparation

Warm up your muscles with some low-intensity activity such as walking or easy jogging.

Instructions

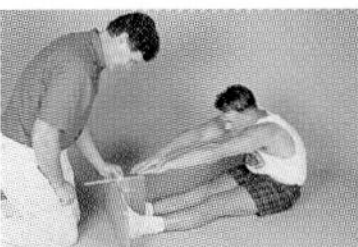

The sit-and-reach test.

1. Remove your shoes, and sit facing the flexibility box with your knees fully extended and your feet about 4 inches apart. Your feet should be flat against the box.
2. Reach as far forward as you can, with palms down and one hand placed on top of the other. Hold the position of maximum reach for 1–2 seconds. Keep your knees locked at all times.
3. Repeat the stretch two times. Your score is the most distant point reached with the fingertips of both hands on the third trial, measured to the nearest quarter of an inch.

Footline of your box: ____________ in. Score of third trial: ____________

Rating Your Flexibility

Find your score in the table below to determine your flexibility rating.

Rating: ____________

Ratings for Sit-and-Reach Test

	Rating/Score (in.)*			
Men	*Very Poor*	*Poor*	*Moderate*	*High*
Age: 15–19	Below 5.25	5.25–6.75	7.00–8.75	9.00–10.75
20–29	Below 5.50	5.50–7.00	7.25–8.75	9.00–11.00
30–39	Below 4.75	4.75–6.50	6.75–8.50	8.75–10.25
40–49	Below 2.75	2.75–5.00	5.25–6.75	7.00–9.25
50–59	Below 2.00	2.00–5.00	5.25–6.50	6.75–9.25
60 and over	Below 1.75	1.75–3.25	3.50–5.25	5.50–8.50
Women				
Age: 15–19	Below 7.25	7.25–8.75	9.00–10.50	10.75–12.25
20–29	Below 6.75	6.75–8.50	8.75–10.00	10.25–11.50
30–39	Below 6.50	6.50–8.00	8.25–9.50	9.75–11.50
40–49	Below 5.50	5.50–7.25	7.50–8.75	9.00–10.50
50–59	Below 5.50	5.50–7.25	7.50–8.50	8.75–10.75
60 and over	Below 4.75	4.75–6.00	6.25–7.75	8.00–9.25

*Footline is set at 6 inches.

Source: Adapted from Fitness Canada. 1986. *CSTF Operations Manual*, 3d ed. Ottowa: Fitness and Amateu
Fitness was developed by, and is reproduced with permission of, Fitness Canada, Government of Canada

Lab 5-1 Assessin

DIMENSIONS OF DIVERSITY

Fitness and Disability

Physical fitness and athletic achievement are not limited to the able-bodied. People with disabilities can also attain high levels of fitness and performance, as shown by the elite athletes who compete in the Paralympics. The premier event for athletes with disabilities, the Paralympics is held in the same year and city as the Olympics. The athletes who participate include people with cerebral palsy, people with visual impairments, paraplegics, quadriplegics, and others. They compete in wheelchair races and wheelchair basketball, tandem cycling, in which a blind cyclist pedals with a sighted athlete, and other events. The performance of these skilled athletes makes it clear that people with disabilities can be active, healthy, and extraordinarily fit.

Paralympians point out that able-bodied athletes and athletes with disabilities have two important things in common—both are striving for excellence, and both can serve as role models. One athlete commented, "I'd like to let kids who have a disability know there is a sports option. The possibilities are endless."

Currently, between 34 and 43 million Americans are estimated to have chronic, significant disabilities. Some disabilities are the result of injury, such as spinal cord injuries sustained in car crashes. Other disabilities result from illness, such as the blindness that sometimes occurs as a complication of diabetes or the joint stiffness that accompanies arthritis. And some disabilities are present at birth, as in the case of congenital limb deformities or cerebral palsy.

Exercise and physical activity are as important for people with disabilities as for able-bodied individuals—if not *more* important. Being active helps prevent secondary conditions that may result from prolonged inactivity, such as circulatory or muscular problems. It also provides an emotional boost that helps support a positive attitude.

People with disabilities don't have to be Olympians to participate in sports and lead an active life. Depending on the nature of the disability, numerous options exist, including tennis, basketball, cycling, swimming, and running. Some fitness centers offer modified aerobics, mild exercise in warm water, and other exercises adapted for people with disabilities.

For those who prefer to get their exercise at home, special aerobic workout videos are available. Most of these videos are produced by hospitals and health associations and are geared to specific disabilities. For example, the Arthritis Foundation produces two videos, at different levels, called "People with Arthritis Can Exercise." There are also workout videos designed especially for individuals with hearing impairments (instructors both speak and sign); for women who have had breast surgery and need to strengthen arm, shoulder, and back muscles; for people confined to wheelchairs; and many others. Some types are designed so that both able-bodied people and people with disabilities can participate.

If you want to try one of these videos or participate in some form of adapted physical activity, check with your physician about what's appropriate for you. Remember that no matter what your level of ability or disability, it's possible to make exercise an integral part of your life.

Sources: U.S. Department of Health and Human Services. 1990. *Healthy People 2000: National Health Promotion and Disease Prevention Objectives.* Washington, D.C.: U.S. Government Printing Office, DHHS Pub. (PHS) 91-50212. Silver, M. 1990. All the right moves. *U.S. News & World Report,* 12 November. Nemeth, M. 1992. Willing and able. *Maclean's,* 7 September.

NEW!
Dimensions of Diversity Boxes

To achieve wellness, students must be able to identify and overcome special challenges that they face because of who they are, either as individuals or as members of groups. Wellness-related differences among people can be related to both biological and cultural influences, such as gender, age, socioeconomic status, and race/ethnicity. Boxes with the Dimensions of Diversity label describe areas where individual and group differences are important for wellness, and they help students respond appropriately. This box from Chapter 2 describes the importance of exercise for people with disabilities.

Clear and Accessible

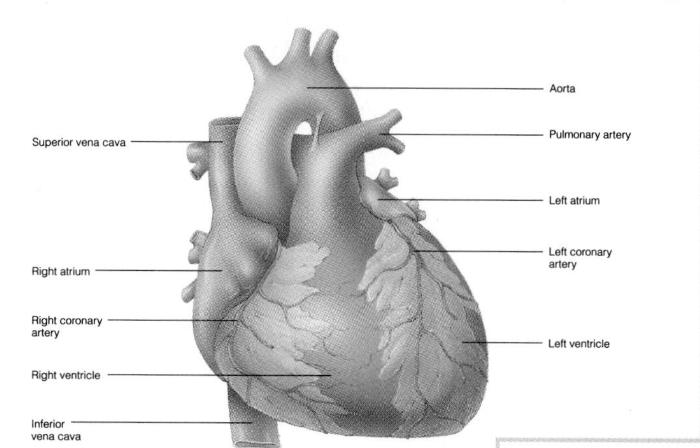

Figure 11-3 ***Blood supply to the heart.***

Major Risk Factors That Can Be Changed

The American Heart Association has identified four major risk factors for CVD that can be eliminated or controlled through lifestyle: tobacco use, high blood pressure, unhealthy blood cholesterol levels, and physical inactivity.

Tobacco Use Pack-a-day smokers have twice the heart attack risk of nonsmokers; smoking two or more packs daily triples the risk. And when smokers do have heart attacks, they are up to four times more likely than nonsmokers to die from them. Women who smoke and use oral contraceptives are up to 39 times more likely to have a heart attack and up to 22 times more likely to have a stroke than those who neither smoke nor take birth control pills.

Smoking has several harmful effects on the cardiovascular system. It can reduce levels of the "good" cholesterol in the bloodstream. Nicotine, the drug in tobacco, is a central nervous system stimulant that causes blood pressure and heart rate to rise. The carbon monoxide in cigarette smoke displaces oxygen in the blood, reducing the amount of oxygen available to the heart and other parts of the body. Cigarette smoking also causes the **platelets** in the blood to become sticky and cluster, thereby shortening platelet survival, decreasing clotting time, and thickening the blood. All these effects increase the risk of CVD.

It is not necessary to be effects of smoking. **Env (ETS)**—"secondhand sm has also been linked to the disease. Living or working riod can be a significant C

Regardless of how long who quit lower their risk o Ten years after quitting, a day or less has about the s has never smoked.

High Blood Pressure H **tension,** is a risk factor fo disease but is also consider blood pressure occurs whe flow of blood through the of blood from the heart. T the harder the heart has t ward. Over time, a straine enlarge, which weakens it sure also scars and harde elastic. Heart attacks, stro ney failure can result.

High blood pressure u signs, so yearly tests of b Diet, weight control, exerc

Colorful, Informative Illustrations

Innovative graphics and illustrations add visual appeal to the text and help students understand important concepts. This drawing of the heart from Chapter 11 shows students the importance of the coronary arteries in cardiovascular health and disease.

? COMMON QUESTIONS ANSWERED

How long must I weight train before I begin to see changes in my body? You will increase strength very rapidly during the early stages of a weight training program, primarily the result of muscle learning (the increased ability of the nervous system to recruit muscle fibers to exert force). Actual changes in muscle size usually begin after about 6–8 weeks of training.

I am concerned about my body composition. Will I gain weight if I do resistance exercises? Your weight probably will not change as a result of a recreational-type weight training program: 3 sets of 10 repetitions of 5–10 exercises. You will tend to increase lean body mass (muscle) and lose body fat, so your weight will stay about the same. (Men will tend to build larger muscles than women because of the tissue-building effects of male hormones.) Increased muscle mass will help you control body fat. Muscle increases your metabolism, which means you burn up more calories every day. If you combine resistance exercises with endurance exercises, you will be on your way to developing a lean, healthy-looking body. Concentrate on fat loss rather than weight loss.

Do I need more protein in my diet when I train with weights? No. While there is some evidence that power athletes involved in heavy training have a higher-than-normal protein requirement, there is no reason for most people to consume extra protein. Most Americans take in more protein than they need, so even if there is an increased protein need during heavy training, it is probably supplied by the average diet.

Are there any supplements or drugs that will help me gain larger and more rapid increases in strength and endurance? No nutritional supplement or drug will change a weak, untrained person into a strong, fit person. Those changes require regular training. Supplements or drugs that are promoted as instant or quick "cures" usually don't work and are either dangerous or expensive, or both. **Anabolic steroids**—the drugs most often taken in an effort to build strength and power—have dangerous side effects, described in the box "Effects of Anabolic Steroids." You are better off staying with proven principles of nutrition and a steady, progressive fitness program.

What causes muscle soreness the day or two following a weight training workout? The muscle pain you feel a day or two after a heavy weight training workout is caused by injury to the muscle fibers and surrounding connective tissue. Contrary to popular belief, delayed-onset muscle soreness is not caused by lactic acid buildup. Scientists believe that injury to muscle fibers causes the release of excess calcium into muscles. The calcium causes the release of substances called **proteases,** which break down part of the muscle tissue and cause pain. After a bout of intense exercise that causes muscle injury and delayed-onset muscle soreness, the muscles produce protective proteins that prevent soreness during future workouts. If you don't work out regularly, you lose these protective proteins and become susceptible to muscle soreness again.

Are there any special exercises I can do to improve speed and power for sports? Plyometric exercises are particularly beneficial for developing speed and power. Also, when performing weight-lifting exercises, try to lift the weights explosively. This will help increase speed and power for sports.

Will I improve faster if I train every day? No. Your muscles need time to recover between training sessions. Doing resistance exercises every day will cause you to become overtrained, which will increase your chance of injury and impede your progress.

If I stop weight training, will my muscles turn to fat? No. Fat and muscle are two different kinds of tissue, and one cannot turn into the other. Muscles that aren't used become smaller (atrophy), and body fat may increase if caloric intake exceeds calories burned. Although the result of inactivity may be smaller muscles and more fat, the change is caused by two separate processes.

TERMS

anabolic steroids Synthetic male hormones taken to enhance athletic performance and body composition.

proteases Enzymes that break down proteins.

SUMMARY

- Improvements in muscular strength and endurance lead to enhanced physical performance, protection against injury, improved body composition, better self-image, and improved muscle and bone health with aging.
- Muscular fitness is particularly important in preventing low-back pain and raising metabolic rates.
- Muscular strength can be assessed by determining the amount of weight that can be lifted in one repetition of an exercise; muscular endurance can be assessed by determining the number of repetitions of a particular exercise that can be performed.
- Hypertrophy, increased muscle fiber size, occurs when weight training causes the number of myofibrils to increase; total muscle size thereby increases. Strength also increases through muscle learning.
- Isometric exercises (contraction without movement) are most useful when a person is recovering from an injury or surgery or needs to overcome weak points in a range of motion.

Common Questions Answered

Sections labeled Common Questions Answered address practical concerns of special interest to students. Expanded for the second edition, these sections now appear in Chapters 2 through 14. This Common Questions Answered section from Chapter 4 addresses students' questions and concerns about weight training, including issues of body composition, muscle soreness, and training frequency.

Running Glossary

Important new terms appear in boldface type in the text and are defined in a running glossary on the same page.

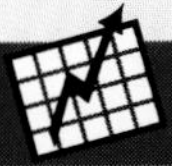

VITAL STATISTICS

TABLE 1-1 Ten Leading Causes of Death in the United States

Rank	Cause of Death	Number	Percent of Total Deaths	Lifestyle Factors
1	Heart disease	734,090	32.1	I D S
2	Cancer	536,866	23.4	I D S A
3	Stroke	154,350	6.7	I D S
4	Chronic obstructive lung disease	101,870	4.5	S
5	Accidents	90,140	3.9	S A
	(Motor vehicle)	(40,735)	(1.8)	
	(All others)	(49,415)	(2.1)	
6	Pneumonia and influenza	82,090	3.6	S
7	Diabetes mellitus	55,390	2.4	I D
8	HIV infection	41,930	1.8	
9	Suicide	32,410	1.4	A
10	Chronic liver disease and cirrhosis	25,730	1.1	A
	All causes	2,286,000	100.0	

Key: I Cause of death in which an inactive lifestyle plays a part.
D Cause of death in which diet plays a part.
S Cause of death in which smoking plays a part.
A Cause of death in which exc

Estimated data for 1995.

Source: National Center for Health Statist

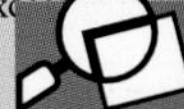

A CLOSER LOOK

Exercise Machines Versus Free Weights

Exercise Machines

Advantages

- Safe
- Convenient
- Don't require spotters
- Provide variable resistance
- Require less skill
- Make it easy to move from one exercise to the next
- Allow easy isolation of individual muscle groups

Disadvantages

- Limited availability
- Inappropriate for performing dynamic movements
- Allow a limited number of exercises

Free Weights

Advantages

- Allow dynamic movements
- Allow the user to develop control of the weights
- Allow a greater variety of exercises
- Widely available
- Truer to real-life situations; strength transfers to daily activities

Disadvantages

- Not as safe
- Require spotters
- Require more skill
- Cause more blisters and calluses

Vital Statistics Tables and Figures

Tables and figures marked with the Vital Statistics icon display information in a highly accessible format, helping students grasp important concepts quickly. This Vital Statistics table from Chapter 1 lists the ten leading causes of death among Americans and clearly links them with controllable lifestyle factors.

Box Program

Fit and Well has five different types of boxes, all aimed at highlighting areas of particular interest and importance to students. The five box types are Tactics and Tips, Critical Consumer, Wellness Connection, Dimensions of Diversity—all described earlier—and A Closer Look. This A Closer Look box from Chapter 4 describes the advantages and disadvantages of exercise machines versus free weights.

Custom Teaching Package

Available with *Fit and Well* is a comprehensive teaching and learning package that will help both you and your students succeed.

Instructor's Resource Binder

The binder contains nearly everything you will need to teach your course:

- An *Instructor's Manual* with extended chapter outlines and objectives; lists of additional resources including videos, software, and other multimedia; and a summary of the transparencies and labs
- A *Test Item File* containing over 1,000 questions, about 65 per chapter
- 42 *Additional Laboratory Activities,* formatted for easy duplication
- 64 *Transparency Masters*

Transparency Acetates

Fifty transparency acetates, half in color, are included to help you teach the course. The acetates do *not* duplicate the Transparency Masters in the Instructor's Resource Binder.

Computerized Test Bank

Microtest III, developed by Chariot Software Group, allows you to design tests using the test questions included with *Fit and Well* and/or to incorporate your own questions. Microtest is available in both Windows and Macintosh formats.

Fit and Well Lab Software

Labs are included in this software package for students. Self-assessment and fitness test results can be calculated and printed out. This disk can be shrinkwrapped with the text for an additional $3.

Daily Fitness Log

This 48-page booklet will help students track their fitness progress. The booklet is free when shrinkwrapped with the text.

Videos, Software, and other Multimedia

Videos and other multimedia—including software on nutrition, menu planning, and fitness—are available to qualified adopters.

If you have any questions concerning the teaching package, please call your local Mayfield sales representative or our Marketing and Sales Department at 800-433-1279.

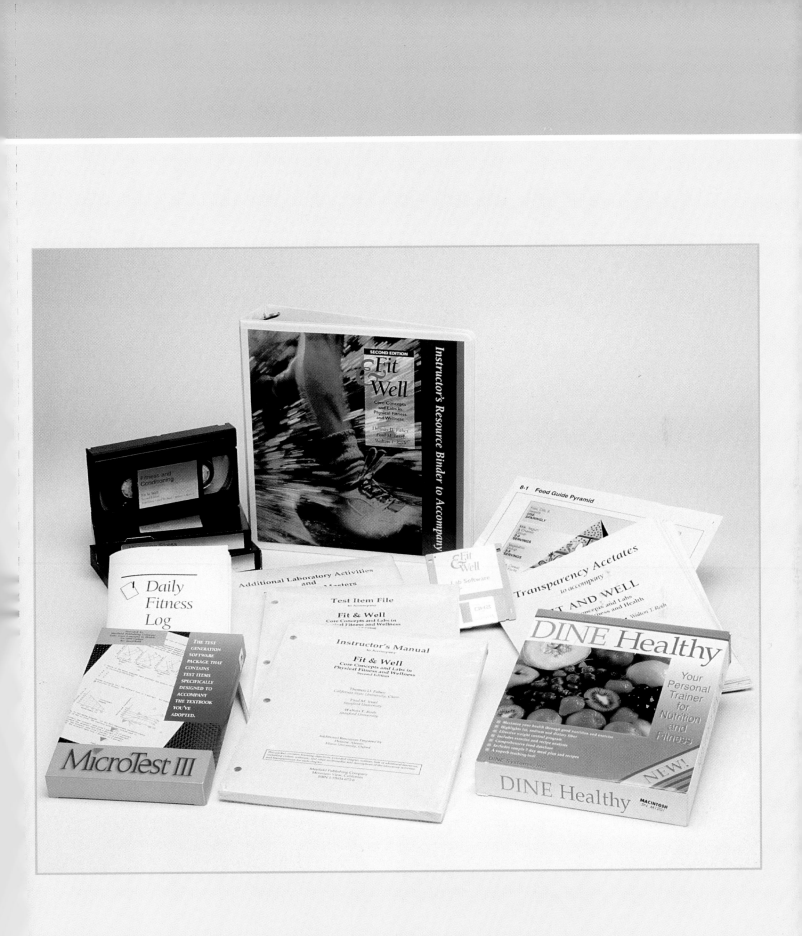

Instructor's Resource Binder to Accompany
SECOND EDITION
Fit & Well
Core Concepts and Labs in Physical Fitness and Wellness
Fitness and Conditioning
8-1 Food Guide Pyramid
Fit & Well
Lab Software
Transparency Acetates
to accompany
Daily Fitness Log
Additional Laboratory Activities and
Test Item File
Fit & Well
Instructor's Manual
to Accompany
Fit & Well
Core Concepts and Labs in Physical Fitness and Wellness
Second Edition
THE TEST GENERATION SOFTWARE PACKAGE THAT CONTAINS TEST ITEMS SPECIFICALLY DESIGNED TO ACCOMPANY THE TEXTBOOK YOU'VE ADOPTED.
MicroTest III
DINE Healthy
Your Personal Trainer for Nutrition and Fitness
NEW!
DINE Healthy
MACINTOSH

Fit and Well

Core Concepts and Labs in Physical Fitness and Wellness

SECOND EDITION

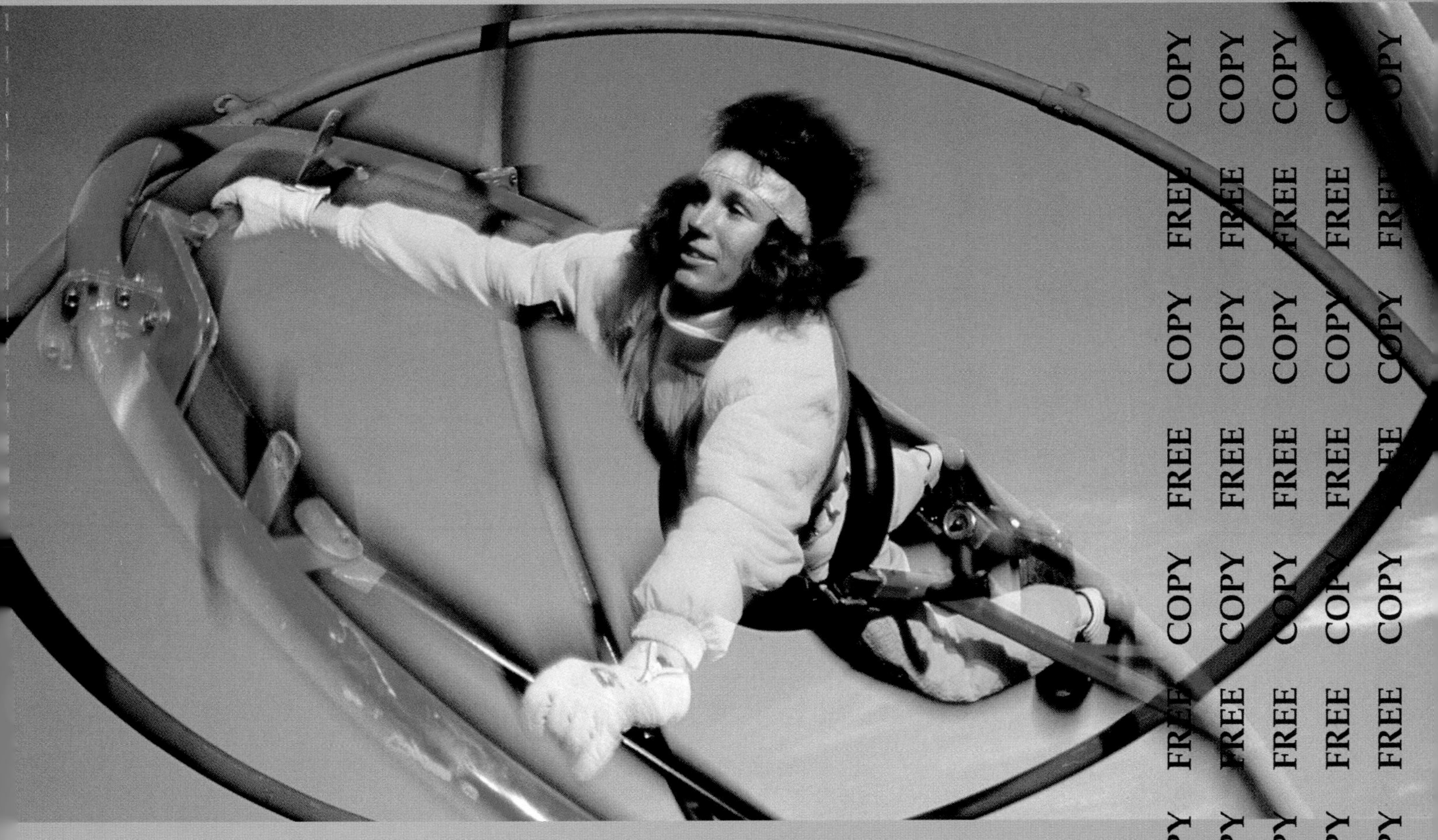

Thomas D. Fahey
California State University, Chico

Paul M. Insel • Walton T. Roth
Stanford University

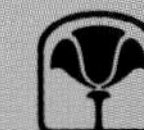

Mayfield Publishing Company
Mountain View, California
London • Toronto

Library of Congress Cataloging-in-Publication Data
Fahey, Thomas D. (Thomas Davin)
Fit and well: core concepts and labs in physical fitness and wellness / Thomas D. Fahey, Paul M. Insel, Walton T. Roth. — 2nd ed.
p. cm.
Includes index.
ISBN 1-55934-672-8
1. Physical fitness. 2. Health. I. Insel, Paul M. II. Roth, Walton T. III. Title.
GV481.F26 1996
613.7′043—dc20 96–6863
CIP

Manufactured in the United States of America
10 9 8 7 6 5 4 3 2 1

Mayfield Publishing Company
1280 Villa Street
Mountain View, California 94041

Sponsoring editor, Serina Beauparlant; *developmental editors,* Kirstan Price and Kathleen Engelberg; *production editor,* Lynn Rabin Bauer; *manuscript editor,* Betsy Dilernia; *art director and cover designer,* Jeanne M. Schreiber; *text designer,* Detta Penna; *art manager,* Jean Mailander; *illustrators,* Willa Bower, Dale Glasgow and Associates, Judith Ogus, Kevin Somerville, Pamela Drury Wattenmaker; *photo researchers,* Brian Pecko and Melissa Kreischer; *manufacturing manager,* Randy Hurst. This text was set in 10.5/12 Berkeley Book by GTS Graphics and printed on 45# Chromatone LG by Banta Company.

Text Credits

Pages 44, 94, 95, 98, 100, 149: Based on norms from The Physical Fitness Specialist Manual, The Cooper Institute for Aerobics Research, Dallas, Texas, revised 1996; used with permission.

Page 227, Critical Consumer box: Reprinted from June 1994 *Mayo Clinic Health Letter* with permission of Mayo Foundation for Medical Education and Research, Rochester, Minnesota 55905. For subscription information, call 1-800-333-9037.

Page 265, Wellness Connection box: From *Anger Kills* by Dr. Redford Williams. Copyright © 1993 by Dr. Redford Williams. Reprinted by permission of Times Books, a division of Random House, Inc.

Page 354, Wellness Connection box: Adapted from *Mental Medicine Update: The Mind/Body Health Newsletter,* Winter 1993 (Center for Health Sciences, P.O. Box 381069, Cambridge, MA 02238-1069, 1-800-222-4745).

Photo Credits

Cover © Gary Nolton/Tony Stone Images

Title Page © Peter Ginter/The Image Bank

Chapter 1 p. 1, © Jeff Greenberg/The Picture Cube, Inc.; p. 6, © Sam Forencich; p. 13, © David Madison 1995

Chapter 2 p. 19, © David Madison; p. 20, © Jon Feingersh/The Stock Market; p. 25, © David Madison

Chapter 3 p. 37, © David Stoecklein/The Stock Market; p. 39, © David Madison 1992; p. 49, © Bob Daemmrich/Stock Boston; exercise photos on pp. 44, 60, courtesy Shirlee Stevens

Chapter 4 p. 65, © Pedro Coll/The Stock Market; pp. 93, 94, photos furnished by Universal Gym Equipment, Inc., Cedar Rapids, Iowa; exercise photos on pp. 70, 71, 75, 80 (top), 82 (bottom), 83, 84 (bottom), 86 (bottom), 87 (bottom), 89 (top), 95, 97, 98, 99, courtesy Neil A. Tanner; exercise photos on pp. 80 (bottom), 81, 82 (top), 84 (top), 85, 86 (top), 87 (top), 88, 89 (bottom), courtesy Shirlee Stevens

Chapter 5 p. 103, © David Madison 1991; exercise photos on pp. 107, 108, 109, 110 (bottom), 111, 112 (top), 116, 117, 118 (top), 123, courtesy Shirlee Stevens; exercise photos on pp. 110 (top and middle), 112 (bottom), 115, 118 (bottom), 124, courtesy Neil A. Tanner

Chapter 6 p. 131, © David Madison; p. 138, © David Madison; exercise photos on pp. 136, 146, courtesy Shirlee Stevens

Chapter 7 p. 153, © David Madison; p. 154, © David Madison; p. 158, © Linda Musick/Photo 20-20; p. 161, © David Madison

Chapter 8 p. 179, © Mark Antman/The Image Works; p. 187, © L. Dardelet/Explorer/Photo Researchers, Inc.; p. 198, © Bob Daemmrich/Stock Boston

Chapter 9 p. 217, © David Madison; p. 221, © Alán Gallegos; p. 223, © Karen Preuss/The Image Works; p. 226, © Jonathan A. Meyers/JAM Photography

Chapter 10 p. 239, © Tony Savino/The Image Works; p. 242, © Bob Daemmrich/Stock Boston; p. 245, © Tony Freeman/PhotoEdit; p. 246, © Bonnie Kamin

Chapter 11 p. 257, © Matthew McVay/Stock Boston; p. 261, © J. Griffin/The Image Works; p. 264, © Alán Gallegos; p. 270, © David Madison

Chapter 12 p. 277, © Cecil Fox/Science Source/Photo Researchers, Inc.; p. 279, © Kindra Clineff/The Picture Cube, Inc.; p. 286, © David Austen/Stock Boston; p. 293, © Blair Seitz/Photo Researchers, Inc.

Chapter 13 p. 299, © Bob Daemmrich/The Image Works; p. 302, © Richard Elkins/Gamma Liaison; p. 307, © Stacy Pick/Stock Boston; p. 311, © Owen Franken/Stock Boston

Chapter 14 p. 327, © Mark Phillips/Photo Researchers, Inc.; p. 332, © Jonathan Meyers/JAM Photography; p. 337, © Esbin-Anderson/Photo 20-20; p. 339, © David R. Frazier/Photo Researchers, Inc.

Chapter 15 p. 347, © Linda Musick/Photo 20-20; p. 348, © Joseph Gianetti/Stock Boston; p. 353, © Alán Gallegos; p. 359, © Tom and Pat Leeson/Photo Researchers, Inc.

Preface

For today's fitness-conscious student, *Fit and Well* combines the best of two worlds. In the area of physical fitness, *Fit and Well* offers expert knowledge based on the latest findings in exercise physiology and sports medicine, along with tools for self-assessment and guidelines for becoming fit. In the area of wellness, it offers accurate, current information on today's most important health-related topics and issues, again with self-tests and guidelines for achieving wellness. To create this book, we have drawn on our combined expertise and experience in exercise physiology, athletic training, personal health, scientific research, and teaching.

OUR AIMS

Our aims in writing this book can be stated simply:

- To show students that becoming fit and well greatly improves the quality of their lives
- To show students how they can become fit and well
- To motivate students to make healthy choices and to provide them with tools for change

The first of these aims means helping students see how their lives can be enhanced by a fit and well lifestyle. This book offers convincing evidence of a simple truth: To look and feel our best, to protect ourselves from degenerative diseases, and to enjoy the highest quality of life, we need to place fitness and wellness among our top priorities. *Fit and Well* makes clear both the imprudence of our modern, sedentary lifestyle and the benefits of a wellness lifestyle.

Our second aim is to give students the tools and information they need to become fit and well. This book provides students with everything they need to create their own personal fitness programs, including instructions for fitness tests, explanations of the components of fitness and guidelines for developing them, descriptions and illustrations of exercises, model programs, and so on. In addition, *Fit and Well* provides accurate, up-to-date, scientifically based information about the most important topics in wellness, including nutrition, weight management, stress, cardiovascular health, cancer, drugs, alcohol, STDs, and a multitude of others.

In providing this material, we have pooled our efforts. Thomas Fahey has contributed his knowledge as an exercise physiologist, teacher, and author of numerous exercise science textbooks. Paul M. Insel and Walton T. Roth have contributed their knowledge of current topics in health as the authors of the leading personal health textbook, *Core Concepts in Health.*

Because we know this expert knowledge can be overwhelming, we have balanced the coverage of complex topics with student-friendly features designed to make the book accessible. Written in a straightforward, easy-to-read style and presented in a colorful, open format, *Fit and Well* invites the student to read, learn, and remember. Boxes, labs, tables, figures, artwork, photographs, and other features add interest to the text and highlight areas of special importance.

Our third aim is to involve students in taking responsibility for their health. *Fit and Well* makes use of interactive features to get students thinking about their own levels of physical fitness and wellness. We offer students assessment tools and laboratory activities to evaluate themselves in terms of each component of physical fitness and each major health area, ranging from cardiorespiratory endurance and muscular strength to heart disease, cancer, and STDs.

We also show students how they can make difficult lifestyle changes by using the principles of behavioral self-management. Chapter 1 contains a step-by-step description of this simple but powerful tool for change. The chapter not only explains the six-step process but also offers a wealth of tips for ensuring success. Behavior management aids, including personal contracts, behavior checklists, and self-tests, appear throughout the book. *Fit and Well's* combined emphasis on self-assessment, self-development in each area of wellness, and behavioral self-management ensures that students not only are inspired to become fit and well but also have the tools to do so.

When students use these tools to make significant lifestyle changes, they begin to realize that they are in charge of their health—and their lives. From this realization comes a sense of competence and personal power. Perhaps our overriding aim in writing *Fit and Well* is to convey the fact that virtually everyone has the ability to understand, monitor, and make changes in his or her own level of fitness and wellness. By making healthy choices from an early age, individuals can minimize the amount of professional medical care they will ever require. Our hope is that *Fit and Well* will help people make this exciting discovery—that they have the power to shape their own futures.

CONTENT AND ORGANIZATION OF THE SECOND EDITION

The basic content of *Fit and Well* remains unchanged in the second edition. Chapter 1 provides an introduction to fitness and wellness and explains the principles of behavioral self-management. Chapters 2–7 focus on the various areas of physical fitness. Chapter 2 provides an overview, discussing the five components of fitness, the principles of physical training, and the factors involved in designing a well-rounded, personalized exercise program. Chapter 3 addresses the most important component of fitness—cardiorespiratory endurance—and discusses the elements of a successful cardiorespiratory fitness program. Chapters 4, 5, and 6 look at muscular strength and endurance, flexibility, and body composition, respectively. Chapter 7 "puts it all together," describing the nature of a complete fitness program that develops all the components of fitness. This chapter also includes several sample exercise programs for developing overall fitness.

Chapters 8, 9, and 10 treat three important areas of wellness promotion: nutrition, weight management, and stress management, respectively. It is in these areas that individuals have some of the greatest opportunities for positive change. Chapters 11 and 12 focus on two of the most important reasons for making lifestyle changes: cardiovascular disease and cancer. Students learn the basic mechanisms of these diseases, how they are related to lifestyle, and what individuals can do to prevent them. Chapters 13 and 14 focus on other important wellness issues—the use and abuse of tobacco, alcohol, and other drugs (Chapter 13) and sexually transmissible diseases (Chapter 14). Finally, Chapter 15 looks at four additional wellness topics: intimate relationships, aging, using the health care system, and environmental health.

For the second edition, each chapter was carefully reviewed, revised, and updated. The latest information from scientific and wellness-related research is incorporated in the text, and newly emerging topics are discussed. The following list gives a sample of some of the new and updated material included in the second edition of *Fit and Well:*

- The 1995 edition of the Dietary Guidelines for Americans
- Exercise recommendations from the American College of Sports Medicine and the Centers for Disease Control and Prevention
- Emotional and psychological benefits of exercise
- Binge drinking among college students
- Aging
- The role of exercise in preventing osteoporosis and osteoporosis-related injuries
- *Healthy People 2000* objectives and our progress toward achieving them
- Smokeless tobacco
- The role of exercise and diet in preventing and managing diabetes
- The relationships between diet and cancer
- Stress-management techniques
- Genetics and weight management

In addition to these specific topic areas, four important themes of the first edition of *Fit and Well* receive increased attention throughout the second edition: total wellness, diversity, behavior management, and critical thinking.

Research in the areas of health and wellness is ongoing, with new discoveries, advances, trends, and theories reported nearly every week. For this reason, no wellness book can claim to have the final word on every topic. Yet within these limits, *Fit and Well* does present the latest available information and scientific thinking on important wellness topics. Taken together, the chapters of the book provide students with a complete, up-to-date guide to maximizing their well-being, now and through their entire lives.

FEATURES OF THE SECOND EDITION

This edition of *Fit and Well* builds on the features that attracted and held our readers' interest in the first edition. These features are designed to help students increase their understanding of the key concepts of wellness and to make better use of the book.

Laboratory Activities

To help students apply the principles of fitness and wellness to their own lives, *Fit and Well* includes **laboratory activities** for classroom use. These hands-on activities give students the opportunity to assess their current level of fitness and wellness, to create plans for changing their lifestyle to reach wellness, and to monitor their progress. They can assess their level of cardiorespiratory endurance, for example, or their daily energy balance; they can design a program to improve muscular strength or meet weight loss goals; they can explore their risk of developing cardiovascular disease or cancer; and they can examine their attitudes and behaviors in relation to drug use and STDs. For the second edition, labs have been placed at the end of each chapter; they are perforated for easy use.

Illustrated Exercise Sections

To ensure that students understand how to perform important exercises and stretches, *Fit and Well* includes three separate **illustrated exercise sections,** one in Chapter 4 and two in Chapter 5. The section in Chapter 4 covers a total of 20 exercises for developing muscular strength and endurance, as performed both with free weights and on Nautilus equipment. One section in Chapter 5 presents 12 stretches for flexibility, and the other presents 10 exercises to stretch and strengthen the lower back. Each exercise is illustrated with one or more full-color photographs showing proper technique.

Sample Programs

To help students get started, Chapter 7 offers six complete **sample programs** designed to develop overall fitness. The programs are built around popular cardiorespiratory endurance activities: bicycling, swimming, and walking/jogging/running; they also include weight training and stretching exercises. Each one includes detailed information and guidelines on equipment and technique; target intensity, duration, and frequency; recommended time spent warming up and cooling down; calorie cost of the activity; record keeping; and adjustments to make as fitness improves. The chapter also includes general guidelines for putting together a personal fitness program—setting goals; selecting activities; setting targets for intensity, duration, and frequency; making and maintaining a commitment; and recording and assessing progress.

Boxes

Boxes are used in *Fit and Well* to explore a wide range of current topics in greater detail than is possible in the text itself. Boxes fall into five different categories, each marked with a special icon and label. Three of the box categories are new to *Fit and Well:* Wellness Connection, Dimensions of Diversity, and Critical Consumer. The boxes in these new categories focus on important themes of the second edition.

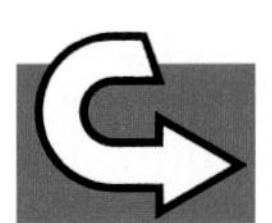

Tactics and Tips boxes distill from the text the practical advice students need to apply information to their own lives. By referring to these boxes, students can easily find information about such topics as proper running technique, preventing athletic injuries, exercising in hot weather, proper weight training technique, bicycling safety, reducing fat in the diet, responsible drinking behavior, preventing and treating STDs, and many others.

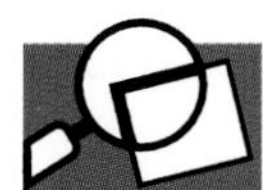

A Closer Look boxes highlight current topics and issues of particular interest to students. These boxes focus on such topics as anabolic steroids, exercise machines versus free weights, diabetes, eating disorders, health implications of obesity, sleep, osteoporosis, and many others.

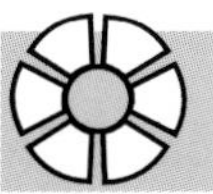

Wellness Connection boxes are a key part of the second edition's increased emphasis on the theme of total wellness. These boxes highlight important links among the different dimensions of wellness—physical, emotional, social/interpersonal, intellectual, spiritual, and environmental—and emphasize that all the dimensions must be developed in order for an individual to achieve optimal health and well-being. Included in Wellness Connection boxes are topics such as how exercise improves mood and mental functioning, how stress affects the immune system, and how helping others can provide physical, emotional, and spiritual benefits.

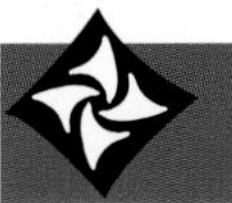

Dimensions of Diversity boxes focus on another important theme of the second edition: diversity. Most wellness issues are universal; we all need to exercise and eat well, for example. However, certain differences among people—based on gender, socioeconomic status, ethnicity, age, and other factors—do have important implications for wellness. Dimensions of Diversity boxes give students the opportunity to identify special wellness concerns that affect them because of who they are, as individuals or as members of a group. Topics of Dimensions of Diversity boxes include fitness for people with disabilities, gender differences in cardiorespiratory endurance, ethnic diets and cuisines, and the relationship between poverty and cancer risk.

Critical Consumer boxes, new to the second edition of *Fit and Well,* emphasize the key theme of critical thinking. These boxes are designed to help students develop and apply critical thinking skills, thereby enabling them to make sound choices related to health and well-being. Critical Consumer boxes provide specific guidelines for choosing fitness centers, exercise footwear and equipment, and health insurance; for evaluating health news and commercial weight loss programs; and for using food labels to make informed dietary choices.

Vital Statistics

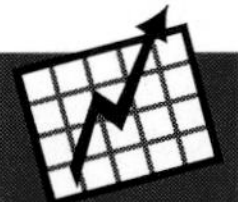

Vital Statistics tables and figures highlight important facts and figures in an accessible format. From tables and figures marked with the Vital Statistics icon and label, students learn about such matters as the leading causes of death for Americans and the factors that play a part in each one; the relationship between level of physical fitness and mortality; what Americans eat compared to what they should eat; incidence of cancer by site and gender; routes of HIV infection; and a wealth of other information. For students who learn best when material is displayed graphically or numerically, Vital Statistics tables and figures offer a way to grasp information quickly and directly.

Common Questions Answered

For the second edition of *Fit and Well,* the sections called **Common Questions Answered** have been expanded; they now appear at the ends of Chapters 2–14. In these student-friendly sections, the answers to the most-often-asked questions are presented in easy-to-understand terms. Included are such questions as, Are there any stretching exercises I shouldn't do? Do I need more protein in my diet when I train with weights? If I stop weight training, will my muscles turn to fat? Does drinking benefit health? How can I safely gain weight? and, Who should have an HIV test?

Behavior Change Activities

Coverage of behavioral self-management has been expanded in the second edition of *Fit and Well* with the inclusion of new chapter-ending **Behavior Change Activities.** Each activity focuses on a particular aspect of behavior change, allowing students to work through each step in a behavior change program in greater detail and to develop strategies for dealing with common obstacles to behavior change. Activities include examining attitudes toward a target behavior, boosting motivation and commitment, breaking behavior chains, managing time successfully, and overcoming peer pressure.

Quick-Reference Appendixes

Included at the end of the book are three appendixes containing vital information in an easy-to-use format. **Appendix A, Injury Prevention and Personal Safety,** is a reference guide to preventing and treating common injuries, whether at home, at work, at play, or on the road. It includes such information as how to treat poisoning, choking, and burns; how to prevent injuries from falls, fires, and motor vehicle crashes; how to be safe when walking, jogging, and biking; and how to protect oneself from assault and rape, including acquaintance rape. It also provides information on giving emergency care when someone else's life is in danger. A chart shows proper technique for administering the Heimlich maneuver and performing rescue breathing.

Appendix B, Nutritional Content of Common Foods, allows students to assess their daily diet in terms of 11 nutrient categories, including protein, fat, saturated fat, fiber, added sugar, cholesterol, and sodium. Keyed to the software available with the text, this guide puts vital nutritional information at students' fingertips.

Appendix C, Nutritional Content of Popular Items from Fast-Food Restaurants, provides a breakdown of the nutritional content of the most commonly ordered menu items at eight popular fast-food restaurants. Especially useful are the facts about fat and sodium in different items and about the proportion of fat calories to total calories. Appendix C was completely updated for the second edition.

LEARNING AIDS

Several specific learning aids have been incorporated in *Fit and Well.* At the beginning of each chapter, under the heading **Looking Ahead,** five or six questions preview the main points of the chapter for the student and serve as learning objectives. Within each chapter, important terms appear in boldface type and are defined on the same page of text in a **running glossary,** helping students handle new vocabulary.

Chapter summaries offer students a concise review and a way to make sure they have grasped the most important concepts in the chapter. Also found at the end of chapters are **selected bibliographies** and sections called **For More Information.** These sections list books, journal articles, and newsletters that may be of interest to students, as well as further resources that can often be found on campus or in the community.

TEACHING TOOLS

Available with the second edition of *Fit and Well* is a comprehensive package of supplementary materials designed to enhance teaching and learning. Included in the package are the following items:

- Instructor's Resource Binder
- Transparency acetates
- Computerized test bank
- Videotapes
- Nutritional analysis software
- Daily fitness log
- *Fit and Well* lab software

The **Instructor's Resource Binder** contains a variety of helpful teaching materials in an easy-to-use form. The **Instructor's Manual** includes learning objectives; extended lecture outlines; lists of additional resources, including videos, software, Internet sites, and other multimedia tools; and descriptions of the transparencies and labs. The **Test Item File** contains over 1000 test questions, revised and updated for the second edition. Also included in the Instructor's Resource Binder are 42 **Additional Laboratory Activities,** formatted and perforated for easy duplication and distribution, and 64 **Transparency Masters.**

The set of **transparency acetates** available with *Fit and Well* has been expanded for the second edition. The package now includes 50 acetates, half of which are in color. The transparency acetates provide material suitable for lecture and demonstration purposes and complement the transparency masters in the Instructor's Resource Binder.

The **computerized test bank** (Microtest III from Chariot Software Group) allows instructors to design tests using the questions in the test item file and/or their own questions. It is available for Macintosh and Windows.

Videotapes available to qualified adopters give instructors the opportunity to expand their classroom treatment of fitness and wellness topics. For more information about the videos, contact your Mayfield representative or call 1-800-433-1279.

Nutritional analysis software from DINE Systems, Inc., allows students to assess their current daily diet, evaluate menus, and compare their diets to nutritional guidelines. Students receive a printout that includes an easy-to-understand scoring system and suggestions for improving food choices.

New to the second edition are two practical items for students that can be shrinkwrapped with the textbook. The first is the **Daily Fitness Log,** a 48-page booklet that contains logs for students to plan and track the progress of their fitness program for up to 40 weeks. The second new student supplement is the ***Fit and Well* lab software** package, which presents laboratory activities from the text in an electronic format. The *Fit and Well* software calculates and prints out the results of self-assessment and fitness tests. It is available for Macintosh and Windows.

Other software, video, and multimedia options are available to qualified adopters. For more information, contact your local representative or call Mayfield at 1-800-433-1279.

A NOTE OF THANKS

Many people have contributed to the production of *Fit and Well.* The book has benefited from their thoughtful commentaries, expert knowledge, and helpful suggestions. We are deeply grateful for their participation in the project. Academic reviewers of the first edition:

Liz Applegate, University of California, Davis
E. Harold Blackwell, Lamar University
Laura L. Borsdorf, Ursinus College
Vicki Boye, Concordia College
William J. Considine, Springfield College
Arlene Crosman, Linn-Benton Community College
Robert Cross, Salisbury State University
Jean F. Dudney, San Antonio College
Eunice Goldgrabe, Concordia College
Susan J. Hibbs, Bloomsburg University of Pennsylvania
William Hottinger, Wake Forest University
Kenneth W. Kambis, College of William and Mary
Russell R. Pate, University of South Carolina
Charles J. Pelitera, Canisius College
Margaret A. Peterson, Central Oregon Community College
Jacalyn J. Robert, Texas Tech University
Rob Schurrer, Black Hills State University
Eugenia S. Scott, Butler University
Charles R. Seager, Miami-Dade Community College
J. L. Sexton, Fort Hays State University
Jack Stovall, Salisbury State University
Karen Teresa Sullivan, Marymount University
Glenn R. West, Transylvania University
Anthony Zaloga, Frostburg State University

Academic reviewers of the second edition:

Viviane L. Avant, University of North Carolina-Charlotte
Elaine H. Blair, Indiana University of Pennsylvania
Susan Brown, Johnson County Community College
Arlene Crosman, Linn Benton Community College
Todd Crowder, U.S. Military Academy
Michael A. Dupper, University of Mississippi
Richard J. Fopeano, Rowan College of New Jersey
Mike Johnson, Berea College
Patricia A. Miller, Anderson University
Roland J. Schick, Tyler Junior College
Rob Schurrer, Black Hills State University
Mark G. Urtel, Indiana University-Purdue University-Indianapolis
Ann Ward, University of Wisconsin-Madison
Christopher J. Womack, Longwood College

We are also grateful to the staff of Mayfield Publishing Company and the *Fit and Well* book team, without whose efforts the book could not have been published. Special thanks to Serina Beauparlant, sponsoring editor; Kirstan Price and Kate Engelberg, developmental editors; Lynn Rabin Bauer, production editor; Jeanne M. Schreiber, art director; Jean Mailander, art manager; Pam Trainer, permissions editor; Brian Pecko and Melissa Kreischer, photo researchers; Randy Hurst, manufacturing manager; Larisa North, production assistant; Michelle Rodgerson, marketing manager; and Jonathan Silvers, product manager.

Thomas D. Fahey
Paul M. Insel
Walton T. Roth

Brief Contents

Contents

CHAPTER 3
CARDIORESPIRATORY ENDURANCE 37

Chapter 3 describes the benefits of cardiorespiratory endurance and provides complete instructions for developing a cardiorespiratory endurance program and for preventing exercise injuries.

NEW Expanded coverage of the psychological and emotional benefits of cardiorespiratory endurance exercise.

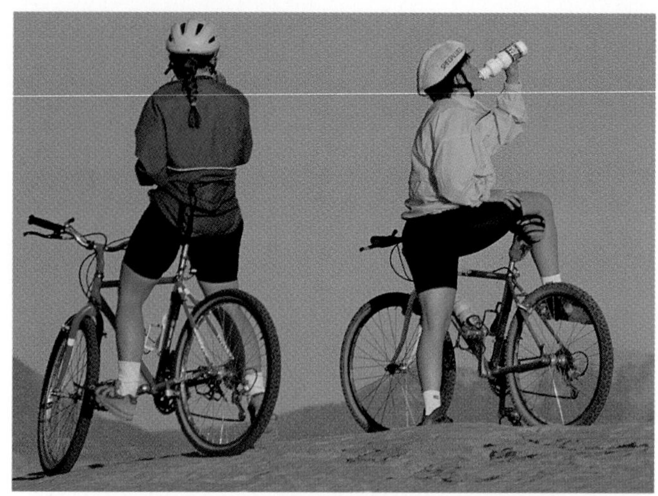

CHAPTER 4
MUSCULAR STRENGTH AND ENDURANCE 65

Chapter 4 includes the information students need to create a safe and successful weight training program. Fully-illustrated sample programs are included for both free weights and weight machines.

NEW Updated and expanded discussion of the lifetime wellness benefits of muscular strength and endurance.

CHAPTER 5 FLEXIBILITY 103

Chapter 5 describes the benefits of flexibility and low-back health, and it presents guidelines and fully-illustrated sample exercise programs for achieving both.

NEW Expanded coverage of how to prevent and manage low-back pain.

CHAPTER 6 BODY COMPOSITION 131

Chapter 6 highlights the links between body composition and overall wellness, and it helps students set a realistic, healthy goal for body composition.

NEW The 1995 federal weight guidelines, the relationship between body composition and diabetes risk, the effects of exercise on body image, and the results of recent studies on body composition and health.

CHAPTER 7 PUTTING TOGETHER A COMPLETE FITNESS PROGRAM 153

Chapter 7 describes how to create a personalized fitness program that develops all the components of fitness. It also includes sample exercise programs built around popular cardiorespiratory endurance activities.

NEW Complementary material on strength training and stretching in the sample programs; discussion of how to choose appropriate exercise footwear.

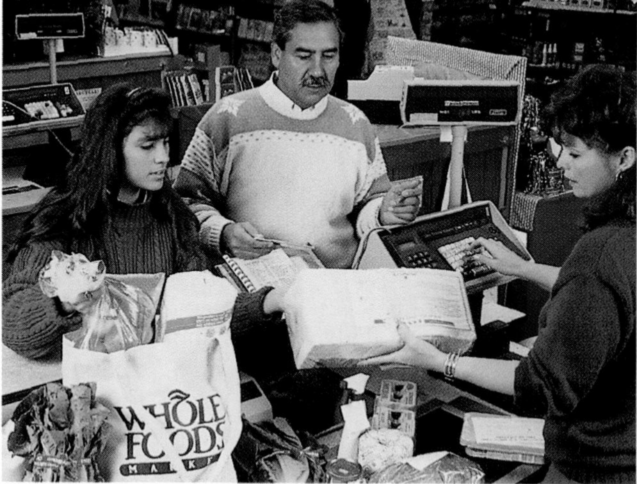

CHAPTER 8 NUTRITION 179

Chapter 8 provides the basic nutrition information students need to choose a healthy diet.

NEW Recommendations from the 1995 version of the Dietary Guidelines for Americans; updated coverage of food labeling, vegetarian diets, vitamin and mineral supplements, osteoporosis, antioxidants, and trans fatty acids.

CHAPTER 9
WEIGHT MANAGEMENT 217

Chapter 9 looks at the factors that influence body weight and composition, and it helps students create and implement a plan for successful weight management.

NEW Updated and expanded coverage of genetics, metabolism, weight cycling, safe methods of gaining weight, and the roles of reduced-fat foods and exercise in weight management.

CHAPTER 10
STRESS 239

Chapter 10 describes how stress affects people in both the short-term and long-term, and it outlines a wide variety of strategies for managing stress.

NEW Expanded discussion of stress management techniques and the relationship between stress and disease.

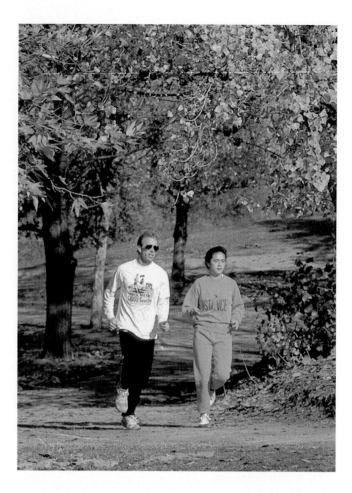

CHAPTER 13 SUBSTANCE USE AND ABUSE 299

Chapter 13 describes how the use of tobacco, alcohol, and other psychoactive drugs can affect wellness. Personal responsibility and decision making are stressed throughout the chapter.

NEW Expanded coverage of binge drinking, environmental tobacco smoke, and smokeless tobacco.

CHAPTER 14 SEXUALLY TRANSMISSIBLE DISEASES 327

Chapter 14 looks at the causes, symptoms, and effects of common STDs. Specific information on how students can protect themselves from STDs is also included.

NEW HIV testing and the efficacy of different contraceptive methods for STD protection; updated material on HIV infection.

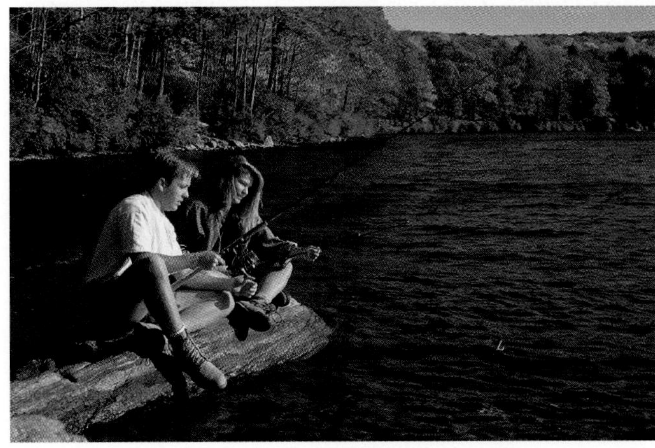

CHAPTER 15
WELLNESS FOR LIFE 347

Chapter 15 introduces additional wellness topics—intimate relationships, using the health care system, and environmental health. Guidelines are provided for achieving wellness in each of these areas.

NEW A section on aging that describes the process of aging and how individuals can protect their health and well-being as they age.

Appendix A Injury Prevention and Personal Safety A-1

Appendix A is a reference guide to preventing and treating common injuries, including those from falls, fires, poisonings, and bicycle and motor vehicle crashes. It also provides information on giving emergency care when someone's life is in danger.

NEW Expanded coverage of how to protect oneself from violence and intentional injuries, including assault and rape.

Appendix B Nutritional Content of Common Foods A-11

Appendix B provides a nutritional breakdown of over 400 common foods and allows students to assess their daily diet in terms of important nutrient categories such as protein, fat, fiber, and sodium. Keyed to the software available with the text, this guide puts vital nutritional information at students' fingertips.

Appendix C Nutritional Content of Popular Items from Fast-Food Restaurants A-22

Appendix C gives a breakdown of the nutritional content of commonly ordered menu items at eight popular fast-food restaurants.

BOXES

Tactics and Tips

Tactics and Tips boxes present the practical advice students need to apply information from the text to their own lives.

A Closer Look

A Closer Look boxes highlight current topics and issues of particular interest to students.

Wellness Connection

NEW Wellness Connection boxes highlight important links among the different dimensions of wellness and emphasize that all must be developed in order for an individual to achieve optimal health and well-being.

Critical Consumer

NEW Critical Consumer boxes are designed to help students develop and apply critical thinking skills, thereby enabling them to make sound choices related to wellness.

Dimensions of Diversity

NEW Dimensions of Diversity boxes emphasize the key theme of diversity by giving students the opportunity to identify special wellness concerns that affect them because of who they are, either as individuals or as members of a group.

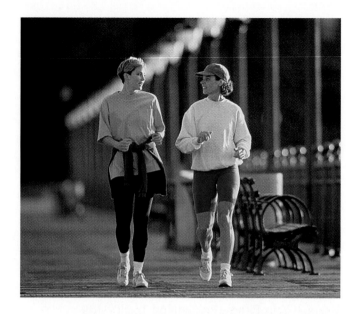

BEHAVIOR CHANGE ACTIVITIES

NEW Each activity focuses on a particular aspect of behavior change, allowing students to work through each step in a behavior change program in greater detail and to develop strategies for overcoming common obstacles to behavior change.

LABORATORY ACTIVITIES

These hands-on activities give students the opportunity to assess their current level of wellness, to create plans for changing their lifestyle to reach wellness, and to monitor their progress.

NEW An easier-to-use format; labs appear at the ends of the chapters on perforated pages.

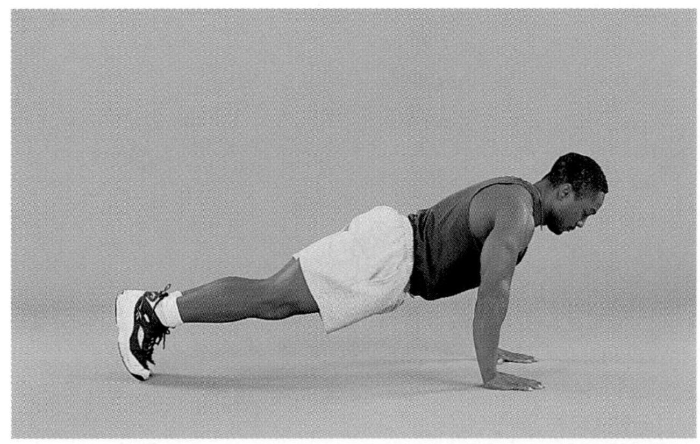

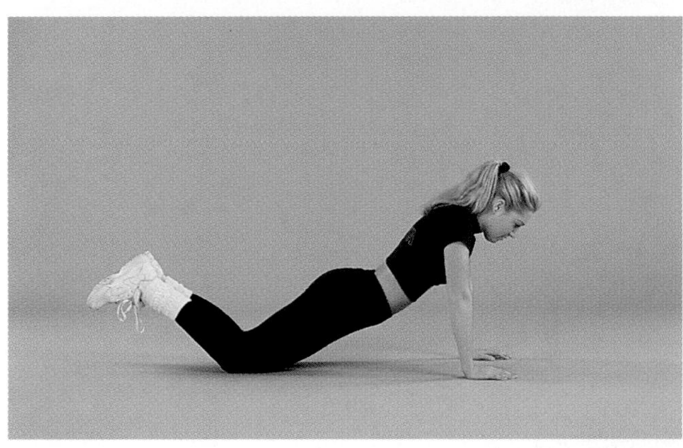

1

Introduction to Fitness, Wellness, and Lifestyle Management

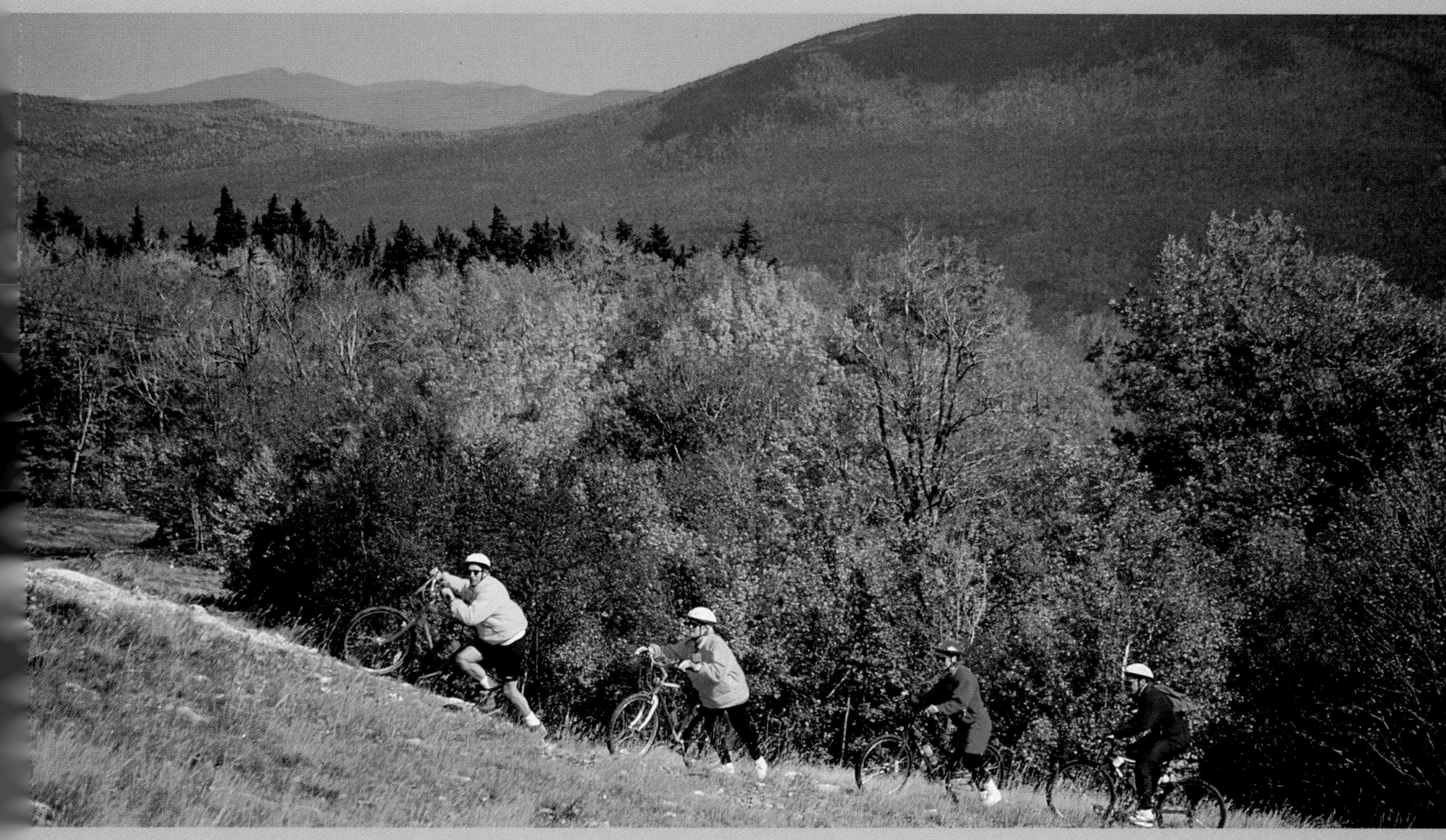

LOOKING AHEAD

After reading this chapter, you should be able to answer these questions about fitness, wellness, and behavioral self-management:

- What are the major health problems in the United States today, and what are their principal causes?
- What changes have occurred in people's health-related attitudes and behaviors in the last 20–30 years?
- What is physical fitness, and why is it important to good health?
- What is wellness?
- What behaviors are part of a fit and well lifestyle?
- What are the components of a behavioral self-management program?

An out-of-shape college student begins riding her bike across town instead of driving. A hard-working business executive enrolls in a stress-management seminar. A former smoker anticipates his impulse to start smoking again and joins a smoking-cessation support group. What do these people have in common? They've all made a commitment to take charge of their health.

Today, many people are striving for optimal health. They are changing their diets, getting more exercise, and having their blood pressure and cholesterol levels checked regularly. They realize that medical science can prolong their lives but that their own choices and behaviors determine how healthy and full those lives will be. They want not just to live long but also to live well—to be healthy throughout their entire lives (Figure 1-1).

A century ago, such a goal was unknown; people considered themselves lucky just to survive. Someone born in 1895, for example, could expect to live only about 40 years. Many children succumbed to **infectious diseases,** such as smallpox, diphtheria, measles, mumps, and polio. Those people who avoided childhood diseases still risked death from tuberculosis, typhus, dysentery, and other diseases. In 1918 alone, 20 million people died in a worldwide influenza epidemic. Contributing to the spread and deadliness of all these diseases were poor sanitation, inadequate food-handling practices, and air pollution from coal-burning furnaces and factories.

The picture today is quite different. Over the past 100 years, the average life span has nearly doubled—to more than 70 years. With the development of vaccines, antibiotics, genetic interventions, and better environmental practices, such as food refrigeration and sewage treatment, most infectious diseases—with the notable exception of HIV/AIDS—have been brought under control. A sense of control over serious health threats has replaced the fatalism that prevailed in the last century.

But with people living longer and most infectious diseases under control, other concerns have come to the fore. The biggest health problems in our society today aren't caused by bacteria or viruses; they're caused by neglect and abuse of our bodies. Sedentary lifestyles, high-fat diets, smoking and drinking, ineffective ways of dealing with stress—all of these behaviors damage our bodies and contribute to the development of **chronic diseases,** including cardiovascular disease (CVD), hypertension (high blood pressure), atherosclerosis (hardening of the arteries), diabetes, cirrhosis of the liver, and cancer.

Of these diseases, the most widespread and devastating are CVD and cancer, the two leading causes of death for Americans today (Table 1-1). CVD—disease of the heart and blood vessels—claims one life every 34 seconds. More Americans die from CVD than from cancer, injuries, emphysema, pneumonia, influenza, suicide, and AIDS combined. In fact, almost half of all Americans living today will die from CVD. Although we often think of heart disease as primarily affecting men and the elderly, heart attack is the number-one killer of American women, and 45% of all heart attacks occur in people younger than 65 years of age.

Cancer, though not as common as CVD, is probably the most dreaded noninfectious disease. Over 1 million Americans are diagnosed with cancer each year. More than half will be cured, but about 40 percent will eventually die of their cancer. About one in three Americans now living—roughly 85 million people—will eventually develop cancer.

The good news is that people have some control over whether they develop CVD, cancer, and other degenerative diseases. People make choices every day that either increase or decrease their risks for these diseases. In fact, since many Americans began making important lifestyle

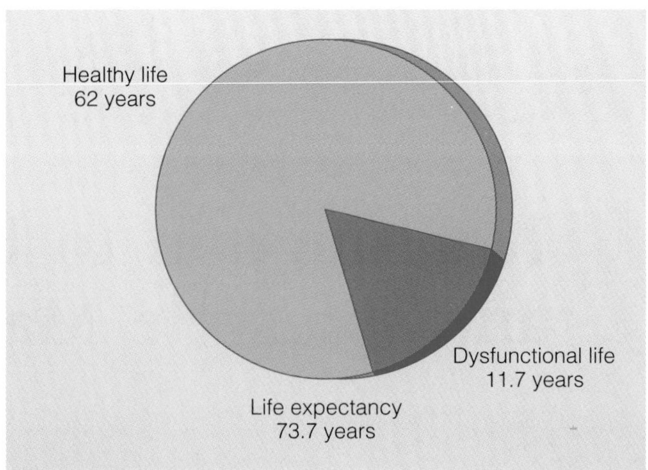

VITAL STATISTICS

Figure 1-1 ***Quantity of life versus quality of life.*** Due to improved medical and environmental practices, the average life expectancy of Americans increased greatly during the twentieth century. But quality of life is also an important consideration, and the typical American currently maintains good health for only about 85% of his or her life. Developing and maintaining a healthy lifestyle can both increase longevity and decrease the number of years of unhealthy life. *Source:* Adapted from National Center for Health Statistics. 1994. *Healthy People 2000 Review, 1993.* Hyattsville, Md.: Public Health Service, DHHS Pub. (PHS) 94-1232-1.

TERMS

infectious disease A disease that is communicable from one person to another.

chronic disease A disease that develops and continues over a long period of time; usually caused by a variety of factors, including lifestyle factors.

risk factor A condition, state, or quality that increases a person's chances of becoming ill or injured.

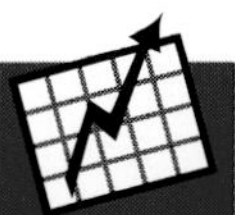

VITAL STATISTICS

TABLE 1-1 Ten Leading Causes of Death in the United States

Rank	Cause of Death	Number	Percent of Total Deaths	Lifestyle Factors
1	Heart disease	734,090	32.1	I D S
2	Cancer	536,866	23.4	I D S A
3	Stroke	154,350	6.7	I D S
4	Chronic obstructive lung disease	101,870	4.5	S
5	Accidents	90,140	3.9	S A
	(Motor vehicle)	(40,735)	(1.8)	
	(All others)	(49,415)	(2.1)	
6	Pneumonia and influenza	82,090	3.6	S
7	Diabetes mellitus	55,390	2.4	I D
8	HIV infection	41,930	1.8	
9	Suicide	32,410	1.4	A
10	Chronic liver disease and cirrhosis	25,730	1.1	A
	All causes	2,286,000	100.0	

Key: I Cause of death in which an inactive lifestyle plays a part.
D Cause of death in which diet plays a part.
S Cause of death in which smoking plays a part.
A Cause of death in which excessive alcohol consumption plays a part.

Estimated data for 1995.

Source: National Center for Health Statistics.

changes in the 1970s, the incidence of some chronic diseases has declined. Since 1979, the death rate from heart attack has fallen 30%, and deaths from strokes have dropped by 31.5%. Death rates from cancer also appear to be leveling off or decreasing, with the exception of lung cancer in women—a trend that parallels the increased rate of smoking among women in the past 20 years.

What are the most important lifestyle choices and changes people can make to enhance their health? Probably the single most important choice is to exercise regularly. Exercise appears to be a significant factor in preventing many chronic diseases. Studies have shown that people with active lifestyles have far fewer health problems and significantly lower death rates from CVD and other chronic diseases than people with sedentary lifestyles. Several recent studies that followed large groups of men and women for as long as 26 years found that regular vigorous exercise decreased their chance of dying from all causes by at least 10% in any given year throughout the life span. And in 1992, the American Heart Association added sedentary lifestyle to the ranks of major **risk factors** for CVD, putting it on a par with smoking, high blood pressure, and unhealthy cholesterol levels. Previously, lack of exercise had been considered only a contributing factor to CVD.

People make other important health-related choices in the areas of nutrition, weight management, stress management, sexual behavior, safety, and the use of tobacco, alcohol, and other drugs. A lifestyle based on good choices and healthy behaviors maximizes the quality of life. It helps people avoid disease, remain strong and fit, and maintain their physical and mental health as long as they live. In short, a healthy lifestyle helps people achieve optimal health, or wellness.

This chapter provides an overview of physical fitness and wellness. It also describes a method that can help people make lasting changes in their lives to promote good health. The chapters that follow provide more detailed information about fitness and the various components of wellness. The book as a whole is designed to be used in a very real way, to help you take charge of your behavior and improve the quality of your life—to become fit and well.

PHYSICAL FITNESS

What exactly is physical fitness, and why is it so important to health? The answers to these questions lie in a closer look at our physical makeup. The human body is

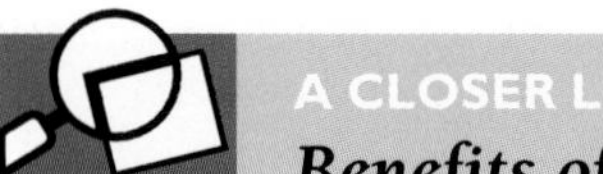

A CLOSER LOOK

Benefits of Regular Exercise and Physical Fitness

Physical Benefits

- Increased life expectancy
- Decreased risk of developing and dying from cardiovascular disease and stroke
- Decreased risk of developing and dying from certain cancers, particularly colon and rectal cancer
- Decreased risk of adult-onset diabetes
- Decreased risk of bone fractures from osteoporosis
- Improved cardiac function
- Control of blood pressure levels
- Improved blood fat concentrations
- Improved regulation of blood clotting
- Improved ability to deliver oxygen to tissues
- Improved body chemistry
- Increased protection against the physiological effects of stress
- Quicker recovery from illness and injury
- Increased resistance to fatigue
- Improved posture and body mechanics
- Strengthened tendons, ligaments, bones, and muscles
- Increased lean body mass
- Decreased body fat
- Decreased risk of injury
- Reduced risk for low-back pain
- Improved joint health
- Decreased postexercise muscle soreness
- Improved performance in sport, work, and recreational activities

Mental Health Benefits

- Tension relief
- Reduced symptoms of stress
- Improved sleeping habits
- Increased energy levels and resistance to mental fatigue
- Increased opportunities for positive interaction with others
- Improved appearance
- Improved self-image
- Improved quality of life

designed to work best when it is physically active. It readily adapts to practically any level of activity and exertion; in fact, **physical fitness** is defined as the ability of the body to adapt to the demands and stresses of physical effort. The more we ask of our bodies—our muscles, bones, heart, lungs—the stronger and more fit they become. However, the converse is also true: The less we ask of them, the less they can do. When our bodies are not kept active, they begin to deteriorate. Bones lose their density, joints stiffen, muscles become weak, and cellular energy systems begin to degenerate. To be truly well, human beings must be active.

Unfortunately, physical activity is no longer part of our daily lives the way it was for our great-grandparents. We use modern technology—cars, elevators, escalators, remote controls—to get through each day with very little physical effort. To develop and maintain physical fitness, we have to make a special effort to incorporate exercise into our lives. Currently, only about 24% of all adult Americans exercise regularly, a level that has remained unchanged since 1985.

The benefits of physical fitness are both physical and mental, immediate and long term. Refer to the box "Benefits of Regular Exercise and Physical Fitness" for specific examples of these benefits. In the short term, being physically fit makes it easier to do everyday tasks, such as lifting; it provides reserve strength for emergencies; and it helps people look and feel good. In the long term, being physically fit confers protection against disease. As described above, physically fit individuals are less likely to develop heart disease, respiratory disease, high blood pressure, and diabetes (Figure 1-2). Their cardiorespiratory systems tend to resemble those of people 10 or more years younger than themselves. As they get older, they may be able to avoid weight gain, muscle and bone loss, fatigue, memory loss, and other problems associated with aging. With healthy hearts, strong muscles, lean bodies, and a repertoire of physical skills they can call on for recreation and enjoyment, fit people can maintain their physical and mental well-being throughout their entire lives.

WELLNESS

As important as it is, physical fitness is not the only component of good health. A person who gets enough exercise but smokes cigarettes, eats a high-fat diet, or drives under the influence of alcohol does not have a healthy lifestyle. The concept of **wellness**—optimal health and

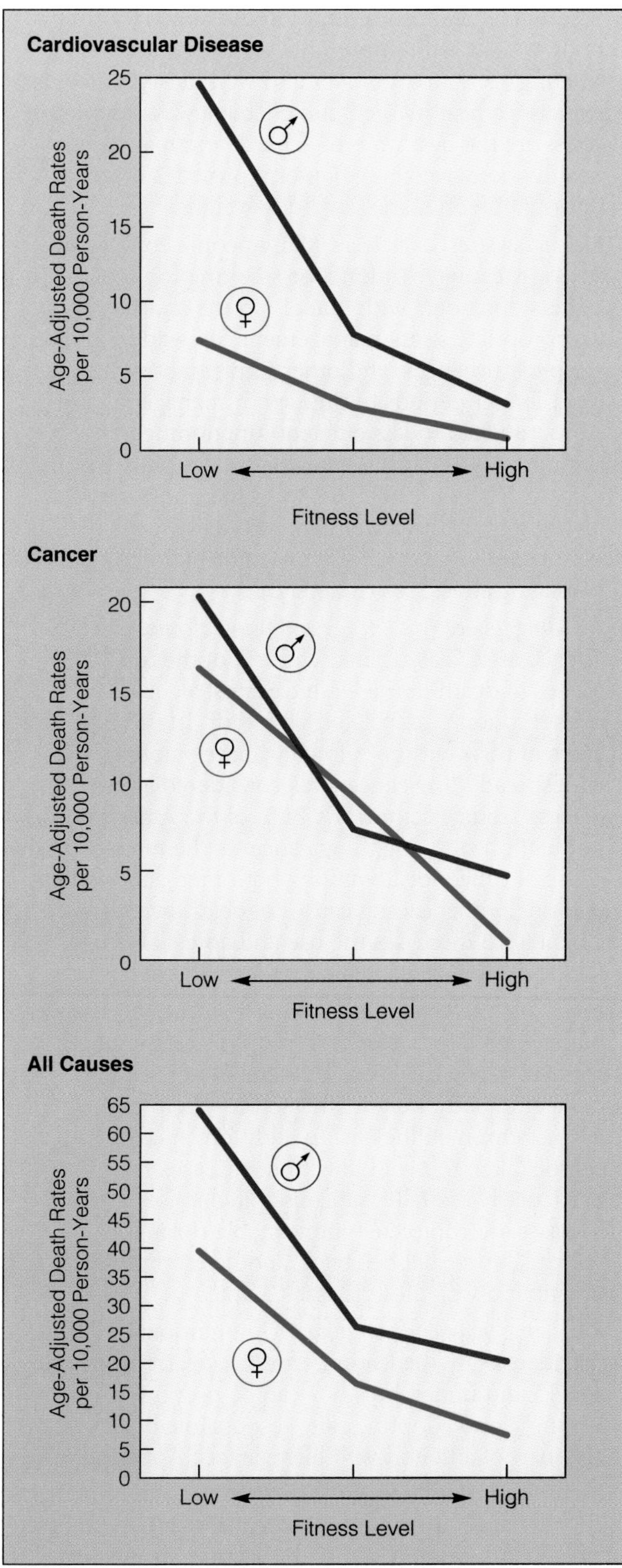

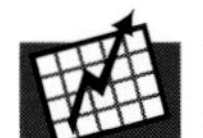

VITAL STATISTICS

Figure 1-2 ***Level of physical fitness and mortality rates.*** *Source:* Blair, S. N., H. W. Kohl, R. S. Paffenbarger, D. G. Clark, K. H. Cooper, and L. W. Gibbons. 1989. Physical fitness and all-cause mortality: A prospective study of healthy men and women. *Journal of the American Medical Association* 262:2395–2401.

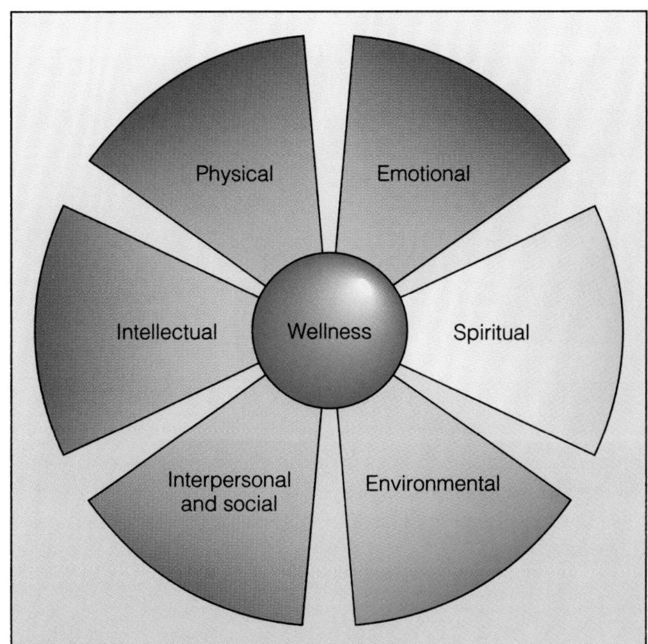

Figure 1-3 ***Components of wellness.***

vital well-being—includes physical fitness but also encompasses several other dimensions (Figure 1-3). Wellness involves an awareness of all these dimensions, an understanding of their importance in well-being, and a conscious effort to develop and balance them. The following have been identified as important dimensions of wellness:

- *Physical:* Maintaining the body's health by eating well, exercising, avoiding unhealthy habits, making responsible decisions about sex, being aware of the symptoms of disease, having regular checkups, and taking steps to prevent injuries.
- *Emotional:* Maintaining a positive self-concept, dealing constructively with feelings, developing such qualities as optimism, trust, and self-confidence.
- *Intellectual:* Keeping an active, curious, open mind with the ability to think critically about issues, pose questions, identify problems, and find solutions.
- *Spiritual:* Developing faith in something beyond yourself as well as the capacity for compassion, altruism, joy, and forgiveness; finding meaning and purpose in life, whether through religion, meditation, art, nature, service to others, or some other practice.

TERMS

physical fitness The ability of the body to respond or adapt to the demands and stress of physical effort.

wellness Optimal health and vitality, encompassing physical, emotional, intellectual, spiritual, interpersonal, social, and environmental well-being.

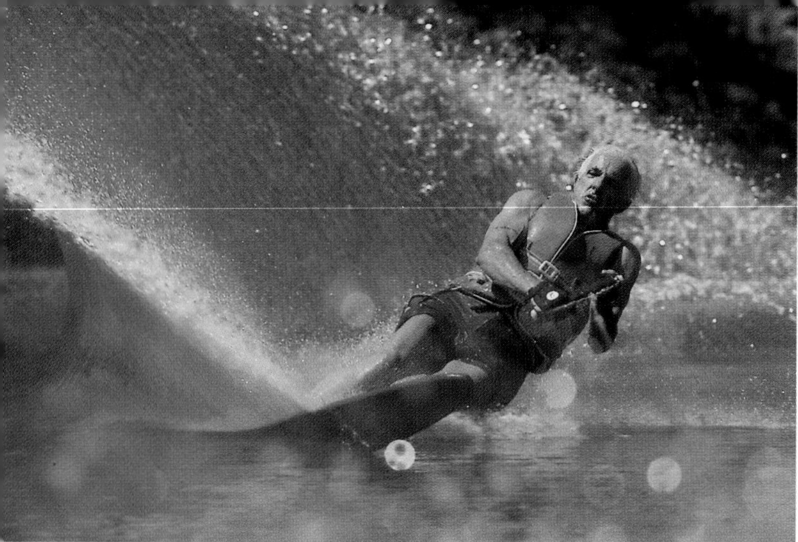

A lifetime of healthy choices makes it possible for this 60-year-old man to water-ski like a 30-year-old. To enjoy health and vigor later in life, people have to cultivate wellness while they are young.

- *Interpersonal and social:* Developing meaningful relationships, cultivating a network of supportive friends and family members, and contributing to the community.
- *Environmental:* Protecting yourself from environmental hazards and minimizing the negative impact of your behavior on the environment.

All of these dimensions are interconnected; making a change in one often affects some or all of the others. For example, regular exercise (developing the physical dimension of wellness) can increase feelings of well-being and self-esteem (emotional wellness), which in turn can increase feelings of confidence in social interactions and one's achievements at work or school (interpersonal and social wellness). Every positive change is a step toward total wellness. Some of the key links among different dimensions of wellness are highlighted in this text in boxes labeled Wellness Connection.

Behaviors Contributing to Wellness

In addition to regular exercise, other behaviors that contribute to wellness include the following:

- *Choosing a healthful diet.* Many Americans have a diet that is too high in calories, fat, and sugar and too low in fiber and complex carbohydrates. This diet is linked to a number of chronic diseases, including heart disease, stroke, and certain kinds of cancer. A better diet is one that provides necessary nutrients and sufficient energy without also providing too much of those substances linked to disease. The basics of a healthy diet are presented in Chapter 8.
- *Maintaining a healthy body weight.* Overweight and obesity are associated with a number of disabling and potentially fatal conditions and diseases. Healthy body weight is an important part of wellness—but "dieting" is not part of a fit and well lifestyle. Regular exercise, a healthy diet, and effective ways to manage stress are the best ways to achieve and maintain a healthy body weight. Chapter 9 provides more information on managing body weight.
- *Managing stress effectively.* Many people cope with stress by eating, drinking, or smoking too much. Others don't deal with it at all. In the short term, inappropriate stress management can lead to fatigue, sleep disturbances, and other unpleasant symptoms. Over longer periods of time, poor management of stress can lead to less efficient functioning of the immune system and increased susceptibility to disease. There *are* effective ways to handle stress; learning to incorporate them into daily life is part of a fit and well lifestyle. For more information on managing stress, see Chapter 10.
- *Avoiding tobacco and drugs and using alcohol wisely.* Tobacco use is associated with six of the top 10 causes of death in the United States; alcohol consumption is associated with four. In the early years of this century, before cigarette smoking was widespread, lung cancer was considered a rare disease. Today, with nearly 30% of the American population smoking, lung cancer is the most common cause of cancer death among both men and women and one of the leading causes of death overall. Chapter 13 discusses the use and abuse of drugs, including tobacco and alcohol, in more detail.
- *Protecting yourself from disease.* The most effective way of dealing with disease is to prevent it. Many of the lifestyle strategies discussed here—exercising, managing body weight, and so on—help protect you against chronic illnesses. In addition, specific steps can be taken to avoid infectious diseases, particularly sexually transmissible diseases. These diseases are completely preventable through responsible sexual behavior, another component of a fit and well lifestyle (see Chapter 14).
- *Protecting yourself from injury.* Unintentional injuries (accidents) are the leading cause of death for people age 45 and under, but they can be prevented. Learning and adopting safe, responsible behaviors is also part of a fit and well lifestyle (see Appendix A).

Other important behaviors in a fit and well lifestyle include developing meaningful relationships, planning ahead for successful aging, becoming knowledgeable about the health care system, and acting responsibly in relation to the environment. More information about these facets of wellness is included in Chapter 15. Lab 1-1 will help you evaluate your behaviors as they relate to wellness.

The Role of Other Factors in Health

Of course, behavior isn't the only factor involved in good health. Heredity, the environment, and access to adequate health care are other important influences. These factors can interact in ways that raise or lower the quality of a person's life and the risk of developing particular diseases. For example, a sedentary lifestyle combined with a genetic predisposition for diabetes can greatly increase a person's risk for developing the disease. If this person also lacks adequate health care, he or she is much more likely to suffer dangerous complications from diabetes and have a lower quality of life. (For a discussion of how different factors affect people as members of groups, see the box "Wellness Issues for Diverse Populations," p. 8.)

But in many cases, behavior can tip the balance toward health even if inheritance or environment is a negative factor. Breast cancer, for example, can run in families, but it also may be associated with overweight and a sedentary lifestyle. A woman with a family history of breast cancer is less likely to die from the disease if she controls her weight, exercises, performs regular breast self-exams, and consults with her physician about mammograms. By taking appropriate action, this woman can influence the effects of heredity on her health.

Looking Toward the Year 2000

You may think of health and wellness as personal concerns, goals that you strive for on your own for your own benefit. But the U.S. government also has a vital interest in the health of all Americans. A healthy population is the nation's greatest resource, the source of its vigor and wealth. Poor health, in contrast, drains the nation's resources and raises national health care costs. As the embodiment of our society's values, the federal government also has a humane interest in people's health.

In 1990, the U.S. Department of Health and Human Services published a report entitled *Healthy People 2000: National Health Promotion and Disease Prevention Objectives.* The work of thousands of health professionals, this 700-page document sets forth health goals for the United States to be achieved by the year 2000. The broad national goals proposed by *Healthy People 2000* are to increase the span of healthy life for all Americans, to reduce health disparities among Americans, and to secure access to preventive health services for all Americans. Giving substance to these broad goals are hundreds of specific objectives—measurable targets for the year 2000—in many different priority areas that relate to health and wellness. These objectives encompass individual actions as well as larger-scale changes in environmental and medical services.

Examples of individual health promotion objectives from *Healthy People 2000,* and estimates of how we are tracking toward the goals, appear in Table 1-2 (p. 9). As you can see, the objectives are tied closely to the wellness lifestyle described in this chapter. The principal topics covered in this book parallel the priority concerns of *Healthy People 2000,* and the approach of *Fit and Well* is based on the report's premise that personal responsibility is a key to achieving wellness. In many ways, personal health goals are not very different from national aspirations.

REACHING WELLNESS THROUGH LIFESTYLE MANAGEMENT

The picture drawn here of a fit and well lifestyle may seem complex and out of reach to you right now. Many people fall into a lifestyle that puts them at risk. Some aren't aware of the damage they're doing, others don't want to or know how to change, and still others want to change but can't seem to get started. These are all very real problems, but they aren't insurmountable. If they were, there would be no ex-smokers, recovering alcoholics, or people who have successfully lost excess body weight. People can and do make difficult changes in their lives.

What are the important components of successful lifestyle management? First, *knowledge* is required. You need facts and information about health and wellness, answers to basic questions: How much fat should you eat? How much exercise will keep your heart and lungs healthy? What are the risks of not wearing a seat belt? You also need knowledge about yourself: What are your strengths and your weaknesses? What conditions or diseases are you at risk for? What are you already doing well? What could you do better? Finally, you need specific information about how to make lasting changes in your life.

As important as knowledge is, however, knowledge alone isn't usually enough to make someone act. Millions of people smoke even though they know it's bad for their health. *Motivation* is another prerequisite for change. Although some people are motivated by long-term goals, such as the desire not to have heart disease at 50, most are inspired by shorter-term, more personal goals. Looking better, feeling better, having more energy, being more popular, improving at a sport or game, and making a good impression on job interviews are all examples of common motivators.

But motivation, too, can be inadequate when hard choices have to be made. A person may want to look good in a bathing suit next summer and also want to eat a hot fudge sundae right now. In situations like this, immediate gratification often wins out over long-term goals. By itself, motivation usually is no more effective at changing behavior than is knowledge alone. Motivation has to be built on *commitment,* the resolve to stick with a plan no matter what temptations come along. A person who is committed can work very hard to change a situation. When a habit is deeply rooted, however, it can take some

DIMENSIONS OF DIVERSITY

Wellness Issues for Diverse Populations

When it comes to striving for wellness, most differences among people are insignificant. We all need to exercise, eat well, and manage stress. We need to know how to protect ourselves from heart disease, cancer, sexually transmissible diseases, and injuries.

But some of our differences—differences among us both as individuals and as members of groups—do have implications for wellness. Some of us, for example, have grown up eating foods that increase our risk of obesity or heart disease. Some of us have inherited predispositions for certain health problems, such as osteoporosis or high cholesterol levels. These health-related differences among individuals and groups can be biological—determined genetically, or cultural—acquired as patterns of behavior through daily interactions with our family, community, and society. Many health conditions are a function of biology and culture combined.

When we talk about wellness issues as they relate to diverse populations, we face two related dangers. The first is the danger of stereotyping, of talking about people as groups rather than as individuals. The second is that of overgeneralizing, of ignoring the extensive biological and cultural diversity that exists among people who may be grouped together because of their gender, socioeconomic status, or ethnicity. Every person is an individual with his or her own unique genetic endowment as well as unique experiences in life. However, many of these influences are shared with others of similar genetic and cultural backgrounds. Information about group similarities relating to wellness issues can be useful; for example, it can alert people to areas that may be of special concern for them and their families.

Wellness-related differences among groups can be identified and described along several different dimensions, including the following:

- *Gender.* Men and women have different life expectancies and different incidences of many diseases, including heart disease, cancer, and osteoporosis. They also differ in body composition and certain aspects of physical performance.
- *Socioeconomic status.* People with low income levels have higher rates of many conditions and diseases, including overweight, alcohol and drug abuse, heart disease, and HIV infection.
- *Race/ethnicity.* A genetic predisposition for a particular health problem can be linked to ethnicity as a result of each ethnic group's relatively distinct history. Diabetes is more prevalent among individuals of Native American or Latino heritage, for example, and African Americans have higher rates of hypertension. Ethnic groups may also vary in other ways that relate to wellness: traditional diets; patterns of family and interpersonal relationships; and attitudes toward using tobacco, alcohol, and other drugs, to name just a few.

These are just some of the "dimensions of diversity"—differences among people and groups that are associated with different wellness concerns. Other factors, too, such as age, educational attainment, and disability, can present challenges as an individual strives for wellness. In this book, topics and issues relating to wellness that affect different American populations are given special consideration in boxes labeled Dimensions of Diversity. All of these discussions are designed to deepen our understanding of the concepts of wellness and vitality in the context of ever-growing diversity.

time to build up to the level of commitment required to tackle the problem.

Perhaps the most important element in changing behavior is *attitude*—the firm conviction that it is possible to successfully manage one's lifestyle and develop wellness. **Locus of control** refers to the figurative "place" where a person locates the source of responsibility for the events in his or her life. People who believe they are in control of their own lives are said to have an internal locus of control. Those who believe that factors beyond their control—heredity, friends and family, the environment, fate, luck, or other outside forces—are more important in determining the events of their lives are said to have an external locus of control. Most people are not purely "internalizers" or "externalizers"; their locus of control changes in response to the situation.

For lifestyle management, an internal locus of control is an advantage because it reinforces motivation and commitment. An external locus of control can actually sabotage efforts to change behavior. For example, if you believe you will inevitably develop heart disease because your father had a heart attack, you may view a healthy diet and regular exercise as pointless. Examine your attitudes carefully. If you find yourself attributing too much influence to outside forces, gather more information about your health-related behaviors. Make a list of all the ways that making lifestyle changes will improve your health. If you believe you'll succeed, and if you recognize and accept that you are in charge of your life, then you're well on your way to successful lifestyle management.

Remember, most behaviors are habits that have been learned. They may be deeply ingrained, long-standing habits, but they're still habits. You can unlearn them the same way you learned them. The key is to approach them in a systematic way. *Behavioral self-management* has proven effective in helping people make changes in their

TABLE 1-2 *Selected* Healthy People 2000 *Objectives*

Objective	Estimate of Current Status	Goal
Increase years of healthy life.	64 years	65 years
Increase the proportion of people age 6 and over who engage regularly, preferably daily, in light to moderate physical activity for at least 30 minutes per day.	24% (5 times/week) 17% (7 times/week)	30%
Increase the proportion of people age 18 and over who engage in vigorous physical activity that promotes the development and maintenance of cardiorespiratory fitness 3 or more days per week for 20 or more minutes per occasion.	14%	20%
Increase the proportion of people age 6 and over who regularly perform physical activities that enhance and maintain muscular strength, endurance, and flexibility.	16%	40%
Reduce dietary fat intake.	34% of calories	30% of calories
Increase the consumption of fruits and vegetables.	2.5 servings/day	5 servings/day
Reduce the prevalence of overweight among people age 20 and over.	34%	20%
Reduce the proportion of people age 18 and over who experience adverse health effects from stress each year.	39.2%	less than 35%
Reduce deaths from coronary heart disease.	114/100,000 people	100/100,000 people
Reverse the rise in cancer deaths to achieve a lower death rate.	133/100,000 people	130/100,000 people
Reduce the prevalence of cigarette smoking among people age 20 and over.	25%	15%
Reduce the proportion of college students engaging in recent occasions of heavy drinking of alcoholic beverages.	40.2%	32%
Increase the proportion of sexually active, unmarried people who used a condom at last sexual intercourse.	19%	50%
Reduce the average amount of solid waste (garbage) produced by each person each day.	4.3 lb/day	3.6 lb/day
Increase the proportion of people who have a specific source of ongoing primary care for coordination of their health care.	85%	95%
Increase the use of helmets by bicyclists.	8%	50%

Sources: U.S. Department of Health and Human Services. 1990. *Healthy People 2000: National Health Promotion and Disease Prevention Objectives.* Washington, D.C.: U.S. Government Printing Office, DHHS Pub. (PHS) 91-50212. National Center for Health Statistics. 1995. *Healthy People 2000 Review, 1994.* Hyattsville, Md.: Public Health Service. Pub. (PHS) 95-1256-1.

lives. Once you have the knowledge, motivation, and commitment, behavioral self-management techniques will give you the means to change your behavior.

Putting Together a Behavioral Self-Management Program

What follows is a self-management model that you can apply to behaviors you want to change. The key to success in this six-step approach is to be both consistent and persistent. Don't skip steps or rush through. You may think you know everything there is to know about your behavior, for example, but people are almost always surprised by patterns they discover through this plan.

TERMS

locus of control The figurative "place" where a person locates the source of responsibility for the events in his or her life.

1. *Monitor your behavior, and gather data.* Begin by isolating a **target behavior** that you wish to change. Concentrate on one behavior at a time; making even a few small changes in your life requires energy and effort. Once you've identified this behavior, keep track of when it occurs and the circumstances surrounding it. Keep your records in a health journal, a small notebook in which you record your observations and comments. Note exactly what the behavior was, when and where it happened, what you were doing, and what your thoughts and feelings were at the time.

   This record helps you identify and get information about the factors in your environment and in yourself that support your target behavior or make it difficult to resist. If your target behavior is eating too many candy bars, for example, you might note that the presence of candy in your home is a factor outside yourself—an environmental factor—that encourages you to indulge. Hunger or anxiety might be a factor within yourself—an internal factor—that also supports this behavior. (Examples of other behaviors a person might wish to change are smoking cigarettes, consuming too much caffeine or alcohol, and not wearing a seat belt or a bicycle helmet.)

   Keep your records for a week or two to get some solid information about the behavior you want to change. You can also use this period to gain information relating to your target behavior: How many calories are there in a candy bar? How much sugar, and how much fat? How does it compare nutritionally with other snacks? And how does it fit into a healthy diet?
2. *Examine the data, and identify patterns.* Now examine your records to discover patterns. When are you most likely to eat a candy bar? What events seem to trigger your desire for candy? What are you doing? Whom are you with? Note any connections between your feelings and environmental factors, such as time of day, location, and the actions of others around you.
3. *Set specific goals.* Whatever your ultimate goal, it's a good idea to break it down into a few small steps. Your plan will seem more manageable, increasing the likelihood that you will stick with it. Breaking it down into pieces will also give you milestones by which to measure your progress and opportunities to reward yourself for the progress you make. For example, if you want to eliminate candy from your diet, plan to work on one part of the day at a time. If you want to lower the fat in your diet by 15%, plan to lower it by 5% at a time. Take the easier steps first and work up to the harder ones.
4. *Make a personal contract.* Once you have set your goals, prepare a personal contract. A serious personal contract clearly states your objective and your commitment to reach it. You may include details of your plan, such as the date you'll begin and the date you expect to reach your final goal; the interim goals and the rewards you've established for reaching them; and the time and resources you've committed to the plan. It often helps to have another person witness the contract, especially someone whose help you're enlisting in the plan. A sample contract is included in Lab 1-2.
5. *Devise a plan of action, and put it into effect.* When you filled in your health journal, you gathered quite a lot of information about your target behavior. Now you can probably trace the chain of events that led to the behavior; you can probably also see points in the chain where other choices are possible. Begin to break this chain by making other choices. For example, if you buy candy bars when you take breaks while studying at the library, try studying in your room for a while. That may be enough to break the habit. For more ideas on interrupting habits, refer to the box "Breaking Behavior Chains."
6. *Keep track of your progress, and revise your plan if necessary.* Use your health journal to keep track of your progress. Record your daily activities and any relevant details. If you don't seem to be making progress, analyze your plan to see what might be causing the problem. Be ready to revise your plan if necessary, and keep at it.

Once you begin a behavioral self-management program, there are ways to increase your likelihood of success. Some of these involve making further environmental changes, and others involve changing your thinking. Refer to the box "Maximizing Your Chances of Success" (p. 12) for some suggestions.

Staying on Track

Barriers, obstacles, and resistance are normal in a behavioral self-management program. In fact, they're inevitable! Most people do not want to change, no matter how much they realize they should. These are some common problems and some suggestions for dealing with them:

- *Insufficient levels of motivation and commitment.* Sometimes the desire to continue a behavior is stronger than the motivation and commitment to change it. If this is the case, a person may have to

TERMS

target behavior An isolated behavior selected as the basis for a behavior change program.

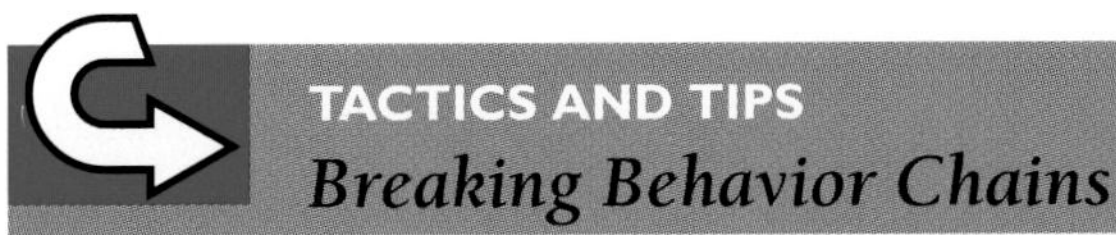

TACTICS AND TIPS
Breaking Behavior Chains

Strategy	Examples
Control environmental stimuli that provoke the behavior.	If you always buy candy when you walk by a certain vending machine, change your route. If you often skip your afternoon jogs because you join your roommate in watching TV, try jogging in the morning, or change into jogging clothes some place other than your room.
Change habits or behaviors that are associated with your target behavior.	If you usually eat when you watch TV, turn on the radio instead.
Place new cues in your environment that trigger your new, healthy behaviors.	Place a picture of a cyclist or a runner on your refrigerator or TV. Keep your jogging or aerobic dance shoes next to the front door.
Make a list of your activities and favorite events to use as rewards.	A new CD, a ticket to a sporting event or concert, a walk in the woods, a study break with a friend. Rewards should be special, inexpensive, and preferably unrelated to food or alcohol.
Set up a system of instant, real rewards for your good behaviors.	If you follow your exercise program all week, go to a movie on Friday night. If you avoid candy snacks all day, take a study break and call a friend.
Get your family members and friends actively involved.	Ask your roommate to go running with you, or ask your friends not to offer you sweet snacks.

wait until the behavior becomes more annoying or worrisome. Many smokers, for example, do not succeed in quitting until their third or fourth attempt. By then, their levels of frustration, disgust, embarrassment, and anger are high enough to override their craving for nicotine.

- *Inadequate support.* The support of family members and friends can be enormously helpful in changing behavior, but sometimes family members or friends don't really want a person to change. Lack of support, especially if it's hidden, can undermine behavior change efforts. If this occurs, the person may want to look elsewhere for support, perhaps in an organized support group.
- *Wrong approach.* A person who needs structure and group support shouldn't choose running as a way to improve physical fitness; an aerobics class would probably be better. If a plan isn't working, the specific approach or technique should be reexamined to see if it really suits the particular individual.
- *Stress barrier.* High levels of stress can make it difficult to pursue a behavioral self-management program. If the stress is temporary, such as a term paper deadline, it makes sense to wait until the event is over before continuing the behavior change program. If the stress is ongoing, the person should develop effective techniques for handling stress first, and then tackle the target behavior. Sometimes a bad habit—drinking, smoking, overeating—is itself being used as a way of dealing with stress. Giving up the habit means losing an important coping mechanism and having to deal with increased stress. When this is the case, it's especially important to work on stress-management techniques (see Chapter 10).
- *Procrastinating, rationalizing, and blaming.* All of these mental games tend to transfer responsibility away from the individual. At their root may lie conflicting feelings and motives about the target behavior. Individuals who put things off, make excuses, or blame others for their inability to change will benefit from looking closely at their feelings, refocusing on the real problem, and accepting responsibility for their actions.
- *Need for outside help.* Some behaviors are too deeply rooted to be changed with a self-management approach. Nicotine, alcohol, and other drug addictions and excessive overeating may fall into this category. Many programs exist to help people with these problems, including self-help groups like Weight Watchers and Alcoholics Anonymous, community services, and private agencies. They can be located through the yellow pages, the local health department, or United Way.

A Behavior Change Activity appears at the end of each chapter in this text. Completing these activities will give you the opportunity to work through each step of behav-

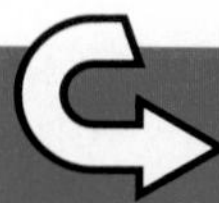

TACTICS AND TIPS
Maximizing Your Chances of Success

- *Make your efforts cost-effective and time-effective.* Be sure your new behavior has a real and lasting value for you personally. Be realistic about the amount of time and energy you can put into it. Choose a strategy or approach that works for you. For example, many activities—from walking to bicycle racing—lead to physical fitness; for long-term success, you need to choose one that you enjoy and that fits smoothly into your existing schedule.
- *Find a buddy.* A buddy can provide support, encouragement, and motivation. The fear of letting your buddy down makes it less likely that you'll take a day off, and in a crisis, your buddy can help overcome an urge to slip (and vice versa). You can probably find a buddy who shares your goal from among your friends, family members, and classmates; alternatively, try joining a group such as Weight Watchers for a ready-made set of buddies.
- *Use a role model.* Find individuals who reached the goal you're striving for, and talk to them about how they did it. What strategies worked for them? What can you borrow from their experience?
- *Prepare for problem situations.* If you know in advance that you're going to be in a situation that will trigger your target behavior, rehearse what you'll do. If you don't want to drink too much at a party, decide on your drink limit ahead of time, and switch to a soft drink when you reach your limit.
- *Expect success.* Change your ideas about yourself as you change your behavior. Drop your old self-image and start thinking of yourself in a new way—as a jogger, a nonsmoker, a person in control.
- *Realize that lasting change takes time.* Major life changes involve giving up a familiar and comfortable part of your life in exchange for something new and unknown. They happen one day at a time, with lots of ups and downs.
- *Forgive and forget.* If you slip—miss a workout or eat a bag of candy—focus on discovering what triggered the slip and how to deal with it next time. Don't waste time blaming yourself. Keeping up your self-esteem will help you stay with your plan; negative feelings will get in your way.

ioral self-management and to devise additional strategies for overcoming potential obstacles to your program's success.

Being Fit and Well for Life

Your first attempts at making behavior changes may never go beyond the project stage. Those that do may not all succeed. But as you experience some success, you'll start to have more positive feelings about yourself. You may discover physical activities you enjoy; you may encounter new situations and meet new people. Perhaps you'll surprise yourself by accomplishing things you didn't think were possible—breaking a nicotine habit, competing in a race, climbing a mountain, developing a lean, muscular body. Most of all, you'll discover the feeling of empowerment that comes from taking charge of your health.

Once you've started, don't stop. Assume that health improvement is forever. Take on the easier problems first, and then use what you learn to tackle more difficult problems later. Periodically review what you've accomplished to make sure you don't fall into old habits. And keep informed about the latest health news and trends. Research is constantly providing new information that directly affects daily choices and habits.

This book will introduce you to the main components of a fit and well lifestyle, show you how to assess your current health status, and help you put together a program that will lead to wellness. You can't control every aspect of your health—there are too many unknowns in life for that to be possible. But you can create a lifestyle that minimizes your health risks and maximizes your enjoyment of life and well-being. You can take charge of your health in a dramatic and meaningful way. *Fit and Well* will show you how.

SUMMARY

- People today have more control over their health than ever before. A lifestyle based on good choices and healthy behaviors contributes to optimal health, or wellness. Poor lifestyle choices can lead to chronic, degenerative diseases like cardiovascular disease and cancer.
- Physical fitness, defined as the ability of the body to adapt to the demands of physical effort, is one of the most important components of wellness.
- Physical activity is a requirement for health; inactivity leads to physical deterioration. Physical fitness provides short-term benefits as well as long-term protection from disease.
- The dimensions of wellness—physical, emotional, intellectual, spiritual, interpersonal and social, and environmental—all need to be developed and balanced in a fit and well lifestyle.

- Behaviors that promote wellness include exercising regularly, choosing a healthful diet, maintaining a healthy body weight, managing stress effectively, avoiding tobacco and drugs and using alcohol wisely, and protecting yourself against disease and injury.
- In addition to behavior, good health is influenced by heredity, environment, and access to health care.
- People can move toward wellness by applying a six-step behavioral self-management program to behaviors they wish to change.
- Each small success in a behavior change program leads to more positive feelings about oneself and a sense of empowerment about one's health. Although some aspects of life are beyond individual control, people can take charge of their health to become fit and well for life.

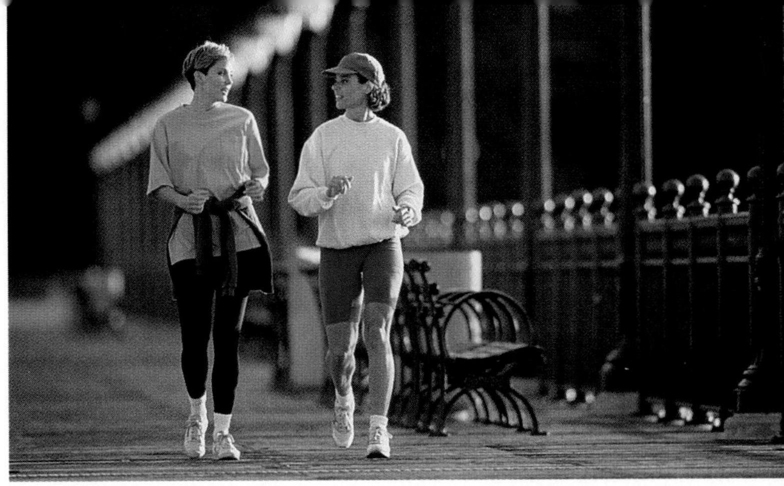

A beautiful day, an enjoyable activity, a supportive friend—all help to make walking a satisfying form of exercise for these women. Choosing the right activity and doing it the right way are important elements in a successful behavioral self-management program.

BEHAVIOR CHANGE ACTIVITY

Gathering Health Information

Gathering accurate, pertinent information about health behaviors is a crucial first step in adopting a wellness lifestyle. You need to get the facts if you are to make considered, informed decisions about your behavior. Health information can also help convince you of the need to change unhealthy behaviors. You can use information from this text, from the resources listed in the For More Information section at the end of each chapter, and from other reliable sources.

Use the lifestyle assessment in Lab 1-1 (pp. 15–16) and what you know about your own health and the health history of your family to choose a target behavior. Then take a closer look at what that behavior means to your health, now and in the future. How is it affecting your level of health and wellness? What diseases or conditions does this behavior place you at risk for? What will changing this behavior mean to you?

Health behaviors have short-term and long-term benefits and costs associated with them. For example, in the short term, an inactive lifestyle allows for more time to watch TV and hang out with friends but leaves a person less able to participate in recreational activities. In the long term, it increases risk for cardiovascular disease, cancer, and death. Fill in the blanks below with the benefits and costs of continuing your current behavior and of changing to a new, healthier behavior. Pay close attention to the short-term benefits of the new behavior—these are an important motivating force behind successful behavior change programs.

Current behavior ______________________________

Benefits *Short-Term* ____________________ ____________________ *Long-Term* ____________________ ____________________

Costs *Short-Term* ____________________ ____________________ *Long-Term* ____________________ ____________________

New behavior ______________________________

Benefits *Short-Term* ____________________ ____________________ *Long-Term* ____________________ ____________________

(continued)

Costs	Short-Term	Long-Term
	____________	____________
	____________	____________

FOR MORE INFORMATION

The following are highly readable monthly or bimonthly newsletters and magazines filled with the latest research and thinking on health-related topics. You can subscribe or get more information by writing to the address given.

Consumer Reports on Health, 101 Truman Ave., Yonkers, NY 10703-1057.

Harvard Health Letter, Palm Coast Data, P.O. Box 420285, Agency Dept., Palm Coast, FL 32142.

Harvard Women's Health Watch, P.O. Box 420234, Palm Coast, FL 32142.

Health (formerly *Hippocrates* and *In Health*), Hippocrates Partners, P.O. Box 56863, Boulder, CO 80322-6863.

Healthline, 830 Menlo Ave., Suite 100, Menlo Park, CA 94025.

HealthNews, P.O. Box 52924, Boulder, CO 80322.

Mayo Clinic Health Letter, Mayo Foundation for Medical Education and Research, Neodata, P.O. Box 2606, Boulder, CO 80322.

Mental Medicine Update: The Mind/Body Health Newsletter, P.O. Box 381065, Boston, MA 02238-1065.

Nutrition Action Health Letter, Center for Science in the Public Interest, 1875 Connecticut Ave., N.W., Suite 300, Washington, DC 20009.

Tufts University Diet & Nutrition Letter, P.O. Box 57857, Boulder, CO 80322.

University of California at Berkeley Wellness Letter, P.O. Box 420148, Palm Coast, FL 32142.

SELECTED BIBLIOGRAPHY

American Cancer Society. 1995. *Cancer Facts and Figures, 1995.* Atlanta: American Cancer Society.

Bensley, R. J. 1991. Defining spiritual health: A review of the literature. *Journal of Health Education* 22(5): 287–290.

Blair, S. N., H. W. Kohl, C. E. Barlow, R. S. Paffenbarger, L. W. Gibbons, and C. A. Macera. 1995. Changes in physical fitness and all-cause mortality: A prospective study of healthy and unhealthy men. *Journal of the American Medical Association* 273(14): 1093–1098.

Blair, S. N., H. W. Kohl, R. S. Paffenbarger, D. G. Clark, K. H. Cooper, and L. W. Gibbons. 1989. Physical fitness and all-cause mortality: A prospective study of healthy men and women. *Journal of the American Medical Association* 262(17): 2395–2401.

Booth, F. W., and B. S. Tseng. 1995. America needs to exercise for health. *Medicine and Science in Sports and Exercise* 27: 462–465.

Caspersen, C. J., and R. K. Merrit. 1995. Physical activity trends among 26 states, 1986–1990. *Medicine and Science in Sports and Exercise* 27:713–720.

Fries, J. F. 1994. *Living Well.* Reading, Mass.: Addison-Wesley.

Haskell, W. L. 1994. J. B. Wolffe Memorial Lecture. Health consequences of physical activity: Understanding and challenges regarding dose-response. *Medicine and Science in Sports and Exercise* 27:649–660.

International Society of Sport Psychology. 1992. Position statement: Physical activity and psychological benefits. *Physician and Sportsmedicine* 20(10): 179–184.

Justice, B. 1988. *Who Gets Sick: How Beliefs, Moods, and Thoughts Affect Your Health.* Los Angeles: Tarcher.

King, A. C., W. L. Haskell, D. R. Young, R. K. Oka, and M. L. Stefanick. 1995. Long-term effects of varying intensities and formats of physical activity on participation rates, fitness, and lipoproteins in men and women aged 50 to 65 years. *Circulation* 91(10): 2596–2604.

Lee, I. M., C. C. Hsieh, and R. S. Paffenbarger. 1995. Exercise intensity and longevity in men. The Harvard Alumni Health Study. *Journal of the American Medical Association* 273(15): 1179–1184.

National Center for Health Statistics. 1994. *Healthy People 2000 Review, 1993.* Hyattsville, Md.: Public Health Service, DHHS Pub. (PHS) 94-1232-1.

National Institutes of Health. 1996. *Physical Activity and Cardiovascular Health. National Institutes of Health Consensus Development Conference Statement, December 18–20, 1995.* Online. Internet. Available at http://text.nlm.gov/nih/cdc/www/101.html

Nicoloff, G., and T. L. Schwenk. 1995. Using exercise to ward off depression. *Physician and Sportsmedicine* 23(9): 44–58.

Nieman, D. C. 1995. *Fitness and Sports Medicine: A Health-Related Approach.* Palo Alto, Calif.: Bull Publishing.

Pate, R. R. 1988. The evolving definition of physical fitness. *Quest* 40:174.

Rippe, J. 1987. The health benefits of exercise. *Physician and Sportsmedicine* 15 (October): 115–132.

Siegel, P. Z., R. M. Brackbill, and G. W. Heath. 1995. The epidemiology of walking for exercise: Implications for promoting activity among sedentary groups. *American Journal of Public Health* 85(5): 706–710.

U.S. Department of Health and Human Services. 1990. *Healthy People 2000: National Health Promotion and Disease Prevention Objectives.* Washington, D.C.: U.S. Government Printing Office, DHHS Pub. (PHS) 91-50212.

Name ______________________ Section ______________ Date ______________

LAB 1-1 *Lifestyle Evaluation*

The following brief test will give you some idea about how your current lifestyle compares to the lifestyle recommended for wellness. For each question, choose the answer that best describes your behavior; then add up your score *for each section*.

Exercise/Fitness

	Almost Always	Sometimes	Never
1. I engage in moderate exercise, such as brisk walking or swimming, for 20–60 minutes, three to five times a week.	4	1	0
2. I do exercises to develop muscular strength and endurance at least twice a week.	2	1	0
3. I spend some of my leisure time participating in individual, family, or team activities, such as gardening, bowling, or softball.	2	1	0
4. I maintain a healthy body weight, avoiding overweight and underweight.	2	1	0

Exercise/Fitness Score: ____________

Nutrition

	Almost Always	Sometimes	Never
1. I eat a variety of foods each day, including five or more servings of fruits and/or vegetables.	3	1	0
2. I limit the amount of fat and saturated fat in my diet.	3	1	0
3. I avoid skipping meals.	2	1	0
4. I limit the amount of salt and sugar I eat.	2	1	0

Nutrition Score: ____________

Tobacco Use

If you never use tobacco, enter a score of 10 for this section and go to the next section.

	Almost Always	Sometimes	Never
1. I avoid using tobacco.	2	1	0
2. I smoke only low-tar-and-nicotine cigarettes, or I smoke a pipe or cigars, or I use smokeless tobacco.	2	1	0

Tobacco Use Score: ____________

Alcohol and Drugs

	Almost Always	Sometimes	Never
1. I drink no more than 1–2 drinks a day, or I avoid alcohol.	4	1	0
2. I avoid using alcohol or other drugs as a way of handling stressful situations or the problems in my life.	2	1	0
3. I am careful not to drink alcohol when taking medications (such as cold or allergy medications) or when pregnant.	2	1	0
4. I read and follow the label directions when using prescribed and over-the-counter drugs.	2	1	0

Alcohol and Drugs Score: ____________

LABORATORY ACTIVITIES

Stress Management

1. I have a job or do other work that I enjoy.	2	1	0
2. I find it easy to relax and express my feelings freely.	2	1	0
3. I manage stress well.	2	1	0
4. I have close friends, relatives, or others whom I can talk to about personal matters and call on for help when needed.	2	1	0
5. I participate in group activities (such as community or church organizations) or hobbies that I enjoy.	2	1	0
Stress-Management Score:	________		

Safety

1. I wear a seat belt while riding in a car.	2	1	0
2. I avoid driving while under the influence of alcohol or other drugs.	2	1	0
3. I obey traffic rules and the speed limit when driving.	2	1	0
4. I read and follow instructions on the labels of potentially harmful products such as household cleaners, poisons, and electrical applicances.	2	1	0
5. I avoid smoking in bed.	2	1	0
Safety Score:	________		

Disease Prevention

1. I know the warning signs of cancer, heart attack, and stroke.	2	1	0
2. I avoid overexposure to the sun and use sunscreen.	2	1	0
3. I get recommended medical screening tests (such as blood pressure checks and Pap tests), immunizations, and booster shots.	2	1	0
4. I practice monthly breast/testicle self-exams.	2	1	0
5. I am not sexually active *or* I have sex with only one mutually faithful, uninfected partner *or* I always engage in "safer sex" (using condoms), *and* I do not share needles to inject drugs.	2	1	0
Disease Prevention Score:	________		

What Your Scores Mean

Scores of 9 and 10 Excellent! Your answers show that you are aware of the importance of this area to your health. More important, you are putting your knowledge to work for you by practicing good health habits. As long as you continue to do so, this area should not pose a serious health risk. It's likely that you are setting an example for your family and friends to follow. Because you got a very high test score on this part of the test, you may want to consider other areas where your scores indicate room for improvement.

Scores of 6 to 8 Your health practices in this area are good, but there is room for improvement. Look again at the items you answered with a "Sometimes" or "Never." What changes can you make to improve your score? Even a small change can often help you achieve better health.

Scores of 3 to 5 Your health risks are showing! Would you like more information about the risks you're facing and about why it's important for you to change these behaviors? Perhaps you need help in deciding how to successfully make the changes you desire. In either case, help is available.

Scores of 0 to 2 Obviously, you were concerned enough about your health to take the test, but your answers show that you may be taking serious and unnecessary risks with your health. Perhaps you are not aware of the risks and what to do about them. You can easily get the information and help you need to improve, if you wish. The next step is up to you.

The behaviors covered in this test are recommended for most Americans, but some may not apply to people with certain chronic diseases or disabilities or to pregnant women, who may require special advice from their physician.

Source: Adapted from *Healthstyle: A Self-Test*, developed by the U.S. Public Health Service.

Name ______________________ Section ______________ Date ______________

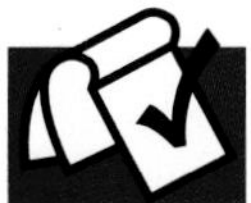

LAB 1-2 *Examining Problem Behaviors and Completing a Contract*

Using your results from Lab 1-1, select three behaviors that you want to change.

The health behaviors I wish to change are:

1. ______________________________

2. ______________________________

3. ______________________________

(Examples: "Smoking cigarettes," "Eating candy bars every night," "Not wearing a seat belt.")

Next, look carefully at the internal factors (thoughts, feelings, moods, etc.) and the external factors (sights, sounds, smells in the environment) that trigger each of your target behaviors. You may also wish to note the consequences of the behaviors, such as a change in mood. Fill in the chain of events and feelings below.

Internal and External Factors →	**Behavior** →	**Consequences**
______________	Target Behavior 1	______________
______________		______________
______________		______________
______________	Target Behavior 2	______________
______________		______________
______________		______________
______________	Target Behavior 3	______________
______________		______________
______________		______________

Examine the behavior chains to identify places you can intervene to break the chains. Complete the sample contract on the next page for one of your target behaviors.

1. I ______________________ agree to ______________________________________
(name) (specify behavior you want to change)

____

____

2. I will begin on ______________ and plan to reach my goal of ______________________
(start date) (specify final goal)

____

by ______________.
(final target date)

3. In order to reach my final goal, I have devised the following schedule of minigoals. For each step in my program, I will give myself the reward listed:

______________________	______________	______________
(minigoal 1)	(target date)	(reward)
______________________	______________	______________
(minigoal 2)	(target date)	(reward)
______________________	______________	______________
(minigoal 3)	(target date)	(reward)

My overall reward for reaching my final goal will be: ______________________________

4. I have analyzed the internal and external factors leading to my target behavior, and I have identified the following actions I can take to change my behavior: ______________________________

____

____

5. I will use the following tools to monitor my progress toward reaching my final goal:

____
(list any charts, graphs, or journals you plan to use)

____

I sign this contract as an indication of my personal commitment to reach my goal.

______________________________________ ______________
(your signature) (date)

I have recruited a helper who will witness my contract and ______________________________

____
(list any way your helper will participate in your program)

______________________________________ ______________
(witness's signature) (date)

2

Basic Principles of Physical Fitness

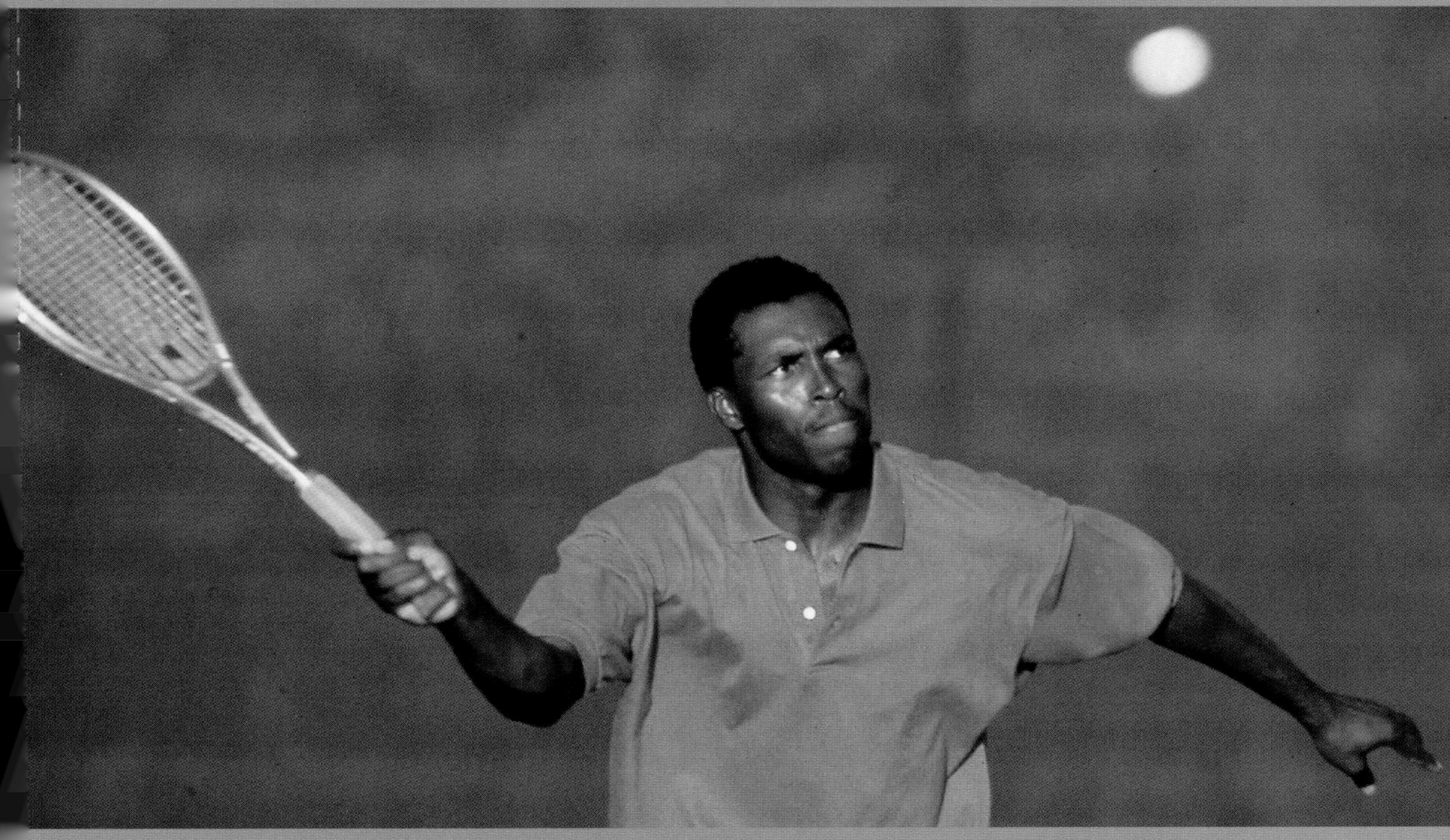

LOOKING AHEAD

After reading this chapter, you should be able to answer these questions about physical fitness:

- What are the components of physical fitness, and how does each one affect wellness?
- What is the goal of physical training, and what are the basic principles of training?
- What principles are involved in designing a well-rounded exercise program? What kinds of activities should be included?
- What steps can be taken to make an exercise program safe, effective, and successful?
- What is the difference between exercising for health and exercising for fitness?

A young mother of twins joins a health club with a weight room, exercise classes, and child care. Every Monday, Wednesday, and Friday, she takes the twins to the club and attends the 7 A.M. low-impact aerobics class. The class includes a warm-up, a 25-minute workout, exercises for major muscle groups, stretches, and a relaxation exercise. By 8:30 A.M. this young woman is exhilarated and ready for the rest of the day.

An engineering student with a heavy workload and an active social life plays tennis for exercise. He likes to play at 6 P.M. when most people are eating dinner. After a fast, hard hour of tennis with his regular partner, he does some stretching exercises. Twice a week he works out at the gym, with particular attention to keeping his arms strong and his joints limber. On weekends he often goes on a hike with two or three friends.

Another student is on the varsity soccer team. She follows a rigorous exercise regimen established by her soccer coach. Practice is two hours long, four days a week, with warm-ups, drills, and a scrimmage. Games are on Saturdays. This athletic woman also enjoys long bicycle rides and recreational swimming when she gets the chance.

There are as many different physical fitness programs as there are different individuals. Each of the people described above has worked an adequate or more-than-adequate fitness program into a busy daily routine. You, too, can incorporate exercise into your life and enjoy the benefits of being physically fit.

Any list of these benefits would be impressive. Exercise helps you generate more energy, control your weight, manage stress, and boost your immune system. It provides psychological and emotional benefits, contributing to your sense of competence and well-being. It offers protection against heart disease, diabetes, high blood pressure, osteoporosis, cancer, and perhaps even premature death. Exercise increases your physical capacity so that you are better able to meet the challenges of daily life with more energy and vigor. Although people vary greatly in the levels of fitness and performance they can ultimately achieve, the benefits of physical fitness are available to everyone. (For more on the benefits of exercise, see the box "A Runner's Rationale.")

This chapter provides an overview of physical fitness. It explains the components of fitness, the basic principles of physical training, and the essential elements of a well-rounded exercise program. Chapters 3–7 provide an in-depth look at each of the elements of a fitness program.

TERMS

cardiorespiratory endurance The ability of the body to perform prolonged, large-muscle, dynamic exercise at moderate-to-high levels of intensity.

muscular strength The amount of force a muscle can produce with a single maximum effort.

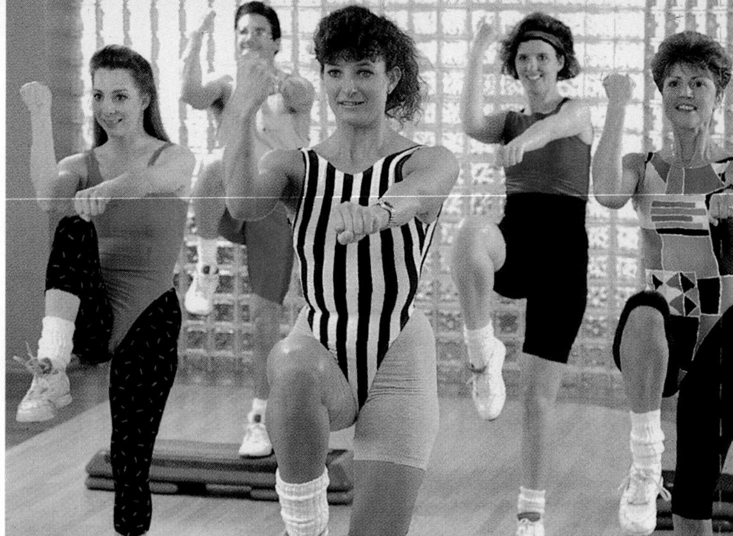

Cardiorespiratory endurance is the most important component of health-related fitness. The members of this step aerobics class are conditioning their hearts and lungs as well as gaining many other health benefits.

COMPONENTS OF PHYSICAL FITNESS

As mentioned in Chapter 1, physical fitness is defined as the ability of the body to adapt to the demands of physical effort—that is, to perform moderate-to-vigorous levels of physical activity without becoming overly tired. Physical fitness has many components, some related to general health and others related more specifically to particular sports or activities. The five components of fitness most important for health are cardiorespiratory endurance, muscular strength, muscular endurance, flexibility, and body composition (proportion of fat to lean body mass).

Cardiorespiratory endurance is the ability to perform prolonged, large-muscle, dynamic exercise at moderate-to-high levels of intensity. It depends on such factors as the ability of the lungs to deliver oxygen from the environment to the bloodstream, the heart's capacity to pump blood, the ability of the nervous system and blood vessels to regulate blood flow, and the capability of the body's chemical systems to use oxygen and process fuels for exercise. When levels of cardiorespiratory fitness are low, the heart has to work very hard during normal daily activities and may not be able to work hard enough to sustain high-intensity physical activity in an emergency. As cardiorespiratory fitness improves, the heart begins to function more efficiently. It doesn't have to work as hard at rest or during low levels of exercise. The heart pumps more blood per heartbeat, resting heart rate slows down, blood volume increases, blood supply to the tissues improves, the body is better able to cool itself, and resting blood pressure decreases. A healthy heart can better withstand the strains of everyday life, the stress of occasional emergencies, and the wear and tear of time. Endurance training also improves the functioning of the chemical systems, particularly in the muscles and liver, thereby enhancing the body's ability to use energy supplied by food.

WELLNESS CONNECTION
A Runner's Rationale

Much of the attention surrounding exercise focuses on its benefits for physical health. But for many exercisers, improved health and longevity are only part of the reason they begin and continue to train. In this selection, long-time *Runner's World* columnist George Sheehan highlights the diverse and interconnected nature of the wellness benefits of exercise.

When I lecture, I often begin with a short film on running. The opening scene is the start of the Boston Marathon. Thousands of runners stream toward the camera, while the narrator remarks that these marathoners are only the visible elite of millions of runners now surging along the world's roads and filling its parks. "The nonrunner watches," he says, "and wonders—*why?*"

The audience almost always laughs at that question. To the people in the film, running is normal; to those in my audience, running—especially marathon running—is a mystery. When the film ends and the lights go on, I ascend the stage and address the question, Why do people run?

My answer is direct: Their lives depend upon it. People begin running for any number of motives, but we stick to it for one basic reason—to find out who we really are. Running or some other form of exercise is essential in the drive to become and perpetuate the ultimate self, because finding out who we are means finding out what our limits are—and we have to *test* ourselves to do that.

I run because my life in all its aspects depends upon it. The length of my life, certainly; the hours in my day, just as surely. The person I am, my productivity, my creativity, my pursuit of happiness—all are conditioned and determined by my hours on the road.

Most non-exercisers are unaware of this global, whole-life effect of athletic training. The experts—physicians, psychologists, sociologists, teachers, even philosophers—carve out discrete territories in which they operate. They focus on certain parts of our lives, but not life in its totality—not Life with a capital *L*.

The physician tells me that my lifespan is related to my lifestyle. When I began running, my coronary risk factors practically disappeared. I stopped smoking, my weight returned to what it had been in college, and my blood pressure didn't rise as I got older. Running also added hours to my day. My physical work capacity is far greater than it was when I was 38 years old and (presumably) in my prime. Clearly, my body benefits from fitness.

But my mind does, too. The psychologist tells me that. The negative feelings—anxiety and depression, anger and hostility—are all reduced by training. While these destructive feelings diminish, constructive ones such as self-esteem and self-confidence rise.

And the public me benefits also: The sociologist argues that my professional success is linked to the fitness I earn from running. It is no longer simply survival of the fittest, it is also success to the fittest. Fit people occupy the upper echelons in education, position, and salary.

The educator views my running and racing as a laboratory where I learn about such things as sacrifice and solitude, courage and cooperation, victory and defeat. And the philosopher reminds me that creative thinking requires the inner and outer solitude that running confers.

So it goes: Each specialist sees the role of exercise through the prism of that particular specialty. I explain this fragmentation to the audience, and then I tell them that no one piece of the puzzle is enough. Each of these experts sees only a bit of me. But I am not a cholesterol level, I am not a Rorschach profile. I am not an ergometer reading or an IQ. I am a physician, a student, a problem solver. I am also a parent, a sibling, a lover, a friend.

But none of these entirely defines me. "I absolutely deny," wrote D. H. Lawrence, "that I am a soul, or a body or an intelligence, or a nervous system or a bunch of glands, or any of the rest of the bits of me. The whole is greater than the sum of my parts. . . . I am a total living human being."

I look out over the audience and ask them, "Are you content with this total living person you are now?" American writer Lewis Mumford once remarked that today might be a fair sample of eternity. If so, who you are today would be the eternal you, the final product of your years on earth. If this were your last day, would you be satisfied?

There it is—my *why* of running, my reason for exercise—no less than the creation of the human being I become. [1986]

Cardiorespiratory endurance is considered the most important component of health-related fitness because the functioning of the heart and lungs is so essential to overall good health. A person simply can't live very long or very well without a healthy heart. Low levels of cardiorespiratory fitness are linked with heart disease, the leading cause of death in the United States.

Muscular strength is the amount of force a muscle can produce with a single maximum effort. Strong muscles are important for the smooth and easy performance of everyday activities, such as carrying groceries, lifting boxes, and climbing stairs, as well as for emergency situations. They help keep the skeleton in proper alignment, preventing back and leg pain and providing the support necessary for good posture. Muscular strength has obvious importance in recreational activities. Strong people can hit a tennis ball harder, kick a soccer ball farther, and ride a bicycle uphill more easily. Muscle tissue is an important element of overall body composition. Greater muscle mass (or lean body mass) means a higher rate of **metabolism** and faster energy use. Maintaining strength and muscle mass is vital for healthy aging. Older people tend to lose muscle cells, and many of the remaining muscle cells become nonfunctional because they lose their attachment to the nervous system. Strength training helps maintain muscle mass and function in older people, which greatly enhances their quality of life and prevents life-threatening injuries.

Muscular endurance is the ability to sustain a given level of muscle tension—that is, to hold a muscle contraction for a long period of time or to contract a muscle over and over again. Muscular endurance is important for good posture and for injury prevention. For example, if abdominal and back muscles aren't strong enough to hold the spine correctly, the chances of low-back pain and back injury are increased. Muscular endurance helps people cope with the physical demands of everyday life and enhances performance in sports and work. It is also important for most leisure and fitness activities.

Flexibility is the ability to move the joints through their full range of motion. Although range of motion isn't a significant factor in everyday activities for most people, inactivity causes the joints to become stiffer with age. Stiffness often causes older people to assume unnatural body postures, and it can lead to back pain. The majority of Americans, some 60–80%, experience low-back pain at some time in their lives, often because of stiff joints. Stretching exercises can help ensure a normal range of motion for all major joints.

Body composition refers to the relative amounts of **lean body tissue** (muscle, bone, and water) and fat in the body. Healthy body composition involves a high proportion of lean body tissue and an acceptably low level of body fat, adjusted for age and gender. A person with excessive body fat is more likely to experience a variety of health problems, including heart disease, high blood pressure, stroke, joint problems, diabetes, gallbladder disease, cancer, and back pain. The best way to lose fat is through a lifestyle that includes a sensible diet and exercise. The best way to add lean body tissue is through weight training, also known as strength or resistance training.

In addition to these five health-related components of physical fitness, physical fitness for a particular sport or activity might include any or all of the following: coordination, speed, reaction time, agility, balance, and skill. Sport-specific skills are best developed through practice. The skill and coordination needed to play basketball, for example, are developed by playing basketball.

PRINCIPLES OF PHYSICAL TRAINING

As mentioned above, the human body is very adaptable. The greater the demands made on it, the more it adjusts to meet the demands. Over time, immediate, short-term adjustments translate into long-term changes and improvements. When breathing and heart rate increase during exercise, for example, the heart gradually develops the ability to pump more blood with each beat. Then, during exercise, it doesn't have to beat as fast to meet the cells' demands for oxygen. The goal of **physical training** is to bring about these long-term changes and improvements in the body's functioning. Although people differ in the maximum levels of physical fitness and performance they can achieve through training, the wellness benefits of exercise are available to everyone (see the box "Fitness and Disability").

Particular types and amounts of exercise are most effective in developing the various components of fitness. To put together an effective exercise program, a person should first understand the basic principles of physical training. Three important principles are specificity, progressive overload, and reversibility.

Specificity

To develop a particular fitness component, exercises must be performed that are specifically designed for that component. This is the principle of **specificity.** Weight training, for example, develops muscular strength, not car-

TERMS

metabolism The sum of all the vital processes by which food energy and nutrients are made available to and used by the body.

muscular endurance The ability of a muscle or group of muscles to remain contracted or to contract repeatedly for a long period of time.

flexibility The range of motion in a joint or group of joints; flexibility is related to muscle length.

body composition The relative proportion of lean body tissue (muscle, bone, and water) and fat in the body.

lean body tissue The nonfat component of the human body, consisting of skeletal muscle, bone, and water.

physical training The performance of different types of activities that cause the body to adapt and improve its level of fitness.

specificity The training principle according to which the body adapts to the particular type and amount of stress placed on it.

progressive overload The training principle according to which increasing amounts of stress are placed on the body, causing adaptations that improve fitness.

DIMENSIONS OF DIVERSITY
Fitness and Disability

Physical fitness and athletic achievement are not limited to the able-bodied. People with disabilities can also attain high levels of fitness and performance, as shown by the elite athletes who compete in the Paralympics. The premier event for athletes with disabilities, the Paralympics is held in the same year and city as the Olympics. The athletes who participate include people with cerebral palsy, people with visual impairments, paraplegics, quadriplegics, and others. They compete in wheelchair races and wheelchair basketball, tandem cycling, in which a blind cyclist pedals with a sighted athlete, and other events. The performance of these skilled athletes makes it clear that people with disabilities can be active, healthy, and extraordinarily fit.

Paralympians point out that able-bodied athletes and athletes with disabilities have two important things in common—both are striving for excellence, and both can serve as role models. One athlete commented, "I'd like to let kids who have a disability know there is a sports option. The possibilities are endless."

Currently, between 34 and 43 million Americans are estimated to have chronic, significant disabilities. Some disabilities are the result of injury, such as spinal cord injuries sustained in car crashes. Other disabilities result from illness, such as the blindness that sometimes occurs as a complication of diabetes or the joint stiffness that accompanies arthritis. And some disabilities are present at birth, as in the case of congenital limb deformities or cerebral palsy.

Exercise and physical activity are as important for people with disabilities as for able-bodied individuals—if not *more* important. Being active helps prevent secondary conditions that may result from prolonged inactivity, such as circulatory or muscular problems. It also provides an emotional boost that helps support a positive attitude.

People with disabilities don't have to be Olympians to participate in sports and lead an active life. Depending on the nature of the disability, numerous options exist, including tennis, basketball, cycling, swimming, and running. Some fitness centers offer modified aerobics, mild exercise in warm water, and other exercises adapted for people with disabilities.

For those who prefer to get their exercise at home, special aerobic workout videos are available. Most of these videos are produced by hospitals and health associations and are geared to specific disabilities. For example, the Arthritis Foundation produces two videos, at different levels, called "People with Arthritis Can Exercise." There are also workout videos designed especially for individuals with hearing impairments (instructors both speak and sign); for women who have had breast surgery and need to strengthen arm, shoulder, and back muscles; for people confined to wheelchairs; and many others. Some types are designed so that both able-bodied people and people with disabilities can participate.

If you want to try one of these videos or participate in some form of adapted physical activity, check with your physician about what's appropriate for you. Remember that no matter what your level of ability or disability, it's possible to make exercise an integral part of your life.

Sources: U.S. Department of Health and Human Services. 1990. *Healthy People 2000: National Health Promotion and Disease Prevention Objectives.* Washington, D.C.: U.S. Government Printing Office, DHHS Pub. (PHS) 91-50212. Silver, M. 1990. All the right moves. *U.S. News & World Report,* 12 November. Nemeth, M. 1992. Willing and able. *Maclean's,* 7 September.

diorespiratory endurance or flexibility. Specificity also applies to the skill-related fitness components—to improve at tennis, you must practice tennis—and to the different parts of the body—to develop stronger arms, you must exercise your arms. A well-rounded exercise program includes exercises geared to each component of fitness, to different parts of the body, and to specific activities or sports.

Progressive Overload

The body adapts to the demands of exercise by improving its functioning. When the amount of exercise (also called overload or stress) is progressively increased, fitness continues to improve. This is the principle of **progressive overload.**

The amount of overload is very important. Too little exercise will have no effect on fitness; too much may cause injury. For every type of exercise, there is a training threshold at which fitness benefits begin to occur, a zone within which maximum fitness benefits occur, and an upper limit of safe training (Figure 2-1). The amount of exercise needed depends on the individual's current level of fitness, his or her fitness goals, and the component being developed. A novice, for example, might experience fitness benefits from jogging a mile in 10 minutes, but this level of exercise would cause no physical adaptations in a trained distance runner. Beginners should start at the lower end of the fitness benefit zone; fitter individuals will make more rapid gains by exercising at the higher end of the maximum zone.

The amount of overload needed to maintain or improve a particular level of fitness is determined in terms of three dimensions: exercise frequency (how often), intensity (how hard), and duration (how long).

- *Frequency.* Developing fitness requires regular exercise. Optimum exercise frequency, expressed in number of days per week, varies with the component being developed and the individual's fitness goals. Most fitness components require a minimum of 3–5

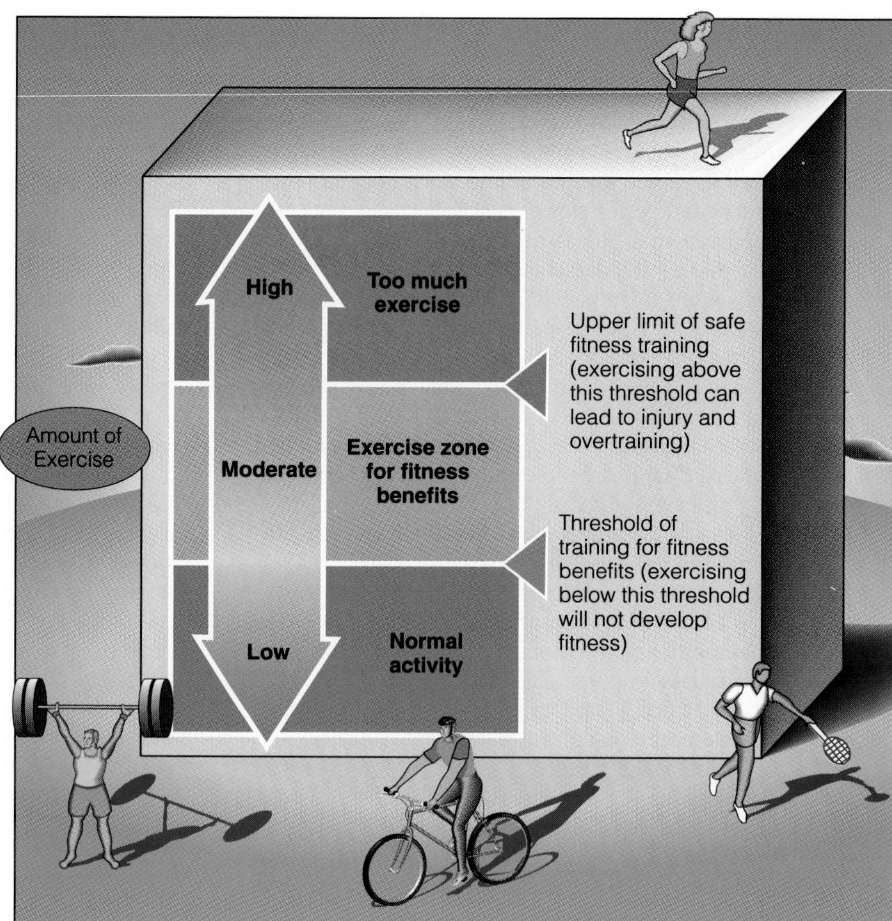

Figure 2-1 ***Amount of exercise for fitness benefits.***

days per week. Once fitness goals have been reached, a lower frequency—2 or 3 days per week—may be sufficient to maintain fitness.

- *Intensity.* Fitness benefits occur when a person exercises harder than his or her normal level of activity. The appropriate exercise intensity varies with each fitness component. To develop cardiorespiratory endurance, for example, a person must raise his or her heart rate above normal; to develop muscular strength, the person must lift a heavier weight than normal; to develop flexibility, the person must stretch the muscles beyond their normal length.
- *Duration.* If fitness benefits are to occur, exercise sessions must last for an extended period of time. For cardiorespiratory endurance exercise, a duration of 20–60 minutes is recommended. (You can improve cardiorespiratory endurance by training at very high intensities for 5–10 minutes. However, you greatly increase the risk of injury, and you are less likely to continue to exercise regularly because high-intensity training can be very uncomfortable.) For muscular strength, muscular endurance, and flexibility, similar amounts of time are advisable, but these exercises are more commonly organized in terms of a specific number of repetitions (50 sit-ups, 30 leg lifts, and so on).

Reversibility

Fitness is a reversible adaptation. The body adjusts to lower levels of physical activity the same way it adjusts to higher levels. This is the principle of **reversibility.** When a person stops exercising, up to 50% of fitness improvements are lost within 2 months. If a training schedule must be curtailed temporarily, fitness improvements are best maintained if exercise intensity is kept constant and frequency and/or duration is reduced.

DESIGNING YOUR OWN EXERCISE PROGRAM

Physical training works best when you have a plan. The plan helps you make gradual but steady progress toward your goals in all five areas of health-related fitness. The basic idea of a workout or training session is to introduce a stress powerful enough to cause adaptation but not so severe as to cause injury.

Assessment

The first step in creating a successful fitness program is to assess your current level of fitness for each of the five health-related fitness components. The results of the assessment tests will help you set specific fitness goals and plan your fitness program. Lab 2-1 gives you the opportunity to assess your current overall level of activity. Assessment tests in Chapters 3, 4, 5, and 6 will help you evaluate your cardiorespiratory endurance, muscular strength, muscular endurance, flexibility, and body composition.

Setting Goals

The ultimate goal of every health-related fitness program is the same—wellness that lasts a lifetime. Is this goal inspiring enough to motivate you to begin and stay with a program of regular exercise? Think carefully about your goals and your reasons for exercising. You may want to exercise to improve your body composition, have more energy, or lower your blood pressure; you may want to be able to run a 10K road race or ski a more advanced slope; or you may just want to feel better about yourself.

Whatever your goals, they must be important enough to you to keep you motivated. Studies have shown that exercising for yourself, rather than for the impression you think you'll make on others, is more likely to lead to long-lasting commitment. After you complete the assessment tests in Chapters 3–6, you will be able to set goals directly related to each fitness component, such as working toward a 3-mile jog or doing 20 push-ups. First, though, think carefully about your overall goals, and be clear about why you are starting a program.

Choosing Activities

A health-related exercise program should center on cardiorespiratory endurance exercises, but it should also include activities to develop muscular strength and endurance, flexibility, and healthy body composition.

- Cardiorespiratory endurance is developed by activities that involve continuous rhythmic movements of large muscle groups like those in the legs. Walking, jogging, cycling, cross-country skiing, and aerobic dance are all good activities for developing cardiorespiratory endurance. Although less effective than continuous types of exercise, start-and-stop activities such as tennis, racquetball, and soccer can develop endurance if skill level is high enough. Training for cardiorespiratory endurance is discussed in Chapter 3.
- Muscular strength and endurance can be developed by training with weights or by performing calisthenic exercises such as push-ups and sit-ups. Training for muscular strength and endurance is discussed in Chapter 4.
- Flexibility is developed by stretching the major muscle groups, regularly and with proper technique. Flexibility is discussed in Chapter 5.
- Healthy body composition can be developed by combining a sensible diet and a program of regular exercise. Endurance exercise is best for reducing body fat. Strength exercises build muscle mass, which helps increase metabolism (the rate of energy expenditure). Body composition is discussed in Chapter 6.

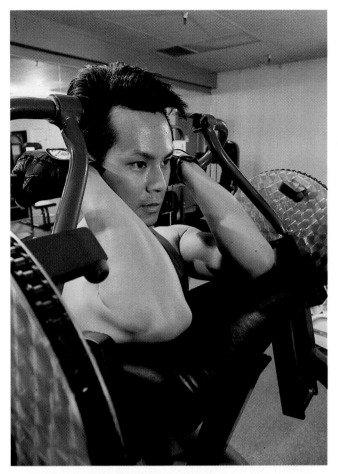

An important principle of exercising is to train the way you want your body to change. By working out on weight training equipment, this young man is increasing the strength and definition of specific muscles and improving the overall appearance of his body.

Fitness training is easier if you enjoy the activity. Many sports provide good conditioning—including volleyball, tennis, cross-country skiing, alpine skiing, water skiing, and windsurfing—and can be used to supplement an exercise program. Chapter 7 contains guidelines for choosing activities and putting together a complete exercise program.

Guidelines for Training

The following guidelines will make your exercise program more effective and successful:

TERMS

reversibility The training principle according to which fitness improvements are lost when demands on the body are lowered.

- *Train the way you want your body to change.* Stress your body such that it adapts in the desired direction. To have a more muscular build, lift weights. To be more flexible, do stretching exercises. To improve performance in a particular sport, practice that sport or the movements used in it.
- *Train regularly.* The optimal workout schedule for endurance training is 3–5 days per week. Exercising fewer than three times a week increases the risk of injury, because the body never gets the chance to adapt fully to the training. And, because adaptations are reversible, fitness improvements are lost if too much time is allowed to pass between exercise sessions.
- *Get in shape gradually.* Give your body time to adapt to the stress of exercise. As you progress, increase duration and frequency before increasing intensity. If you train too much or too intensely, you are more likely to suffer injuries or become **overtrained,** a condition characterized by lack of energy, aching muscles and joints, and decreased physical performance. Injuries and overtraining slow down an exercise program and impede rather than enhance motivation. The goal is not to get in shape as quickly as possible but to gradually become and remain physically fit.
- *Warm up before exercising, and cool down afterward.* Warming up decreases the chances of injury by helping the body gradually progress from rest to activity. A warm-up should include low-intensity movements similar to those used in the activity that will follow. Stretching exercises are also often recommended. Cooling down after exercise is important for restoring circulation to its normal resting condition. Cool down by continuing to exercise but at a lower level of intensity.
- *Listen to your body.* Don't insist on exercising if it doesn't feel right. Sometimes you need a few days of rest to recover enough to train with the intensity required for improving fitness. On the other hand, you can't train sporadically either. If you listen to your body and it always tells you to rest, you won't make any progress. You have to work to improve fitness, so try to maintain a structured—but flexible—workout program.
- *Try training with a partner.* Training partners can motivate and encourage each other through hard spots and help each other develop proper exercise techniques. Training with a partner can make exercising easier and more fun.
- *Train your mind.* This is one of the most difficult skills to acquire, but it is critical for achieving and maintaining fitness. Becoming fit requires commitment, discipline, and patience. These qualities come from understanding the importance of exercise and having clear and reachable goals. Use the lifestyle management techniques discussed in Chapter 1 to keep your program on track. Believe in yourself and your potential—and you *will* achieve your goals!
- *Keep your exercise program in perspective.* As important as physical fitness is, it is only part of a well-rounded life. You have to have time for work and school, family and friends, relaxation and hobbies. Some people become overinvolved in exercise and neglect other parts of their lives. They think of themselves as runners, dancers, swimmers, or triathletes rather than as people who participate in those activities. Balance and moderation are the key ingredients of a fit and well life.

TERMS

overtraining A condition caused by training too much or too intensely, characterized by lack of energy, decreased physical performance, fatigue, depression, aching muscles and joints, and susceptibility to injury.

exercise stress test A test usually administered on a treadmill or stationary bicycle that involves analysis of the changes in electrical activity in the heart from an electrocardiogram (EKG or ECG) taken during exercise. Used to determine if any heart disease is present and to assess current fitness level.

FITNESS BENEFITS VERSUS HEALTH BENEFITS

To become physically fit, it's best to be active almost every day. The American College of Sports Medicine (ACSM) has established guidelines for creating an exercise program that will develop physical fitness (Table 2-1). Based on years of carefully conducted research into how people respond to exercise training, the ACSM recommendations represent a consensus among leading experts in medicine and exercise science. An exercise program developed in line with these guidelines will lead to the fitness benefits described in Chapter 1.

You can gain health benefits from smaller amounts of exercise, however. Low- to moderate-intensity activities like gardening, cleaning, and strolling have been shown to lower the risk of heart disease if they are performed regularly, for long durations, over a period of years. In 1995, the Centers for Disease Control and Prevention (CDC) and the ACSM jointly issued a "moderate activity prescription" aimed at the more than 75% of the American population that is completely sedentary. They recommend that everyone accumulate at least 30 minutes of moderate-intensity physical activity over the course of each day. This advice is not a contradiction of the ACSM guidelines for developing physical fitness; rather, it stresses that moderate levels of activity lead to significant health benefits. People who are completely sedentary and

TABLE 2-1 Recommended Quantity and Quality of Exercise for Healthy Adults

Mode of activity	Cardiorespiratory endurance exercises such as running-jogging, walking-hiking, swimming, skating, bicycling, rowing, cross-country skiing, rope skipping, and various game activities; resistance training; flexibility training.
Frequency of training	3–5 days per week.
Intensity of training	60–90% of maximum heart rate or 50–85% of maximal oxygen uptake.
Duration of training	20–60 minutes of continuous aerobic activity.
Resistance training	At least one set of 8–12 repetitions of 8–10 exercises that condition the major muscle groups; recommended minimum frequency: at least 2 days per week.
Flexibility training	Statically stretch the major muscle groups for 5 repetitions of 15–30 seconds, at least three times per week. Use caution when performing exercises that require substantial skill or flexibility, particularly if you are older, less flexible, or less experienced.

Sources: American College of Sports Medicine. 1995. *Guidelines for Exercise Testing and Prescription,* 5th ed. Baltimore: Williams & Wilkins. American College of Sports Medicine. 1990. Position Stand on the Recommended Quantity and Quality of Exercise for Developing and Maintaining Cardiorespiratory and Muscular Fitness in Healthy Adults. *Medicine and Science in Sports and Exercise* 22:265–274.

for whom the ACSM recommendations seem out of reach should begin by trying to meet the CDC/ACSM moderate activity prescription.

One recent, widely publicized study of Harvard University alumni seemed to indicate that only "vigorous" exercise leads to significant health benefits. However, researchers generally view the relationship between exercise intensity and health benefits as a continuum. The conclusions of the Harvard study must be considered in light of problems that can result from the different ways in which people report their physical activity to researchers and the difficulty in defining what constitutes "moderate" and "vigorous" activity. For example, some activities the Harvard study rated as vigorous—walking at the rate of 4 mph, for example—would be classified as moderate by the CDC/ACSM criteria.

Most studies have shown health benefits of even very low-intensity exercise, especially when compared with a completely sedentary lifestyle. For example, one study examining the number of calories burned each week in total physical activity—whether in everyday activities like walking and stair climbing or in formal exercise—found that death rates decreased steadily as activity levels increased (Figure 2-2, p. 28). Additional studies may further clarify the relationship between intensity of exercise and health.

The general advice from researchers is that some exercise is better than none, but that more—as long as it does not result in injury or overtraining—is probably better than some. Exercising for fitness benefits is the type of activity most recommended, but lower-intensity exercise is also an important part of a fit and well lifestyle. Since activity of any kind has health benefits, try to be active even when you're not exercising. Take the stairs rather than the escalator; walk to the store instead of driving; turn off the TV and go for a hike. You may not become an Olympic athlete by walking for 30 minutes several times a week, but you will be contributing to your health and well-being, now and in the future (see the box "Exercise and Intellectual Wellness," p. 29).

? COMMON QUESTIONS ANSWERED

Is exercise safe for me? If you are male and under 40 or female and under 50 and in good health, exercise is probably safe for you. If you are over these ages or have health problems (especially high blood pressure, heart disease, muscle or joint problems, or obesity), see your physician before starting a vigorous exercise program. The British Columbia Ministry of Health has developed a questionnaire called PAR-Q to determine exercise safety. This questionnaire is included in Lab 2-2. Completing it should alert you to any potential problems you may have.

If a physician isn't sure whether exercise is safe for you, he or she may recommend an **exercise stress test** to see whether you develop symptoms of heart disease during exercise. For most people, however, it's far safer to exercise than to remain sedentary.

You must also consider your physical safety when exercising. If you ride a bicycle or run on public streets, make sure you wear clothing that can be seen easily. Bicyclists should always wear helmets. Even though you may have the right-of-way, give cars plenty of leeway; in a collision, a car will usually sustain less damage than a bicycle or your unprotected body. Don't train in isolated areas

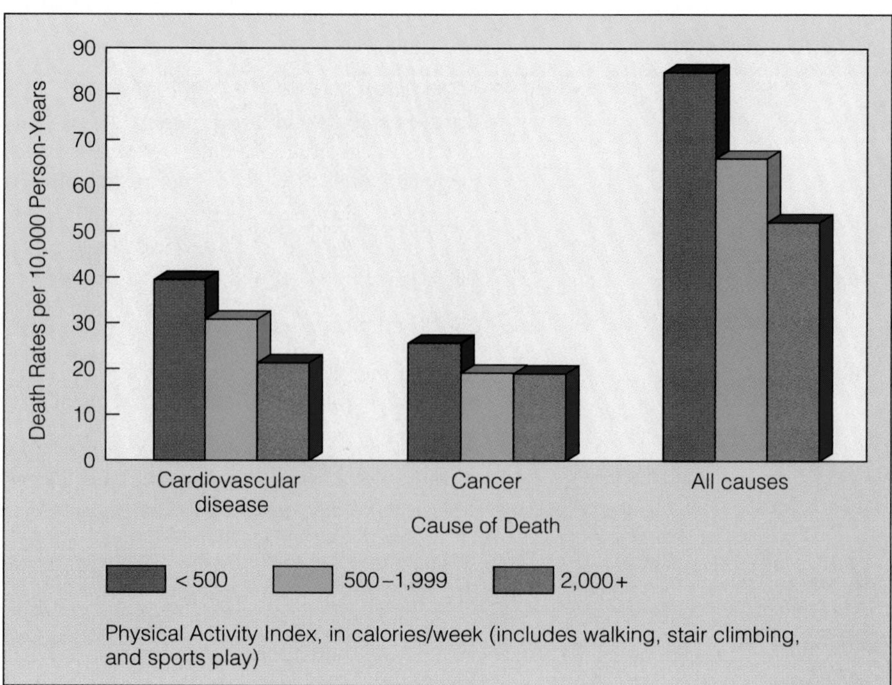

Figure 2-2 ***The relationship between physical activity and health.***

unless you're with a friend. Exercising alone, you could easily be injured or become a crime victim. (See Appendix A for more information on personal safety.)

Where can I get help and advice about exercise? Because fitness is essential to a wellness lifestyle, you need to learn as much as you can about exercise. One of the best places to get help is to take an exercise class. There, expert exercise instructors can help you learn the basics of training and answer your questions. Read articles by credible experts in fitness magazines. Because of fierce competition among publications, these magazines include articles by leading experts in exercise science written at a layperson's level.

A qualified personal trainer can also be helpful in getting you started in an exercise program or a new form of training. Make sure this person has proper qualifications, such as a college degree in exercise physiology or physical education or ACSM certification. Don't seek out a person for advice simply because he or she looks fit.

Should I follow my exercise program if I'm sick? No. You shouldn't train when you're ill—especially if you have a fever—or injured. Doing so could seriously compromise your recovery and may even be dangerous. In too many cases, people have to give up favorite activities because they don't allow their injuries to heal properly. Specific types of injuries and how to handle them are discussed in Chapter 3.

Is there a limit to how strong, powerful, flexible, or skilled I can become? Yes. All people are not created equal when it comes to the maximum level of physical fitness and performance they can achieve. Some people are able to run longer distances, or lift more weight, or kick a soccer ball more skillfully than others will ever be able to, no matter how much they train. There are limits on the adaptability—the potential for improvement—of any human body. The body's ability to transport and use oxygen, for example, can be improved by only about 20% through training. An endurance athlete must therefore inherit a large lung capacity in order to reach competitive performance levels.

However, an individual doesn't have to be an Olympic sprinter to experience health benefits from running. Physical training improves fitness regardless of heredity. For the average person, the body's adaptability is enough to achieve all fitness goals. An improvement of 20% in oxygen consumption can mean the difference between lifelong health and the development of a chronic disease.

How can I fit my exercise program into my day? Good time management is an important skill in creating and maintaining an exercise program. Choose a regular time to exercise, preferably the same time every day. Don't tell yourself you'll exercise "sometime during the day" when you have some free time—that free time may never come. Schedule your workout into your day, and make it a priority. Include alternative plans in your program to account for circumstances like bad weather or vacations.

WELLNESS CONNECTION
Exercise and Intellectual Wellness

Although most people don't typically associate exercise with mental skills, physical activity has been shown to have positive effects on cognitive functioning in both the short term and the long term. Exercise triggers the release of several key neurotransmitters, including epinephrine and norepinephrine, that are known to boost alertness. Many people report that they feel more alert after a session of exercise and that they can study more attentively. Exercise also appears to improve memory and intellectual functioning, particularly for tasks that are complex and require a significant amount of mental effort. There is no evidence that exercise can actually boost intelligence, but it can help you to perform cognitive tasks at your peak level.

Exercise may also boost creativity. In a study of college students, those who ran regularly or took aerobic dance classes scored significantly higher on standard psychological tests of creativity than students who remained sedentary. The improvement in creativity was seen after only 4 months of regular exercise.

Over the long term, regular physical activity can have even more dramatic effects. Studies have shown that exercise can slow and possibly even reverse certain age-related declines in cognitive performance, including slowed reaction time and loss of short-term memory and nonverbal reasoning skills. Regular exercise helps improve cerebral blood flow by controlling high blood pressure and improving blood fat levels and platelet activity. Exercise activates the brain and enhances cerebral metabolic demands. All of these physical effects help sustain cognitive abilities as we age. Exercise also has a positive effect on self-esteem and helps control stress and anxiety, all of which are associated with improvements in cognitive function. Several studies have shown that physically fit older people react to both simple and complicated mental challenges just as quickly as unfit individuals 30 years younger.

The message from these studies is that exercise is a critical factor in developing *all* the dimensions of wellness—not just physical health. A lifetime of physical activity can leave you with a healthier body and a sharper, more creative mind.

Sources: Exercise can go to your head. 1995. *Consumer Reports on Health,* September. Chollar, S. Psychological benefits of exercise. *American Health,* June. Rogers, R., J. Meyer, and K. Mortel. 1990. After reaching retirement age physical activity sustains cerebral perfusion and cognition. *Journal of the American Geriatrics Society* 38:123–128.

Research has shown that people who exercise in the morning are least likely to miss their workouts. They complete their program early and have the rest of the day ahead of them. People who plan to exercise at lunchtime or in the evening are more likely to miss their sessions because of unexpected schedule conflicts. However, if afternoon or evening fits into your schedule better, plan to exercise then. Choose the time of day that works best for you.

You don't have to work on all fitness components in the same exercise session. You can jog and stretch in one session and lift weights in another. The important thing is to have a regular schedule. (You'll have the chance to develop strategies for successful time management and maintaining an exercise program while away from home in the Behavior Change Activities in Chapters 10 and 12.)

Where can I work out? Identify accessible and pleasant places to work out. For running, find a field or park with a soft surface. For swimming, find a pool that's open at times convenient for you. For cycling, find an area with minimal traffic and air pollution. Make sure the place you exercise is safe and convenient.

If you join a health club or fitness center, choose one close to your home or place of work. You'll be less likely to go to the club if it's farther away. Choose a club with an atmosphere that fits with your personality and offers the activities you want. For guidelines, refer to the box "Choosing a Fitness Center" (p. 30).

SUMMARY

- Everyone can incorporate exercise into a daily or weekly routine and enjoy the benefits of fitness.
- The five components of physical fitness most important for health are cardiorespiratory endurance, muscular strength, muscular endurance, flexibility, and body composition.
- Physical fitness for a particular sport or activity might include coordination, speed, reaction time, agility, balance, and/or skill.
- Physical training is the process of bringing about long-term improvements in the body's functioning through exercise. Three important principles of training are specificity, progressive overload, and reversibility.
- Progressive overload is quantified in terms of frequency, intensity, and duration of exercise.
- Important steps in designing an exercise program include assessing your current level of fitness, setting

CRITICAL CONSUMER
Choosing a Fitness Center

If you're thinking of becoming a member of a health club or fitness center, the following guidelines will help you make a final choice:

1. Does the center provide programs that are appropriate for you and at convenient times? You may wish to consult with a physician about your specific exercise needs.
2. Ask members and former members about the operation, services, staff, and programs. Names should be available upon request. Avoid clubs that refuse to comply with your request.
3. Visit the club at the time of day when you plan to use it. Are the classes crowded, or are there long lines for the equipment you plan to use?
4. Check the atmosphere of the club. Are personnel friendly, enthusiastic, attentive, and well-informed? Do instructors have special training? Is there a fitness supervisor who has a degree in exercise science or certification from the ACSM or another recognized organization?
5. Observe the facility. Is it clean, well-ventilated, and properly maintained? Is the equipment in good condition? Is there shock-absorbent flooring for aerobics workouts? Is safety information provided for using weight machines? Are dressing rooms and showers available and clean?
6. Find out about the different types of memberships and payment plans the club offers. Ask for a short-term trial membership. Don't be rushed into signing a long-term contract. Before signing any contract, ask for a few days to think it over; a reputable facility will let you consider joining without applying pressure.
7. Read the contract carefully before signing, or get a knowledgeable person to read it. Be sure you understand the provisions and agreements. Don't hesitate to ask questions.
8. Understand what happens if you wish to cancel the membership. What type of refund policy does the club have?
9. Find out how long the club has been in your area. The longer the better, and if under the same management, that's another plus. Beware of new clubs offering "pre-opening" membership discounts.
10. Find out if the club belongs to the Association of Physical Fitness Centers or the International Racquet Sports Association. These trade associations have established standards to help protect consumer health, safety, and rights. You can also check with the Better Business Bureau to see if any complaints have been filed against the club.

In addition, be wary of promotion gimmicks and high-pressure sales techniques. Be alert to practices such as special reduced prices, free visits, reservation forms, and guarantees of fitness improvements or weight loss. Get all the facts before making a decision. If you feel any excessive amount of pressure, leave or at least ask for more time. Under no circumstances should you feel badgered, embarrassed, or threatened. You want to find a facility that you feel comfortable with and that meets your needs.

Sources: Adapted from Health clubs: The right choice for you? 1996. *Consumer Reports,* January, 27–30; Cornacchia, H. 1994. How to choose a fitness center. *Healthline,* April. Krucoff, C. 1989. Joining the club. *Washington Post Health,* 5 September, 20.

realistic goals, and choosing activities that develop all the components of fitness.

- Guidelines that can make an exercise program more effective include training the way you want your body to change, training regularly, getting in shape gradually, warming up and cooling down, maintaining a structured but flexible program, training with a partner, training your mind, and keeping exercise in perspective.
- Activity at a level too low to produce physical adaptations can nevertheless provide health benefits. Activity should be incorporated into daily life as much as possible.
- Exercise is safe for most people, but men over 40, women over 50, and anyone with a health problem should consult a physician before beginning a vigorous exercise program.
- Accurate information about exercise can be obtained from exercise class leaders, fitness magazines, and qualified personal trainers.
- Exercise is not recommended when a person is ill or has an injury.
- Individual differences mean that people will vary in the maximum level of fitness or performance they can achieve. However, every person is capable of reaching personal fitness goals.
- Good time management is an essential skill in maintaining an exercise program. The place chosen for exercising should be pleasant, safe, and convenient.

BEHAVIOR CHANGE ACTIVITY

Monitoring Behavior

To develop a successful behavior change program, you need detailed information about your own behavior patterns. Using your health journal, develop a system of record keeping, geared toward your target behavior. Depending on your behavior change goals, you may want to monitor a single behavior, such as your diet, or you may want to keep daily activity records to determine how you could make time for exercise or another new behavior. Consider tracking factors such as the following:

- The behavior
- When it occurs
- Where it occurs
- What else you were doing at the time
- Who you were with, and how they influenced you
- Your thoughts and feelings
- How strong your urge for the behavior was (for example, how hungry you were, or how much you wanted to watch TV)

Figure 2-3 (p. 32) is a sample health journal record of eating behavior for part of a day.

Keep records for a week or two to help you identify patterns in your behavior. Once you've developed a plan for changing your behavior, you may want to continue keeping records in order to monitor your progress.

FOR MORE INFORMATION

American College of Sports Medicine. 1995. *Guidelines for Exercise Testing and Prescription,* 5th ed. Baltimore: Williams & Wilkins. *Includes the ACSM guidelines for safety of exercising, a basic discussion of exercise physiology, and information about fitness testing and prescription.*

Bouchard, C., et al., eds. 1990. *Exercise, Fitness, and Health: A Consensus of Current Knowledge.* Champaign, Ill.: Human Kinetics. *A complete and up-to-date summary of the relationships among exercise, fitness, and health.*

Brooks, G. A., T. D. Fahey, and T. P. White. 1996. *Exercise Physiology: Human Bioenergetics and Its Applications,* 2d ed. Mountain View, Calif.: Mayfield. *Comprehensive coverage of exercise physiology, including information on fitness testing, nutrition, and disease prevention.*

Golding, L. A., C. R. Myers, and W. E. Sinning, eds. 1989. *Y's Way to Physical Fitness: The Complete Guide to Fitness Testing and Instruction.* Champaign, Ill.: Human Kinetics. *A basic discussion of exercise physiology and descriptions and worksheets for completing a battery of fitness assessment tests.*

Nieman, D. C. 1995. *Fitness and Sports Medicine: An Introduction.* 3d ed. Menlo Park, Calif.: Bull Publishing. *Comprehensive discussions of fitness testing, exercise and disease, nutrition and physical performance, and exercise prescription.*

Wilmore, J. H., and D. L. Costill. 1994. *Physiology of Sport and Exercise.* Champaign, Ill.: Human Kinetics. *A superb summary of the physiological basis of sport and exercise written by two highly respected exercise physiologists.*

Additional sources for information and programs include campus physical education departments, exercise physiology labs, and adult fitness programs; private health clubs; and YMCAs, YWCAs, and other community organizations.

SELECTED BIBLIOGRAPHY

American College of Sports Medicine. 1990. Position stand on the recommended quantity and quality of exercise for developing and maintaining cardiorespiratory and muscular fitness in healthy adults. *Medicine and Science in Sports and Exercise* 22:265–274.

American College of Sports Medicine. 1995. *Guidelines for Exercise Testing and Prescription,* 5th ed. Baltimore: Williams & Wilkins.

American Heart Association. 1991. *Exercise Standards: A Statement for Health Professionals.* Dallas: American Heart Association.

Blair, S. N., H. W. Kohl, C. E. Barlow, R. S. Paffenbarger, L. W. Gibbons, and C. A. Macera. 1995. Changes in physical fitness and all-cause mortality: A prospective study of healthy and unhealthy men. *Journal of the American Medical Association* 273(14): 1093–1098.

Blair, S. N., and H. W. Kohl. 1988. Physical activity or physical fitness: Which is more important for health? *Medicine and Science in Sports and Exercise* 20:S8.

Brooks, G. A., T. D. Fahey, and T. P. White. 1996. *Exercise Physiology: Human Bioenergetics and Its Applications,* 2d ed. Mountain View, Calif.: Mayfield.

Centers for Disease Control and Prevention. 1993. Public health focus: Physical activity and the prevention of coronary heart disease. *Journal of the American Medical Association* 270(13): 1529–1530.

Centers for Disease Control and Prevention. 1995. Prevalence of recommended levels of physical activity among women—Behavioral Risk Factor Surveillance System, 1992. *Journal of the American Medical Association* 273(13): 986–987.

Fahey, T. D. 1997. *Basic Weight Training for Men and Women,* 3d ed. Mountain View, Calif.: Mayfield.

Date November 5 Day M (TU) W TH F SA SU

Time of day	M/S	Food eaten	Cals.	H	Where did you eat?	What else were you doing?	How did someone else influence you?	What made you want to eat what you did?	Emotions and feelings?	Thoughts and concerns?
7:30	M	1 C Crispix cereal 1/2 C skim milk coffee, black 1 C orange juice	110 40 — 120	3	dorm cafeteria	reading newspaper	eating w/ friends, but I ate what I usually eat	I always eat cereal in the morning	a little keyed up & worried	thinking about quiz in class today
10:30	S	1 apple	90	1	library	studying	alone	felt tired & wanted to wake up	tired	worried about next class
12:30	M	1 C chili 1 roll 1 pat butter 1 orange 2 oatmeal cookies 1 soda	290 120 35 60 120 150	2	cafeteria terrace	talking	eating w/ friends; we decided to eat at the cafeteria	wanted to be part of group	excited and happy	interested in hearing every-one's plans for the weekend

M/S = Meal or snack H = Hunger rating (0-3)

Figure 2-3 ***A sample health journal record of eating behavior for part of a day.***

Haskell, W. L. 1994. J. B. Wolffe Memorial Lecture. Health consequences of physical activity: Understanding and challenges regarding dose-response. *Medicine and Science in Sports and Exercise* 26(6): 649–660.

Haskell, W. L., H. J. Montoye, and D. Orenstein. 1985. Physical activity and exercise to achieve health-related physical fitness components. *Public Health Reports* 100(2): 202–212.

How hard do you *really* need to exercise? Interview with J. M. Rippe. 1995. *Tufts University Diet & Nutrition Letter* 13(5): 4–6.

King, A. C., W. L. Haskell, D. R. Young, R. K. Oka, and M. L. Stefanick. 1995. Long-term effects of varying intensities and formats of physical activity on participation rates, fitness, and lipoproteins in men and women aged 50 to 65 years. *Circulation* 91(10): 2596–2604.

Lee, I. M., C. C. Hsieh, and R. S. Paffenbarger. 1995. Exercise intensity and longevity in men. The Harvard Alumni Health Study. *Journal of the American Medical Association* 273(15): 1179–1184.

National Institutes of Health. 1996. *Physical Activity and Cardiovascular Health.* National Institutes of Health Consensus Development Conference Statement, December 18–20, 1995. Online. Internet. Available http://text.nlm.gov/nih/cdc/www/101.html

Nieman, D. C. 1995. *Fitness and Sports Medicine: A Health-Related Approach,* 3d ed. Palo Alto, Calif.: Bull Publishing.

Paffenbarger, R. S., et al. 1986. Physical activity, all-cause mortality, and longevity of college alumni. *New England Journal of Medicine* 314:605–613.

Pate, R. R., M. Pratt, S. N. Blair, W. L. Haskell, C. A. Macera, C. Bouchard, D. Buchner, W. Ettinger, G. W. Heath, and A. C. King. 1995. Physical activity and public health: A recommendation from the Centers for Disease Control and Prevention and the American College of Sports Medicine. *Journal of the American Medical Association* 273(5): 402–407.

Pollock, M. L., J. H. Wilmore, and S. M. Fox. 1984. *Exercise in Health and Disease.* Philadelphia: Saunders.

Rosenberg, I. H. 1994. Keys to a longer, healthier, more vital life. *Nutrition Review* 52(8 Pt 2): S50–51.

Shephard, R. J., and P. N. Shek. 1995. Cancer, immune function, and physical activity. *Canadian Journal of Applied Physiology* 20(1): 1–25.

Siegel, P. Z., R. M. Brackbill, and G. W. Heath. 1995. The epidemiology of walking for exercise: Implications for promoting activity among sedentary groups. *American Journal of Public Health* 85(5): 706–710.

Name ______________________ Section ______________ Date ______________

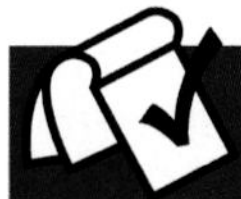

LAB 2-1 *Calculating Your Activity Index*

Answer the questions below to assess your overall level of activity.

1. Frequency: How often do you exercise?

If you exercise:	Your frequency score is:
Less than 1 time a week	0
1 time a week	1
2 times a week	2
3 times a week	3
4 times a week	4
5 or more times a week	5

2. Duration: How long do you exercise?

If each session continues for:	Your duration score is:
Less than 5 minutes	0
5–14 minutes	1
15–29 minutes	2
30–44 minutes	3
45–59 minutes	4
60 minutes or more	5

3. Intensity: How hard do you exercise?

If exercise results in:	Your intensity score is:
No change in pulse from resting level	0
Little change in pulse from resting level (slow walking, bowling, yoga)	1
Slight increase in pulse and breathing (table tennis, active golf with no golf cart)	2
Moderate increase in pulse and breathing (leisurely bicycling, easy continuous swimming, rapid walking)	3
Intermittent heavy breathing and sweating (tennis singles, basketball, squash)	4
Sustained heavy breathing and sweating (jogging, cross-country skiing, rope skipping)	5

To assess your activity index, multiply your three scores:

Frequency ______ × Duration ______ × Intensity ______= Activity index ______

To assess your activity index, refer to the following table:

If your activity index is:	Your estimated level of activity is:
Less than 15	Sedentary
15–24	Low active
25–40	Moderate active
41–60	Active
Over 60	High active

LABORATORY ACTIVITIES

LABORATORY ACTIVITIES

If your activity level is in one of the lower categories, review the components of your score (frequency, duration, intensity) to see how you can raise your score. Add to your current exercise program, or devise a new one.

To monitor your progress toward your goal, enter the results of this lab in the Preprogram Assessment column of Lab 15-2. After several weeks of an exercise program, do this lab again, and enter the results in the Postprogram Assessment column of Lab 15-2. How do the results compare?

Source: Kusinitz, I., and M. Fine. 1995. *Your Guide to Getting Fit,* 3d ed. Mountain View, Calif.: Mayfield.

Name ______________________ Section ____________ Date ______________

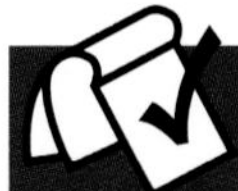

LAB 2-2 *Safety of Exercise Participation*

To determine whether exercise is safe for you, complete the general PAR-Q questionnaire in Part 1. If you have had a complete physical examination and are familiar with your medical history, complete the longer health history questionnaire in Part 2, asking you to identify specific medical conditions or risk factors that could make exercise unsafe for you.

LABORATORY ACTIVITIES

Part 1. Physical Activity Readiness Questionnaire (PAR-Q)

If you answer yes to any question, vigorous exercise or exercise testing should be postponed; medical clearance may be necessary.

Yes	No	
_____	_____	Has your physician ever said you have heart trouble?
_____	_____	Do you frequently suffer from pains in your chest?
_____	_____	Do you often feel faint or have spells of severe dizziness?
_____	_____	Has your physician ever said your blood pressure was too high?
_____	_____	Has a physician ever told you that you have a bone or joint problem, such as arthritis, that has been or could be aggravated by exercise?
_____	_____	Is there a good physical reason not mentioned here why you should not follow an activity program even if you wanted to? If yes, explain. ______________________________
_____	_____	Are you over age 65 and not accustomed to vigorous exercise?

Part 2. Health History Questionnaire

If any of the following apply to you, vigorous exercise or exercise testing should be postponed; medical clearance may be necessary.

Do you currently have any of the following conditions?

Yes	No	
_____	_____	Resting systolic blood pressure of 160 mm Hg or more
_____	_____	Resting diastolic blood pressure of 90 mm Hg or more
_____	_____	Total cholesterol level above 240 mg/dl
_____	_____	Cigarette smoking
_____	_____	Diabetes mellitus
_____	_____	Sickle-cell disease
_____	_____	Blood-clotting abnormalities
_____	_____	Systemic or pulmonary embolus
_____	_____	Obesity (over 25% body fat for men or over 32% body fat for women)
_____	_____	Heart murmur
_____	_____	Abnormal resting or stress EKG
_____	_____	Thrombophlebitis
_____	_____	Arthritis, rheumatism, or other joint problems
_____	_____	Chronic low-back pain
_____	_____	Anorexia or bulimia
_____	_____	Chronic infectious disease (HIV infection, hepatitis, mononucleosis, etc.)
_____	_____	Advanced pregnancy

LABORATORY ACTIVITIES

Have you ever suffered from any of the following?

Yes	No	
_____	_____	Heart attack
_____	_____	Coronary artery disease
_____	_____	Stroke
_____	_____	Congestive heart failure
_____	_____	Rheumatic or congenital heart disease

Do you experience any of the following symptoms?

_____	_____	Pain or discomfort in your chest during physical exertion or emotional stress
_____	_____	Shortness of breath with mild exertion
_____	_____	Dizziness or fainting
_____	_____	Swelling in the ankles
_____	_____	Skipped or racing heartbeats
_____	_____	Leg pains that increase in severity with increased exercise intensity
_____	_____	Are you currently taking prescription medication?
_____	_____	Did either of your parents or a brother or sister suffer from heart disease before age 55?

Do you have any other concerns about the safety of exercise for you? If so, explain:

____

____

____

3

Cardiorespiratory Endurance

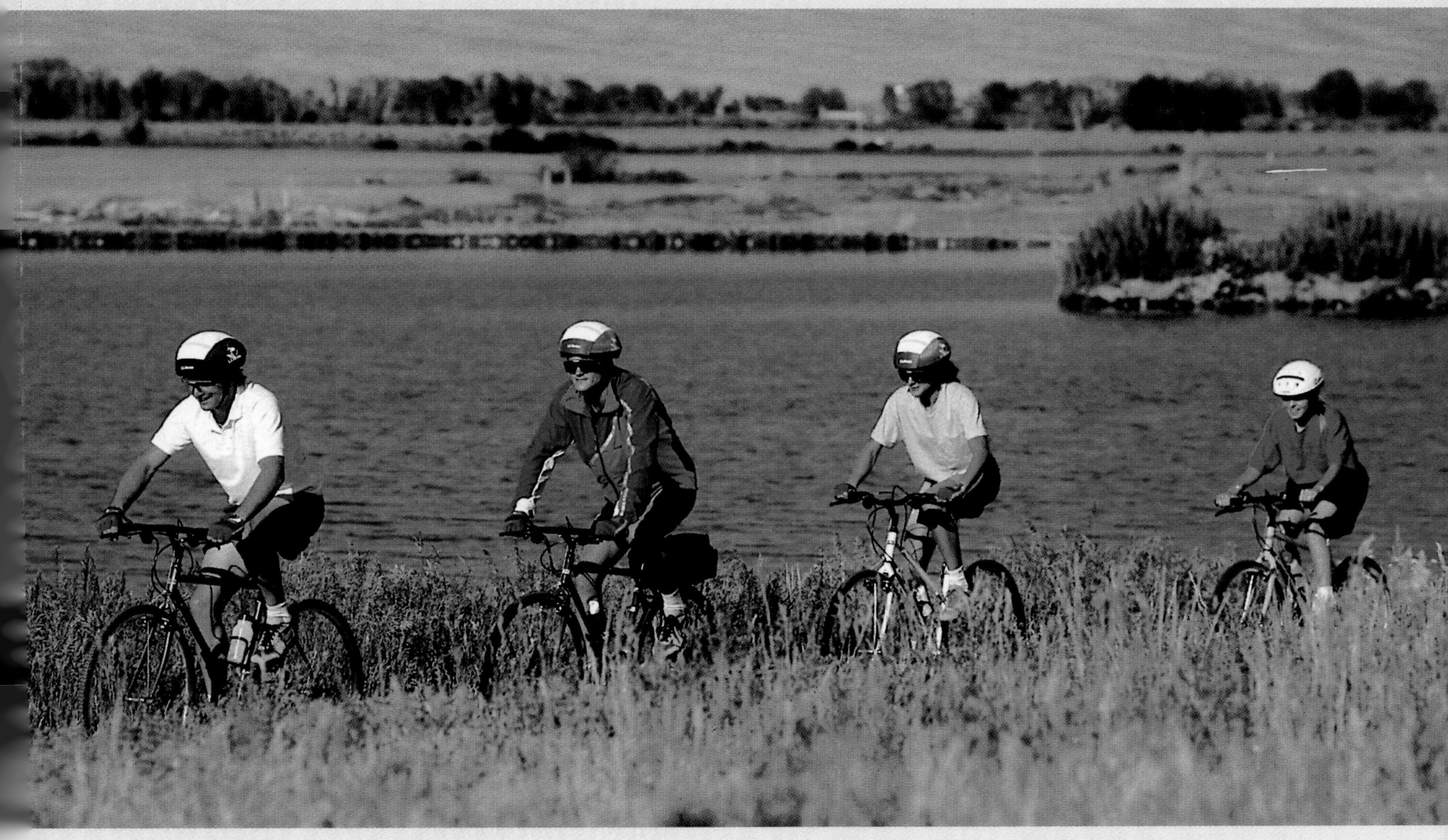

LOOKING AHEAD

After reading this chapter, you should be able to answer these questions about cardiorespiratory endurance:

- What are the major health benefits of cardiorespiratory endurance exercise?
- How is cardiorespiratory endurance measured?
- What tests can be used to assess cardiorespiratory endurance?
- How do type, intensity, duration, and frequency of exercise affect the development of cardiorespiratory endurance?
- What elements go into a successful cardiorespiratory fitness program?
- What are the best ways to prevent and treat exercise injuries?

Cardiorespiratory endurance—the ability of the body to perform prolonged, large-muscle, dynamic exercise at moderate-to-high levels of intensity—is the most important health-related component of fitness. As explained in Chapter 2, a healthy heart is essential to high levels of fitness and wellness, as well as to a long and healthy life.

This chapter reviews and explains the numerous benefits of cardiorespiratory fitness. It then describes several tests that are commonly used to assess cardiorespiratory fitness. Finally, it provides guidelines for creating your own cardiorespiratory endurance program, one that is geared to your current level of fitness and built around activities you enjoy.

BENEFITS OF CARDIORESPIRATORY ENDURANCE

Cardiorespiratory endurance exercise helps the body become more efficient and better able to cope with physical challenges. Regular endurance exercise produces two principal groups of physiological adaptations:

- Improved cardiorespiratory functioning
- Improved metabolism

Endurance exercise also leads to other positive changes:

- Better control of blood fat levels
- Better control of body fat
- Improved immune function
- Protection against some types of cancer
- Improved psychological and emotional well-being

Improved Cardiorespiratory Functioning

Every time a person takes a breath, some of the oxygen in the air that goes to the lungs is picked up by red blood cells and transported to the heart. From there, this oxygenated blood is pumped by the heart throughout the body to organs and tissues that use it. During exercise, the cardiorespiratory system (heart, lungs, and circulatory system) must work harder to meet the body's increased demand for oxygen. Regular endurance exercise improves heart function and the ability of the cardiorespiratory system to carry oxygen to the body's tissues. These improvements reduce the effort required to carry out everyday activities and make the body better able to cope with physical challenges. Regular training also reduces the risk of cardiovascular disease.

Endurance training enhances the health of the heart by maintaining or increasing its oxygen supply, decreasing work and oxygen demand by the heart, increasing the function of the heart muscle, and increasing the electrical stability of the heart. The trained heart is more efficient and subject to less stress. It pumps more blood per beat, so heart rate is lower at rest and during exercise. The resting heart rate of a fit person is often 10–20 beats per minute lower than that of a sedentary person; this translates into as many as 10 million fewer beats in the course of one year. Improved heart efficiency results because endurance training improves heart contraction strength, increases heart cavity size, and increases blood volume so that the heart pushes more blood into the circulation system during each of its contractions. Training also tends to reduce blood pressure, so the heart does not have to work as hard when it contracts.

Endurance training also helps maintain the flow of oxygenated blood to the heart itself. Exercise helps prevent, or possibly even reverse, the development of fatty deposits that can block blood flow to the heart and cause a heart attack. Many research studies have shown conclusively that exercise not only affects the risk factors for heart disease (for example, blood pressure and levels of blood fats) but also directly interferes with the disease process itself. As discussed in Chapter 1, fit people have much lower rates of cardiovascular disease than do sedentary people.

Improved Metabolism

Another important effect of endurance exercise is improved metabolism, the process by which food is converted to energy and tissue is built. Much metabolism takes place in the muscles, which do the body's work. Although, as noted in Chapter 2, people have different aerobic capacities, regular exercise increases the number of capillaries in the muscles, supplying them with more oxygen and fuel. Regular exercise also trains the muscles to make the most of available oxygen and fuel so that they work more efficiently.

Exercise increases the size and number of cellular energy centers called **mitochondria.** These structures contain important chemicals called enzymes that help convert the energy in foods to energy you can use to exercise

TERMS

mitochondria Intracellular structures containing enzymes used in the chemical reactions that convert the energy in food to a form the body can use.

free radicals Highly reactive compounds that can damage cells by taking electrons from key cellular components such as DNA or the cell membrane; produced by normal metabolic processes and through exposure to environmental factors, including sunlight.

glycogen A complex carbohydrate stored principally in the liver and skeletal muscles; the major fuel source during most forms of intense exercise.

lactic acid A metabolic acid resulting from the metabolism of glucose and glycogen; an important source of fuel for many tissues of the body, its accumulation may produce fatigue.

lipids Fats or fatlike substances such as cholesterol or triglycerides that are insoluble in water.

lipoproteins Substances in blood, classified according to size, density, and chemical composition, that transport fats.

and carry on cell functions. This increase in mitochondria contributes to wellness because mitochondria help your body process fuels better, thereby giving you more energy to carry out your daily activities.

Exercise also helps protect your cells from chemical damage. Many scientists believe that aging is caused by cell damage by substances called **free radicals** that are produced during normal metabolism. Training activates antioxidant enzymes that prevent free radical damage to cell structures, thereby enhancing health.

Training also improves the functional stability of cells and tissues by improving the regulation of salts and fluids in the cells. Exercise increases the activity and density of cellular pumps that regulate the interior environment of cells. This regulation is particularly important in the heart, where instability can lead to cardiac arrest and death. In other tissues, these cellular pumps help maintain an optimal internal environment, which contributes to ensuring the health and well-being of the cells.

Exercise also improves the functions of many of the body's hormone systems. For example, insulin sensitivity is enhanced with training, which in turn improves the metabolism of carbohydrates, fats, and protein. Training reduces the body's response to stress hormones such as epinephrine and cortisol, which are produced when the body has physical and emotional challenges. Hormone overreaction has been implicated in heart disease and the suppression of immune function.

During intense exercise, muscles use the carbohydrate **glycogen** as their principal energy source. Fat is a secondary fuel source but is used more efficiently to carry out body processes during periods of rest and light activity. A person who is not fit will not have a sufficient supply of oxygen to the muscles to metabolize the amount of fuel needed for periods of intense activity. Glycogen will be used very rapidly and metabolic acids, particularly **lactic acid,** will be produced. When glycogen is depleted and lactic acid accumulates, the body is fatigued and requires rest.

Endurance training not only prevents glycogen depletion but also improves the muscles' ability to use lactic acid and fat as fuel. Fitness programs that best develop metabolic efficiency are characterized by both long-duration, moderately intense endurance exercise and brief periods of more intense exercise. For example, climbing a small hill while jogging or cycling introduces the kind of intense exercise that leads to more efficient use of lactic acid and fats.

Better Control of Blood Fat Levels

In addition to these two major adaptations, cardiorespiratory endurance exercise has an impact on levels of fats in the blood. High concentrations of **lipids,** or blood fats, such as cholesterol and triglycerides, are linked to heart disease because they contribute to the formation of fatty deposits on the lining of the arteries that supply blood to the heart. When these coronary arteries are clogged or blocked, a heart attack or stroke can occur.

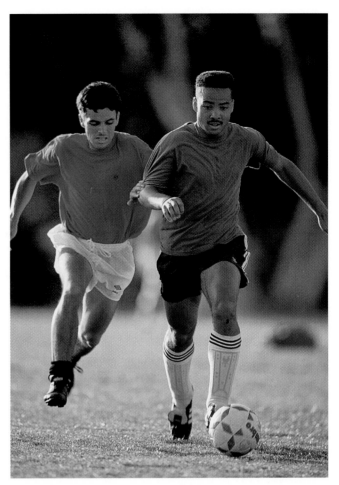

Exercise offers both long-term health benefits and immediate pleasures. Many popular sports and activities, including soccer, develop cardiorespiratory endurance.

Cholesterol is carried in the blood by **lipoproteins,** which are classified according to size and density. Low-density lipoproteins (LDLs) are often referred to as "bad" cholesterol because they carry cholesterol from the liver (where it is made) to the parts of the body that need it. If LDLs transport more cholesterol than the body can use, the excess is deposited in the blood vessels, where it accumulates. One particular form of LDL, smaller than other types, is associated with severe coronary artery disease. High-density lipoproteins (HDLs), or "good" cholesterol, carry unused cholesterol back to the liver for recycling. High LDL levels and low HDL levels are associated with a high risk of cardiovascular disease (CVD). Low levels of LDL and high levels of HDL are associated with lower risk.

More information about cholesterol and heart disease is provided in Chapter 11. For our purposes in this chapter, it is important to know only that endurance exercise influences blood lipid levels in a positive way—lowering levels of LDL, including dangerous small LDL, and raising

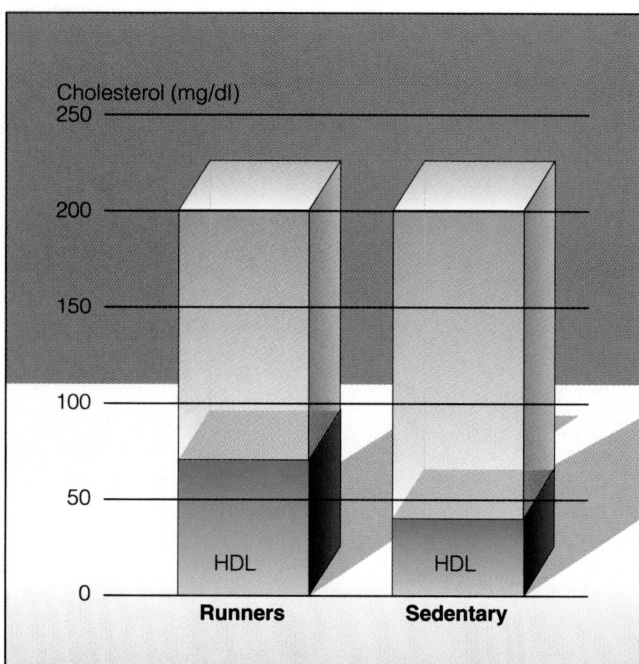

Figure 3-1 *HDL blood levels for runners and sitters.*

levels of HDL—and thereby helps reduce the risk of CVD (Figure 3-1).

Better Control of Body Fat

Endurance exercise also influences body chemistry by regulating energy balance. A diet that provides all the nutrients the body needs for essential functioning can be relatively high in calories, especially for a sedentary person. Regular exercise increases daily calorie expenditure so that a healthy diet does not lead to weight gain. Endurance exercise burns calories directly and continues to do so by raising resting metabolic rate for up to 12 hours following an exercise session.

Endurance exercise also helps people maintain a high proportion of lean body mass (though strength training is more effective). Trying to lose body fat through changes in diet alone leads to a loss of as much lean body mass as fat. One study found that when dieters didn't exercise, as much as 40% of their weight loss was lean body mass. Loss of lean body mass means that metabolism slows down and fewer calories are burned. A lower metabolic rate makes it much easier to regain the lost weight when normal eating patterns are resumed, and it can also make future weight loss more difficult.

Improved Immune Function

Exercise can have either positive or negative effects on the immune system, the physiological processes that protect us from disease. It appears that moderate endurance exercise boosts immune function, while excessive training (overtraining) depresses it. Physically fit people get fewer colds and upper respiratory tract infections than people who are not fit. In addition to regular exercise, the immune system can be strengthened by eating a well-balanced diet rich in vitamins and minerals from whole grains, fruits, vegetables, and low-fat dairy and meat products; managing stress; and getting 7–8 hours of sleep every night.

Protection Against Some Types of Cancer

Cancer is the second leading cause of death in the United States, and cancer rates have been increasing steadily since the 1950s (rates of heart disease and stroke dropped during this period). Some studies have shown a relationship between increased physical activity and a reduction in a person's risk for all types of cancer, but these findings are not conclusive. There is good evidence that exercise reduces the risk of colon cancer, and promising data that it reduces the risk of cancer of the breast and reproductive organs in women. Exercise may decrease the risk of colon cancer by speeding the movement of food through the gastrointestinal tract, enhancing immune function, and reducing blood fats. The protective mechanism in the case of reproductive system cancers is less clear.

Improved Psychological and Emotional Well-Being

Most people who participate in regular endurance exercise experience social, psychological, and emotional benefits. Performing physical activities provides proof of skill mastery and self-control, thus enhancing self-image. Recreational sports provide an opportunity to socialize, have fun, and strive to excel.

Endurance exercise also provides protection against the effects of stress that have been linked to poor cardiorespiratory health. Psychological stress causes increased secretion of **epinephrine** and **norepinephrine,** the so-called fight-or-flight hormones, which are thought to speed the development of atherosclerosis, or hardening of the arteries. Excessive hostility is also associated with the risk of heart disease. Endurance exercise decreases the secretion of hormones triggered by emotional stress. It can diffuse hostility and alleviate depression and anxiety by providing an emotional outlet and inducing feelings of relaxation (see the box "Exercise, Mood, and Mental State"). Regular exercise can also relieve sleeping problems.

Endurance exercise also seems to increase the secretion of **endorphins,** a group of substances resembling morphine that are secreted by the brain. Endorphins play a role in decreasing pain, in producing euphoria, and in suppressing fatigue; and some researchers credit them with the "runner's high" sometimes experienced during exercise. Research to determine the precise nature of endorphins and their role in a person's sense of well-being is ongoing.

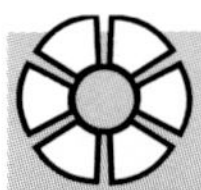

WELLNESS CONNECTION

Exercise, Mood, and Mental State

Many people report that exercise puts them in a better mood, but studies have also shown that exercise is an effective treatment for mild to moderate cases of depression. Researchers have found that exercise can be as effective as psychotherapy in treating depression, and even more effective when used in conjunction with conventional therapies. This is an important finding because major depression is a common condition among Americans; the estimated lifetime prevalence is about 5% for men and 10% for women. Although depression is a highly treatable condition, only about one-third of affected individuals seek professional help.

The ties among exercise and physical, emotional, and social wellness become clear when one looks at the variety of theories that have been proposed to explain exercise's antidepressant effects:

- Exercise provides a distraction from stressful stimuli.
- Exercise provides a way for people to gain mastery or control over their bodies and lives and enhance their self-esteem.
- Psychological benefits accompany the positive social interaction that can occur during exercise.
- Exercise causes an increase in the activity of certain brain chemicals, including dopamine, serotonin, and norepinephrine (low levels of these substances are linked to depression).

What type of exercise is most effective for treating depression? Cardiorespiratory endurance exercise seems to work the best. In a study of moderately depressed individuals, those involved in endurance training experienced a significant improvement in their condition, compared with individuals involved in a stretching program that did not include endurance exercise. Exercise recommendations for depressed people are similar to those given to the general population: a program of regular, moderate endurance exercise that is fun, convenient, and includes lots of opportunities for positive feedback.

How does exercise affect mood and depression levels in the rest of the population, those not suffering from clinical depression? Research indicates that exercise elevates mood in nondepressed people who feel fine or who feel a little bit "down." Physical fitness also seems to have a protective effect. National surveys suggest that sedentary adults have a much higher risk of feeling fatigue and depression than those who are physically active. A study of college students found that among those who were exposed to high levels of life stresses, the students who had low cardiorespiratory fitness subsequently developed more health problems and scored higher on tests measuring depression than those who were more fit.

The bottom line is that exercise is important for your emotional wellness—now and in the future. A program of regular exercise will enhance self-esteem and increase your feelings of well-being and vigor; it will decrease depression, anxiety, and the impact of stressful life events. Exercise is essential for the development of all aspects of wellness.

Sources: Nicoloff, G., and T. L. Schwenk. 1995. Using exercise to ward off depression. *Physician and Sportsmedicine* 23(9):44–58. Nieman, D. 1995. Physical activity and psychological health, in *Fitness and Sports Medicine: A Health-Related Approach.* Menlo Park, Calif.: Bull Publishing.

Additional Benefits

Through regular endurance exercise, bones can maintain density more effectively and are less prone to osteoporosis. Exercise also helps protect against the development of diabetes by making the body more sensitive to insulin. Refer to the box "Benefits of Cardiorespiratory Endurance Exercise" (p. 42) for a summary of specific physiological benefits. As cardiorespiratory fitness is developed, these benefits translate into both greater physical and emotional well-being and a much lower risk of chronic disease.

ASSESSING CARDIORESPIRATORY FITNESS

The body's ability to maintain a level of exertion (exercise) for an extended period of time is a direct reflection of cardiorespiratory fitness. It is determined by the body's ability to take up, distribute, and use oxygen during physical activity. The best quantitative measure of cardiorespiratory endurance is **maximal oxygen consumption,** expressed as $\dot{V}O_{2max}$, the amount of oxygen the body uses when a person reaches maximum ability to supply oxygen during exercise (measured in milliliters of oxygen used per minute for each kilogram of body weight). Maximal oxygen consumption can be measured precisely in

TERMS

epinephrine A hormone secreted in response to stress that stimulates the heart, makes carbohydrates available in the liver and muscles, and releases fat from fat cells.

norepinephrine A stress hormone with many of the same effects as epinephrine.

endorphins Substances resembling morphine that are secreted by the brain and that decrease pain, suppress fatigue, and produce euphoria.

maximal oxygen consumption, expressed as $\dot{V}O_{2max}$ The highest rate of oxygen consumption an individual is capable of during maximum physical effort, reflecting the body's ability to transport and use oxygen; measured in milliliters used per minute for each kilogram of body weight.

A CLOSER LOOK

Benefits of Cardiorespiratory Endurance Exercise

Cardiorespiratory System

Cardiorespiratory endurance exercise tends to increase the following:

- Heart size
- Stroke volume (the amount of blood pumped with each beat)
- Total blood volume
- Number of red blood cells
- Blood concentration of high-density lipoproteins (HDLs)
- Capillary density (associated with the increased ability of cells to extract oxygen from blood)
- Overall efficiency of the delivery of oxygen to the tissues ($\dot{V}O_{2max}$)
- Blood flow to active muscles during exercise

Cardiorespiratory endurance exercise tends to decrease the following:

- Resting heart rate and heart rate at different workloads
- Concentrations of epinephrine and norepinephrine during exercise
- Blood levels of triglycerides and low-density lipoproteins (LDLs)
- Blood pressure
- Platelet stickiness (a factor in coronary artery disease)

Skeletal Muscles

Cardiorespiratory endurance exercise tends to increase the following:

- Number and size of mitochondria (the energy-producing parts of cells)
- Myoglobin content (aids in the delivery of oxygen to the mitochondria)
- Amount of stored glycogen
- Capacity to use fat and lactic acid as fuel

Other

Cardiorespiratory endurance exercise tends to increase the following:

- Lean body mass
- Density and strength of bones, ligaments, and tendons
- Sensitivity to insulin (helps prevent adult-onset diabetes)
- Ability to exercise during hot weather
- Performance in sports, recreational activities, and work
- Feelings of well-being
- Self-concept

Cardiorespiratory endurance exercise tends to decrease the following:

- Total body fat
- Strain associated with stress
- Anxiety and depression
- Risk of death from coronary artery disease, colon cancer, and some types of reproductive cancers (women)

an exercise physiology laboratory through analysis of the air a person inhales and exhales when exercising to a level of exhaustion (maximum intensity). This procedure can be expensive and time-consuming, making it impractical for the average person.

Four Assessment Tests

Fortunately, several simple assessment tests provide good estimates of maximal oxygen consumption. Four methods are described here and presented in Lab 3-1: a 1-mile walk test, a 3-minute step test, a 1.5-mile run-walk test, and the Åstrand-Rhyming bicycle ergometer test. To assess yourself, choose among these methods based on your access to equipment, your current physical condition, and your own preference. Don't take any of these tests without checking with your physician if you are ill or have any of the risk factors for exercise discussed in Chapter 2. Table 3-1 lists the fitness prerequisites and cautions recommended for each test.

You'll get more accurate results from these tests if you avoid strenuous activity the day of the test and don't smoke or eat a heavy meal for up to 3 hours before the test. Record your test results in Lab 3-1, and then use the appropriate formula to calculate your maximal oxygen consumption.

The 1-Mile Walk Test The 1-mile walk test estimates your level of cardiorespiratory fitness (maximal oxygen consumption) based on the amount of time it takes you to complete 1 mile of brisk walking and your exercise heart rate at the end of your walk; age, gender, and body weight are also considered. A fast time and a low heart rate indicate a high level of cardiorespiratory endurance.

TABLE 3-1 Fitness Prerequisites and Cautions for the Cardiorespiratory Endurance Assessment Tests

Note: The conditions for exercise safety given in Chapter 2 apply to all fitness assessment tests. If you answered yes to any question on the PAR-Q in Lab 2-2, see your physician before taking any assessment test. If you experience any unusual symptoms while taking a test, stop exercising, and discuss your condition with your instructor.

Test	Fitness Prerequisites/Cautions
1-mile walk test	Recommended for anyone who meets the criteria for safe exercise. Can be used by individuals who cannot perform other tests because of low fitness level or injury.
3-minute step test	If you suffer from joint problems in your ankles, knees, or hips or are significantly overweight, check with your physician before taking this test.
1.5-mile run-walk test	Recommended for people who are healthy and at least moderately active. If you have been sedentary, you should participate in a 4- to 8-week walk-run program before taking the test. Don't take this test in extremely hot or cold weather if you aren't used to exercising under those conditions.
Åstrand-Rhyming test	Recommended for people who are healthy and at least moderately active. It can be taken by people with some joint problems because body weight is supported by the bicycle.

The 3-Minute Step Test The rate at which the pulse returns to normal after exercise is also a good measure of cardiorespiratory capacity; heart rate recovers faster in people who are more physically fit. For the step test, you step continually at a steady rate for 3 minutes, then monitor your heart rate during recovery.

The 1.5-Mile Run-Walk Test The 1.5-mile run-walk test is considered one of the best indirect measures of cardiorespiratory capacity. Oxygen consumption increases with speed in distance running; a fast time on this test indicates high maximal oxygen consumption.

The Åstrand-Rhyming Bicycle Ergometer Test A bicycle ergometer measures power output, the amount of resistance the bicycle exerts against a person's pedaling. A higher power output means the cyclist is applying more pressure—that is, pedaling harder or faster. The Åstrand-Rhyming test estimates maximal oxygen consumption from the exercise heart rate reached after pedaling a bicycle ergometer for 6 minutes at a constant rate and resistance. A low exercise heart rate after pedaling at a high power output indicates a high maximal oxygen consumption.

Determining Your Heart Rate

Each time your heart beats, it pumps blood into your arteries; this surge of blood causes a pulse that you can feel by holding your fingers against an artery. Counting your pulse to determine your exercise heart rate is a key part of most assessment tests for maximal oxygen consumption. Heart rate can also be used to monitor exercise intensity during a workout. (Intensity is described in more detail in the next section.)

The two most common sites for monitoring heart rate are the carotid artery in the neck and the radial artery in the wrist. To take your pulse, press your index and middle fingers gently on the correct site. You may have to shift position several times to find the best position to feel your pulse. Don't use your thumb to check your pulse; it has a pulse of its own that can confuse your count. Be careful not to push too hard, particularly when taking your pulse in the carotid artery (strong pressure on this artery may cause a reflex that slows the heart rate).

Heart rates are usually assessed in beats per minute (bpm). But counting your pulse for an entire minute isn't practical when you're exercising. And because your heart rate slows rapidly when you stop exercising, it can give inaccurate results. It's best to do a shorter count—say, 15 seconds—and then multiply the result by 4 to get your heart rate in beats per minute. Using a 10- or 6-second count can be less accurate because an inaccuracy of one beat will be magnified by 6 or 10 times, rather than 4 times. As a result, a 15-second count, taken immediately when you stop exercising, is usually recommended for determining exercise heart rate.

The same procedure can be used to take someone else's pulse, as in the bicycle ergometer test.

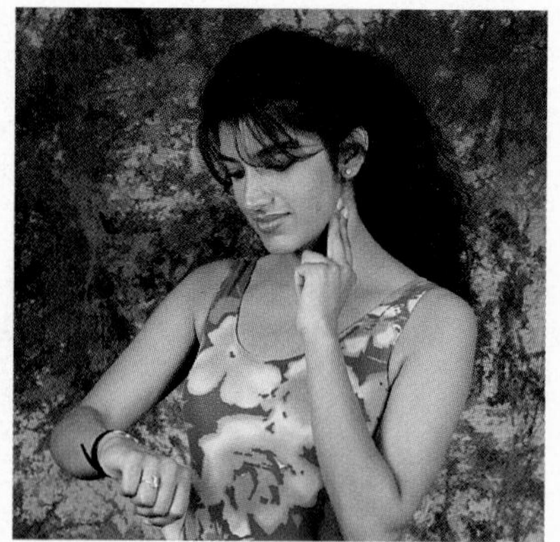
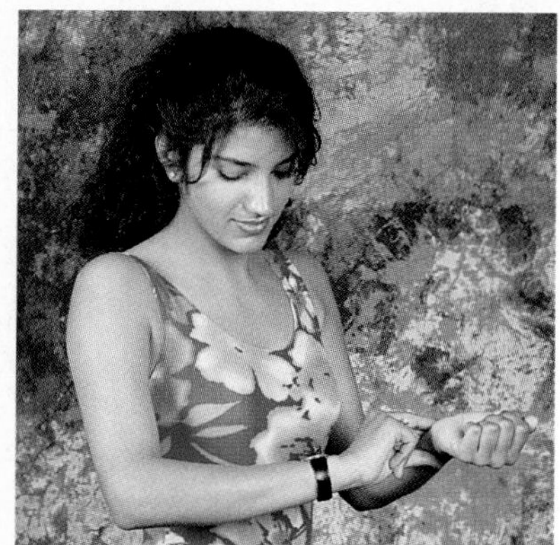

A pulse count can be used to determine exercise heart rate. The pulse can be taken at the carotid artery in the neck (left) or at the radial artery in the wrist (right).

TABLE 3-2 Cardiorespiratory Fitness Classification

	Maximal Oxygen Consumption (ml/kg/min)					
	Very Poor	*Poor*	*Fair*	*Good*	*Excellent*	*Superior*
Women						
Age: 18–29	Below 30.6	30.6–33.7	33.8–36.6	36.7–40.9	41.0–46.7	Above 46.7
30–39	Below 28.7	28.7–32.2	32.3–34.5	34.6–38.5	38.6–43.8	Above 43.8
40–49	Below 26.5	26.5–29.4	29.5–32.2	32.3–36.2	36.3–40.9	Above 40.9
50–59	Below 24.3	24.3–26.8	26.9–29.3	29.4–32.2	32.3–36.7	Above 36.7
60 and over	Below 22.8	22.8–24.4	24.5–27.1	27.2–31.1	31.2–37.4	Above 37.4
Men						
Age: 18–29	Below 37.1	37.1–40.9	41.0–44.1	44.2–48.1	48.2–53.9	Above 53.9
30–39	Below 35.4	35.4–38.8	38.9–42.3	42.4–46.7	46.8–52.4	Above 52.4
40–49	Below 33.0	33.0–36.7	36.8–39.8	39.9–44.0	44.1–50.3	Above 50.3
50–59	Below 30.2	30.2–33.7	33.8–36.6	36.7–40.9	41.0–47.0	Above 47.0
60 and over	Below 26.5	26.5–30.1	30.2–33.5	33.6–38.0	38.1–45.1	Above 45.1

Source: Based on norms from the Cooper Institute for Aerobics Research, Dallas, Texas; used with permission.

Interpreting Your Score

Once you've completed one or more of the assessment tests, use Table 3-2 to determine your level of cardiorespiratory fitness. Find the row that corresponds to your age and gender, and then find the category that contains your score for maximal oxygen consumption. For example, a 19-year-old female with a maximal oxygen consumption score of 36 ml/kg/min would be classified as having fair cardiorespiratory fitness. You can see from Table 3-2 that there are differences in ratings for $\dot{V}O_{2max}$ between men and women; for more on this disparity, see the box "Gender Differences in Cardiorespiratory Endurance."

You can monitor the progress of your fitness program by repeating the cardiorespiratory assessment test(s) from time to time. Because your $\dot{V}O_{2max}$ score will vary somewhat for different types of tests, always compare scores for the *same* test.

DEVELOPING A CARDIORESPIRATORY ENDURANCE PROGRAM

Cardiorespiratory endurance exercises are best for developing the type of fitness associated with good health, so they should serve as the focus of your exercise program. To create a successful endurance exercise program, you must set realistic goals; choose suitable activities; set your starting frequency, intensity, and duration of exercise at appropriate levels; remember to warm up and cool down; and adjust your program as your fitness improves.

Setting Goals

You can use the results of cardiorespiratory fitness assessment tests to set a specific oxygen consumption goal for your cardiorespiratory endurance program. Your goal should be high enough to ensure a healthy cardiorespira-

DIMENSIONS OF DIVERSITY

Gender Differences in Cardiorespiratory Endurance

Research has shown that there are significant differences in the average levels of cardiorespiratory endurance, as measured by maximal oxygen consumption, for men and women. When expressed in absolute terms, maximal oxygen consumption is about 40% higher in men. When this is adjusted for body weight, as it is in Table 3-2, the difference drops to 20%—a smaller difference, but still significant.

Several factors are believed to contribute to this difference. Males tend to be larger than females, and they have larger hearts, in both size and volume. This means that their hearts pump more blood with each beat (stroke volume), thereby delivering more oxygenated blood to working muscles. Females tend to have higher heart rates during exercise, but this higher rate does not entirely compensate for their lower stroke volume.

Men have relatively higher concentrations of hemoglobin in their blood than women. Hemoglobin is a blood protein that transports oxygen throughout the body; higher hemoglobin levels translate into a higher maximal oxygen consumption. Men have higher levels of androgens (steroid hormones), which stimulate their bodies to produce more hemoglobin. And menstrual blood loss contributes to lower hemoglobin levels among women.

Differences in body composition also affect maximal oxygen consumption. Men tend to have relatively more muscle mass, while women's bodies have a higher percentage of fat. (Body composition is discussed in greater detail in Chapter 6.) This additional muscle mass gives men more strength and power in both absolute and relative terms, and it raises maximal oxygen consumption. The relationship between maximal oxygen consumption and lean body mass is so strong that when $\dot{V}O_{2max}$ is expressed in terms of lean body weight instead of total body weight, the gender difference in maximal oxygen consumption drops to about 10%.

One area in which there is no difference between the sexes is in the benefits of training. Both men and women can improve their maximal oxygen consumption by up to 20%. Physical activity is critical for the health and wellness of everyone.

Source: Adapted from Brooks, G. A., T. D. Fahey, and T. P. White. 1996. *Exercise Physiology: Human Bioenergetics and Its Applications,* 2d ed. Mountain View, Calif.: Mayfield.

tory system, but not so high that it will be impossible to achieve. Scores in the fair and good ranges for maximal oxygen consumption should ensure good health; scores in the excellent and superior ranges indicate a high standard of physical performance.

Choosing Sports and Activities

As mentioned in Chapter 2, cardiorespiratory endurance exercises include activities that involve the rhythmic use of large muscle groups over a long period of time, such as jogging, walking, cycling, aerobic dancing, cross-country skiing, and swimming. Start-and-stop sports, such as tennis and racquetball, also qualify, as long as you have enough skill to play continuously and intensely enough to raise your heart rate to target levels. Cardiorespiratory fitness ratings of many common activities are listed in the box "Activities and Sports for Developing Cardiorespiratory Endurance" (p. 46).

Having fun is a strong motivator; select a physical activity that you enjoy, and it will be easier to stay with your program. Consider whether you prefer competitive or individual sports, or whether starting something new would be best. Other important considerations are access to facilities, expense, and the time required to achieve an adequate skill level and workout.

Determining Frequency of Training

To build cardiorespiratory endurance, you should exercise 3–5 days per week. Beginners should start with 3 and work up to 5 days per week. Training more than 5 days per week can lead to injury and isn't necessary for the typical person on an exercise program designed to promote wellness. Training less than 3 days per week won't improve your fitness, and you risk injury because your body never gets a chance to fully adapt to regular exercise training.

Determining Intensity of Training

Intensity is the most important factor in achieving training effects. You must exercise intensely enough to stress your body so that fitness improves. Two methods of monitoring exercise intensity are described below; choose the method that works best for you. Be sure to make adjustments in your intensity levels for environmental or individual factors. For example, on a hot and humid day or on your first day back to your program after an illness, you should decrease your intensity level.

Target Heart Rate Zone One of the best ways to monitor the intensity of cardiorespiratory endurance exercise

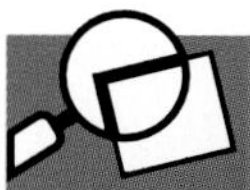

A CLOSER LOOK

Activities and Sports for Developing Cardiorespiratory Endurance

The potential of an activity to develop cardiorespiratory endurance depends primarily upon the intensity, duration, and frequency of training. The ratings given here are general guidelines.

High Potential

- Aerobic dance
- Backpacking
- Badminton (singles)
- Basketball
- Bicycling
- Cross-country skiing
- Cross-country skiing machine
- Field hockey
- Frisbee, ultimate
- Handball (singles)
- Hiking
- Hockey, ice and roller
- In-line skating
- Jogging and running
- Karate
- Lacrosse
- Outdoor fitness trails
- Racquetball (singles)
- Rope skipping
- Rowing
- Rugby
- Soccer
- Squash (singles)
- Stationary bicycle
- Step aerobics
- Swimming
- Tennis (singles)
- Treadmill
- Walking
- Water polo
- Wrestling

Medium Potential

- Ballet
- Ballroom dancing
- Baseball (pitcher and catcher)
- Canoeing and kayaking
- Cheerleading
- Fencing
- Folk and square dancing
- Football, touch
- Horseback riding
- Judo
- Modern dance
- Popular dancing
- Rock climbing
- Skating, ice and roller
- Skiing, alpine
- Slide boarding
- Surfing
- Synchronized swimming
- Table tennis
- Volleyball
- Water aerobics
- Waterskiing

Low Potential

- Archery
- Bowling
- Golf (riding cart)
- Sailing
- Weight training
- Yoga

is by measuring your heart rate. It isn't necessary to exercise at your maximum heart rate to improve maximal oxygen consumption. Fitness adaptations occur at lower heart rates with a much lower risk of injury.

According to the American College of Sports Medicine, your **target heart rate zone**—rates at which you should exercise to experience cardiorespiratory benefits—is between 50 and 85% of your maximum heart rate reserve. This measure of exercise intensity coincides closely with exercise oxygen consumption (metabolism). To calculate your target heart rate zone, follow these steps:

1. Measure your resting heart rate (RHR) by taking your pulse after at least 10 minutes of complete rest. Taking your pulse first thing in the morning (before you get out of bed) is a good way to measure your RHR.
2. Find your maximum heart rate (MHR) by undergoing an exercise stress test (in a physician's office, hospital, or sports medicine laboratory) or by subtracting your age from 220. (The latter method is fairly accurate for most people, but it can be *very* inaccurate for some.)
3. Determine your heart rate reserve (HRR) by subtracting your resting heart rate from your maximum heart rate.
4. Your target heart rate zone for achieving cardiorespiratory fitness benefits is your resting heart rate added to 50–85% of your heart rate reserve.

   For example, a 19-year-old with a RHR of 67 bpm

would use the following numbers to calculate her target heart rate zone:

RHR = 67 bpm

MHR = 220 − 19 = 201 bpm

HRR = 201 − 67 = 134 bpm

Her target heart rate zone is calculated at upper and lower limits:

50% training intensity = 67 + (0.50 × 134) = 134 bpm

85% training intensity = 67 + (0.85 × 134) = 181 bpm

To gain fitness benefits, the young woman in our example would have to exercise at an intensity that raises her heart rate to between 134 and 181 bpm.

You can also estimate your target heart rate zone by calculating 60% and 90% of your maximum heart rate (the percent of MHR method). While slightly less accurate than the HRR method described above, it is much easier to calculate:

1. Determine your MHR as described for the heart rate reserve method.
2. Multiply MHR by 60% and 90% to calculate your target heart rate zone.

The young woman in our example would calculate her target heart rate zone as follows:

MHR = 220 − 19 = 201 bpm

60% training intensity = 0.6 × 201 = 121 bpm

90% training intensity = 0.9 × 201 = 181 bpm

According to the percent of MHR method, this young woman's target heart rate zone is between 121 bpm and 181 bpm.

Use Lab 3-2 to determine your target heart rate zone. If you have been sedentary, start by exercising at the lower end of your target heart rate range (50% training intensity in the HRR method or 60% in the MHR method) for at least 4–6 weeks. Fast gains in fitness (maximal oxygen consumption) can be made as you progress by exercising closer to the top of the range. You *can* achieve significant health benefits by exercising at the bottom of your target range, so don't feel pressured into exercising at an unnecessarily intense level.

To monitor your heart rate during exercise, count your pulse while you're still moving or immediately after you stop exercising. Count beats for 15 seconds, and then multiply that number by 4 to see if your heart rate is in your target zone. If the young woman in our example were aiming for 144 bpm, she would want a 15-second count of 36 beats.

Your resting heart rate will drop in response to endurance training, so you should reassess your target heart rate zone every 8–10 weeks while your fitness level is improving. By monitoring your heart rate (and periodically reassessing your target range), you will always know if you are working hard enough to improve, not hard enough, or too hard.

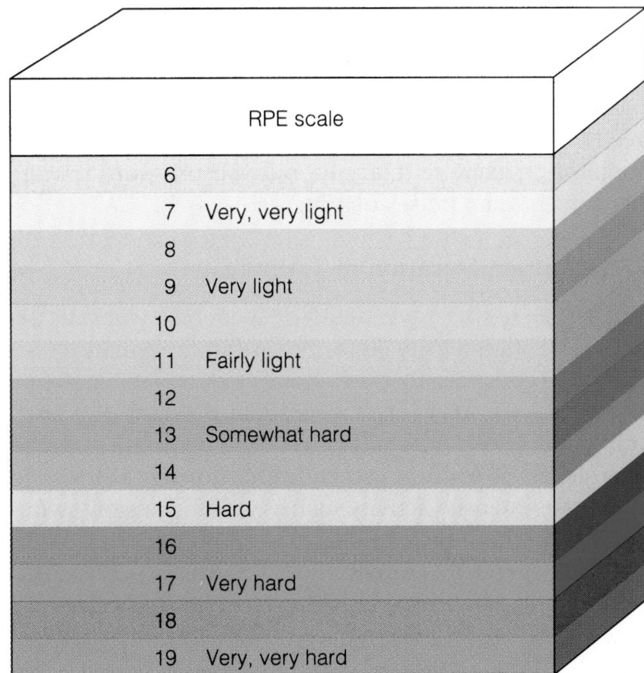

Figure 3-2 ***Ratings of perceived exertion.***

Ratings of Perceived Exertion The second way to monitor intensity is by perceived exertion. Repeated pulse-counting during exercise can become a nuisance if it interferes with the activity. As your exercise program progresses, you will probably become familiar with the amount of exertion required to raise your heart rate to target levels. In other words, you will know how you feel when you have exercised intensely enough. If this is the case, you can use the scale of **ratings of perceived exertion (RPE)** shown in Figure 3-2 to monitor the intensity of your exercise session without checking your pulse.

To use the RPE scale, select a rating that corresponds to your subjective perception of how hard you are exercising when you are training in your target heart rate zone. If your target zone is about 135–155 bpm, exercise intensely enough to raise your heart rate to that level, and then associate a rating—for example, "somewhat hard" or "hard" (14 or 15)—with how hard you feel you are work-

TERMS

target heart rate zone The range of heart rates that should be reached and maintained during cardiorespiratory endurance exercise to obtain training effects.

ratings of perceived exertion (RPE) A system of monitoring exercise intensity based on assigning a number to the subjective perception of target intensity.

ing. To reach and maintain intensity in future workouts, exercise hard enough to reach what you feel is the same level of exertion. You should periodically check your RPE against your target heart rate zone to make sure it's correct. Research has shown RPE to be an accurate means of monitoring exercise intensity, and you may find it more convenient than pulse counting.

Determining Duration of Training

The length of time that should be spent on a workout depends on its intensity. To improve cardiorespiratory endurance, continue to exercise in your target heart rate zone until you have expended about 4 calories for each kilogram of body weight (or 1.8 calories/pound). To reach this level of calorie expenditure during a low- to moderate-intensity activity such as walking or slow swimming, you should exercise for 45–60 minutes. For high-intensity exercise, a duration of 20 minutes is sufficient. Some studies have shown that 5–10 minutes of extremely intense exercise (greater than 90% of maximal oxygen consumption) improves cardiorespiratory endurance. However, training at this intensity increases the risk of injury. Also, because of the discomfort of high-intensity exercise, you are more likely to discontinue your exercise program. Longer duration, low- to moderate-intensity activities generally result in more gradual gains in maximal oxygen consumption. You should start off with less-vigorous activities and only gradually increase intensity.

Warming Up and Cooling Down

It's important to warm up before every session of cardiorespiratory endurance exercise and to cool down afterward. Because the body's muscles work better when their temperature is slightly above resting level, warming up enhances performance and decreases the chance of injury. It gives the body time to redirect blood to active muscles and the heart time to adapt to increased demands. Warming up also helps spread **synovial fluid** throughout the joints, which helps protect their surfaces from injury.

As mentioned in Chapter 2, a warm-up session should include low-intensity movements similar to those in the activity that will follow. Low-intensity movements include walking slowly before beginning a brisk walk, hitting forehands and backhands before a tennis match, and running a 12-minute mile before progressing to an 8-minute one. Some experts also recommend including stretching exercises in your warm-up (see Chapter 5).

Cooling down after exercise is important for returning the body to a nonexercising state. A cool-down, consisting of 5–10 minutes of reduced activity, should follow every workout to allow heart rate, breathing, and circulation to return to normal. Stretching exercises can be part of a cool-down.

The general pattern of a safe and successful workout for cardiorespiratory fitness is illustrated in Figure 3-3.

Maintaining Cardiorespiratory Fitness

Although your fitness level will probably improve quickly at the beginning of your fitness program, this rate of progress will probably slow after 4–6 weeks. The more fit you become, the harder you will have to work to improve. But there is a limit. Increasing intensity and duration indefinitely can lead to injury. Once you reach an acceptable level of fitness, maintain it by continuing to exercise at the same intensity at least 3 nonconsecutive days every week.

EXERCISE INJURIES

Even the most careful physically active person can suffer an injury. Most injuries are annoying rather than serious or permanent. However, an injury that isn't cared for properly can escalate into a chronic problem, sometimes serious enough to permanently curtail the activity. It's important to learn how to deal with injuries so they don't derail your fitness program. Strategies for the care of common exercise injuries appear in Table 3-3 (p. 50); some general guidelines are given below.

When to Call a Physician

Some injuries require medical attention. Consult a physician for head and eye injuries, possible ligament injuries, broken bones, and internal disorders such as chest pain, fainting, elevated body temperature, and intolerance to hot weather. Also seek medical attention for ostensibly minor injuries that do not get better within a reasonable amount of time. You may need to modify your exercise program for a few weeks to allow an injury to heal. A knowledgeable physician can often give you important medical advice that will speed healing and get you back to your program sooner.

Managing Minor Exercise Injuries

For minor cuts and scrapes, stop the bleeding and clean the wound. Treat injuries to soft tissue (muscles and joints) immediately with rest and ice packs. Elevate the affected part of the body, and compress it with an elastic bandage to minimize swelling. Apply ice regularly for 36–48 hours after an injury occurs or until all the swelling is gone. (Don't leave ice on one spot for more than 20 minutes.) Some experts also recommend taking an over-the-counter medication such as aspirin or ibuprofen to decrease inflammation.

TERMS

synovial fluid Fluid found within many joints that provides lubrication and nutrition to the cells of the joint surface.

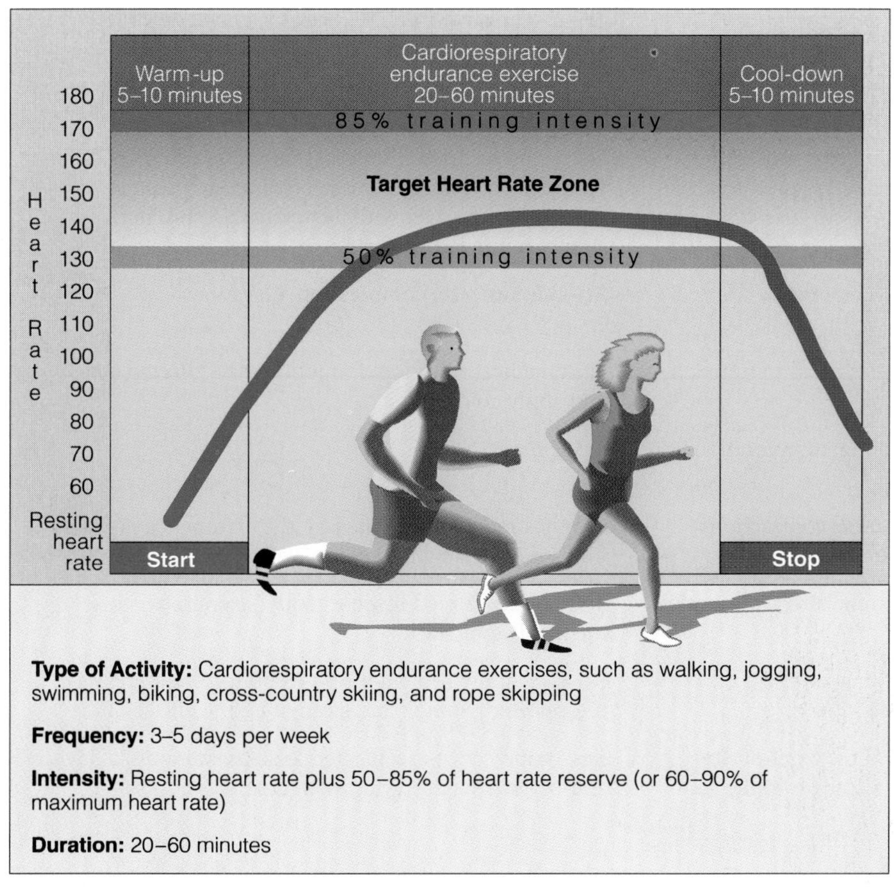

Figure 3-3 *A cardiorespiratory endurance workout.*

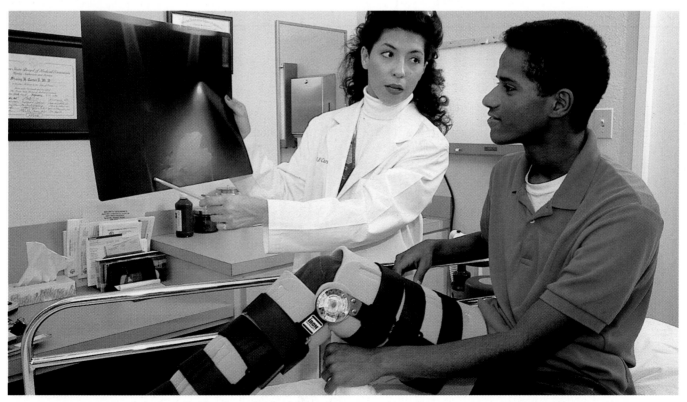

Many exercise injuries can be handled by the individual, but serious injuries, such as broken bones and torn ligaments, require medical attention.

TABLE 3-3 Care of Common Exercise Injuries

Injury	Symptoms	Treatment
Blister	Accumulation of fluid in one spot under the skin	Don't pop or drain it unless it interferes too much with your daily activities. If it does pop, clean the area with antiseptic and cover with a bandage. Do not remove the skin covering the blister.
Bruise (contusion)	Pain, swelling, and discoloration	R-I-C-E: rest, ice, compression, elevation.
Fractures and dislocations	Pain, swelling, tenderness, loss of function, and deformity	Seek medical attention, immobilize the affected area, and apply cold.
Joint sprain	Pain, tenderness, swelling, discoloration, and loss of function	R-I-C-E.
Muscle cramp	Painful, spasmodic muscle contractions	Gently stretch and/or massage the cramped area. Drink fluids if exercising in hot weather.
Muscle soreness or stiffness	Pain and tenderness in the affected muscle	Stretch the affected muscle gently; exercise at a low intensity; apply heat.
Muscle strain	Pain, tenderness, swelling, and loss of strength in the affected muscle	R-I-C-E; apply heat after 36–48 hours if swelling has disappeared. Stretch and strengthen the affected area.
Shin splints	Pain and tenderness on the front of the lower leg; sometimes also pain in the calf muscle	Rest; apply ice to the affected area several times a day and before exercise; wrap with tape for support.
Side stitch	Pain on the side of the abdomen	Decrease the intensity of your workout, or stop altogether; bend over in the direction of the stitch.
Tendinitis	Pain and tenderness of the affected area; loss of use	R-I-C-E; apply heat after 36–48 hours if swelling has disappeared. Stretch and strengthen the affected area.

Sources: Adapted from Fahey, T. D., ed. 1986. *Athletic Training Principles and Practice.* Mountain View, Calif.: Mayfield. Pryor, E., and M. G. Kraines. 1996. *Keep Moving! It's Aerobic Dance,* 3d ed. Mountain View, Calif.: Mayfield.

Don't apply heat to an injury at first because heat draws blood to the area and increases swelling. After the swelling has subsided, apply either moist heat (hot towels, heat packs) or dry heat (heating pads) to speed up healing.

To rehabilitate your body, follow the steps listed in the box "Rehabilitation Following a Minor Athletic Injury."

Preventing Injuries

The best method for dealing with exercise injuries is to prevent them. If you choose activities for your program carefully and follow the training guidelines described here and in Chapter 2, you should be able to avoid most types of injuries. Important guidelines for preventing athletic injuries include the following:

- Train regularly, and stay in condition.
- Gradually increase the intensity, duration, or frequency of your workouts.
- Get proper rest between exercise sessions.
- Warm up thoroughly before you exercise, and cool down afterward.
- Achieve and maintain a good level of flexibility.
- Use proper body mechanics when lifting objects or executing sports skills.
- Don't exercise when you are ill or overtrained.
- Use proper equipment, particularly shoes, and choose an appropriate exercise surface. If you exercise on a grass field, soft track, or wooden floor, you are less likely to be injured than on concrete or a hard track.
- Don't return to your normal exercise program until your athletic injuries have healed.

? COMMON QUESTIONS ANSWERED

What kind of clothing should I wear during exercise? Exercise clothing should be comfortable, let you move freely, and allow your body to cool itself. Avoid clothing that

TACTICS AND TIPS
Rehabilitation Following a Minor Athletic Injury

1. Reduce the initial inflammation using the R-I-C-E principle:

   Rest: Stop using the injured area as soon as you experience pain.

   Ice: Apply ice to the injured area to reduce swelling and alleviate pain. Apply ice immediately for 15–20 minutes, and repeat every few hours until the swelling disappears. Let the injured part return to normal temperature between icings, and do not apply ice to one area for more than 20 minutes. An easy method for applying ice is to freeze water in a paper cup, peel some of the paper away, and rub it on the injured area. If the injured area is large, you can surround it with several bags of crushed ice or ice cubes.

   Compression: Wrap the injured area firmly with an elastic or compression bandage between icings. If the area starts throbbing or begins to change color, the bandage may be wrapped too tightly. Do not sleep with the wrap on.

   Elevation: Raise the injured area above heart level to decrease the blood supply and reduce swelling. Pillows, books, or a low chair or stool can be used to raise the injured area.
2. After 36–48 hours, apply heat if the swelling has completely disappeared. As soon as it's comfortable, begin moving the affected joints slowly. If you feel pain, or if the injured area begins to swell again, reduce the amount of movement. Continue stretching and moving the affected area until you have regained normal range of motion.
3. Gradually begin exercising the injured area to build strength and endurance. Depending on the type of injury, weight training, walking, and resistance training with a partner can all be effective.
4. Gradually reintroduce the stress of an activity until you can return to full intensity. Don't progress too rapidly or you'll reinjure yourself. Before returning to full exercise participation, you should have a full range of motion in your joints, normal strength and balance among your muscles, normal coordinated patterns of movement (with no injury compensation movements, such as limping), and little or no pain.

constricts normal blood flow or is made from nylon or rubberized fabrics that prevent evaporation of perspiration.

What kind of equipment should I buy? Once you have chosen activities to develop cardiorespiratory fitness, carefully consider what equipment you'll need. Good equipment enhances your enjoyment and decreases your risk of injury. The recent surge of interest in physical activity has been accompanied by a wave of new equipment, but some new products are either overpriced or of poor quality. See the box "Choosing Equipment for Fitness and Sport" (p. 52) for ways to make sound decisions about equipment.

Do I need a special diet for my endurance exercise program? No. For most people, a nutritionally balanced diet contains all the energy and nutrients needed to sustain an exercise program. Don't waste your money on unnecessary vitamins, minerals, and protein supplements. (Chapter 8 has information about putting together a healthy diet.)

Should I drink extra fluids during or after exercise? Yes. Your body depends on water to carry out many chemical reactions and to regulate body temperature. Sweating during exercise depletes your body's water supply and can lead to dehydration if fluids aren't replaced. Serious dehydration can cause reduced blood volume, increased heart rate, elevated body temperature, muscle cramps, heat stroke, and other serious problems. Drinking water before and during exercise is important to prevent dehydration and enhance your performance.

Thirst alone isn't a good indication of how much you need to drink because one's sense of thirst is quickly depressed by drinking even small amounts of water. As a rule of thumb, try to drink about 8 ounces of water (more in hot weather) for every 30 minutes of heavy exercise. Bring a water bottle with you when you exercise so you can replace your fluids while they're being depleted. Water, preferably cold, and diluted carbohydrate drinks are the best fluid replacements. Many excellent athletic fluid replacement beverages are available that satisfy fluid, energy, and electrolyte requirements.

What is cross-training? Cross-training is a pattern of training in which your program centers on two or more different cardiorespiratory endurance activities. Alternating activities can help make your exercise program more fun, but it may slow your development of activity-specific adaptations. For example, if you alternate jogging and tennis, you will probably not develop the coordination, speed, and upper-body strength associated with tennis as quickly as if you just played tennis. However, if you are quickly bored with a single activity, you'll be more likely to stick with your exercise program if you alternate activities to make it more interesting.

Is it all right to participate in cardiorespiratory endurance exercise while menstruating? Yes. There is no evidence that exercise during menstruation is unhealthy or that it

CRITICAL CONSUMER

Choosing Equipment for Fitness and Sport

Your choice of exercise equipment often affects your enjoyment, your risk of injury, and the likelihood of your continued participation. Nothing will ruin the joy of an activity more than ill-fitting or defective equipment. Following a few simple principles of equipment selection will greatly enhance your sport and exercise experiences.

Price

Try to purchase the best equipment you can afford. If you shop around, you can often find merchandise of good quality at a discount. Bargains are often available through mail-order companies and discount stores. Look in the back of sports specialty magazines for good prices on items such as tennis rackets, running shoes, and windsurf boards.

Good-quality used equipment can often be purchased at a fraction of the retail price. Used sporting goods shops have become very popular throughout the United States and Canada. Sporting goods are also often listed in newspaper classified ads.

Quality

While price and quality generally go hand in hand, you can often buy good-quality equipment at less than premium prices. Before you invest in a new piece of equipment, investigate it. Ask coaches and instructors if the results are worth the price. Most magazines devoted to individual sports and activities review new equipment, and publications such as *Consumer Reports* also rate exercise equipment. Don't buy without doing some research. It's also a good idea to buy equipment with a money-back guarantee or a free trial period; if the equipment doesn't meet your expectations, you can return it.

Fit

Equipment that fits properly will enhance your enjoyment and prevent injury. Shoes that pinch your feet will make running unbearable. The wrong size grip on a tennis racket can lead to an elbow injury. When shopping for exercise equipment, take your time and get the help you need to ensure a proper fit.

Intended Use

Many people purchase expensive home exercise equipment, only to have it sit in a corner gathering dust. Before buying an expensive home treadmill, stationary bicycle, or stair-climber, try it for several weeks at a local health club or gym. If you really decide you want to own one, buy it for your home.

An important question to ask yourself is how often you'll actually use the equipment. If you honestly will use it regularly, go ahead and buy a home treadmill or stationary bicycle. If you will use a piece of equipment only occasionally, you are better off using one at a gym.

Also consider how intense your workouts will be. If you intend to push your equipment to the limit, buy a model that can handle the stress. There's nothing more frustrating than a tennis racket that breaks the first time you use it, or a treadmill belt that slips when you try to run fast. While heavy-duty equipment tends to cost more, it may be worth the extra money. But take care not to pay extra for features you don't need.

Your Skill Level

Some equipment is designed for people with superior levels of strength, fitness, and skill. Buying "advanced" equipment can actually diminish your enjoyment of an activity. For example, slalom skis designed for a racer would be extremely difficult for a beginning skier to turn. Shoes designed for competitive marathon runners may have less padding to protect the legs and feet from injury, making them inappropriate for a recreational runner. (Chapter 7 contains additional information on choosing footwear.) Buy equipment that is appropriate for your current skill level.

Safety

Don't skimp on safety equipment. For popular sports like in-line skating, failing to buy a helmet and appropriate pads can lead to a serious injury. Check your safety equipment frequently to ensure that it's in good working condition. For example, ski bindings that work perfectly one season may not release properly after sitting in your garage for a year.

---

has negative effects on performance. If you have headaches, backaches, and abdominal pain during menstruation, you may not feel like exercising; for some women, exercise helps relieve these symptoms. Listen to your body, and exercise at whatever intensity is comfortable for you.

Is endurance exercise safe during pregnancy? For most women, there is no reason not to exercise during pregnancy. In the absence of either medical or obstetric complications, pregnant women can continue with an established exercise program and can obtain all the benefits of regular exercise. However, although maternal fitness and a sense of well-being may be enhanced by exercise, no level of exercise during pregnancy has been conclusively demonstrated to be beneficial in improving the outcome of pregnancy.

Consult your physician before continuing or beginning an exercise program. If you were exercising before your pregnancy, you can probably continue with your regular program and modify it as necessary. If you weren't exercising before pregnancy, begin slowly. Throughout pregnancy you should listen to your body and adjust

TACTICS AND TIPS
Exercising During Pregnancy

Women can continue to exercise and derive health benefits from exercise during pregnancy. Recommendations for exercising safely during pregnancy include the following:

- Exercise regularly (at least three times per week) rather than intermittently.
- Avoid exercise in a supine position—lying on your back—after the first trimester. Research indicates that this position restricts blood flow to the uterus. Also avoid prolonged periods of motionless standing.
- Modify the intensity of your exercise according to how you feel. Stop exercising if you feel fatigued, and don't exercise to exhaustion. You may find that non–weight-bearing exercises such as cycling and swimming are more comfortable than weight-bearing activities in the later months of pregnancy; they also minimize the risk of injury.
- Take care when performing any activity in which balance is important or in which losing balance would prove dangerous. Pregnancy shifts your center of gravity. Also avoid any type of exercise that has the potential for even mild abdominal trauma.
- Eat an adequate diet.
- Avoid heat stress, particularly during the first trimester, by drinking an adequate amount of fluids, wearing appropriate clothing, and avoiding exercise in hot and humid weather.
- Resume prepregnancy exercise routines gradually. Many of the changes of pregnancy persist 4–6 weeks postpartum.
- If you experience any unusual symptoms, stop exercising, and consult your physician.

Source: Adapted from American College of Obstetricians and Gynecologists. 1994. Exercise during pregnancy and the postpartum period. *ACOG Technical Bulletin Number 189*. February.

your exercise program to keep it comfortable. Follow the general pattern for cardiorespiratory endurance exercise described in this chapter. Be sure to warm up, cool down, and drink plenty of fluids. General guidelines for exercise during pregnancy are summarized in the box "Exercising During Pregnancy."

Is it safe to exercise in hot weather? Prolonged, vigorous exercise can be dangerous in hot and humid weather. Heat from exercise is released in the form of sweat, which cools the skin and the blood circulating near the body surface as it evaporates. The hotter the weather, the more water the body loses through sweat; the more humid the weather, the less efficient the sweating mechanism is at lowering body temperature. If you lose too much water or if your body temperature rises too high, you may suffer from a heat disorder such as heat exhaustion or heat stroke. Use caution when exercising if the temperature is above 80°F or if humidity is above 60%. To exercise safely, watch for the signals of heat disorder, regardless of the weather, and follow the tips given in the box "Exercising in Hot Weather" (p. 54).

Is it safe to exercise in cold weather? If you dress warmly in layers and don't stay out in very cold temperatures for too long, exercise can be safe even in subfreezing temperatures. Take both the temperature and the wind-chill factor into account when choosing clothing. Dress in layers so you can subtract them as you warm up and add them if you get cold. In subfreezing temperatures, protect the areas of your body most susceptible to frostbite—fingers, toes, ears, nose, and cheeks—with warm socks, mittens or gloves, and a cap, hood, or ski mask. For exercising in rain or snow, be sure to wear clothing that "breathes" to avoid being overheated by trapped perspiration.

Is it safe to exercise in a smoggy city? Do not exercise outdoors during a smog alert or if air quality is very poor (symptoms of poor air quality include eye and throat irritation and respiratory discomfort). If you have any type of cardiorespiratory difficulty, you should avoid exertion outdoors when air quality is poor. You can avoid smog and air pollution by exercising in parks, near water (riverbanks, lakeshores, and ocean beaches), or in residential areas with less traffic (areas with stop-and-go traffic will have lower air quality than areas where traffic moves quickly). Air quality is usually better in the early morning and late evening.

How can I keep long-distance travel from having a negative effect on my body and my exercise regimen? Inexpensive air travel makes it likely that you will participate in sports and exercise great distances from your home. Going on a skiing or hiking vacation may force you to endure a long airplane ride. Long trips may inhibit your ability to exercise by disturbing normal living habits and altering biological rhythms.

Jet lag is characterized by fatigue, malaise, sluggishness, decreased reaction time, and disorientation. This condition is caused by factors such as loss of sleep due to the excitement of travel, irregular and unfamiliar meals, dehydration, and disturbance of the biological clock from

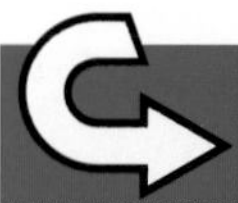

TACTICS AND TIPS

Exercising in Hot Weather

- Use caution when exercising in extreme heat or humidity (over 80°F and/or 60% humidity).
- Expose yourself gradually to exercise in hot and humid environments; work up slowly to your usual levels of intensity and duration.
- Exercise in the early morning or evening, when temperatures are lowest.
- Drink a glass or two of fluids before you begin exercising, and drink 4–8 ounces of fluid every 10–15 minutes during exercise (more frequently during high-intensity activities).
- Wear clothing that "breathes," allowing air to circulate and cool the body. Wearing white or light colors will help by reflecting, rather than absorbing, heat. A hat can help keep direct sun off your face. Do not wear rubber, plastic, or other nonporous clothing.
- Rest frequently in the shade.
- Keep a record of your morning body weight to track whether weight lost through sweating is restored.
- Slow down or stop if you begin to feel uncomfortable. Watch for the signs of heat disorders listed below; if they occur, act appropriately.

Problem	Symptoms	Treatment
Heat cramps	Muscle cramps, usually in the muscles most used during exercise.	Stop exercising, drink fluids, and stretch cramped muscles.
Heat exhaustion	Paleness; headache; nausea; fainting; dizziness; profuse sweating; weakness; cold, clammy skin; and a rapid, weak pulse.	Cool the body: Stop exercising, get out of the heat, remove excess clothing, drink cold fluids, and apply cool and/or damp towels to the body.
Heat stroke	Hot, flushed skin (skin may be dry or sweaty); rapid pulse; high body temperature; dizziness; disorientation; vomiting; diarrhea; unconsciousness.	Get immediate medical attention, and try to lower your body temperature: Get out of the heat, remove excess clothing, drink cold fluids, and apply cool and/or damp towels or immerse the body in cold water.

switching between time zones. You may get stiff muscles or become constipated from sitting for prolonged periods.

Eastbound travel seems to cause the most problems because it has the greatest effect on sleep. Proper travel scheduling can help alleviate the symptoms. If possible, schedule your trip for evening arrival, so you can get a full night's sleep. Several days before the trip is scheduled, gradually shift your hours for eating and sleeping toward the time schedule of your destination. Be well rested before the beginning of the journey.

Traveling in an airplane can lead to dehydration. Airplane cabin air is extremely dry, so you tend to lose a lot of body water. Drink more water than normal both before and during the trip to prevent this problem. In addition, constipation can often be prevented by ensuring adequate fluid intake.

Guidelines for preventing jet lag include the following:

- Make eastbound flights during daylight hours, leaving as early as possible—earlier as the distance increases.
- Make westbound flights late in the day, arriving as close to your retiring hour as possible.
- Drink plenty of water during the trip.
- Eat light meals, and avoid fatty foods.
- At regular intervals, get up from your seat and stretch or walk.

You can minimize the negative effects of travel by planning the trip well and adhering to your normal schedule as much as possible.

SUMMARY

- The primary health benefits of cardiorespiratory endurance exercise are improvements in heart and lung functioning and in metabolic efficiency.
- Improved blood fat levels, increased calorie burning, creation of lean body mass, improved immune function, and protection from cancer are additional health benefits of endurance exercise. Psychological benefits also accrue, as well as protection against osteoporosis and diabetes.
- Cardiorespiratory fitness is measured by maximal oxygen consumption, expressed as $\dot{V}O_{2max}$. Direct measurement of $\dot{V}O_{2max}$ is performed in scientific laboratories. Indirect assessment methods include the 1-mile walk test, the 3-minute step test, the 1.5-mile walk-run test, and the Åstrand-Rhyming bicycle ergometer test.
- A successful endurance exercise program sets realistic goals; includes suitable activities; sets starting frequency, intensity, and duration at appropriate

levels; includes warm-up and cool-down activities; and is adjusted as fitness improves.

- Intensity of training, the most important factor in achieving cardiorespiratory benefits, can be measured through target heart rate zone and ratings of perceived exertion.
- Serious injuries require medical attention. Application of the R-I-C-E principle (rest, ice, compression, elevation) is appropriate for treating muscle or joint injuries.

BEHAVIOR CHANGE ACTIVITY

Setting Goals

For your behavior change program to succeed, you must set meaningful, realistic goals. In addition to an ultimate goal, also set some intermediate goals—milestones that you can strive for on the way to your final objective. For example, if your overall goal is to run a 5K road race, an intermediate goal might be to successfully complete 2 weeks of your fitness program. If you set a final goal of eating five servings of fruits and vegetables every day, an intermediate goal would be to increase your intake from two to three servings.

Choose goals that are both meaningful and realistic; don't strive for perfection. Allow an adequate amount of time to reach each of your goals.

Intermediate Goals	Target Date
______________________________	______________
______________________________	______________
______________________________	______________
______________________________	______________
______________________________	______________
Final Goal	
______________________________	______________

FOR MORE INFORMATION

American College of Sports Medicine. 1992. *ACSM Fitness Book.* Champaign, Ill.: Human Kinetics. *Includes assessment tests for cardiorespiratory endurance, along with step-by-step instructions for creating a personal exercise program.*

Kusinitz, I., and M. Fine. 1995. *Your Guide to Getting Fit,* 3d ed. Mountain View, Calif.: Mayfield. *Includes assessment tests and a step-by-step guide to developing a cardiorespiratory endurance exercise program.*

Johnson, R., and B. Tulin. 1995. *Travel Fitness.* Champaign, Ill.: Human Kinetics. *A comprehensive guide to staying fit and well while traveling.*

The Melpomene Institute for Women's Health Research. 1990. *The Bodywise Woman.* Champaign, Ill.: Human Kinetics. *A comprehensive look at the relationship between women's health and physical activity.*

Shephard, R. J. 1994. *Aerobic Fitness and Health.* Champaign, Ill.: Human Kinetics. *A comprehensive review of the research on aerobic fitness.*

YMCA of the USA and T. W. Hanlon. 1995. *Fit for Two: The Official YMCA Prenatal Exercise Guide.* Champaign, Ill.: Human Kinetics. *A practical guide to safe exercise during pregnancy.*

Tippett, S. R. 1989. *Coaches' Guide to Sport Rehabilitation.* Champaign, Ill.: Human Kinetics. *A concise guide to rehabilitation techniques for common sports injuries. Topics include evaluation and care of injuries, life-support techniques, and guidelines for injury rehabilitation.*

Refer to the books listed in Chapter 2 for resources on exercise physiology and fitness testing. Chapter 7 lists sources of information about sports and activities that develop cardiorespiratory endurance and other fitness components.

Additional sources of information and programs include the YMCA, and campus or private sports medicine centers, for fitness testing; health clubs for places to exercise and training advice; and physical education departments for activity classes.

SELECTED BIBLIOGRAPHY

American College of Sports Medicine. 1990. The recommended quantity and quality of exercise for developing and maintaining cardiorespiratory and muscular fitness in healthy adults. *Medicine and Science in Sports and Exercise* 22: 265–274.

American College of Sports Medicine. 1995. *Guidelines for Exercise Testing and Prescription,* 5th ed. Baltimore: Williams & Wilkins.

American Heart Association. 1991. *Exercise Standards: A Statement for Health Professionals.* Dallas: American Heart Association.

Berg, A., I. Frey, M. W. Baumstark, M. Halle, and J. Keul. 1994. Physical activity and lipoprotein lipid disorders. *Sports Medicine* 17:6–21.

Bijnen, F. C., C. J. Caspersen, and W. L. Mosterd. 1994. Physical inactivity as a risk factor for coronary heart disease: A WHO and International Society and Federation of Cardiology position statement. *Bulletin of the World Health Organization* 72(1): 1–4.

Blair, S. N., H. W. Kohl, C. E. Barlow, R. S. Paffenbarger, L. W. Gibbons, and C. A. Macera. 1995. Changes in physical fitness and all-cause mortality: A prospective study of healthy and unhealthy men. *Journal of the American Medical Association* 273(14): 1093–1098.

Blair, S. N., H. W. Kohl, R. S. Paffenbarger, D. G. Clark, K. H. Cooper, and L. W. Gibbons. 1989. Physical fitness and all-cause mortality: A prospective study of healthy men and women. *Journal of the American Medical Association* 262(17): 2395–2401.

Borg, G. A. V. 1982. Psychophysical bases of perceived exertion. *Medicine and Science in Sports and Exercise* 14:377–381.

Brooks, G. A. 1985. Anaerobic threshold: Review of the concept and directions for future research. *Medicine and Science in Sports and Exercise* 17:22.

Brooks, G. A., T. D. Fahey, and T. P. White. 1996. *Exercise Physiology: Human Bioenergetics and Its Applications,* 2d ed. Mountain View, Calif.: Mayfield.

Centers for Disease Control and Prevention. 1993. Public health focus: Physical activity and the prevention of coronary heart disease. *Journal of the American Medical Association* 270:1529–1530.

Coyle, E. F. 1995. Substrate utilization during exercise in active people. *American Journal of Clinical Nutrition* 61 (4 Suppl): 968S–979S.

Despres, J. P., and B. Lamarche. 1994. Low-intensity endurance exercise training, plasma lipoproteins and the risk of coronary heart disease. *Journal of Internal Medicine* 236:7–22.

Fahey, T. D. 1986. *Athletic Training: Principles and Practice.* Mountain View, Calif.: Mayfield.

Fletcher, G. F., et al. 1992. Statement on exercise benefits and recommendations for physical activity programs for all Americans. *Circulation* 86:340–344.

Gillette, C. A., R. C. Bullough, and C. L. Melby. Postexercise energy expenditure in response to acute aerobic or resistive exercise. 1994. *International Journal of Sport Nutrition* 4:347–360.

Haskell, W. L., H. J. Montoye, and D. Orenstein. 1985. Physical activity and exercise to achieve health-related physical fitness components. *Public Health Reports* 100:202–212.

Holloszy, J. O. 1975. Adaptation of skeletal muscle to endurance exercise. *Medicine and Science in Sports and Exercise* 7:155.

Israel, R. G., M. J. Sullivan, R. H. Marks, R. S. Cayton, and T. C. Chenier. 1994. Relationship between cardiorespiratory fitness and lipoprotein (a) in men and women. *Medicine and Science in Sports and Exercise* 26:425–431.

King, A. C., W. L. Haskell, D. R. Young, R. K. Oka, and M. L. Stefanick. 1995. Long-term effects of varying intensities and formats of physical activity on participation rates, fitness, and lipoproteins in men and women aged 50 to 65 years. *Circulation* 91:2596–2604.

Klissouras, V., F. Pirnay, and J.-M. Petit. 1976. Adaptation to maximal effort: Genetics and age. *Journal of Applied Physiology* 1:195.

Nieman, D. C., et al. 1990. Reducing-diet and exercise-training effects on serum lipids and lipoproteins in mildly obese women. *American Journal of Clinical Nutrition* 52:640–645.

Noakes, T. 1991. *Lore of Running,* 3d ed. Champaign, Ill.: Leisure Press.

Noakes, T. 1993. Fluid replacement during exercise. *Science and Sports Reviews* 21:297–330.

Pollock, M. L. 1977. Submaximal and maximal working capacity of elite distance runners: Part 1, Cardiovascular aspects. *Annals of the New York Academy of Science* 301:361.

Rodriguez, B. L., J. D. Curb, C. M. Burchfiel, R. D. Abbott, H. Petrovitch, K. Masaki, and D. Chiu. 1994. Physical activity and 23-year incidence of coronary heart disease morbidity and mortality among middle-aged men. The Honolulu Heart Program. *Circulation* 89:2540–2544.

Shephard, R. J. 1988. PAR-Q, Canadian Home Fitness Test and exercise screening alternatives. *Sports Medicine* 5:188–195.

Shephard, R. J., and P. N. Shek. 1995. Cancer, immune function, and physical activity. *Canadian Journal of Applied Physiology* 20:1–25.

Shephard, R. J., T. Kavanagh, D. J. Mertens, S. Qureshi, and M. Clark. 1995. Personal health benefits of Masters athletics competition. *British Journal of Sports Medicine* 29:35–40.

Siegel, P. Z., R. M. Brackbill, and G. W. Heath. 1995. The epidemiology of walking for exercise: Implications for promoting activity among sedentary groups. American Journal of Public Health 85:706–710.

Tuomi, K. 1994. Characteristics of work and life predicting coronary heart disease. Finnish research project on aging workers. *Social Science Medicine* 38:1509–1519.

U.S. Department of Health and Human Services. 1990. *Healthy People 2000: National Health Promotion and Disease Prevention Objectives.* Washington, D.C.: U.S. Government Printing Office, DHHS Pub. (PHS) 95-50213.

Viru, A., and T. Smirnova. 1995. Health promotion and exercise training. *Sports Medicine* 19:123–136.

Webster, D. L., J. C. Mason, and T. M. Keating. 1992. *Guidelines for Professional Practice in Athletic Training.* Canton, Ohio: Professional Reports Corporation.

Wells, C. L. 1991. *Women, Sports, and Performance.* Champaign, Ill.: Human Kinetics.

Name ______________________ Section ____________ Date ____________

LAB 3-1 *Assessing Your Current Level of Cardiorespiratory Endurance*

Before taking any of the cardiorespiratory endurance assessment tests, refer to the fitness prerequisites and cautions given in Table 3-1. For best results, don't exercise strenuously the day of the test, and don't smoke or eat a heavy meal within about 3 hours of the test.

The 1-Mile Walk Test

Equipment

1. A track or course that provides a measurement of 1 mile
2. A stopwatch, clock, or watch with a second hand
3. A weight scale

Preparation

Measure your body weight (in pounds) before taking the test.

Body weight: __________ lb

Instructions

1. Warm up before taking the test. Do some walking, easy jogging, or calisthenics and some stretching exercises.
2. Cover the 1-mile course as quickly as possible. Walk at a pace that is brisk but comfortable. You must raise your heart rate above 120 bpm.
3. As soon as you complete the distance, note your time and take your pulse for 15 seconds.

   Walking time: __________ min __________ sec

   15-second pulse count: __________ beats
4. Cool down after the test by walking slowly for several minutes.

Determining Maximal Oxygen Consumption

1. Convert your 15-second pulse count into a value for exercise heart rate by multiplying it by 4.

   Exercise heart rate: __________ × 4 = __________ bpm
   15-sec pulse count
2. Convert your walking time from minutes and seconds to a decimal figure. For example, a time of 14 minutes and 45 seconds would be 14 + (45/60), or 14.75 minutes.

   Walking time: __________ min + (__________ sec ÷ 60 sec/min) = __________ min
3. Insert values for your age, gender, weight, walking time, and exercise heart rate in the following equation, where

   W = your weight (in pounds)

   A = your age (in years)

   G = your gender (male = 1; female = 0)

   T = your time to complete the 1-mile course (in minutes)

   H = *your exercise heart rate (in beats per minute)*

   $\dot{V}O_{2max} = 132.853 - (0.0769 \times W) - (0.3877 \times A) + (6.315 \times G) - (3.2649 \times T) - (0.1565 \times H)$

LABORATORY ACTIVITIES

For example, a 20-year-old, 190-pound male with a time of 14.75 minutes and an exercise heart rate of 152 **bpm** would calculate maximal oxygen consumption as follows:

$\dot{V}O_{2max} = 132.853 - (0.0769 \times 190) - (0.3877 \times 20) + (6.315 \times 1) - (3.2649 \times 14.75) - (0.1565 \times 152) =$ 45 ml/kg/min

$\dot{V}O_{2max} = 132.853 - (0.0769 \times \underset{\text{weight (lb)}}{\underline{\qquad}}) - (0.3877 \times \underset{\text{age (years)}}{\underline{\qquad}}) + (6.315 \times \underset{\text{gender}}{\underline{\qquad}})$

$- (3.2649 \times \underset{\text{walking time (min)}}{\underline{\qquad}}) - (0.1565 \times \underset{\text{exercise heart rate (bpm)}}{\underline{\qquad}}) =$ ________ **ml/kg/min**

4. Copy this value for $\dot{V}O_{2max}$ into the appropriate place in the chart on the final page of this lab.

The 3-Minute Step Test

Equipment

1. A step, bench, or bleacher step that is 16.25 inches from ground level
2. A stopwatch, clock, or watch with a second hand
3. A metronome

Preparation

Practice stepping up and down from the step before you begin the test. Each step has four beats: up-up-down-down. Males should perform the test with the metronome set for a rate of 96 beats per minute, or 24 steps per minute. Females should set the metronome at 88 beats per minute, or 22 steps per minute.

Instructions

1. Warm up before taking the test. Do some walking, easy jogging, and stretching exercises.
2. Set the metronome at the proper rate. Your instructor or a partner can call out starting and stopping times; otherwise, have a clock or watch within easy viewing during the test.
3. Begin the test, and continue to step at the correct pace for 3 minutes.
4. Stop after 3 minutes. Remain standing, and count your pulse for the 15-second period from 5 to 20 seconds into recovery.

   15-second pulse count: ____________ beats
5. Cool down after the test by walking slowly for several minutes.

Determining Maximal Oxygen Consumption

1. Convert your 15-second pulse count to a value for recovery heart rate by multiplying by 4.

   Recovery heart rate: $\underset{\text{15-sec pulse count}}{\underline{\qquad\qquad}} \times 4 =$ ____________ bpm
2. Insert your recovery heart rate in the equation below, where

   H = recovery heart rate (in beats per minute)
   Males: $\dot{V}O_{2max} = 111.33 - (0.42 \times H)$
   Females: $\dot{V}O_{2max} = 65.81 - (0.1847 \times H)$
   For example, a man with a recovery heart rate of 162 bpm would calculate maximal oxygen consumption as follows:

   $\dot{V}O_{2max} = 111.33 - (0.42 \times 162) = 43$ ml/kg/min

   Males: $\dot{V}O_{2max} = 111.33 - (0.42 \times \underset{\text{recovery heart rate (bpm)}}{\underline{\qquad}}) =$ ________ **ml/kg/min**

   Females: $\dot{V}O_{2max} = 65.81 - (0.1847 \times \underset{\text{recovery heart rate (bpm)}}{\underline{\qquad}}) =$ ________ **ml/kg/min**
3. Copy this value for $\dot{V}O_{2max}$ into the appropriate place in the chart on the final page of this lab.

The 1.5-Mile Run-Walk Test

Equipment

1. A running track or course that is flat and provides exact measurements of up to 1.5 miles
2. A stopwatch, clock, or watch with a second hand

Preparation

You may want to practice pacing yourself prior to taking the test to avoid going too fast at the start and becoming prematurely fatigued. Allow yourself a day or two to recover from your practice run before taking the test.

Instructions

1. Warm up before taking the test. Do some walking, easy jogging, and stretching exercises.
2. Try to cover the distance as fast as possible, at a pace that is comfortable for you. If possible, monitor your own time, or have someone call out your time at various intervals of the test to determine whether your pace is correct.
3. Record the amount of time, in minutes and seconds, it takes for you to complete the 1.5-mile distance.

   Running-walking time: ____________ min ____________ sec
4. Cool down after the test by walking or jogging slowly for about 5 minutes.

Determining Maximal Oxygen Consumption

1. Convert your running time from minutes and seconds to a decimal figure. For example, a time of 14 minutes and 25 seconds would be 14 + (25/60), or 14.4 minutes.

   Running-walking time: ________ min + (_________ sec ÷ 60 sec/min) = ________ min
2. Insert your running time in the equation below, where

   T = running time (in minutes)

   $\dot{V}O_{2max} = (483 \div T) + 3.5$

   For example, a person who completes 1.5 miles in 14.4 minutes would calculate maximal oxygen consumption as follows:

   $\dot{V}O_{2max} = (483 \div 14.4) + 3.5 = 37$ ml/kg/min

   $\dot{V}O_{2max} = (483 \div$ _______ $) + 3.5 =$ _______ **ml/kg/min**

   run-walk time (min)
3. Copy this value for $\dot{V}O_{2max}$ into the appropriate place in the chart on the final page of this lab.

The Åstrand-Rhyming Bicycle Ergometer Test

Equipment

1. Bicycle ergometer that allows for regulation of power output in kilopounds per meter (kpm)
2. A stopwatch, clock, or watch with a second hand
3. Weight scale
4. Metronome or meter on bicycle to measure pedal revolutions
5. Partner to monitor heart rate

Preparation

Weigh yourself before taking the test. Adjust the seat height of the bicycle so that your knees are almost completely extended as your foot goes through the bottom of the pedaling cycle. Practice pedaling the bicycle ergometer at the speed of 50 pedal revolutions per minute. Each revolution includes a downstroke with each foot, so set your metronome at 100 beats per minute.

Body weight: ________ lb

Instructions

1. Warm up before taking the test. Do some walking, easy jogging, and stretching exercises. A few minutes' practice on the bicycle ergometer can also be part of your warm-up.
2. Set up the metronome to monitor your pace. If you aren't using a metronome, have a partner call out times at regular intervals.
3. Set the power output between 300 and 1200 kpm. If you are small or have been sedentary, a setting of 300–600 kpm is appropriate. If you are larger or fitter, try a setting of 600–900 kpm. Find a setting high enough to raise your heart rate to between 125 and 170 bpm, but not so high that you can't continue pedaling for 6 minutes.

   Note: If your heart rate goes above 170 or you experience any unusual symptoms, stop pedaling the bicycle, rest for 15–20 minutes, and then repeat the test at a lower workload.
4. Ride the bicycle ergometer for 6 minutes at a rate of 50 pedal revolutions per minute. Your partner should monitor your heart rate by counting your pulse for the last 15 seconds of each minute of your ride (see the photograph). Your heart rate should rise to a level in the target range (125–170 bpm) and then level off, staying relatively constant during the last few minutes of your ride. If your exercise heart rate stays below 125 bpm, rest for 15–20 minutes, then repeat the test at a higher workload. If your heart rate gets too high or if it continues to rise throughout your ride (not leveling off in the last few minutes), rest for 15–20 minutes, and repeat the test at a lower workload.

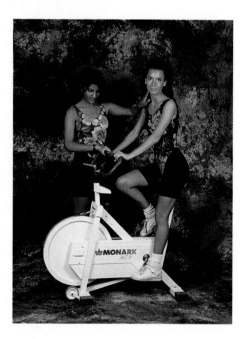

During the bicycle ergometer test, a partner monitors heart rate for the last 15 seconds of every minute.

5. If your heart rate levels off within the target range (125–170 bpm), your partner should make a final count during the last 15 seconds of the sixth minute of your ride.

   15-second pulse count: ___________ beats

   Power output: ___________ kpm
6. Cool down after the test by pedaling, walking, or jogging slowly for several minutes.

Determining Maximal Oxygen Consumption

1. Calculate your exercise heart rate by multiplying your final 15-second count by 4.

   Exercise heart rate: ___________ × 4 = ___________ bpm
   15-sec pulse count
2. On the nomogram, connect the point that represents your exercise heart rate with the point that represents the power output you used (on the scale for your sex). Read your total oxygen uptake score (in liters) at the point where the line you've drawn crosses the maximal oxygen consumption line.

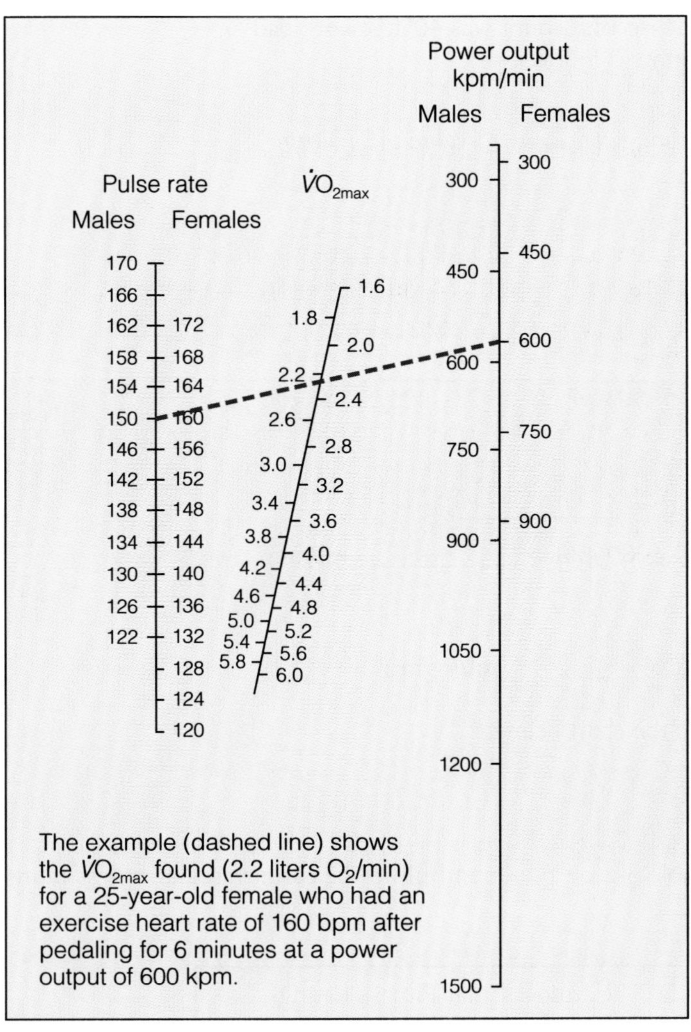

Nomogram for use with the Åstrand-Rhyming bicycle ergometer test.

Maximal oxygen consumption (from nomogram): __________ l/min

3. Adjust your maximal oxygen consumption score for your age by multiplying it by the appropriate age-correction factor in the table below:

Age	15	20	25	30	35	40	45	50	55	60	65
Factor	1.10	1.05	1.0	0.94	0.87	0.83	0.78	0.75	0.71	0.68	0.65

$\dot{V}O_{2max}$ corrected for age: ____________ l/min × ____________ = ____________ l/min
($\dot{V}O_{2max}$) (age-correction factor)

4. Convert your score to one for maximal oxygen consumption (in milliliters of oxygen per minute per kilogram of body weight):
   a. Convert your weight from pounds to kilograms by dividing it by 2.2.
   b. Multiply your $\dot{V}O_{2max}$ by 1000 (to convert from liters to milliliters).
   c. Divide this number by your weight (in kilograms).

LABORATORY ACTIVITIES

For example, a 135-pound, 25-year-old female whose 15-second count was 40 at a workload of 600 kpm would calculate maximal oxygen consumption as follows:

1. 40 beats × 4 = 160 bpm
2. Connecting 600 kpm and 160 bpm on the nomogram gives a $\dot{V}O_{2max}$ value of 2.2 l/min
3. The age-adjustment factor for a 25-year-old is 1.00.
   2.2 l/min × 1.00 = 2.2 l/min
4. To convert 135 pounds to kilograms:
   135 lb ÷ 2.2 lb/kg = 61.4 kg
   To convert liters to milliliters:
   2.2 l/min × 1000 ml/l = 2200 ml/min
   To adjust for weight:
   2200 ml/min ÷ 61.4 kg = 35.8 ml/kg/min

Convert body weight to kg: ____________ lb ÷ 2.2 lb/kg = ____________ kg

Convert from liters to milliliters: ____________ l/min × 1000 ml/l = ____________ ml/min
age-corrected $\dot{V}O_{2max}$

Adjust for weight:

$\dot{V}O_{2max}$ = ____________ ml/min ÷ ____________ kg = ____________ **ml/kg/min**
$\dot{V}O_{2max}$ body weight

5. Copy this value for $\dot{V}O_{2max}$ into the appropriate place in the chart below.

Rating Your Cardiovascular Fitness

Record your $\dot{V}O_{2max}$ score(s) in the chart below. Turn to Table 3-2 on p. 44, and fill in the cardiovascular fitness rating that corresponds to your $\dot{V}O_{2max}$ score.

	$\dot{V}O_{2max}$	Cardiovascular Fitness Rating
1-mile walk test		
3-minute step test		
1.5-mile run-walk test		
Åstrand-Rhyming bicycle ergometer test		

Is your rating as high as you want it to be? If not, what is your goal for $\dot{V}O_{2max}$? ____________

____

To monitor your progress toward your goal, enter the results of this lab in the Preprogram Assessment column of Lab 15-2. After several weeks of a cardiorespiratory endurance exercise program, complete this lab again, and enter the results in the Postprogram Assessment column of Lab 15-2. How do the results compare?

Sources: Kline, G. M., et al. 1987. Estimation of $\dot{V}O_{2max}$ from a one-mile track walk, gender, age, and body weight. *Medicine and Science in Sports and Exercise* 19(3): 253–259. McArdle, W. D., F. I. Katch, and V. L. Katch. 1991. *Exercise Physiology: Energy, Nutrition, and Human Performance.* Philadelphia: Lea and Febiger, pp. 225–226. Brooks, G. A., and T. D. Fahey. 1987. *Fundamentals of Human Performance.* New York: Macmillan. Åstrand, P. O., and I. Rhyming. 1954. A nomogram for calculation of aerobic capacity (physical fitness) from pulse rate during submaximal work. *Journal of Applied Physiology* 7: 218–221.

Name ______________________ Section ______________ Date ______________

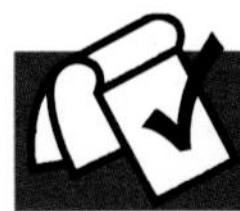

LAB 3-2 *Developing an Exercise Program for Cardiorespiratory Endurance*

1. *Activities.* Refer to the box "Activities and Sports for Developing Cardiorespiratory Endurance" (p. 46) and choose one or more activities for your program. Fill in the activity name and general intensity rating sections on the program plan below.
2. *Duration.* Fill in an appropriate duration for each activity (20–60 minutes).
3. *Intensity.* Determine your exercise intensity, and fill in below.
   a. Resting heart rate: __________ bpm (taken after 10 minutes of complete rest)

   Maximum heart rate: 220 − __________ (age (years)) = __________ bpm

   Heart Rate Reserve Method

   Heart rate reserve: __________ (maximum heart rate) bpm − __________ (resting heart rate) bpm = __________ bpm

   50% training intensity = (__________ (heart rate reserve) bpm × 0.5) + __________ (resting heart rate) bpm = __________ bpm

   85% training intensity = (__________ (heart rate reserve) bpm × 0.85) + __________ (resting heart rate) bpm = __________ bpm

   Target heart rate zone = __________ to __________ bpm

   Maximum Heart Rate Method

   60% training intensity = __________ (maximum heart rate) bpm × 0.60 = __________ bpm

   90% training intensity = __________ (maximum heart rate) bpm × 0.90 = __________ bpm

   Target heart rate zone = __________ to __________ bpm

   b. If you prefer, determine an RPE value that corresponds to your target heart rate range (see p. 47 and Figure 3-2).
4. *Frequency.* Fill in how often you plan to participate in each activity.

Program Plan

Activity	General Intensity Rating (L, M, H)	Duration (min)	Intensity (bpm or RPE)	Frequency (check) M	T	W	Th	F	Sa	Su

5. *Monitoring your program.* Complete a log like the one on the next page to monitor your program and track your progress. Fill in the duration of exercise for each workout. To monitor your progress more closely, you can also track another variable, such as distance. For example, if your cardiorespiratory endurance program includes walking and swimming, you can keep track of miles walked and yards swum in addition to the duration of each exercise session.

Activity/Date													
1	Duration												
2	Duration												
3	Duration												
4	Duration												
5	Duration												

Activity/Date													
1	Duration												
2	Duration												
3	Duration												
4	Duration												
5	Duration												

Activity/Date													
1	Duration												
2	Duration												
3	Duration												
4	Duration												
5	Duration												

4

Muscular Strength and Endurance

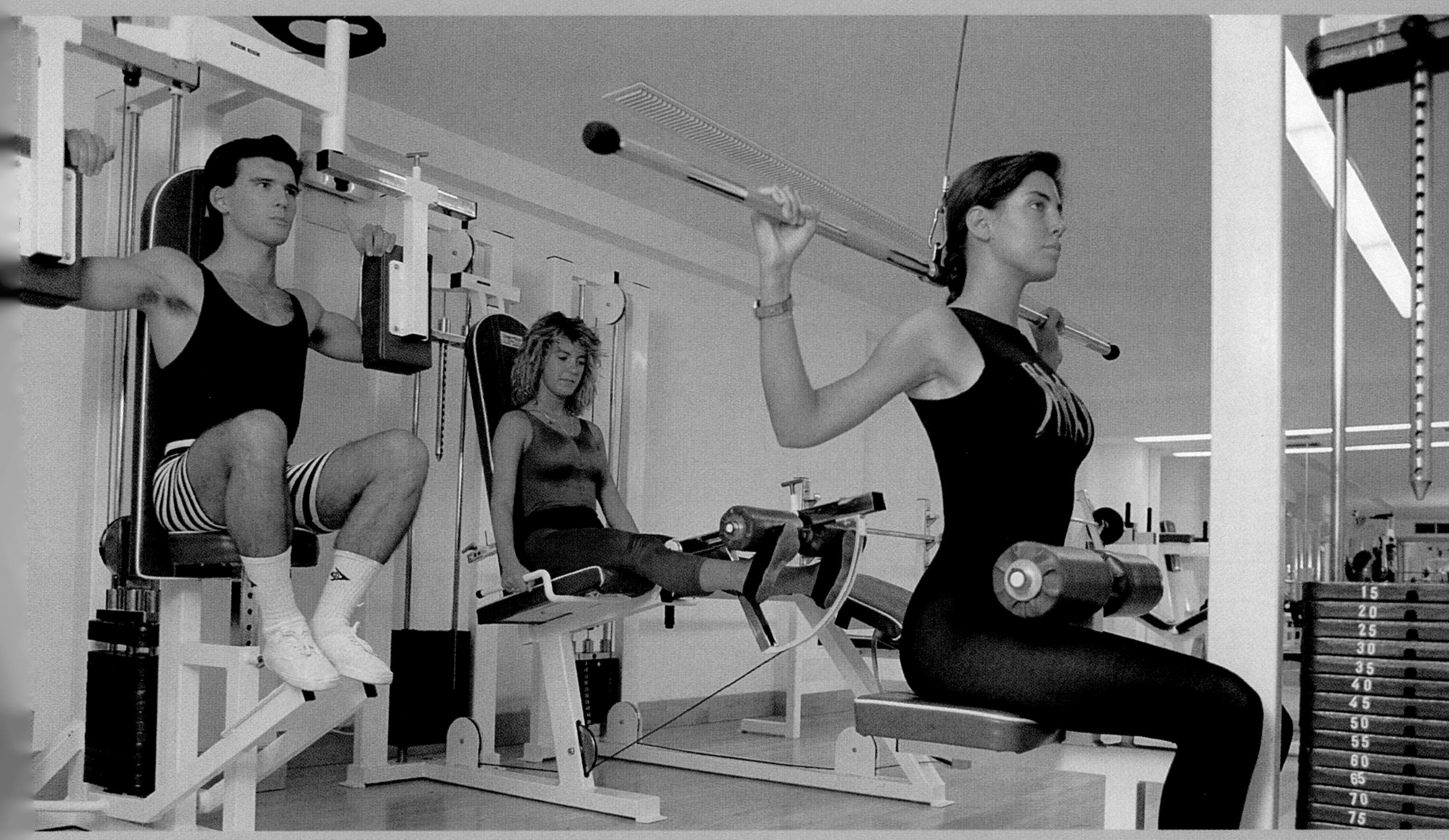

LOOKING AHEAD

After reading this chapter, you should be able to answer these questions about muscular strength and endurance:

- What are muscular strength and endurance, and how do they relate to wellness?
- How can muscular strength and endurance be assessed?
- How do weight training exercises affect muscles?
- What type, frequency, and number of weight training exercises make up a successful program?
- What are the most important strategies for avoiding injuries in a weight training program?
- How are common weight training exercises performed using weight machines and free weights?

Exercise experts have long emphasized the importance of cardiovascular fitness. Other physical fitness factors, such as muscle strength and flexibility, were mentioned almost as an afterthought. As more was learned about how the body responds to exercise, however, it became obvious that these other factors are vital to health, wellness, and overall quality of life. Muscles make up over 40% of your body mass. You depend on them for movement, and, because of their mass, they are the site of a large portion of the energy reactions (metabolism) that take place in your body. Strong, well-developed muscles help you perform daily activities with greater ease, protect you from injury, and enhance your well-being in other ways.

This chapter explains the benefits of strength training and describes methods of assessing muscular strength and endurance. It then explains the basics of weight training and provides guidelines for setting up your own weight training program.

BENEFITS OF MUSCULAR STRENGTH AND ENDURANCE

Enhanced muscular strength and endurance can lead to improvements in the areas of performance, injury prevention, body composition, self-image, and lifetime muscle and bone health.

Improved Performance of Physical Activities

A person with a moderate-to-high level of muscular strength and endurance can perform everyday tasks—such as climbing stairs and carrying books or groceries—with ease. Muscular strength and endurance are also important in recreational activities: People with poor muscle strength tire more easily and are less effective in activities like hiking, skiing, and playing tennis. Increased strength can enhance your enjoyment of recreational sports by making it possible to achieve high levels of performance and to handle advanced techniques.

Injury Prevention

Increased muscle strength provides protection against injury because it helps people maintain good posture and appropriate body mechanics when carrying out everyday activities like walking, lifting, and carrying. Strong muscles in the abdomen, hips, low back, and legs support the back in proper alignment and help prevent low-back pain, which afflicts over 85% of all Americans at some time in their lives. (Prevention of low-back pain is discussed in greater detail in Chapter 5.) Training for muscular strength also makes the **tendons, ligaments,** and joint surfaces stronger and less susceptible to injury.

Improved Body Composition

As Chapter 2 explained, healthy body composition means that the body has a high proportion of lean body mass (primarily composed of muscle) and a relatively small proportion of fat. Strength training improves body composition by increasing muscle mass, thereby tipping the body composition ratio toward lean body mass and away from fat.

Building muscle mass through strength training also helps with losing fat because metabolic rate is directly proportional to lean body mass: The more muscle mass, the higher the metabolic rate. A high metabolic rate means that a nutritionally sound diet will not lead to an increase in body fat.

The combination of diet and weight training causes fat loss, not necessarily weight loss. Because muscle is denser (heavier) than fat, a fitness program often leads to a loss of inches but not weight. And reducing body fat, not body weight, is the most important outcome for wellness.

Enhanced Self-Image

Weight training leads to an enhanced self-image by providing stronger, firmer-looking muscles and a toned, healthy-looking body. Men tend to build larger, stronger, more shapely muscles. Women tend to lose inches, increase strength, and develop greater muscle definition. The larger muscles in men combine with high levels of the hormone **testosterone,** the principal androgen, for a strong tissue-building effect; see the box "Gender Differences in Muscular Strength."

Because weight training provides measurable objectives (pounds lifted, repetitions accomplished), a person can easily recognize improved performance, leading to improved confidence. It's especially satisfying to work on improving one's personal record.

Improved Muscle and Bone Health with Aging

Research has shown that good muscle strength helps people live longer and healthier lives. A lifelong program of

TERMS

tendon A tough band of fibrous tissue that connects a muscle to a bone or other body part and transmits the force exerted by the muscle.

ligament A tough band of tissue that connects the ends of bones to other bones or supports organs in place.

testosterone The principal male hormone, responsible for the development of secondary sex characteristics and important in the increase of muscle size.

osteoporosis A condition in which the bones become extremely thin and brittle.

repetitions maximum (RM) The maximum amount of resistance that can be moved a specified number of times; 1 RM is the maximum weight that can be lifted once.

repetitions The number of times an exercise is performed during one set.

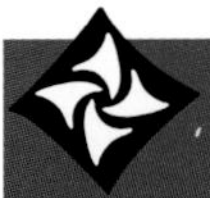

DIMENSIONS OF DIVERSITY

Gender Differences in Muscular Strength

Men are generally stronger than women because they typically have larger bodies overall and larger muscles. But when strength is expressed per unit of cross-sectional area of muscle tissue, men are only 1–2% stronger than women in the upper body and about equal to women in the lower body. (Men have a larger proportion of muscle tissue in the upper body, so it's easier for them to build upper-body strength than it is for women.) Individual muscle fibers are larger in men, but the metabolism of cells within those fibers is the same in both sexes.

Two factors that help explain these disparities between the sexes are androgen levels and the speed of nervous control of muscle. Androgens are naturally occurring male hormones that are responsible for the development of secondary sex characteristics (facial hair, deep voice, and so forth). Androgens also promote the growth of muscle tissue. Androgen levels are about 6–10 times higher in men than in women, so men tend to have larger muscles. Also, because the male nervous system can activate muscles faster, men tend to have more power.

Some women are concerned that they will develop large muscles from weight training. Most studies show that women do not develop big muscles, but the evidence of top women body builders suggests that they can. Some of these women may have taken drugs to increase their muscle size, but many muscular women have not. Evidence suggests, though, that it is difficult for women to gain a large amount of muscle without training intensely over many years.

The bottom line is that both men and women can increase strength through weight training. Women may not be able to lift as much weight as men, but pound for pound of muscle, they have nearly the same capacity to gain strength as men. The lifetime wellness benefits of strength training are available to everyone.

Source: Adapted from Fahey, T. D., and G. Hutchinson. 1992. *Weight Training for Women.* Mountain View, Calif.: Mayfield.

regular strength training prevents muscle and nervous degeneration that can compromise the quality of life and increase the risk of hip fractures and other potentially life-threatening injuries. After age 30, people begin to lose muscle mass. At first they may notice that they can't play sports as well as they could in high school. After more years of inactivity and strength loss, people may have trouble performing even the simple movements of daily life—getting out of a bathtub or automobile, walking up a flight of stairs, or doing yard work. Poor strength makes it much more likely that a person will be injured during the course of everyday activities.

As a person ages, motor nerves can become disconnected from the portion of muscle they control. Muscle physiologists estimate that by age 70, 15% of the motor nerves in most people are no longer connected to muscle tissue. Aging and inactivity also cause muscles to become slower and therefore less able to perform quick, powerful movements. Strength training helps maintain motor nerve connections and the quickness of muscles.

Bone loss, a condition called **osteoporosis,** is common in people over age 55, particularly postmenopausal women. Osteoporosis leads to fractures that can be life-threatening. Hormonal changes from aging account for much of the bone loss that occurs, but lack of bone stress due to inactivity is a contributing factor. Recent research indicates that strength training can lessen bone loss even if it is taken up later in life. (Strategies for preventing osteoporosis are described in greater detail in Chapter 8.)

ASSESSING MUSCULAR STRENGTH AND ENDURANCE

Muscular strength and muscular endurance are distinct but related components of fitness. Muscular strength, the maximum amount of force a muscle can produce in a single effort, is usually assessed by measuring the maximum amount of weight a person can lift one time. This single maximal movement is referred to as one **repetition maximum (RM).** You can assess the strength of your major muscle groups by taking the one-repetition maximum tests for the bench press and the leg press. Refer to Lab 4-1 for guidelines on taking these tests. Grip strength is a reasonably good predictor of the strength of many major muscle groups in the body. Instructions for assessing grip strength using a dynamometer are also included in Lab 4-1. For more accurate results, avoid any strenuous weight training for 48 hours beforehand.

Muscular endurance is the ability of a muscle to exert a submaximal force repeatedly or continuously over time. This ability depends on muscular strength because a certain amount of strength is required for any muscle movement. Muscular endurance is usually assessed by counting the maximum number of **repetitions** of a muscular contraction a person can do (such as in push-ups) or the maximum amount of time a person can hold a muscular contraction (such as in the flexed arm hang). You can test the muscular endurance of major muscle groups in your

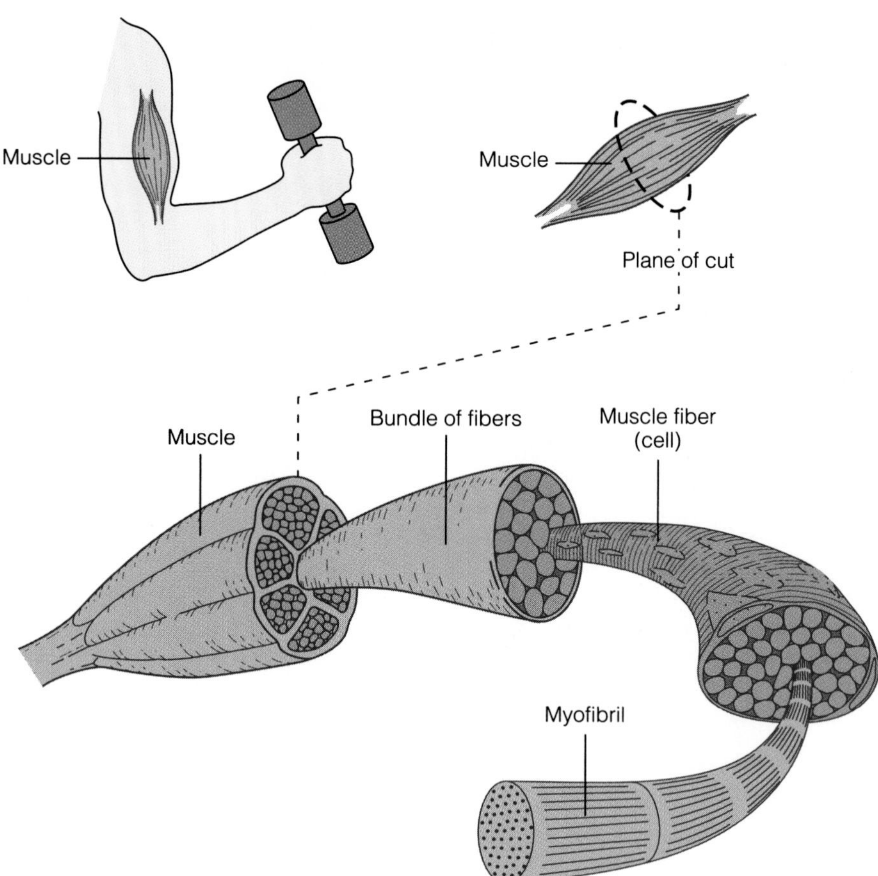

Figure 4-1 ***Components of skeletal muscle tissue.***

body by taking the 60-second sit-up test or the curl-up test and the push-up test. Refer to Lab 4-1 for complete instructions on taking these assessment tests.

Record your results and your fitness ratings from the assessment tests in Lab 4-1. If the results show that improvement is needed, a weight training program will enable you to make rapid gains in muscular strength and endurance.

FUNDAMENTALS OF WEIGHT TRAINING

Weight training develops muscular strength and endurance in the same way that endurance exercise develops cardiovascular fitness: When the muscles are stressed by a greater load than they are used to, they adapt and improve their function. The type of adaptation that occurs depends on the type of stress applied.

Physiological Effects of Weight Training

Muscles move the body and enable it to exert force because they move the skeleton. When a muscle contracts (shortens), it moves a bone by pulling on the tendon that attaches the muscle to the bone. Muscles consist of individual muscle cells, or **muscle fibers,** connected in bundles (Figure 4-1). A single muscle is made up of many bundles of muscle fibers and is covered by layers of connective tissue that hold the fibers together. Muscle fibers, in turn, are made up of smaller units called **myofibrils.** (When your muscles are given the signal to contract, protein filaments within the myofibrils slide across one another, causing the muscle fiber to shorten.) Weight training causes the size of individual muscle fibers to increase by increasing the number of myofibrils. Larger muscle fibers mean a larger and stronger muscle. The development of large muscle fibers is called **hypertrophy.**

Muscle fibers are classified as fast-twitch or slow-twitch fibers according to their strength, speed of contraction, and energy source. **Slow-twitch fibers** are relatively fatigue-resistant, but they don't contract as rapidly or strongly as fast-twitch fibers. The energy system that fuels slow-twitch fibers is **aerobic**, meaning it requires oxygen. **Fast-twitch fibers** contract more rapidly and forcefully than slow-twitch fibers but fatigue more quickly. Although oxygen is important in the energy system that fuels fast-twitch fibers, they rely more on **anaerobic** metabolism, which occurs in the absence of oxygen, than do slow-twitch fibers.

Most muscles contain a mixture of slow-twitch and fast-twitch fibers. The type of fibers that acts depends on the type of work required. Endurance activities like jogging tend to use slow-twitch fibers, while strength and **power** activities like sprinting use fast-twitch fibers.

TABLE 4-1 Physiological Changes and Benefits from Weight Training

Change	Benefits
Increased muscle mass*	Increased muscular strength Improved body composition Higher rate of metabolism Toned, healthy-looking muscles
Increased utilization of motor units during muscle contractions	Increased muscular strength and power
Improved coordination of motor units	Increased muscular strength and power
Increased strength of tendons, ligaments, and bones	Lower risk of injury to these tissues
Increased storage of fuel in muscles	Increased resistance to muscle fatigue
Increased size of fast-twitch muscle fibers (from a high-resistance program)	Increased muscular strength and power
Increased size of slow-twitch muscle fibers (from a high-repetition program)	Increased muscular endurance
Increased blood supply to muscles (from a high-repetition program)	Increased delivery of oxygen and nutrients Increased elimination of wastes

*Due to genetic and hormonal differences, men will build more muscle mass than women.

Weight training can increase the size and strength of both fast-twitch and slow-twitch fibers.

To exert force, the body recruits one or more motor units to contract. A **motor unit** is made up of a nerve connected to a number of muscle fibers. When a motor nerve calls upon its fibers to contract, all the fibers contract to their maximum capacity. The number of motor units recruited depends on the amount of strength required: When a person picks up a small weight, he or she uses fewer motor units than when picking up a large weight. Training with weights improves the body's ability to recruit motor units—a phenomenon called muscle learning—which increases strength even before muscle size increases.

In summary, weight training increases muscle strength because it increases the size of muscle fibers and improves the body's ability to call upon motor units to exert force. The physiological changes and benefits that result from weight training are summarized in Table 4-1.

Types of Weight Training Exercises

Weight training exercises are generally classified as isometric or isotonic. Each involves a different way of using and strengthening muscles.

Isometric Exercise Also called static exercise, **isometric** exercise involves applying force without movement. To perform an isometric exercise, a person can use an immovable object like a wall to provide resistance, or the individual can just tighten a muscle while remaining still (for example, tightening the abdominal muscles while sitting at a desk). In isometrics, the muscle contracts, but there is no movement.

Isometric exercises aren't as widely used as isotonic exercises because they develop strength only at or near the joint angle where they are performed, not throughout a joint's entire range of motion. However, isometric exercises are useful in strengthening muscles after an injury or surgery, when movement of the affected joint could delay healing. Isometrics are also used to overcome weak points in an individual's range of motion. Isometrically strengthening a muscle at its weakest point will allow more weight to be lifted with that muscle during isotonic exercise.

TERMS

muscle fiber A single muscle cell, usually classified according to strength, speed of contraction, and energy source.

myofibrils Protein structures that make up muscle fibers.

hypertrophy An increase in the size of a muscle fiber, usually stimulated by muscular overload.

slow-twitch fibers Red muscle fibers that are fatigue-resistant but have a slow contraction speed and a lower capacity for tension; usually recruited for endurance activities.

aerobic Dependent on the presence of oxygen.

fast-twitch fibers White muscle fibers that contract rapidly and forcefully but fatigue quickly; usually recruited for actions requiring strength and power.

anaerobic Occurring in the absence of oxygen.

power The ability to exert force rapidly.

motor unit A motor nerve (one that initiates movement) connected to one or more muscle fibers.

isometric The application of force without movement; also called static.

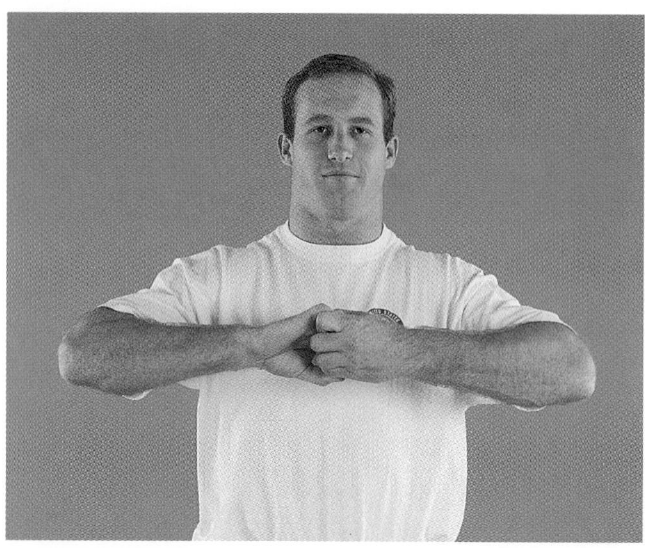

This isometric exercise for the arms and upper back involves locking the hands together and attempting to pull them apart. Isometric contractions involve force without movement.

Isotonic Exercise **Isotonic** (or dynamic) exercise involves applying force with movement. Isotonic exercises are the most popular type of exercises for increasing muscle strength and seem to be most valuable for developing strength that can be transferred to other forms of physical activity. They can be performed with weight machines, free weights, or a person's own body weight (as in sit-ups or push-ups).

There are two kinds of isotonic muscle contractions: concentric and eccentric. A **concentric muscle contraction** occurs when the muscle applies force as it shortens. An **eccentric muscle contraction** occurs when the muscle applies force as it lengthens. For example, in an arm curl, the biceps muscle works concentrically as the weight is raised toward the shoulder and eccentrically as the weight is lowered.

Two of the most common isotonic exercise techniques are constant resistance exercise and variable resistance exercise. Constant resistance exercise uses a constant load (weight) throughout a joint's entire range of motion. Training with free weights is a form of constant resistance exercise. A problem with this technique is that, because of differences in leverage, there are points in a joint's range of motion where the muscle controlling the movement is stronger and points where it is weaker. The amount of weight a person can lift is limited by the weakest point in the range. In variable resistance exercise, the load is changed to provide maximum load throughout the entire range of motion. This form of exercise uses machines that place more stress on muscles at the end of the range of motion, where a person has better leverage and is capable of exerting more force. The Nautilus pullover machine is an example of a variable resistance exercise machine.

Four other kinds of isotonic techniques, used mainly by athletes for training and rehabilitation, are eccentric loading, plyometrics, speed loading, and isokinetics.

- **Eccentric loading** involves placing a load on a muscle as it lengthens. The muscle contracts eccentrically in order to control the weight. Eccentric loading is practiced during most types of resistance training. For example, you are performing an eccentric movement as you lower the weight to your chest during a bench press in preparation for the active movement.
- **Plyometrics** is the sudden eccentric loading and stretching of muscles followed by a forceful concentric contraction. An example would be jumping from a bench to the ground and then jumping back onto the bench. This type of exercise is used to develop explosive strength.
- **Speed loading** involves moving a weight as rapidly as possible in an attempt to approach the speeds used in movements like throwing a softball or sprinting. In the bench press, for example, speed loading might involve doing five repetitions as fast as possible using a weight that is half the maximum load you can lift. You can gauge your progress by timing how fast you can perform the repetitions.
- **Isokinetic** exercise involves exerting force at a constant speed against an equal force exerted by a special strength training machine. The isokinetic machine provides variable resistance at different points in the joint's range of motion, matching the effort applied by the individual, while keeping the speed of the movement constant. In other words, the force exerted by the individual at any point in the range of motion is resisted by an equal force from the isokinetic machine. Isokinetic exercise is used primarily in the rehabilitation of athletic injuries.

Comparing the Different Types of Exercise Isometric exercises require no equipment, so they can be done virtually anywhere and any time. They build strength rapidly and are useful for rehabilitating injured joints. On the other hand, they have to be performed at several different angles for each joint because improvement is specific to each angle. Isotonic exercises can be performed without equipment (calisthenics) or with equipment (weight lifting). They are excellent for building strength and endurance, and they tend to build strength through a joint's full range of motion. They would not be appropriate for rehabilitating a joint, however. Isokinetic exercises are excellent for building strength and endurance, but the equipment is expensive and less commonly available than other kinds of weight machines.

Most people develop muscular strength and endurance using isotonic exercises. Ultimately, the type of exercise a person chooses depends on individual goals, preferences, and access to equipment.

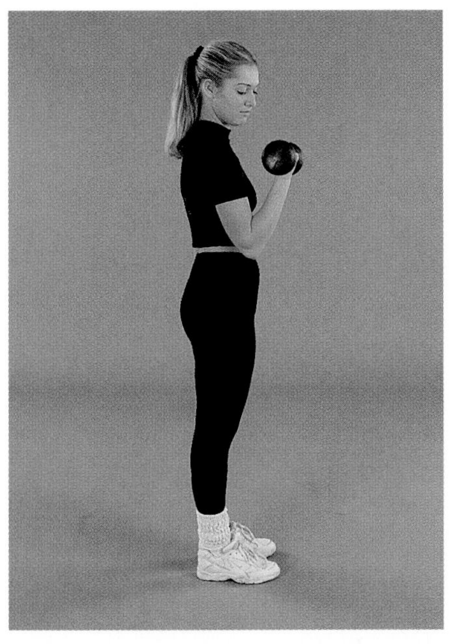

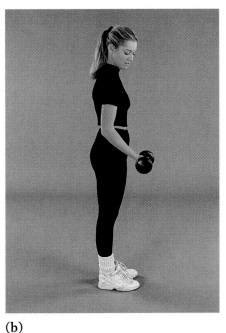

(a)

(b)

(**a**) A concentric contraction: The biceps muscle shortens as the arm lifts a weight toward the shoulder. (**b**) An eccentric contraction: The biceps muscle lengthens as the arm lowers a weight toward the thigh.

CREATING A SUCCESSFUL WEIGHT TRAINING PROGRAM

To get the most out of your weight training program, you must design it to achieve maximum fitness benefits with a low risk of injury. Before you begin, seriously consider the type and amount of training that's right for you.

Choosing Equipment: Weight Machines Versus Free Weights

Your muscles will get stronger if you make them work against a resistance. Resistance can be provided by free weights, by your own body weight, or by sophisticated exercise machines. Weight machines are preferred by many people because they are safe, convenient, and easy to use. You just set the resistance (usually by placing a pin in the weight stack), sit down at the machine, and start working. Machines make it easy to isolate and work specific muscles. You don't need a **spotter,** someone who stands by to assist when free weights are being used, and you don't have to worry about a weight crashing down on you.

Free weights require more care, balance, and coordination to use, but they strengthen your body in ways that are more adaptable to real life. Free weights are also better for developing explosive strength for sports.

Unless you are training seriously for a sport that requires a great deal of strength, training on machines is probably safer, more convenient, and just as effective as training with free weights. However, you can increase strength either way; which to use is a matter of personal preference. The box "Exercise Machines Versus Free Weights" (p. 72) can help you make a decision.

Selecting Exercises

A complete weight training program works all the major muscle groups. It usually takes about 8–10 different exercises to get a complete workout. For overall fitness, you need to include exercises for your neck, upper back, shoulders, arms, chest, abdomen, lower back, thighs, buttocks, and calves. If you are also training for a particular sport, include exercises to strengthen the muscles important for optimal performance *and* the muscles most likely to be injured. A program of weight training exercises for general fitness is presented later in this chapter.

Resistance

The amount of weight (resistance) you lift in weight training exercises is equivalent to intensity in cardiorespiratory

TERMS

isotonic The application of force resulting in movement; also called dynamic.

concentric muscle contraction An isotonic contraction in which the muscle gets shorter as it contracts.

eccentric muscle contraction An isotonic contraction in which the muscle lengthens as it contracts.

eccentric loading Loading the muscle while it is lengthening; sometimes called "negatives."

plyometrics Rapid stretching of a muscle group that is undergoing eccentric stress (the muscle is exerting force while it lengthens), followed by a rapid concentric contraction.

speed loading Moving a load as rapidly as possible.

isokinetic The application of force at a constant speed against an equal force.

spotter A person who assists with a weight training exercise done with free weights.

A CLOSER LOOK

Exercise Machines Versus Free Weights

Exercise Machines

Advantages

- Safe
- Convenient
- Don't require spotters
- Provide variable resistance
- Require less skill
- Make it easy to move from one exercise to the next
- Allow easy isolation of individual muscle groups

Disadvantages

- Limited availability
- Inappropriate for performing dynamic movements
- Allow a limited number of exercises

Free Weights

Advantages

- Allow dynamic movements
- Allow the user to develop control of the weights
- Allow a greater variety of exercises
- Widely available
- Truer to real-life situations; strength transfers to daily activities

Disadvantages

- Not as safe
- Require spotters
- Require more skill
- Cause more blisters and calluses

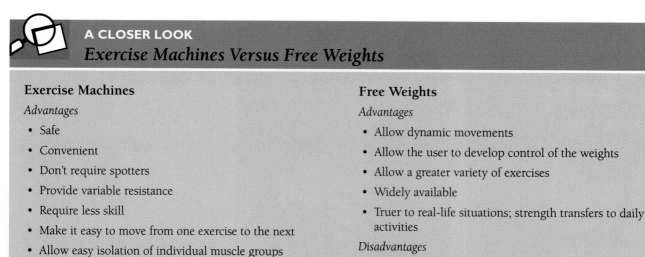

endurance training. It determines the way your body will adapt to weight training and how quickly these adaptations will occur. Choose weights based on your current level of muscular fitness and your fitness goals. To build strength rapidly, you should lift weights as heavy as 80% of your maximum capacity (1 RM). If you're more interested in building endurance, choose a lighter weight, perhaps 40–60% of 1 RM. For example, if your maximum capacity for the leg press is 160 pounds, you might choose a weight of 130 pounds to build strength and a weight of 80 pounds to build endurance. For a general fitness program to develop both strength and endurance, choose a weight in the middle of this range, perhaps 70% of 1 RM.

Because it can be tedious and time-consuming to continually reassess your maximum capacity for each exercise, you might find it easier to choose a weight based on the number of repetitions of an exercise you can perform with a given resistance.

Repetitions and Sets

In order to improve fitness, you must do enough repetitions of each exercise to fatigue your muscles. The number of repetitions needed to cause fatigue depends on the amount of resistance: the heavier the weight, the fewer repetitions to reach fatigue. In general, a heavy weight and a low number of repetitions (1–5) build strength, while a light weight and a high number of repetitions (20–25) build endurance (Figure 4-2). For a general fitness program to build both strength and endurance, try to do 8–12 repetitions of each exercise. (A few exercises, such as abdominal crunches and calf raises, may require more.) Choose a weight heavy enough to fatigue your muscles but light enough for you to complete the repetitions.

In weight training, a **set** refers to a group of repetitions of an exercise followed by a rest period. You should perform a minimum of one set of each exercise; doing three sets of each exercise is recommended for optimal fitness gains. The rest period after each set allows your muscles to work at a high enough intensity during the next set to increase fitness. The length of the rest interval between sets depends on the goal of your weight training program. If your goal is to develop a combination of strength and endurance for fitness and wellness, then rest 1–3 minutes between sets. However, if your goal is to develop maximum strength (and you are lifting heavier loads), rest 3–5 minutes between sets. You can save time in your workouts if you alternate sets of different exercises. Each muscle group can rest between sets while you work on other muscles.

The Warm-Up and Cool-Down

As with cardiorespiratory endurance exercise, you should warm up before every weight training session and cool down afterward. You should do both a general warm-up—several minutes of walking or easy jogging—and a warm-up for the weight training exercises you plan to perform. For example, if you plan to do three sets of 10 repetitions of bench presses with 125 pounds, you might do one set of 10 repetitions with 50 pounds as a warm-up. Do similar warm-up exercises for each exercise in your program.

To cool down after weight training, relax for 5–10 minutes after your workout. Including a period of post-exercise stretching may help prevent muscle soreness;

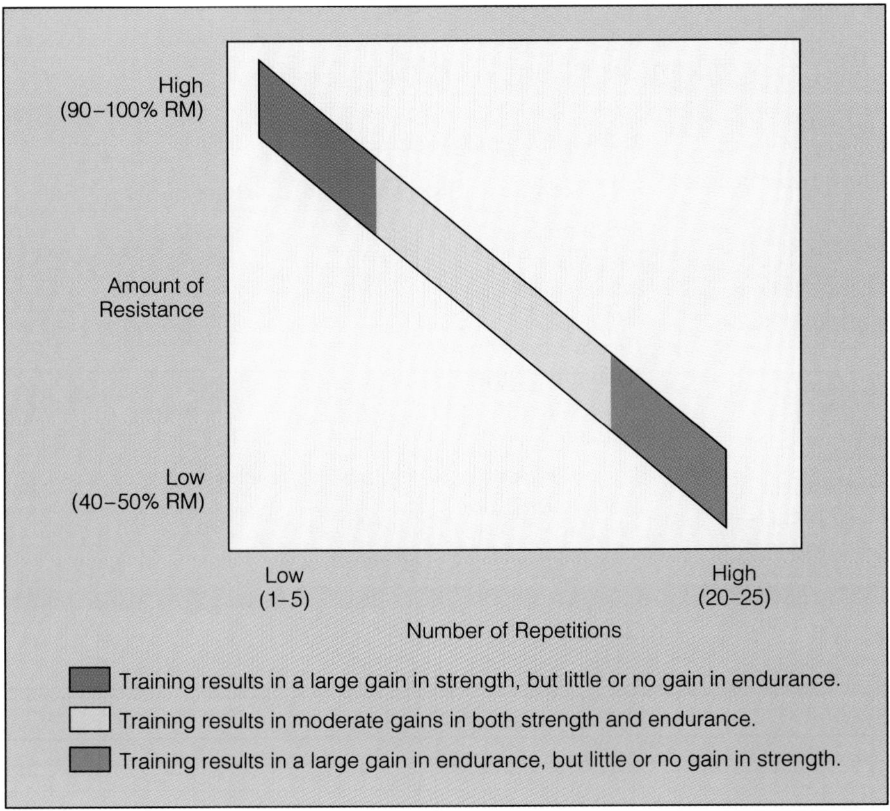
High
(90–100% RM)
Amount of
Resistance
Low
(40–50% RM)
Low
(1–5)
High
(20–25)
Number of Repetitions
Training results in a large gain in strength, but little or no gain in endurance.
Training results in moderate gains in both strength and endurance.
Training results in a large gain in endurance, but little or no gain in strength.

Figure 4-2 ***Training for strength versus training for resistance.***

warmed-up muscles and joints make this a particularly good time to work on flexibility.

Frequency of Exercise

You should train with weights 2–4 days per week. Two days per week is the minimum needed to gain strength; 3 days per week is optimal for most people. Allow your muscles a day of rest between workouts; if you train too often, your muscles won't be able to work at a high enough intensity to improve their fitness, and soreness and injury are more likely to result. If you enjoy weight training and would like to train more often, try working different muscle groups on alternate days. For example, work your arms and upper body one day, your lower body the next day, and then return to upper-body exercises on the third day. Refer to the box "Sample Weight Training Program for General Fitness" (p. 74) for suggestions on beginning a program.

Making Progress

The first few weeks of weight training should be devoted to learning the exercises. You need to learn the movements, and your nervous system needs to practice communicating with your muscles so you can develop strength effectively. To start, choose a weight that you can move easily through 8–12 repetitions, and do only one set of each exercise. Gradually add weight and sets to your program over the first few weeks until you are doing three sets of 10 repetitions of each exercise.

As you progress, add weight when you can do more than 12 repetitions of an exercise. If adding weight means you can do only 7 or 8 repetitions, stay with that weight until you can again complete 12 repetitions per set. If you can do only 4–6 repetitions after adding weight, you've added too much and should take some off.

You can expect to improve rapidly during the first 6 weeks of training: a 10–30% increase in the amount of weight lifted. Gains will then come more slowly. Your rate of improvement will depend on how hard you work and your genetic disposition to improving from resistance exercise.

Your ultimate goal depends on you. If you are training for a sport that requires great strength, you must push yourself consistently to achieve high levels of strength. After you have achieved the level of strength and muscularity that you want, you can maintain your gains by training 2–3 days per week.

You can monitor the progress of your program by recording the amount of resistance and the number of repetitions and sets you perform on a workout card like the one shown in Figure 4-3 (p. 74).

TERMS

set A group of repetitions followed by a rest period.

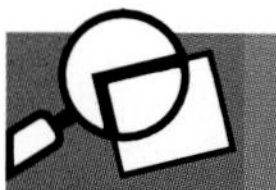

A CLOSER LOOK

A Sample Weight Training Program for General Fitness

Guidelines

Type of activity 8–10 weight training exercises that focus on major muscle groups

Frequency 2–4 days per week

Resistance Weights heavy enough to cause muscle fatigue when performed for the selected number of repetitions

Repetitions 8–12 of each exercise (one set)

Sets 1 (minimum) to 3 (recommended)

Sample Program

1. Warm-up (5–10 minutes): includes a general warm-up and a set of exercises using low resistance for each muscle group that will be trained during the workout.
2. Weight training exercises:

Exercise	Resistance (lb)	Repetitions	Sets
Bench press	60	10	3
Lat pulls	40	10	3
Lateral raises	5	10	3
Biceps curls	25	10	3
Triceps extensions	15	10	3
Abdominal curls	—	30	3
Leg presses	30	10	3
Calf raises	25	15	3

3. Cool-down (5–10 minutes): relax after each weight training session.

WORKOUT CARD FOR *Scott Peterson*

Exercise/Date		9/14	9/16	9/18	9/21	9/23	9/25	9/28	9/30	10/2	10/5	10/7	10/9	10/12	10/14	10/16									
Bench press	Wt.	70	70	70	75	75	75	80	80	80	90	90	95	105	105	110									
	Sets	1	2	3	3	3	3	3	3	3	3	3	3	3	3	3									
	Reps.	10	10	10	10	10	10	10	10	10	10	10	10	10	10	.10									
Lat pulls	Wt.	50	50	50	60	60	60	60	60	60	70	70	70	80	80	80									
	Sets	1	2	3	3	3	3	3	3	3	3	3	3	3	3	3									
	Reps.	10	10	10	10	10	10	10	10	10	10	10	10	10	10	10									
Lateral raises	Wt.	5	5	5	7.5	7.5	7.5	7.5	7.5	7.5	7.5	7.5	7.5	10	10	10									
	Sets	1	2	3	3	3	3	3	3	3	3	3	3	3	3	3									
	Reps.	10	10	10	10	10	10	10	10	10	10	10	10	10	10	10									
Biceps curls	Wt.	35	35	35	40	40	40	45	45	45	50	50	50	50	50	50									
	Sets	1	2	3	3	3	3	3	3	3	3	3	3	3	3	3									
	Reps.	10	10	10	10	10	10	10	10	10	10	10	10	10	10	10									
Triceps Extensions	Wt.	20	20	20	30	30	30	30	30	30	30	30	30	40	40	40									
	Sets	1	2	3	3	3	3	3	3	3	3	3	3	3	3	3									
	Reps.	10	10	10	10	10	10	10	10	10	10	10	10	10	10	10									
Abdominal curls	Wt.	–	–	–	–	–	–	–	–	–	–	–	–	–	–	–									
	Sets	1	2	3	3	3	3	3	3	3	3	3	3	3	3	3									
	Reps.	20	20	20	20	20	20	25	25	25	30	30	30	30	30	30									
Squats	Wt.	–	–	–	45	45	85	85	105	115	125	135	135	145	145	145									
	Sets	1	2	3	3	3	3	3	3	3	3	3	3	3	3	3									
	Reps.	10	10	10	10	10	10	10	10	10	10	10	10	10	10	10									
Calf raises	Wt.	–	–	–	45	45	85	85	105	115	125	135	135	145	145	145									
	Sets	1	2	2	3	3	3	3	3	3	3	3	3	3	3	3									
	Reps.	15	15	15	15	15	15	15	15	15	15	15	15	15	15	15									

Figure 4-3 ***A sample workout card.***

Weight Training Safety

Injuries do happen in weight training. Maximum physical effort, elaborate machinery, rapid movements, and heavy weights can combine to make the weight room a dangerous place if proper precautions aren't taken. To help ensure that your workouts are safe and productive, follow the guidelines in the box "Safe Weight Training" and the suggestions given below.

Use Proper Lifting Technique Every exercise has a proper technique that is important for obtaining maximum benefits and preventing injury. Your instructor or weight room attendant can help explain the specific techniques for performing different exercises and using different weight machines. Perform exercises smoothly and with good form. Lift or push the weight forcefully during the active phase of the lift, then lower it slowly with control. Perform all lifts through the full range of motion.

Use Spotters and Collars with Free Weights Spotters are necessary when an exercise has potential for danger: A weight that is out of control or falls can cause a serious injury. A spotter can assist you if you cannot complete a lift,

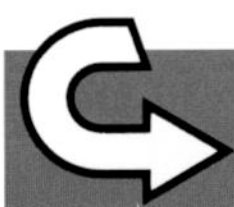

TACTICS AND TIPS
Safe Weight Training

- Lift weights from a stabilized body position.
- Be aware of what's going on around you. Stay away from other people when they're doing exercises. If you bump into someone, you could cause an accident or injury.
- Don't use defective equipment. Report any equipment malfunctions immediately.
- Protect your back by maintaining control of your spine (protect your spine from dangerous positions). Observe proper lifting techniques, and use a weight lifting belt when doing heavy lifts.
- Don't hold your breath while doing weight training exercises.
- Always warm up before training, and cool down afterward.
- Don't exercise if you're ill, injured, or overtrained.

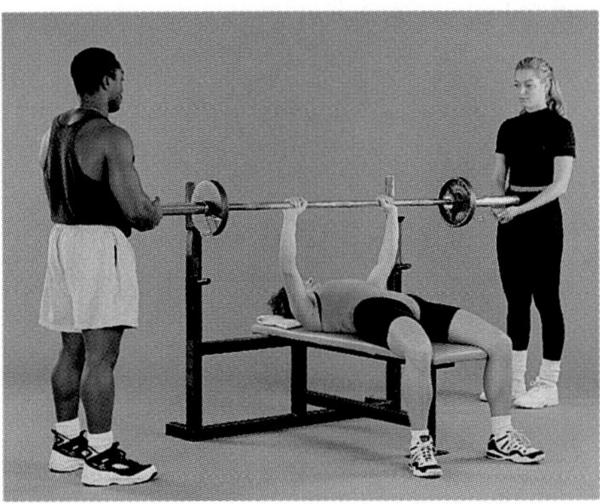

(a)

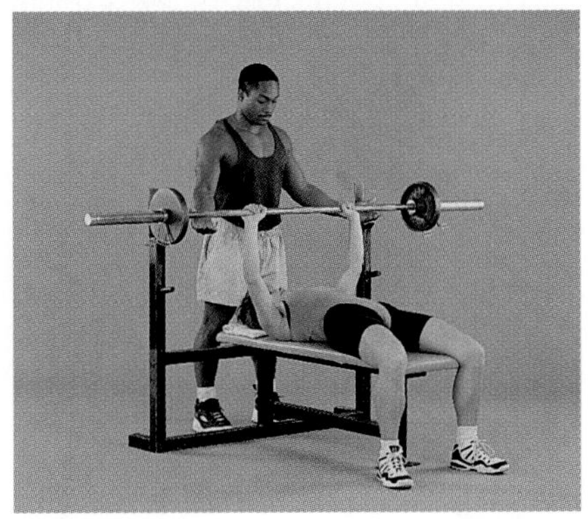

(b)

Spotters should always be present when a person trains with free weights. **(a)** If two spotters are used, one spotter should stand at each end of the barbell. **(b)** If one spotter is present, he or she should stand behind the lifter.

or if the weight tilts. A spotter can also help you move a weight into position before a lift and provide help or additional resistance during a lift. Spotting requires practice and coordination between the lifter and spotter(s).

Collars are devices that secure weights to a barbell or dumbbell. Although people lift weights without collars, doing so is dangerous. It is easy to lose your balance or to raise one side of the weight faster than the other. Without collars, the weights on one side of the bar will slip off, and the weights on the opposite side will crash to the floor.

Proper lifting technique for free weights also includes the following:

- Keep weights as close to your body as possible.
- Do most of your lifting with your legs. Keep your hips and buttocks tucked in.
- When you pick a weight up from the ground, keep your back straight and your head level or up. Don't bend at the waist with straight legs.
- Don't twist your body while lifting.
- Lift weights smoothly and slowly; don't jerk them. Control the weight through the entire range of motion.
- Don't bounce weights against your body during an exercise.
- Never hold your breath when you lift. Exhale when exerting the greatest force, and inhale when moving the weight into position for the active phase of the lift. (Holding your breath causes a decrease in blood returning to the heart and can make you become dizzy and faint.)
- Rest between lifts. (Fatigue hampers your ability to obtain maximum benefits from your program and is a prime cause of injury.) If your goal is to improve strength and endurance, rest 1–3 minutes between sets. When you are using more weight and are trying to maximize strength increases, rest 3–5 minutes between sets.
- When lifting barbells and dumbbells, wrap your thumbs around the bar when gripping it. You can easily drop the weight when using a "thumbless" grip.
- Gloves are not mandatory but may prevent calluses on your hands.
- When doing standing lifts, maintain a good posture so that you protect your back.
- Don't lift beyond the limits of your strength.

Use Common Sense When Exercising on Weight Machines Although notable for their safety, weight machines are not completely danger-free. The following strategies can help prevent injuries:

- Keep away from moving weight stacks. Pay attention when you're changing weights. Someone may jump

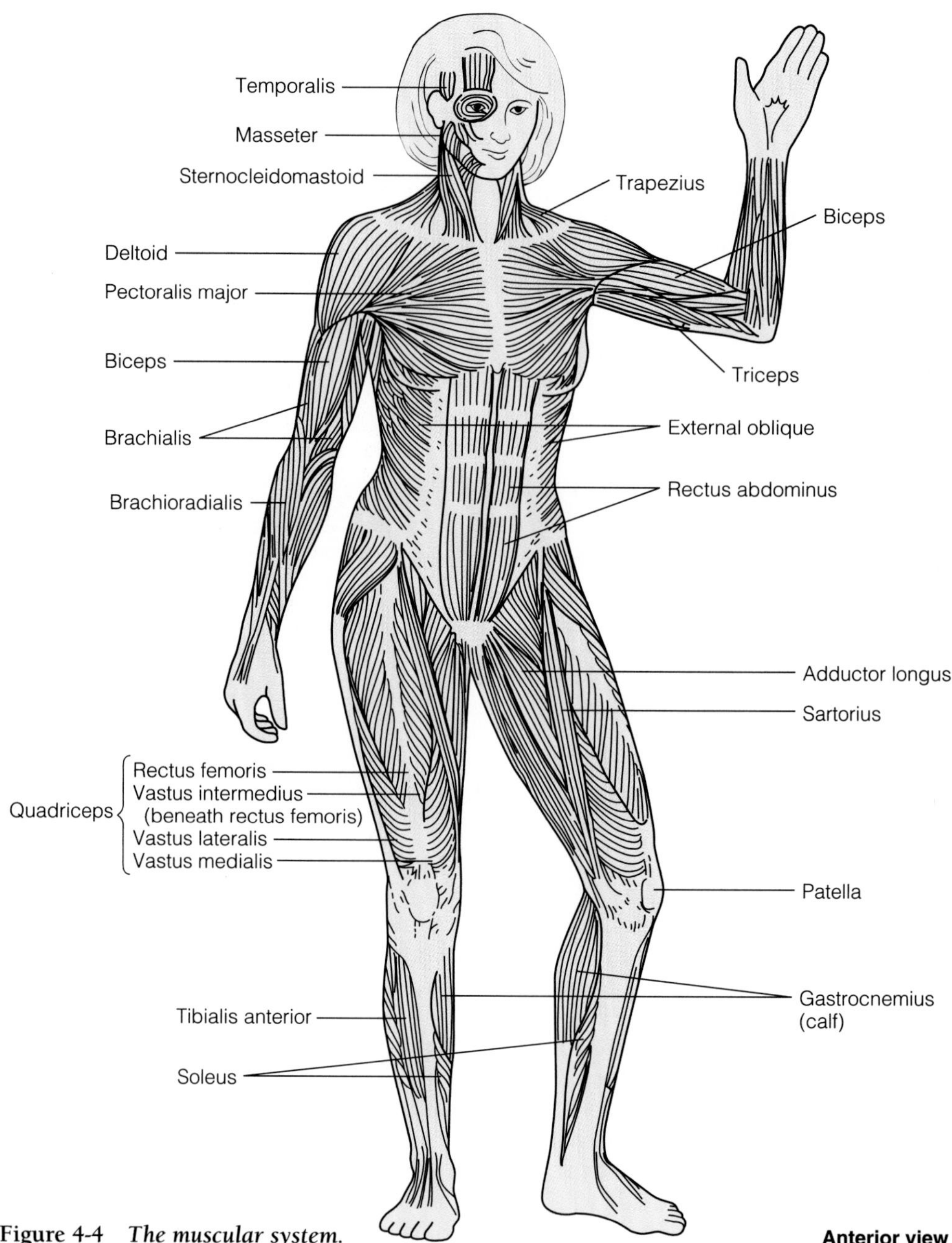

Figure 4-4 *The muscular system.*

on the machine ahead of you and begin an exercise while your fingers are close to the weight stack.

- Stay away from moving parts of the machine that could pinch your skin.
- Adjust each machine for your body so that you don't have to work in an awkward position. Lock everything in place before you begin.
- Beware of broken bolts, frayed cables, broken chains, or loose cushions that can give way and cause serious injury. If you notice a broken or frayed part, tell an instructor immediately.
- Make sure the machines are clean. Dirty vinyl is a breeding ground for germs that can cause skin diseases. Carry a towel around with you and place it on the machine where you will sit or lie down.
- Be aware of what's happening around you. Talking between sets is a great way to relax and have fun, but inattention can lead to injury.

Be Alert for Injuries Report any obvious muscle or joint injuries to your instructor or physician, and stop exercising the affected area. Training with an injured joint or muscle can lead to a more serious injury. Make sure you get the necessary first aid. Even minor injuries heal faster if you use the R-I-C-E principle of treating injuries described in Chapter 3.

Consult a physician if you're having any unusual symptoms during exercise, or if you're uncertain whether weight training is a proper activity for you. Conditions such as heart disease and high blood pressure can be aggravated during weight training. Symptoms such as

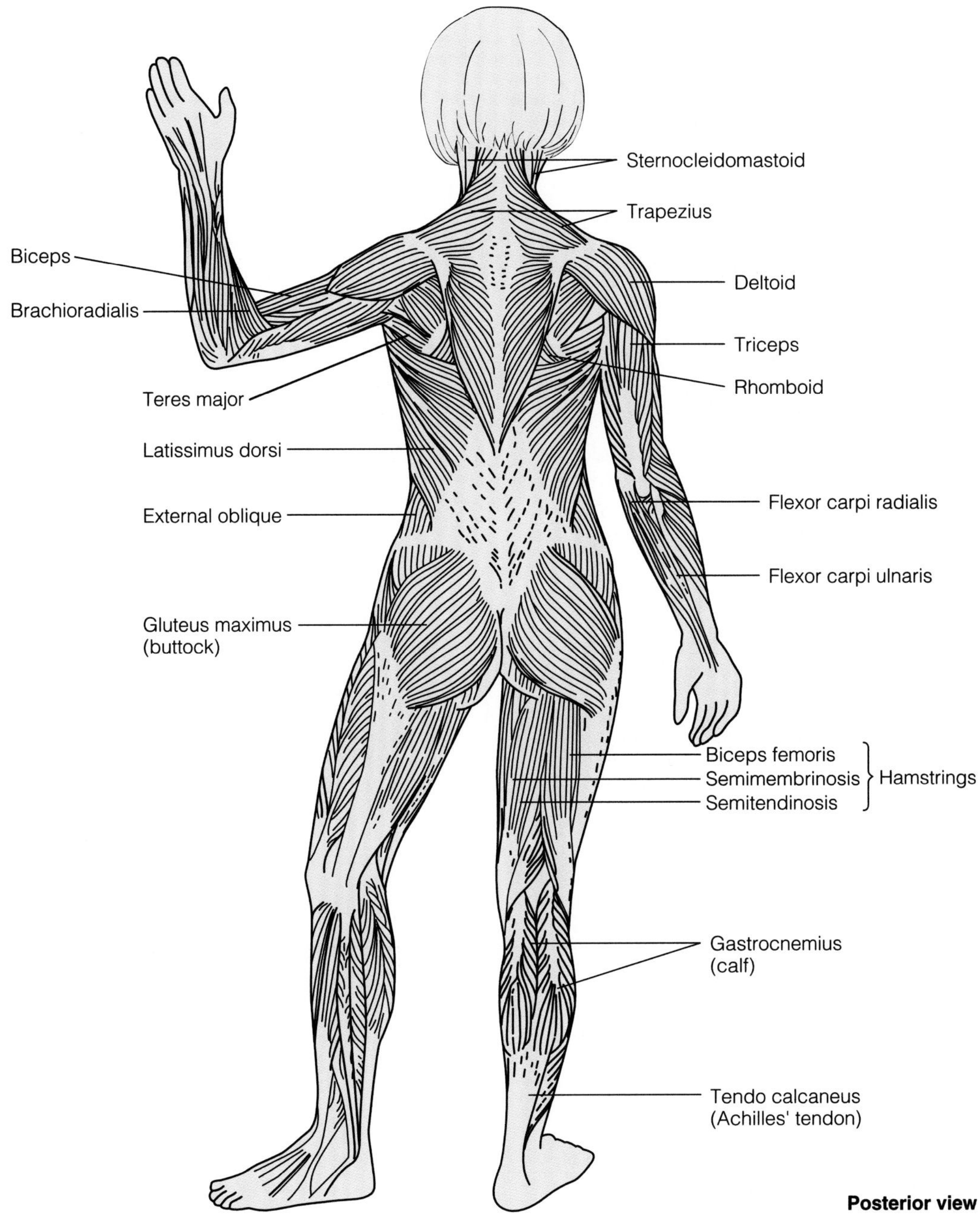

headaches, dizziness, labored breathing, numbness, visual disturbances, and chest, neck, or arm pains should be reported immediately.

Weight Training Exercises

A general book on fitness and wellness cannot include a detailed description of all weight training exercises. Here we present a basic program for developing muscular strength and endurance for general fitness using free weights and Nautilus weight machines. Instructions for each exercise are accompanied by photographs and a listing of the muscles being trained. (Figure 4-4 is a diagram of the muscular system.) Table 4-2 (p. 78) lists alternative and additional exercises that can be performed on Nautilus or Universal machines or with free weights. If you are interested in learning how to do these exercises, ask your instructor or coach for assistance.

If you want to develop strength for a particular activity, your program should contain exercises for general fitness, exercises for the muscle groups most important for the activity, and exercises for muscle groups most often injured. To create a weight training program for your favorite sport or activity, choose from among the exercises listed in Table 4-3 (p. 79), as well as from those listed in Table 4-2. Regardless of the goals of your program or the type of equipment you use, your program should be structured so that you obtain maximum results without risking injury. You should train 2–4 days per week, and each exercise session should contain a warm-up, a series of sets of 8–12 repetitions of 8–10 exercises, and a period of rest.

TABLE 4-2 Weight Training Exercises for Machines and Free Weights

Body Part	Nautilus	Universal Gym	Free Weights
Neck	4-way neck	Neck conditioning station	Neck harness Manual exercises
Trapezius ("Traps")	Overhead press Lateral raise Reverse pullover Compound row Shoulder shrug Rowing back	Shoulder press Shoulder shrug Upright row Bent-over row Rip-up Front raise Pull-up	Overhead press Lateral raise Shoulder shrug Power clean Upright row
Deltoids	Lateral raise Overhead press Reverse pullover Double chest 10° chest 50° chest Seated dip Bench press Compound row Rotary shoulder	Bench press Shoulder shrug Shoulder press Upright row Rip-up Front raise Pull-up	Raise Bench press Shoulder press Upright row Pull-up
Biceps	Biceps curl Lat pull	Biceps curl Lat pull	Biceps curl Lat pull Pull-up
Triceps	Triceps extension Seated dip Triceps exten. (lat machine) Bench press Overhead press	French curl Dip Triceps exten. (lat machine) Bench press Seated press	French curl Dip Triceps exten. (lat machine) Bench press Military press
Latissimus dorsi ("Lats")	Pullover Behind neck Torso arm Lat pull Seated dip Compound row	Pull-up Lat pull Bent-over row Pull-over Dip	Pull-up Pull-over Dip Bent-over row Lat pull
Abdominals	Abdominal Rotary torso	Hip flexor Leg raise Crunch Sit-up Side-bend	Hip flexor Leg raise Crunch Sit-up Side-bend Isometric tightener
Lower back	Lower back	Back extension Back leg raise	Back extension Good-morning
Thigh and buttocks	Leg press Leg extension Leg curl Hip adductor Hip abductor	Leg press Leg curls Leg extension Adductor kick Abductor kick Back hip extension	Squat Leg press Leg extension Leg curl Power clean Snatch Dead lift
Calf	Seated calf Heel raise: multiexercise	Calf press	Heel raise

TABLE 4-3 Weight Training for Sports and Activities

Emphasize these body parts when training for the following sports and activities. While it is important to condition all major muscle groups, specific activities require extra conditioning in specific muscles.

Activity or Sport	Neck	Shoulders	Chest	Arms	Forearms	Upper Back	Lower Back	Abdominals	Thighs	Hamstrings	Calves
Badminton		✔	✔	✔	✔	✔			✔	✔	✔
Basketball		✔	✔	✔		✔	✔	✔	✔	✔	✔
Billiards		✔		✔	✔	✔	✔				
Canoeing		✔	✔	✔	✔	✔	✔	✔			
Cycling		✔		✔	✔	✔	✔	✔	✔	✔	✔
Dancing							✔	✔	✔	✔	✔
Fishing				✔	✔				✔	✔	✔
Field hockey		✔	✔	✔	✔	✔	✔	✔	✔	✔	✔
Football	✔	✔	✔	✔	✔	✔	✔	✔	✔	✔	✔
Golf		✔		✔	✔	✔	✔	✔	✔	✔	✔
Gymnastics	✔	✔	✔	✔	✔	✔	✔	✔	✔	✔	✔
Jogging		✔		✔		✔	✔	✔	✔	✔	✔
Rock climbing		✔	✔	✔	✔	✔	✔	✔	✔	✔	✔
Skating, in-line		✔				✔	✔	✔	✔	✔	✔
Skiing, cross-country		✔		✔	✔	✔	✔	✔	✔	✔	✔
Skiing, downhill		✔		✔		✔	✔	✔	✔	✔	✔
Scuba diving				✔		✔	✔	✔	✔	✔	
Squash		✔	✔	✔	✔	✔	✔	✔	✔	✔	✔
Swimming		✔	✔	✔	✔	✔	✔	✔	✔	✔	
Table tennis		✔		✔	✔	✔			✔	✔	✔
Tennis		✔	✔	✔	✔	✔	✔	✔	✔	✔	✔
Triathlon		✔	✔	✔	✔	✔	✔	✔	✔	✔	✔
Volleyball		✔	✔	✔	✔	✔	✔	✔	✔	✔	✔
Water skiing	✔	✔		✔	✔	✔	✔	✔	✔	✔	✔
Wrestling	✔	✔	✔	✔	✔	✔	✔	✔	✔	✔	✔

WEIGHT TRAINING EXERCISES
Free Weights

EXERCISE 1

Neck Flexion and Lateral Flexion (Isometric Exercises)

Muscles developed: Sternocleidomastoids, scaleni

Instructions:

Flexion: **(a)** Place your hand on your forehead with fingertips pointed up. Using the muscles at the back of your neck, press your head forward and resist the pressure with the palm of your hand.

Lateral flexion: **(b)** Place your hand on the right side of your face, fingertips pointed up. Using the muscles on the left side of your neck, press your head to the right and resist the pressure with the palm of your hand. Repeat on the left side.

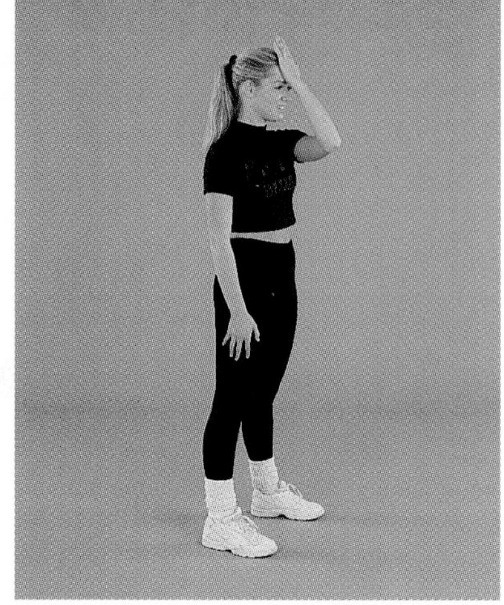

(a)

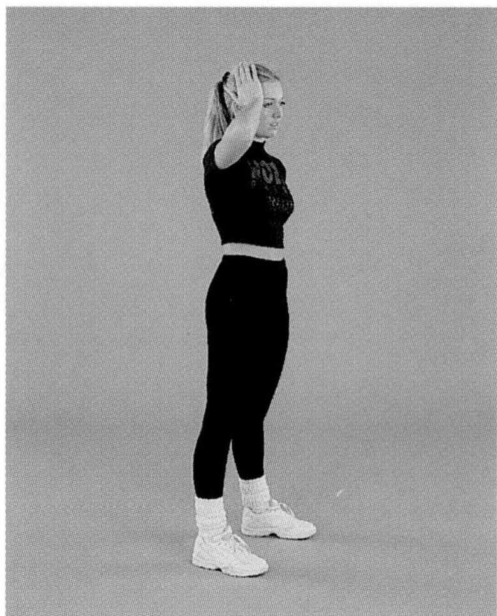

(b)

EXERCISE 2

Lat Pull

Muscles developed: Latissimus dorsi, biceps

Instructions: Begin in a seated or kneeling position, depending on the type of lat machine and the manufacturer's instructions. **(a)** Grasp the bar of the machine with arms fully extended. **(b)** Slowly pull the weight down until it reaches the back of your neck. Slowly return to the starting position.

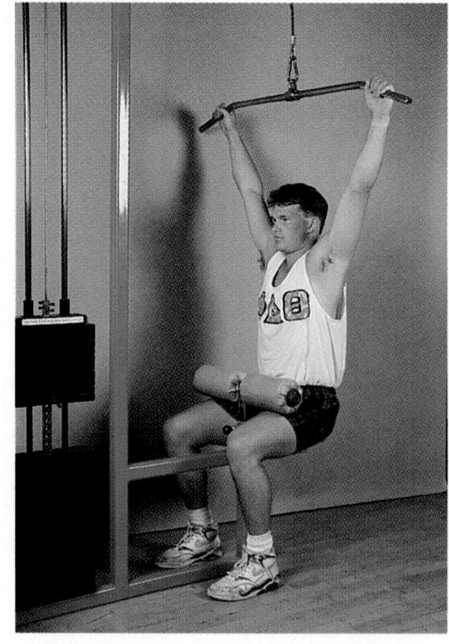

(a)

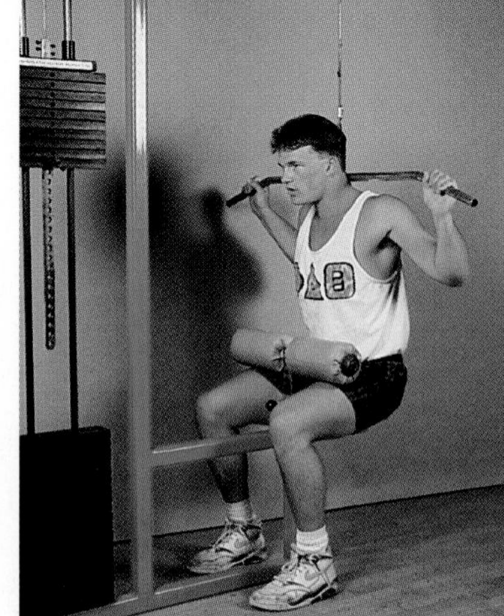

(b)

EXERCISE 3

Shoulder Press (Overhead or Military Press)

Muscles developed: Deltoids, triceps, trapezius

Instructions: This exercise can be done standing or seated, with dumbbells or barbells. The shoulder press begins with the weight at your chest, preferably on a rack. **(a)** Grasp the weight with your palms facing away from you. **(b)** Push the weight overhead until your arms are extended. Then return to the starting position (weight at chest). Be careful not to arch your back excessively.

If you are a more advanced weight trainer, you can "clean" the weight to your chest (lift it from the floor to your chest). The clean should be attempted only after instruction from a knowledgeable coach; otherwise, it can lead to injury.

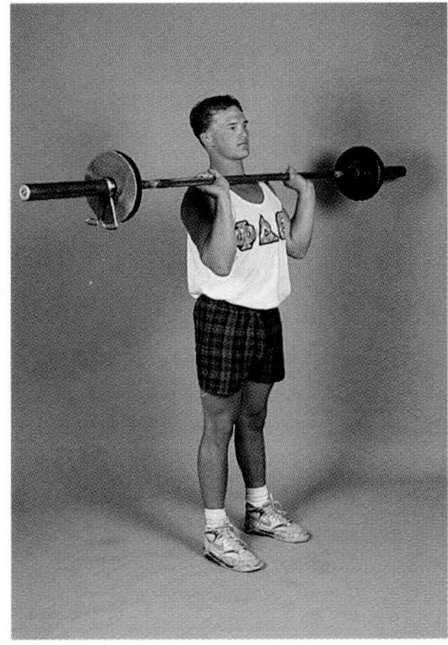

(a)

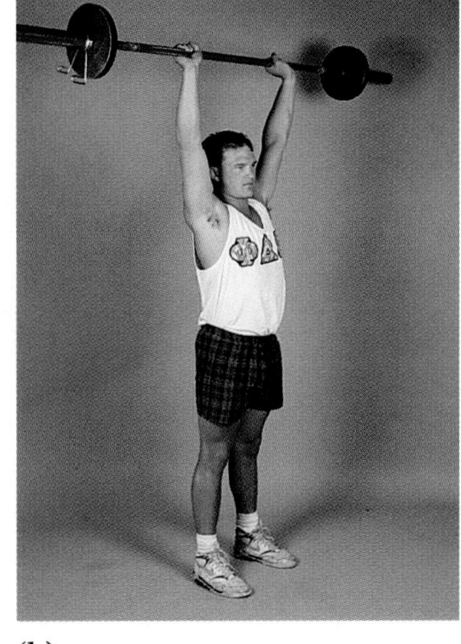

(b)

EXERCISE 4

Curl

Muscles developed: Biceps, brachialis

Instructions: **(a)** From a standing position, grasp the bar with your palms upward and your hands shoulder-width apart. **(b)** Keeping your upper body rigid, flex (bend) your elbows until the bar reaches a level slightly below the collarbone. Return the bar to the starting position.

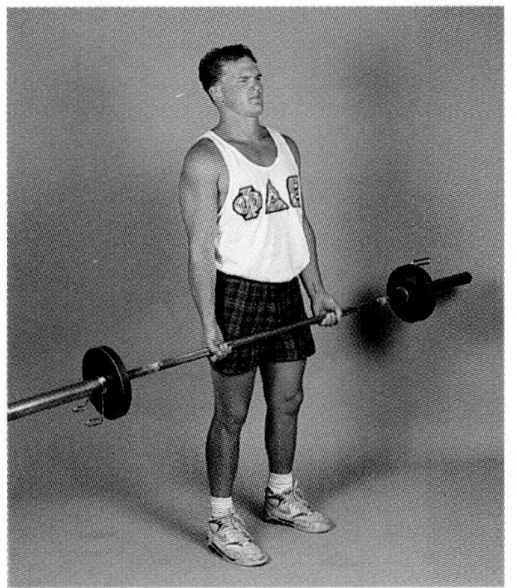

(a)

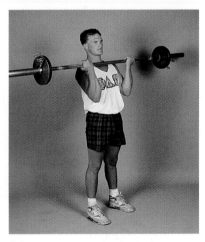

(b)

Although a spotter does not appear in these demonstration photographs, spotters should always be used in any exercises with free weights.

EXERCISE 5

Bench Press

Muscles developed: Pectoralis major, triceps, deltoids

Instructions: **(a)** Lying on a bench on your back with your feet on the floor, grasp the bar with palms upward and hands shoulder-width apart. **(b)** Lower the bar to your chest. Then return it to the starting position. The bar should follow an elliptical path, during which the weight moves from a low point at the chest to a high point over the chin. If your back arches too much, try doing this exercise with your feet on the bench.

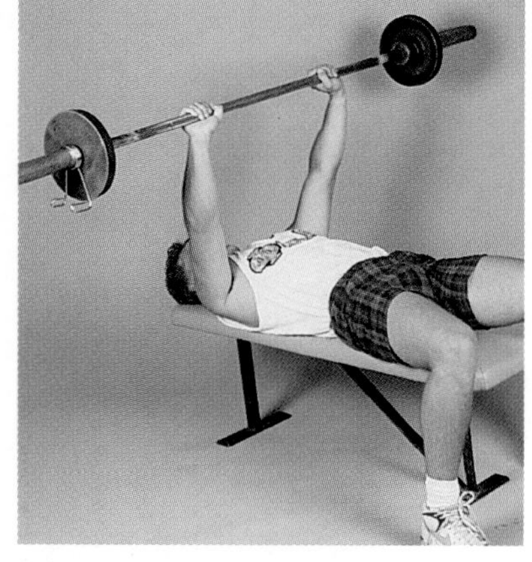
(a)

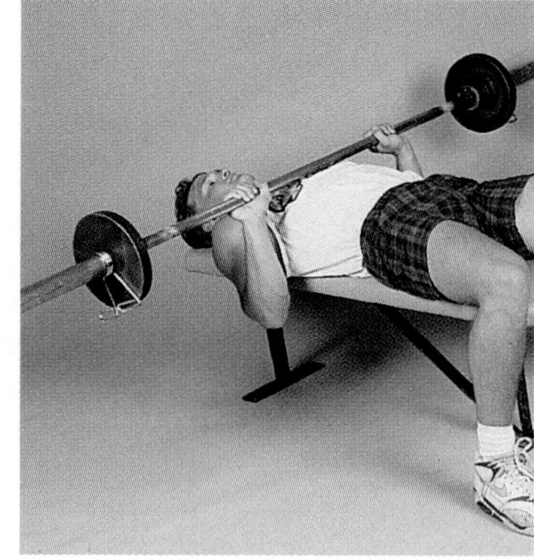
(b)

EXERCISE 6

Curl-Up or Crunch

Muscles developed: Rectus abdominis, obliques

Instructions: **(a)** Lie on your back on the floor with your arms folded across your chest and your feet on the floor or on a bench. **(b)** Curl your trunk up and forward by raising your head and shoulders from the ground. Lower to the starting position.

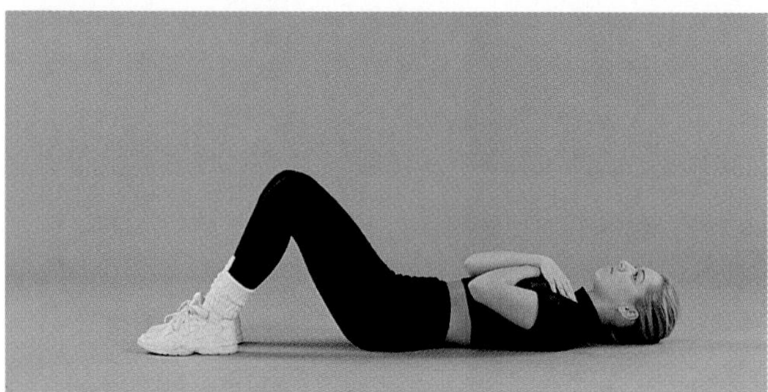
(a)

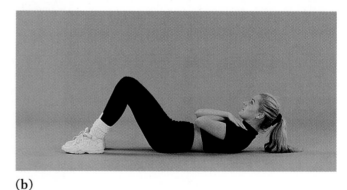

(b)

EXERCISE 7

Squat

Muscles developed: Quadriceps, gluteus maximus, hamstrings, gastrocnemius

Instructions: Stand with feet shoulder-width apart and toes pointed slightly outward. **(a)** Rest the bar on the back of your shoulders, holding it there with hands facing forward. **(b)** Keeping your head up and lower back straight, squat down until your thighs are almost parallel with the floor. Drive upward toward the starting position, keeping your back in a fixed position throughout the exercise.

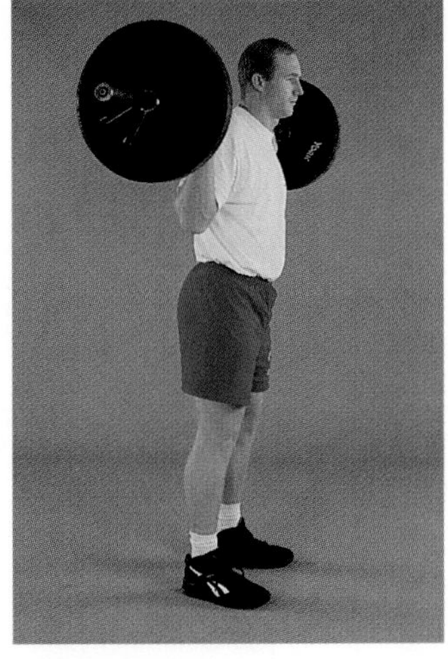
(a)

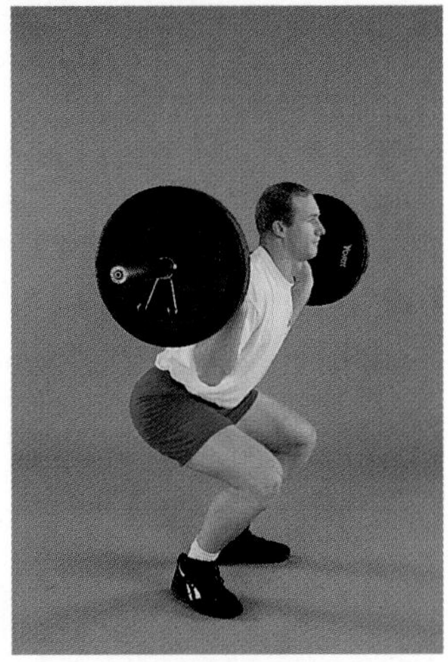
(b)

EXERCISE 8

Toe Raise

Muscles developed: Gastrocnemius, soleus

Instructions: Stand with feet shoulder-width apart and toes pointed straight ahead. **(a)** Rest the bar on the back of your shoulders, holding it there with hands facing forward. **(b)** Press down with your toes while lifting your heels. Return to the starting position.

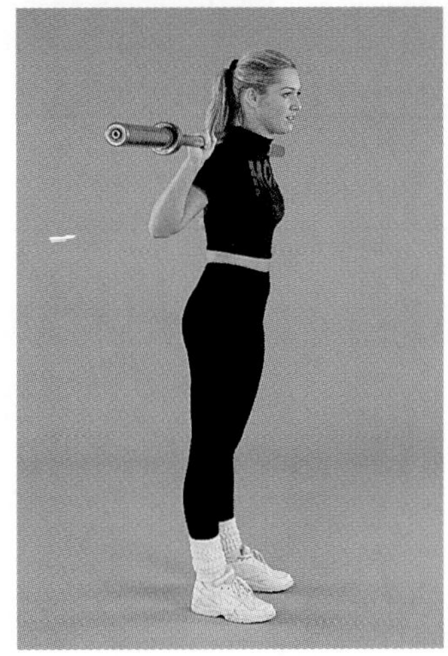
(a)

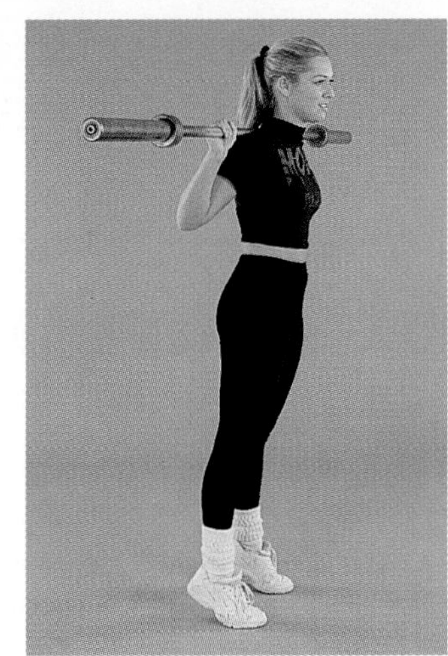
(b)

Although a spotter does not appear in these demonstration photographs, spotters should always be used in any exercises with free weights.

Nautilus Weight Machines

EXERCISE 1

Four-Way Neck Machine

Muscles developed: sternocleidomastoids, scaleni (flexion and lateral flexion); splenius capitus, splenius cervicus, trapezius (extension)

Instructions:

Flexion: **(a)** Adjust the seat so the front of your forehead rests in the center of the two pads. Bend your head forward as far as possible, using your neck muscles, then return to the starting position.

Lateral flexion: **(b)** Adjust the seat so the side of your head rests in the center of the two pads. Bend your head sideways toward your shoulder as far as possible, then return to the starting position. Perform the exercise for both the right and left sides of your head.

Extension: **(c)** Adjust the seat so the back of your head rests in the center of the two pads. Bend your head backward as far as possible, then return to the starting position.

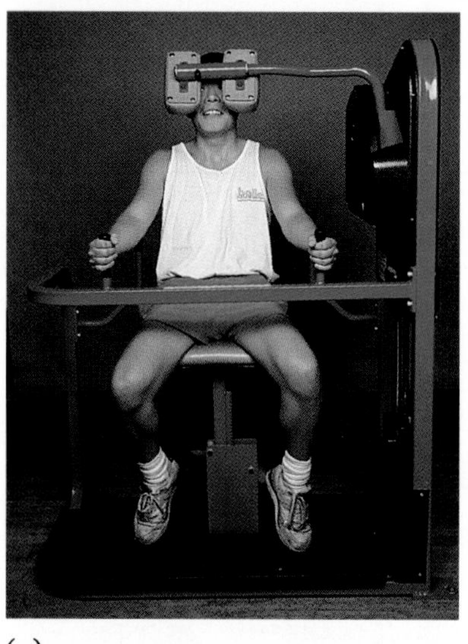

(a)

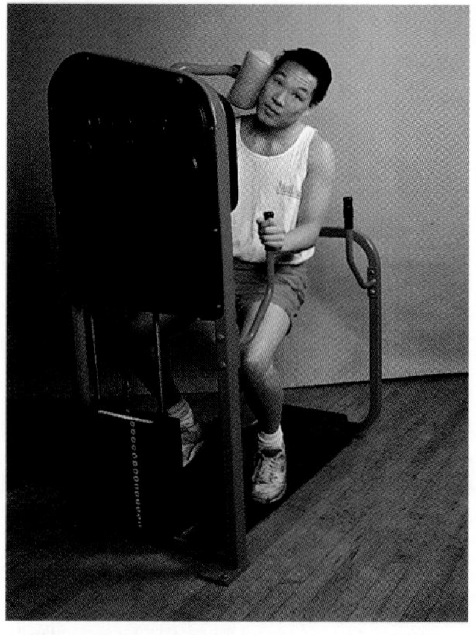

(b)

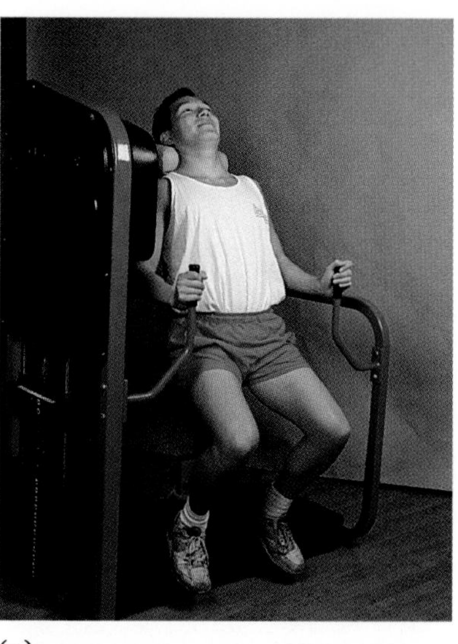

(c)

EXERCISE 2

Pullover

Muscles developed: Latissimus dorsi, pectoralis major and minor, triceps, abdominals

Instructions: Adjust the seat so your shoulders are aligned with the cams. Push down on the foot pads with your feet to bring the bar forward until you can place your elbows on the pads. Rest your hands lightly on the bar. If possible, place your feet flat on the floor. **(a)** To get into the starting position, let your arms go backward as far as possible. **(b)** Pull your elbows forward until the bar almost touches your abdomen. Return to the starting position.

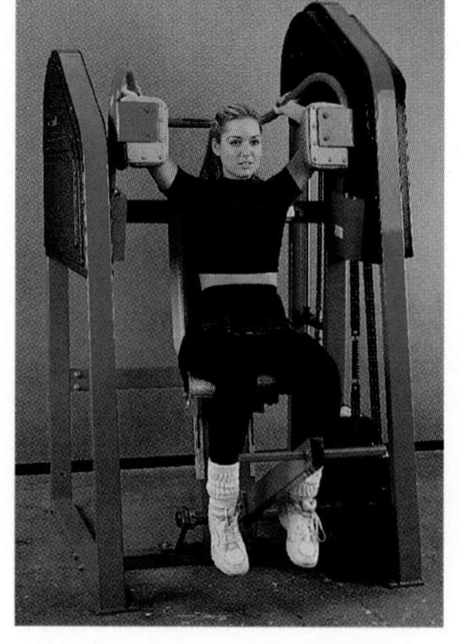

(a)

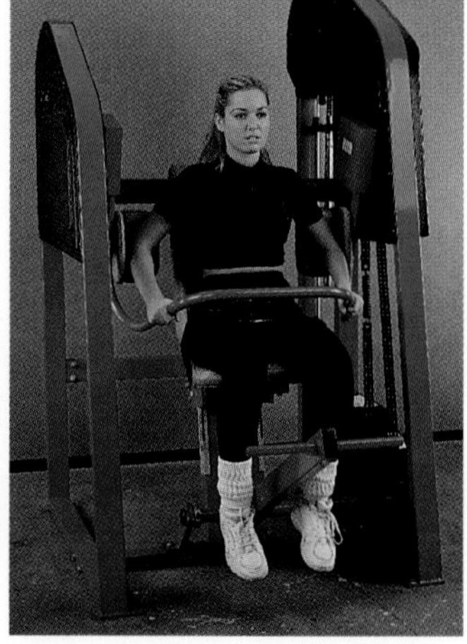

(b)

EXERCISE 3

Overhead Press (Shoulder Press)

Muscles developed: Deltoids, trapezius, triceps

Instructions: Adjust the seat so the two bars are slightly above your shoulders. **(a)** Sit down, facing away from the machine, and grasp the bars with your palms facing inward. **(b)** Press the weight upward until your arms are extended. Return to the starting position.

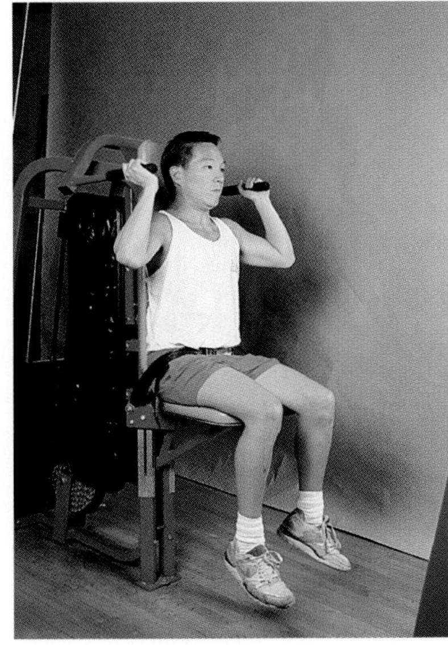

(a)

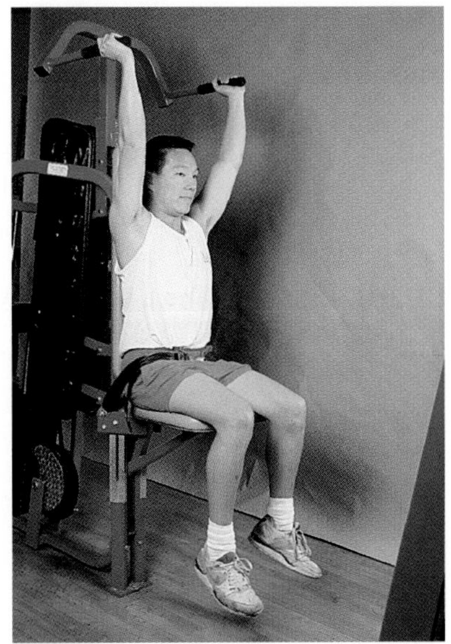

(b)

EXERCISE 4

Lateral Raise

Muscles developed: Deltoids, trapezius

Instructions: **(a)** Adjust the seat so the pads rest just above your elbows when your upper arms are at your sides, your elbows are bent, and your forearms are parallel to the floor. **(b)** Lightly grasp the handles and push outward and up with your arms until the pads are shoulder height. Lead with your elbows rather than trying to lift the bars with your hands. Return to the starting position.

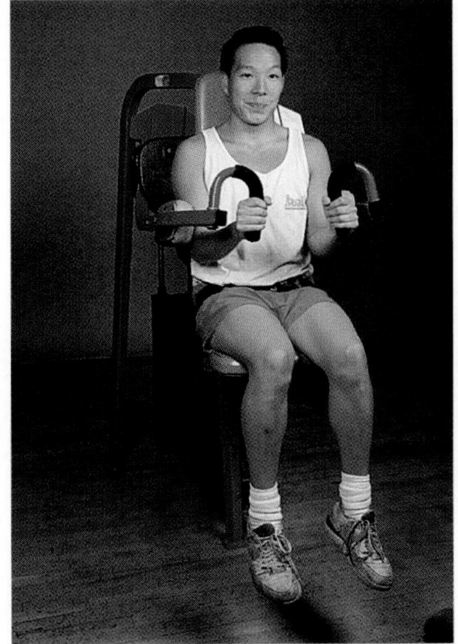

(a)

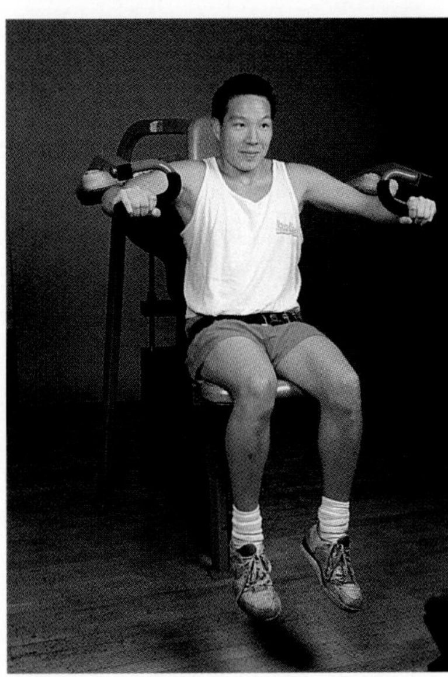

(b)

EXERCISE 5

Multitriceps

Muscles developed: Triceps

Instructions: Adjust the seat so your elbows are slightly lower than your shoulders when you sit down. **(a)** Place your elbows on the support cushions and your forearms on the bar pads. **(b)** Extend your elbows as much as possible. Return to the starting position.

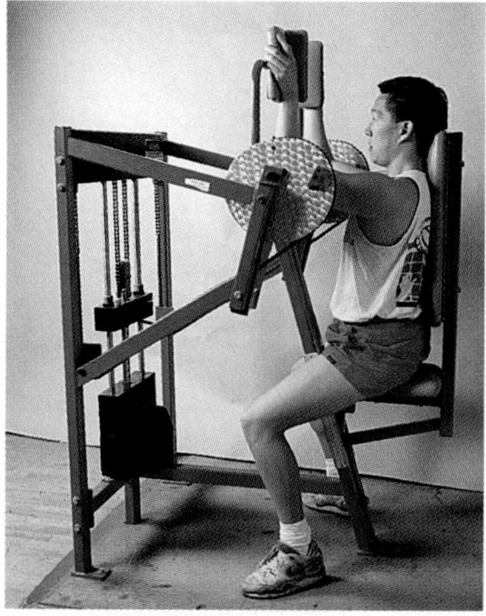

(a)

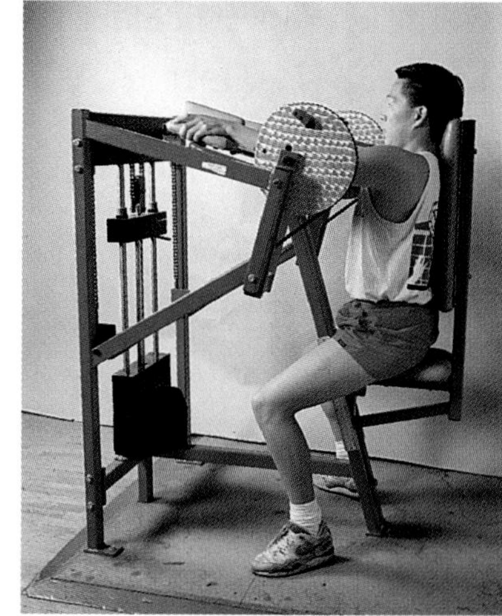

(b)

EXERCISE 6

Bench Press

Muscles developed: Pectoralis major, anterior deltoids, triceps

Instructions: Lie on the bench so the tops of the handles are aligned with the tops of your armpits. Place your feet flat on the floor; if they don't reach, place them on the bench. **(a)** Grasp the handles with your palms facing away from you. **(b)** Push the bars until your arms are fully extended. Return to the starting position.

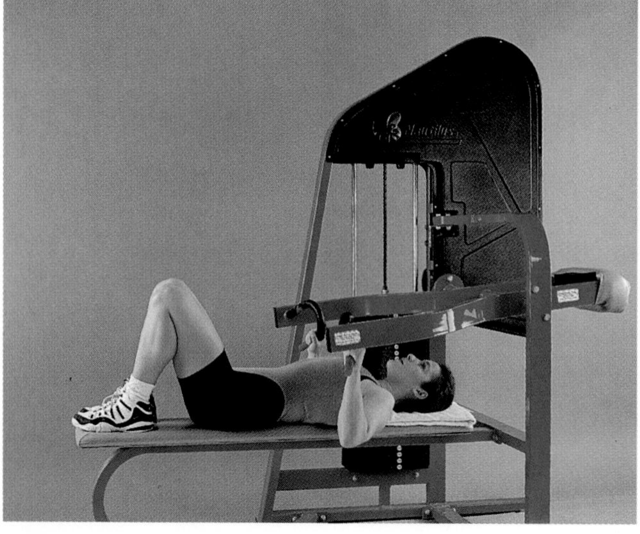

(a)

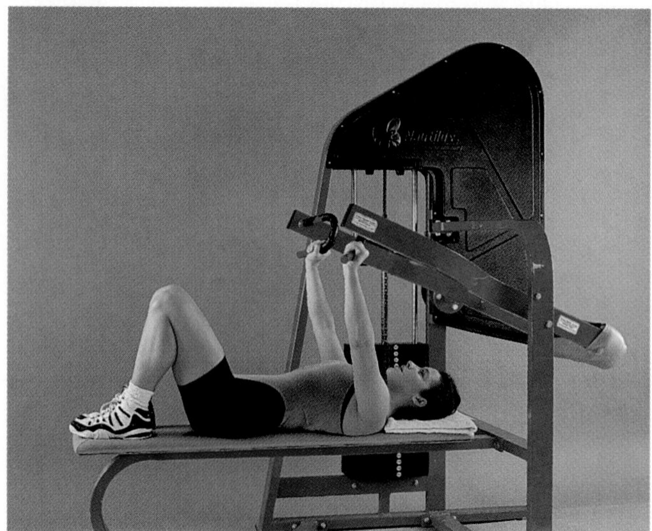

(b)

EXERCISE 7

Abdominal Curl

Muscles developed: Rectus abdominis, internal and external obliques

Instructions: **(a)** Adjust the seat so the machine rotates at the level of your navel, the pad rests on your upper chest, and your feet can rest comfortably on the floor. **(b)** Move your trunk forward as far as possible. Return to the starting position.

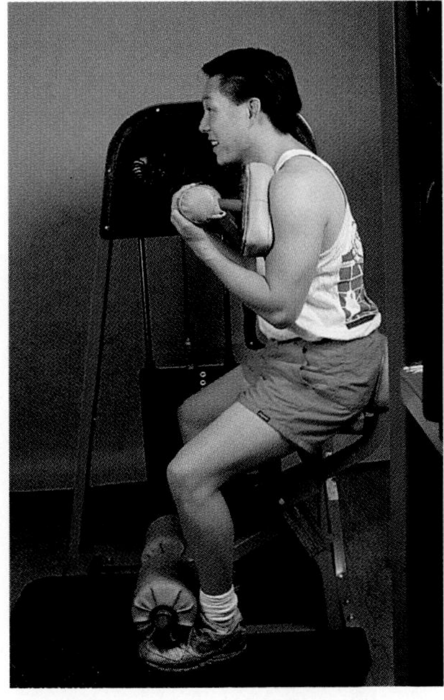

(a)

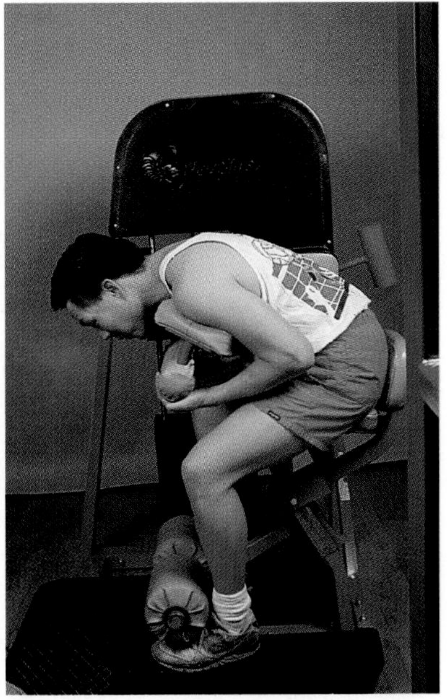

(b)

EXERCISE 8

Low-Back Machine (Back Extensions)

Muscles developed: Erector spinae, quadratus lumborum

Instructions: **(a)** Sit on the seat with your upper legs under the thigh-support pads, your back on the back roller pad, and your feet on the platform. **(b)** Extend backward until your back is straight. Return to the starting position. Try to keep your spine rigid during the exercise.

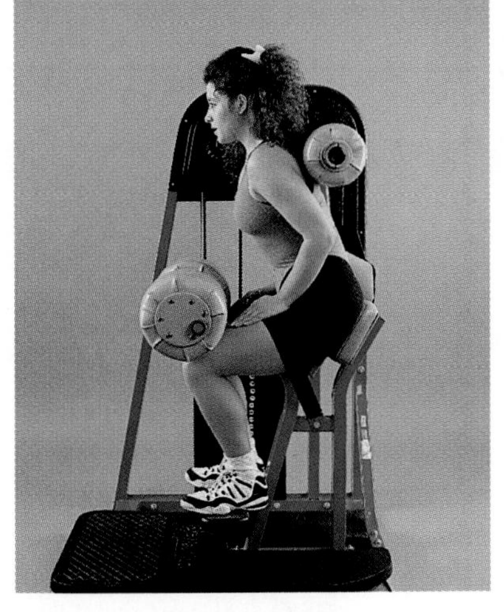

(a)

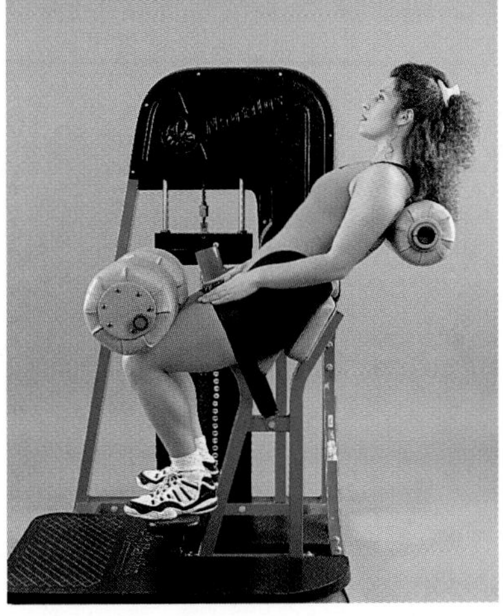

(b)

EXERCISE 9

Leg Press

Muscles developed: Gluteus maximus, quadriceps, hamstrings

Instructions: **(a)** Adjust the seat so your knees are bent at a 90-degree angle. **(b)** Sit with your hands on the side handles, your feet on the pedals, and your legs fully extended. **(c)** From this position, bend your right leg 90 degrees, then forcefully extend it. Repeat with your left leg. Alternate between right and left legs.

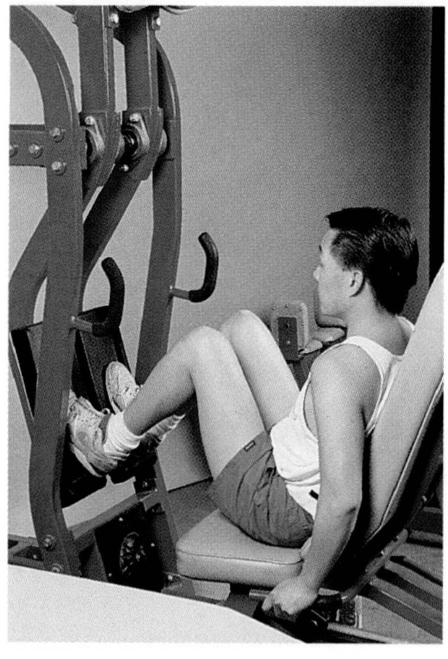

(a)

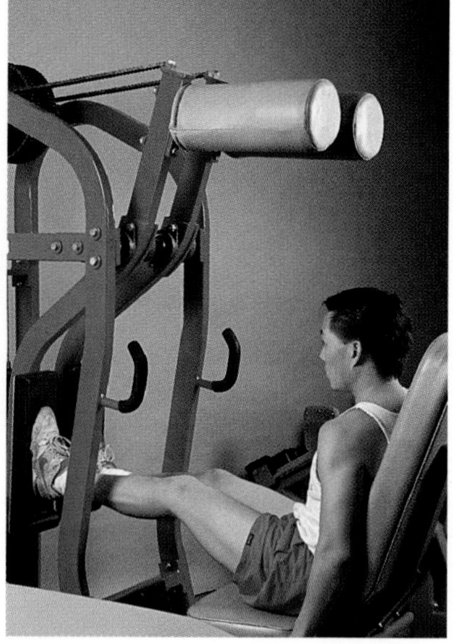

(b)

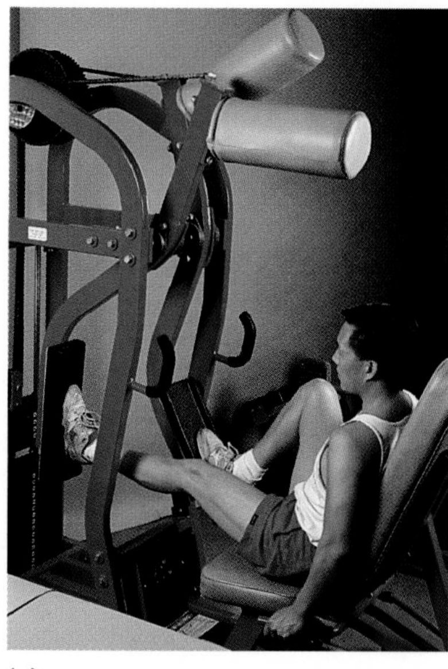

(c)

EXERCISE 10

Leg Extension (Knee Extension)

Muscles developed: Quadriceps

Instructions: **(a)** Sit on the seat with your shins under the knee-extension pads. **(b)** Extend your knees until they are straight. Return to the starting position.

Knee extensions cause kneecap pain in some people. If you have kneecap pain during this exercise, check with an orthopedic specialist before repeating it.

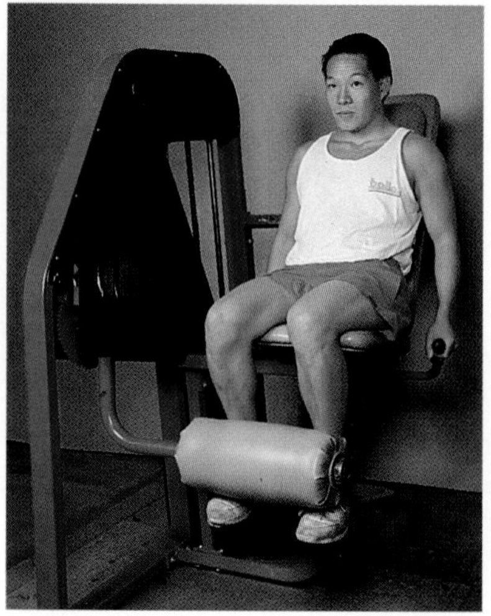

(a)

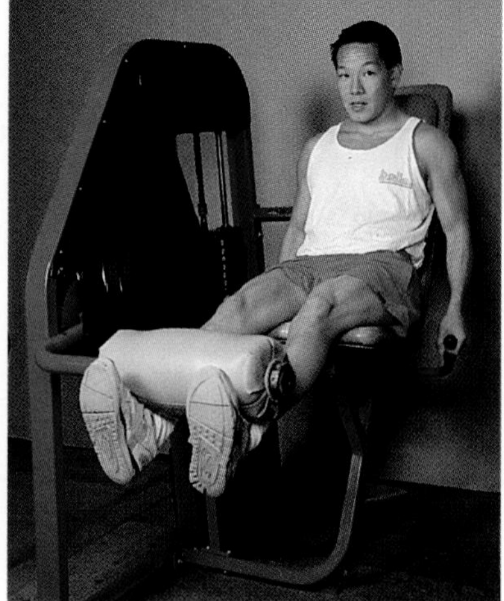

(b)

EXERCISE 11

Prone Leg Curl (Knee Flexion)

Muscles developed: Hamstrings

Instructions: **(a)** Lie on your stomach, resting the pads of the machine just below your calf muscles and with your knees just off the edge of the bench. **(b)** Flex your knees until they approach your buttocks. Return to the starting position.

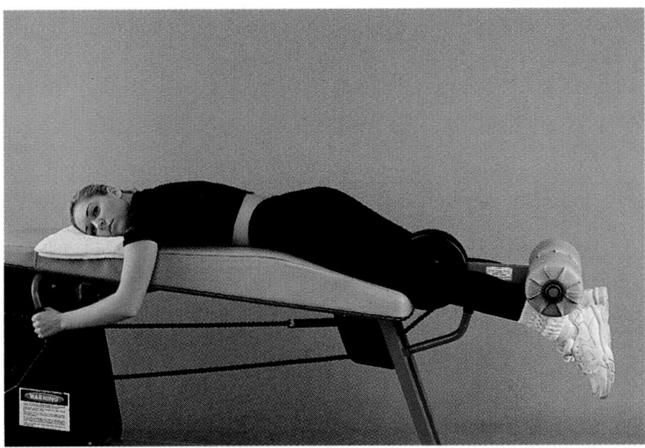

(a)

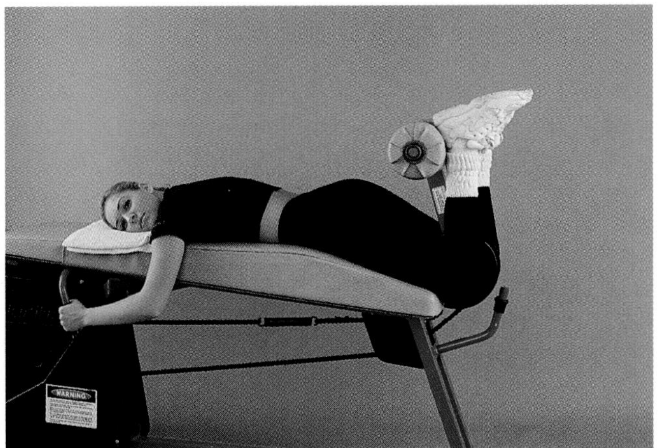

(b)

EXERCISE 12

Toe Raise

Muscles developed: Gastrocnemius, soleus

Instructions: **(a)** Stand with your head between the pads and one pad on each shoulder. **(b)** Press down with your toes while lifting your heels. Return to the starting position. Changing the direction your feet are pointing (straight ahead, inward, and outward) will work different portions of your calf muscles.

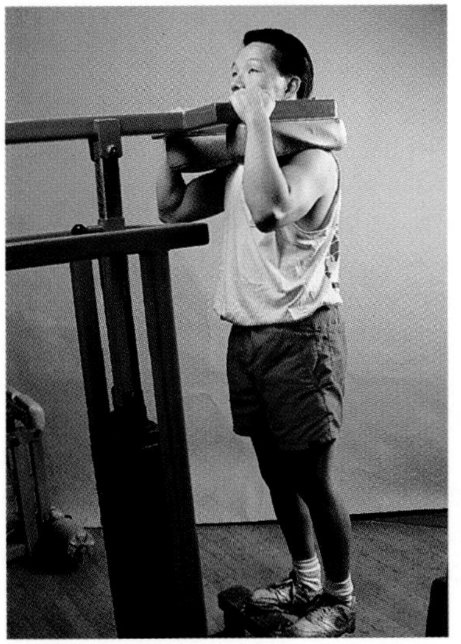

(a)

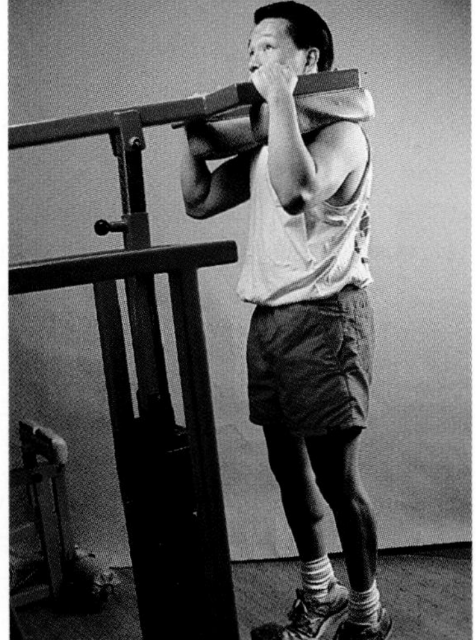

(b)

? COMMON QUESTIONS ANSWERED

How long must I weight train before I begin to see changes in my body? You will increase strength very rapidly during the early stages of a weight training program, primarily the result of muscle learning (the increased ability of the nervous system to recruit muscle fibers to exert force). Actual changes in muscle size usually begin after about 6–8 weeks of training.

I am concerned about my body composition. Will I gain weight if I do resistance exercises? Your weight probably will not change as a result of a recreational-type weight training program: 3 sets of 10 repetitions of 5–10 exercises. You will tend to increase lean body mass (muscle) and lose body fat, so your weight will stay about the same. (Men will tend to build larger muscles than women because of the tissue-building effects of male hormones.) Increased muscle mass will help you control body fat. Muscle increases your metabolism, which means you burn up more calories every day. If you combine resistance exercises with endurance exercises, you will be on your way to developing a lean, healthy-looking body. Concentrate on fat loss rather than weight loss.

Do I need more protein in my diet when I train with weights? No. While there is some evidence that power athletes involved in heavy training have a higher-than-normal protein requirement, there is no reason for most people to consume extra protein. Most Americans take in more protein than they need, so even if there is an increased protein need during heavy training, it is probably supplied by the average diet.

Are there any supplements or drugs that will help me gain larger and more rapid increases in strength and endurance? No nutritional supplement or drug will change a weak, untrained person into a strong, fit person. Those changes require regular training. Supplements or drugs that are promoted as instant or quick "cures" usually don't work and are either dangerous or expensive, or both. **Anabolic steroids**—the drugs most often taken in an effort to build strength and power—have dangerous side effects, described in the box "Effects of Anabolic Steroids." You are better off staying with proven principles of nutrition and a steady, progressive fitness program.

What causes muscle soreness the day or two following a weight training workout? The muscle pain you feel a day or two after a heavy weight training workout is caused by injury to the muscle fibers and surrounding connective tissue. Contrary to popular belief, delayed-onset muscle soreness is not caused by lactic acid buildup. Scientists believe that injury to muscle fibers causes the release of excess calcium into muscles. The calcium causes the release of substances called **proteases,** which break down part of the muscle tissue and cause pain. After a bout of intense exercise that causes muscle injury and delayed-onset muscle soreness, the muscles produce protective proteins that prevent soreness during future workouts. If you don't work out regularly, you lose these protective proteins and become susceptible to muscle soreness again.

Are there any special exercises I can do to improve speed and power for sports? Plyometric exercises are particularly beneficial for developing speed and power. Also, when performing weight-lifting exercises, try to lift the weights explosively. This will help increase speed and power for sports.

Will I improve faster if I train every day? No. Your muscles need time to recover between training sessions. Doing resistance exercises every day will cause you to become overtrained, which will increase your chance of injury and impede your progress.

If I stop weight training, will my muscles turn to fat? No. Fat and muscle are two different kinds of tissue, and one cannot turn into the other. Muscles that aren't used become smaller (atrophy), and body fat may increase if caloric intake exceeds calories burned. Although the result of inactivity may be smaller muscles and more fat, the change is caused by two separate processes.

TERMS

anabolic steroids Synthetic male hormones taken to enhance athletic performance and body composition.

proteases Enzymes that break down proteins.

SUMMARY

- Improvements in muscular strength and endurance lead to enhanced physical performance, protection against injury, improved body composition, better self-image, and improved muscle and bone health with aging.
- Muscular fitness is particularly important in preventing low-back pain and raising metabolic rates.
- Muscular strength can be assessed by determining the amount of weight that can be lifted in one repetition of an exercise; muscular endurance can be assessed by determining the number of repetitions of a particular exercise that can be performed.
- Hypertrophy, increased muscle fiber size, occurs when weight training causes the number of myofibrils to increase; total muscle size thereby increases. Strength also increases through muscle learning.
- Isometric exercises (contraction without movement) are most useful when a person is recovering from an injury or surgery or needs to overcome weak points in a range of motion.

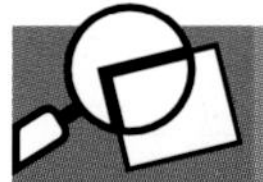

A CLOSER LOOK

Effects of Anabolic Steroids

Physical Effects

- Abnormal bleeding and blood clotting
- Acne
- Breast enlargement in males
- Decreased male hormone levels
- Decreased HDL levels
- Depressed sperm production in men
- Dizziness
- Elevated blood pressure
- Elevated blood sugar
- Gastrointestinal distress
- Growth of facial hair in women
- Hair loss (scalp)
- Increased risk of heart disease
- Impaired immune function
- Increased risk of liver cancer
- Liver toxicity
- Masculinization in females and children
- Menstrual irregularities in females
- Nosebleeds
- Increased risk of prostate cancer in men
- Stunted growth in children
- Tissue swelling

Psychological Effects

- Depression
- Increased aggressiveness
- Mood swings
- Personality changes

Source: Adapted from Fahey, T. D. 1997. *Weight Training for Men and Women,* 3d ed. Mountain View, Calif.: Mayfield.

- Isotonic exercises involve contraction that results in movement. The two most common types are constant resistance (free weights) and variable resistance (weight machines).
- Free weights and weight machines are basically equally effective in producing fitness, although machines are safer and more convenient.
- Lifting heavy weights for only a few repetitions helps develop strength. Lifting lighter weights for more repetitions helps develop muscular endurance.
- A weight training program for general fitness includes three sets of 8–12 repetitions (enough to cause fatigue) of 8–10 exercises, along with warm-up and cool-down periods; the program should be carried out 2–4 times a week.
- Safety guidelines for weight training include using proper technique, using spotters and collars when necessary, using common sense and remaining alert, and taking care of injuries. Regular exercise provides protection against soreness.
- Neither a high-protein diet, nutritional supplements, nor drugs are necessary components of an effective weight training program.

BEHAVIOR CHANGE ACTIVITY

Examining Attitudes

Your attitudes toward your target behavior can determine whether or not your behavior change program will be successful. Consider your attitudes carefully by answering the following questions about how you think and feel about your current behavior and your goal:

1. I like ______________________ because ______________________
(current behavior)
____
____

2. I don't like ______________________ because ______________________
(behavior goal)
____
____

(continued)

3. I don't ____________________ now because ____
(behavior goal)

____

____

4. I would be more likely to ____________________ if ________________________________
(behavior goal)

____

____

If your answers to these questions indicate that you have major reservations about changing your behavior, work to build your motivation and commitment before you begin your program. Look carefully at your objections to changing your behavior. How valid and important are they? What can you do to overcome them? Can you adopt any of the strategies you listed under the last question? Review the facts about your current behavior and your goals.

FOR MORE INFORMATION

Darden, E. 1982. *The Nautilus Bodybuilding Book.* Chicago: Contemporary Books.

Darden, E. 1984. *The Nautilus Advanced Bodybuilding Book.* New York: Simon & Schuster.

Fahey, T. D. 1997. *Basic Weight Training for Men and Women,* 3d ed. Mountain View, Calif.: Mayfield. *A practical guide to developing training programs using free weights tailored to individual needs.*

Fahey, T. D., and G. Hutchinson. 1992. *Weight Training for Women.* Mountain View, Calif.: Mayfield. *A practical guide for women who want to develop an individualized training program using free weights or weight machines.*

Komi, P. V., ed. 1992. *Strength and Power in Sport.* London: Blackwell Scientific. *Explains the scientific basis of strength training, including physiology, biomechanics, injuries, and training programs.*

Yessis, M. 1994. *Body Shaping.* Emmaus, Penn.: Rodale. A basic guide to exercise and weight control.

Information on and programs in weight training are available through physical education and athletics departments, private health clubs, and weight-lifting clubs.

SELECTED BIBLIOGRAPHY

American College of Sports Medicine. 1995. *Guidelines for Exercise Testing and Prescription,* 5th ed. Baltimore: Williams & Wilkins.

Brooks, G. A., T. D. Fahey, and T. White. 1996. *Exercise Physiology: Human Bioenergetics and Its Applications,* 2d ed. Mountain View, Calif.: Mayfield.

Castro, M. J., D. J. McCann, J. D. Shaffrath, and W. C. Adams. 1995. Peak torque per unit cross-sectional area differs between strength-trained and untrained young adults. *Medicine and Science in Sports and Exercise* 27:397–403.

Chilibeck, P. D., D. G. Sale, and C. E. Webber. 1995. Exercise and bone mineral density. *Sports Medicine* 19:103–122.

Enoka, R. M. 1988. Muscle strength and its development. *Sports Medicine* 6:146–168.

Fahey, T. D. 1997. *Basic Weight Training for Men and Women,* 3d ed. Mountain View, Calif.: Mayfield.

Fleck, S. J., and W. J. Kraemer. 1988. Resistance training: Physiological responses. *Physician and Sportsmedicine* 16:68.

Fowler, N. E., Z. Trzaskoma, A. Wit, L. Iskra, and A. Lees. 1995. The effectiveness of a pendulum swing for the development of leg strength and counter-movement jump performance. *Journal of Sports Science* 13:101–108.

Hadley, E. C., et al. 1995. The effects of exercise on falls in elderly patients: A preplanned meta-analysis of the FICSIT Trials. Frailty and Injuries: Cooperative Studies of Intervention Techniques, Province, MA. *Journal of the American Medical Association* 273(17): 1341–1347.

Komi, P. V., ed. 1992. *Strength and Power in Sport.* London: Blackwell Scientific.

Kraemer, W. J., J. F. Patton, S. E. Gordon, E. A. Harman, M. R. Deschenes, K. Reynolds, R. U. Newton, N. T. Triplett, and J. E. Dziados. 1995. Compatibility of high-intensity strength and endurance training on hormonal and skeletal muscle adaptations. *Journal of Applied Physiology* 78:976–989.

Kuramoto, A. K., and V. G. Payne. 1995. Predicting muscular strength in women: A preliminary study. *Research Quarterly for Exercise and Sport* 66:168–172.

McCarthy, J. P., J. C. Agre, B. K. Graf, M. A. Pozniak, and A. C. Vailas. Compatibility of adaptive responses with combining strength and endurance training. 1995. *Medicine and Science in Sports and Exercise* 27:429–436.

Rooney, K. J., R. D. Herbert, and R. J. Balnave. 1994. Fatigue contributes to the strength training stimulus. *Medicine and Science in Sports and Exercise* 26:1160–1164.

Sale, D. G. 1988. Neural adaptations to resistance training. *Medicine and Science in Sports and Exercise* 20:S135–45.

Shangold, M., and G. Mirkin. 1994. *Women and Exercise: Physiology and Sports Medicine,* 2d ed. Philadelphia: F. A. Davis.

Taaffe, D. R., L. Pruitt, J. Reim, G. Butterfield, and R. Marcus. 1995. Effect of sustained resistance training on basal metabolic rate in older women. *Journal of the American Geriatrics Society* 43:465–471.

Treuth, M. S., G. R. Hunter, T. Kekes-Szabo, R. L. Weinsier, M. I. Goran, and L. Berland. 1995. Reduction in intra-abdominal adipose tissue after strength training in older women. *Journal of Applied Physiology* 78:1425–1431.

Welle, S., C. Thornton, and M. Statt. 1995. Myofibrillar protein synthesis in young and old human subjects after three months of resistance training. *American Journal of Physiology* 268:E422–427.

Name ______________________ Section ______________ Date ______________

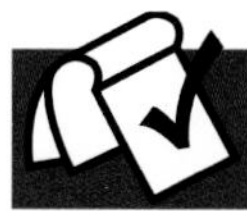

LAB 4-1 *Assessing Your Current Level of Muscular Strength*

For best results, don't do any strenuous weight training within 48 hours of any test.

The Maximum Bench Press Test

Equipment

1. Universal Gym Dynamic Variable Resistance machine
2. Weight scale

The ratings for this test were developed using the Universal Gym Dynamic Variable Resistance machine; results will be somewhat less accurate if the test is performed on another type of machine or with free weights.

If free weights are used, the following equipment is needed:

1. Flat bench (with or without racks)
2. Barbell
3. Assorted weight plates
4. Collars to hold weight plates in place
5. One or two spotters
6. Weight scale

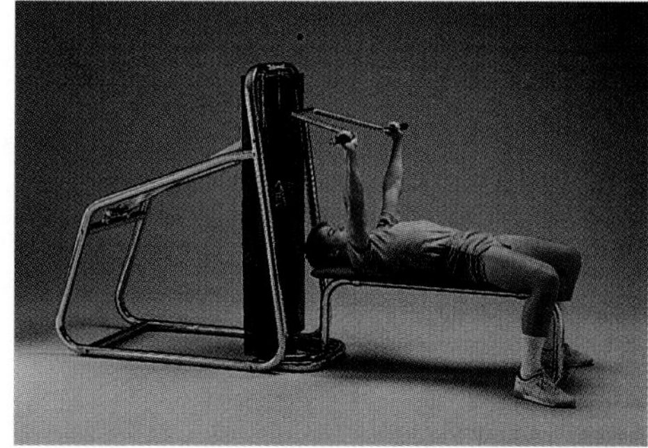

Maximum bench press test.

Preparation

Try a few bench presses with a small amount of weight so you can practice your technique, warm up your muscles, and, if you use free weights, coordinate your movements with those of your spotters. Weigh yourself, and record the results.

Body weight: ____________ lb

Instructions

1. Set the machine (or place weights on the barbell) for a weight that is lower than the amount you believe you can lift.
2. Lie on the bench with your feet firmly on the floor. If you are using a weight machine, grasp the handles with palms away from you; the tops of the handles should be aligned with the tops of your armpits.

   If you are using free weights, grasp the bar at shoulder width with your palms away from you. If you have one spotter, he or she should stand directly behind the bench; if you have two spotters, they should stand to the side, one at each end of the barbell. Lower the bar to your chest in preparation for the lift.
3. Push the bars or barbell until your arms are fully extended. Exhale as you lift. If you are using free weights, the bar should follow an elliptical path, during which the weight moves from a low point at the chest to a high point over the chin. Keep your feet firmly on the floor, don't arch your back, and push the weight evenly with your right and left arms. Don't bounce the weight on your chest.
4. Rest for several minutes, then repeat the lift with a heavier weight. It will probably take several attempts to determine the maximum amount of weight you can lift.

   1 RM: ____________ lb

Rating Your Bench Press Result

1. Divide your 1 RM value by your body weight.

   1 RM ____________ lb ÷ body weight ____________ lb = ____________

2. Find this ratio on the table below to determine your bench press strength rating. Record the result here and on the final page of this lab.

   Bench press strength rating: ___________

Strength Ratings for the Maximum Bench Press Test

	Pounds Lifted/Body Weight (lb)					
Men	*Very Poor*	*Poor*	*Fair*	*Good*	*Excellent*	*Superior*
Age: Under 20	Below 0.89	0.89–1.05	1.06–1.18	1.19–1.33	1.34–1.75	Above 1.75
20–29	Below 0.88	0.88–0.98	0.99–1.13	1.14–1.31	1.32–1.62	Above 1.62
30–39	Below 0.78	0.78–0.87	0.88–0.97	0.98–1.11	1.12–1.34	Above 1.34
40–49	Below 0.72	0.72–0.79	0.80–0.87	0.88–0.99	1.00–1.19	Above 1.19
50–59	Below 0.63	0.63–0.70	0.71–0.78	0.79–0.89	0.90–1.04	Above 1.04
60 and over	Below 0.57	0.57–0.65	0.66–0.71	0.72–0.81	0.82–0.93	Above 0.93
Women						
Age: Under 20	Below 0.53	0.53–0.57	0.58–0.64	0.65–0.76	0.77–0.87	Above 0.87
20–29	Below 0.51	0.51–0.58	0.59–0.69	0.70–0.79	0.80–1.00	Above 1.00
30–39	Below 0.47	0.47–0.52	0.53–0.59	0.60–0.69	0.70–0.81	Above 0.81
40–49	Below 0.43	0.43–0.49	0.50–0.53	0.54–0.61	0.62–0.76	Above 0.76
50–59	Below 0.39	0.39–0.43	0.44–0.47	0.48–0.54	0.55–0.67	Above 0.67
60 and over	Below 0.38	0.38–0.42	0.43–0.46	0.47–0.53	0.54–0.71	Above 0.71

Source: Based on norms from the Cooper Institute for Aerobics Research, Dallas, Texas; used with permission.

The Maximum Leg Press Test

Equipment

1. Universal Gym Dynamic Variable Resistance leg press machine (If you're using a Universal Gym leg press with two sets of pedals, use the lower pedals.)
2. Weight scale

The ratings for this test were developed using the Universal Gym Dynamic Resistance machine; results will be somewhat less accurate if the test is performed on another type of machine.

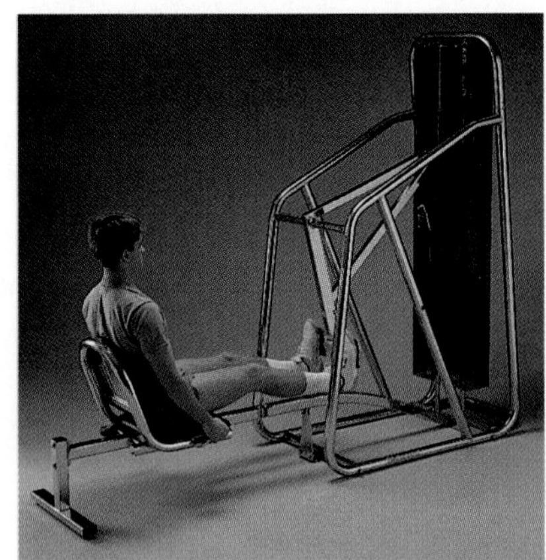

Maximum leg press test.

Preparation

Try a few leg presses with the machine set for a small amount of weight so you can practice your technique and warm up your muscles. Weigh yourself, and record the results.

Body weight: ___________ lb

Instructions

1. Set the machine for a weight that is lower than the amount you believe you can press.
2. Adjust the seat so that your knees are bent at a 70-degree angle to start.
3. Grasp the side handlebars, and push with your legs until your knees are fully extended.
4. Rest for several minutes, then repeat the press with a higher weight setting. It will probably take several attempts to determine the maximum amount of weight you can press.

   1 RM: ___________ lb

Rating Your Leg Press Result

1. Divide your 1 RM value by your body weight.

   1 RM ___________ lb ÷ body weight ___________ lb = ___________

2. Find this ratio on the table below to determine your leg press strength rating. Record the result below and on the final page of this lab.

   Leg press strength rating: ___________

Strength Ratings for the Maximum Leg Press Test

	Pounds Lifted/Body Weight (lb)					
Men	*Very Poor*	*Poor*	*Fair*	*Good*	*Excellent*	*Superior*
Age: Under 20	Below 1.70	1.70–1.89	1.90–2.03	2.04–2.27	2.28–2.81	Above 2.81
20–29	Below 1.63	1.63–1.82	1.83–1.96	1.97–2.12	2.13–2.39	Above 2.39
30–39	Below 1.52	1.52–1.64	1.65–1.76	1.77–1.92	1.93–2.19	Above 2.19
40–49	Below 1.44	1.44–1.56	1.57–1.67	1.68–1.81	1.82–2.01	Above 2.01
50–59	Below 1.32	1.32–1.45	1.46–1.57	1.58–1.70	1.71–1.89	Above 1.89
60 and over	Below 1.25	1.25–1.37	1.38–1.48	1.49–1.61	1.62–1.79	Above 1.79
Women						
Age: Under 20	Below 1.22	1.22–1.37	1.38–1.58	1.59–1.70	1.71–1.87	Above 1.87
20–29	Below 1.22	1.22–1.36	1.37–1.49	1.50–1.67	1.68–1.97	Above 1.97
30–39	Below 1.09	1.09–1.20	1.21–1.32	1.33–1.46	1.47–1.67	Above 1.67
40–49	Below 1.02	1.02–1.12	1.13–1.22	1.23–1.36	1.37–1.56	Above 1.56
50–59	Below 0.88	0.88–0.98	0.99–1.09	1.10–1.24	1.25–1.42	Above 1.42
60 and over	Below 0.85	0.85–0.92	0.93–1.03	1.04–1.17	1.18–1.42	Above 1.42

Source: Based on norms from the Cooper Institute for Aerobics Research, Dallas, Texas; used with permission.

Hand Grip Strength Test

Equipment

Grip strength dynamometer

Preparation

If necessary, adjust the hand grip size on the dynamometer into a position that is comfortable for you.

Instructions

1. Stand erect, and hold the dynamometer parallel to the side of your body, with the dial facing away from you. Squeeze the dynamometer as hard as possible without moving your arm.
2. Perform three trials with each hand. Rest for about a minute between each trial. Record the highest score for each hand. (The score for one hand—your preferred hand—will probably be higher than the score for the other hand.)

   Right hand: ___________ kg

   Left hand: ___________ kg

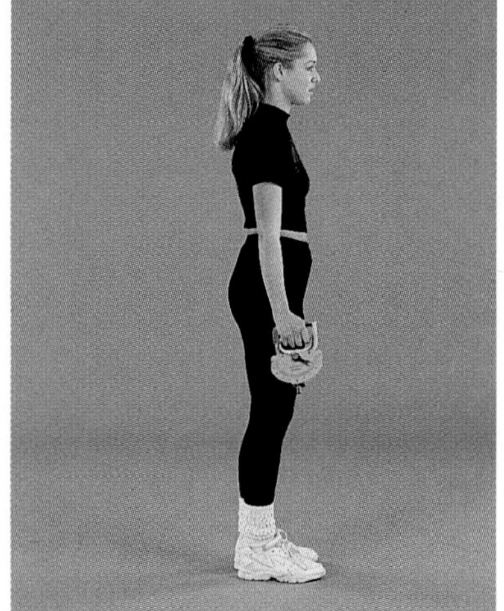

Hand grip strength test.

(Scores on the dynamometer should be given in kilograms. If the dynamometer you are using gives scores in pounds, convert pounds to kilograms by dividing your score by 2.2.)

Rating Your Hand Grip Strength

Refer to the table below for a rating of your grip strength on each hand. Use the Preferred Hand column for the hand for which you obtained the higher value. Record the results below and in the chart below.

Rating for right-hand grip strength: ____________

Rating for left-hand grip strength: ____________

Strength Ratings for the Hand Grip Test

	Rating	Preferred hand Grip Strength (kg)	Other Hand Grip Strength (kg)
Men			
	Excellent	>70	>68
	Good	62–79	56–67
	Average	48–61	43–55
	Poor	41–47	39–42
	Very poor	<41	<39
Women			
	Excellent	>41	>37
	Good	38–40	34–36
	Average	25–37	22–33
	Poor	22–24	18–21
	Very poor	<22	<18

For people over age 50, reduce scores by 10% to adjust for muscle tissue loss due to aging.

Source: Adapted from Haywood, V. H. 1991. *Advanced Fitness Assessment and Exercise Prescription,* 2d ed. Champaign, Ill.: Human Kinetics.

Summary of Results

Maximum bench press test

Weight pressed: ____________ lb Rating: ____________

Maximum leg press test

Weight pressed: ____________ lb Rating: ____________

Hand grip strength test

Right hand: ____________ kg Rating: ____________

Left hand: ____________ kg Rating: ____________

Remember that muscular strength is specific: Your ratings may vary considerably for different parts of your body. You can use these results to guide you in planning a weight training program.

To monitor your progress toward your goal, enter the results of this lab in the Preprogram Assessment column of Lab 15-2. After several weeks of a weight training program, do this lab again, and enter the results in the Postprogram Assessment column of Lab 15-2. How do the results compare?

Name ______________________ Section ______________ Date ______________

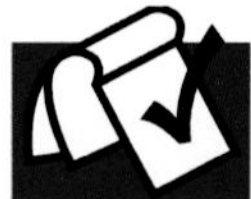

LAB 4-2 *Assessing Your Current Level of Muscular Endurance*

For best results, don't do any strenuous weight training within 48 hours of any test. To assess endurance of the abdominal muscles, perform the sit-up test or the curl-up test. The push-up test assesses endurance of muscles in the upper body.

The 60-Second Sit-Up Test

Do not take this test if you suffer from low-back pain.

Equipment

1. Stopwatch, clock, or watch with a second hand
2. Partner to hold your ankles
3. Mat or towel to lie on (optional)

Preparation

Try a few sit-ups to get used to the proper technique and warm up your abdominal muscles.

Instructions

1. Lie flat on your back on the floor with knees bent, feet flat on the floor, and your fingers interlocked behind your neck. Your partner should hold your ankles firmly so that your feet stay on the floor as you do the sit-ups.
2. When someone signals you to begin, raise your head and chest off the floor until your elbows touch your knees or thighs, then return to the starting position. Keep your neck neutral.
3. Perform as many sit-ups as you can in 60 seconds.

   Note: The norms for this test were established with subjects interlocking their fingers behind their neck; your results will be most accurate if you use this technique. However, some experts feel that sit-ups done in this position can cause injury to the neck, and they recommend that sit-ups and curl-ups be done with the arms crossed over the chest (see exercise 6 on p. 82 or the curl-up test later in this lab). If you perform sit-ups with your hands behind your neck, take care not to force your neck forward, and stop if you feel any pain in your neck.

   Number of sit-ups: ____________

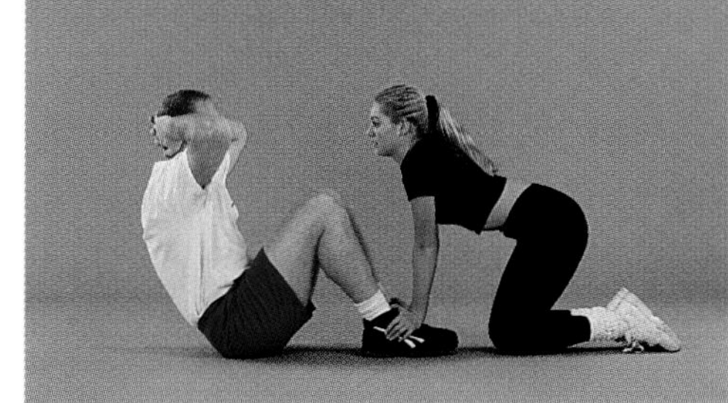

The 60-second sit-up test.

Rating Your Muscular Endurance

Refer to the table below for a rating of your abdominal muscle endurance. Record your rating below and on the final page of this lab.

Rating: ____________

Ratings for the 60-Second Sit-Up Test

	Number of Sit-Ups					
Men	*Very Poor*	*Poor*	*Fair*	*Good*	*Excellent*	*Superior*
Age: Under 20	Below 36	36–40	41–46	47–50	51–61	Above 61
20–29	Below 33	33–37	38–41	42–46	47–54	Above 54
30–39	Below 30	30–34	35–38	39–42	43–51	Above 51
40–49	Below 24	24–28	29–33	34–38	39–47	Above 47
50–59	Below 19	19–23	24–27	28–34	35–43	Above 43
60 and over	Below 15	15–18	19–21	22–29	30–38	Above 38

(continued)

Women	Very Poor	Poor	Fair	Good	Excellent	Superior
Age: Under 20	Below 28	28–31	32–35	36–45	46–54	Above 54
20–29	Below 27	27–31	32–37	38–43	44–50	Above 50
30–39	Below 20	20–24	25–28	29–34	35–41	Above 41
40–49	Below 14	14–19	20–23	24–28	29–37	Above 37
50–59	Below 10	10–13	14–19	20–23	24–29	Above 29
60 and over	Below 3	3–5	6–10	11–16	17–27	Above 27

Source: Based on norms from the Cooper Institute for Aerobics Research, Dallas, Texas; used with permission.

The Curl-Up Test

The curl-up test is preferred by some exercise scientists as a test of abdominal endurance. In a full sit-up, part of the lift is provided by the hip flexor muscles. Curl-ups optimize the use of the abdominal muscles without involving the hip flexors.

Equipment

1. Metronome
2. Heavy tape
3. Large piece of cardboard (optional)
4. Ruler
5. Partner
6. Mat (optional)

Preparation

1. Set the metronome at a rate of 40 beats per minute.
2. Place a tape strip approximately 1 meter long on the floor or mat. Place another strip of tape 12 centimeters away from the first one. Alternatively, cut a piece of cardboard 1 meter by 12 centimeters, and tape it to the floor.

Instructions

1. Start by lying on your back on the floor, arms by your sides, palms down and on the floor, elbows locked, and fingers straight. The longest fingertip of each hand should touch the edge of the near strip of tape or the front edge of the cardboard strip. Your knees should be bent at about 90 degrees, with your feet 12–18 inches away from your buttocks.
2. To perform a curl-up, curl your head and upper back upward, keeping your arms straight. Slide your fingertips forward along the floor until you touch the other strip of tape or the far side of the cardboard strip, 12 centimeters from the starting position. Then curl back down so that your upper back and head touch the floor. Fingers, feet, and buttocks should stay on the floor throughout the curl-up. (For this test, your partner does not hold your feet.) Maintain the 90-degree angle in your knees.

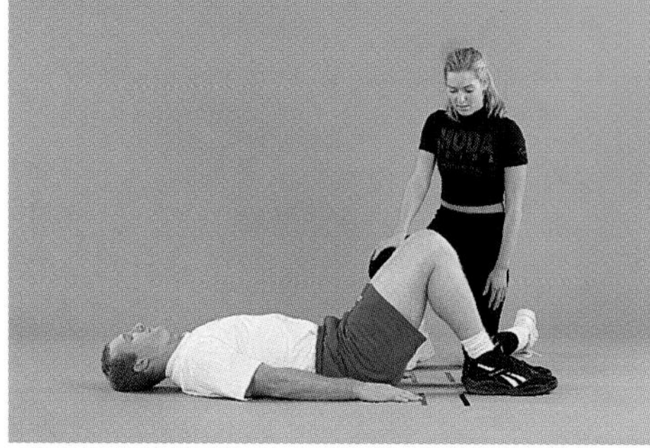

Curl-up test: (a) starting position

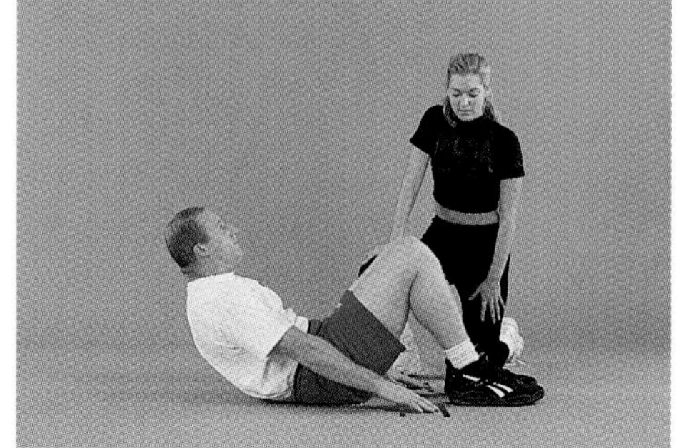

(b) curl-up

3. Start the metronome at the correct cadence. You will perform curl-ups at the steady, continuous rate of 20 per minute. Curl up on one beat and curl down on the next. Your partner counts the number of curl-ups you complete and makes sure that you maintain correct form.
4. Perform as many curl-ups as you can with proper form until you can no longer keep up with the rhythm set by the metronome.

   Number of curl-ups: ___________

Rating Your Muscular Endurance

Your score is the number of completed curl-ups. Refer to the appropriate portion of the table below for a rating of your abdominal muscular endurance. Record your rating below and on the final page of this lab.

Rating: ___________

Ratings for the Curl-Up Test

	Number of Curl-Ups					
Men	*Very Poor*	*Poor*	*Fair*	*Good*	*Excellent*	*Superior*
Age: 18–29	Below 25	25–34	35–44	45–64	65–74	Above 74
30–39	Below 20	20–29	30–39	40–59	60–69	Above 69
40–49	Below 15	15–24	25–34	35–54	55–64	Above 64
50–59	Below 10	10–19	20–29	30–49	50–59	Above 59
60 and over	Below 5	5–9	10–15	25–44	45–54	Above 54
Women						
Age: 18–29	Below 20	20–29	30–39	40–54	55–69	Above 69
30–39	Below 15	15–24	25–34	35–49	50–64	Above 64
40–49	Below 10	10–19	20–29	30–44	45–59	Above 59
50–59	Below 6	6–14	15–24	25–39	40–54	Above 54
60 and over	Below 4	4–12	13–19	20–34	35–49	Above 49

Source: Adapted from the data of Faulkner, R. A., E. J. Springings, A. McQuarrie, and R. D. Bell. 1989. A partial curl-up protocol for adults based on an analysis of two procedures. *Canadian Journal of Sports Science* 14: 135–141.

The Push-Up Test

Equipment

Mat or towel (optional)

Preparation

In this test, you will perform either standard push-ups or modified push-ups, in which you support yourself with your knees. The Cooper Institute developed the ratings for this test with men performing push-ups and women performing modified push-ups. (Biologically, males tend to be stronger than females; the modified technique reduces the need for upper-body strength in a test of muscular endurance.) Therefore, for an accurate assessment of upper-body endurance, men should perform standard push-ups and women should perform modified push-ups.

Instructions

1. *For push-ups:* Start in the push-up position with your body supported by your hands and feet. *For modified push-ups:* Start in the modified push-up position with your body supported by your hands and knees. *For both positions,* your arms and your back should be straight and your fingers pointed forward.

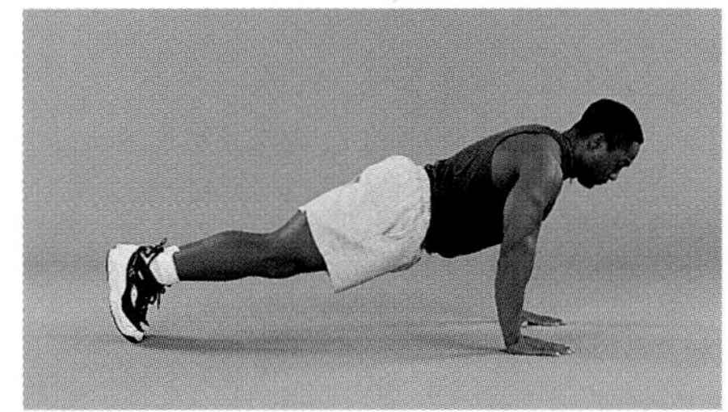

(a) Push-up

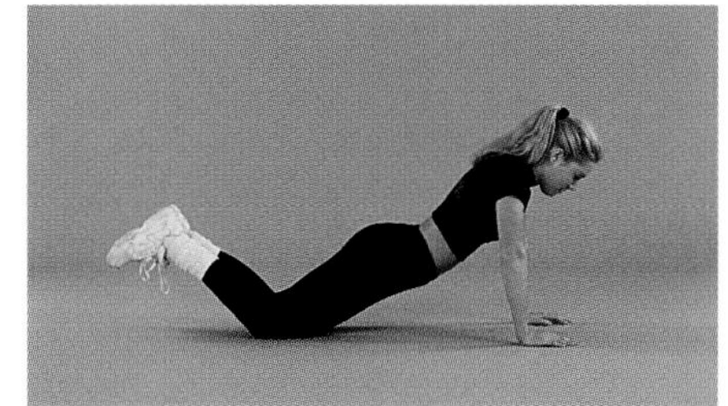

(b) Modified push-up

2. Lower your chest to the floor with your back straight, then return to the starting position.
3. Perform as many push-ups or modified push-ups as you can without stopping.
   Number of push-ups: ____________ or number of modified push-ups: ____________

Ratings for the Push-Up and Modified Push-Up Tests

	Number of Push-Ups					
Men	*Very Poor*	*Poor*	*Fair*	*Good*	*Excellent*	*Superior*
Age: 18–29	Below 22	22–28	29–36	37–46	47–61	Above 61
30–39	Below 17	17–23	24–29	30–38	39–51	Above 51
40–49	Below 11	11–17	18–23	24–29	30–39	Above 39
50–59	Below 9	9–12	13–18	19–24	25–38	Above 38
60 and over	Below 6	6–9	10–17	18–22	23–27	Above 27

	Number of Modified Push-Ups					
Women	*Very Poor*	*Poor*	*Fair*	*Good*	*Excellent*	*Superior*
Age: 18–29	Below 17	17–22	23–29	30–35	36–44	Above 44
30–39	Below 11	11–18	19–23	24–30	31–38	Above 38
40–49	Below 6	6–12	13–17	18–23	24–32	Above 32
50–59	Below 6	6–11	12–16	17–20	21–27	Above 27
60 and over	Below 2	2–4	5–11	12–14	15–19	Above 19

Source: Based on norms from the Cooper Institute for Aerobics Research, Dallas, Texas; used with permission.

Summary of Results

60-second sit-up test

Number of sit-ups: ____________ Rating: ____________

Curl-up test

Number of curl-ups: ____________ Rating: ____________

Push-up test

Number of push-ups: ____________ Rating: ____________

Remember that muscular endurance is specific: Your ratings may vary considerably for different parts of your body. You can use these results to guide you in planning a weight training program.

To monitor your progress toward your goal, enter the results of this lab in the Preprogram Assessment column of Lab 15-2. After several weeks of a weight training program, do this lab again, and enter the results in the Postprogram Assessment column of Lab 15-2. How do the results compare?

Name ______________________ Section ______________ Date ______________

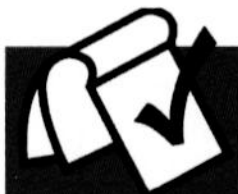

LAB 4-3 *Designing and Monitoring a Weight Training Program*

1. *Set goals.* List the goals of your weight training program. Goals can be general, such as developing greater muscle definition, or specific, such as increasing the power in a golf swing. If your goals involve the development of a specific muscle group, note that also.

1. ______________________________
2. ______________________________
3. ______________________________
4. ______________________________

2. *Choose exercises.* Based on your goals, choose 8–10 exercises to perform during each weight training session. If your goal is general training for wellness, use the sample program in the box "Sample Weight Training Program for General Fitness" on p. 74. If your goals relate to a specific sport, use Table 4-3 to put together a program to develop the important muscle groups. List your exercises and the muscles they develop in the space provided in the program plan below.

3. *Choose starting weights.* Experiment with different amounts of weight until you settle on a good starting weight, one that you can lift easily for 10–12 repetitions. As you progress in your program, you can add more weight. Fill in the starting weight for each exercise on the program plan.

4. *Choose a starting number of sets and repetitions.* The optimal pattern for a weight training workout includes 3 sets of 10 repetitions of each exercise. These are probably good values to start with. (As you add weight, you may have to decrease the number of repetitions slightly until your muscles adapt to the heavier load.) If your program is focusing on strength alone, your sets can contain fewer repetitions using a heavier load. Fill in the starting number of sets and repetitions of each exercise on the program plan.

5. *Choose the number of training sessions per week.* Choose a frequency between 2 and 4 days per week (3 days per week is recommended), and add it to your program plan.

6. *Monitor your progress.* Use the workout card on the next page to monitor program progress and keep track of exercises, weights, sets, and repetitions.

Exercise	Muscle(s) Developed	Weight (lb)	Repetitions	Sets	Frequency (check ✓)						
					M	T	W	Th	F	Sa	Su

LABORATORY ACTIVITIES

WORKOUT CARD FOR ____________________

Exercise/Date																												
	Wt																											
	Sets																											
	Reps																											
	Wt																											
	Sets																											
	Reps																											
	Wt																											
	Sets																											
	Reps																											
	Wt																											
	Sets																											
	Reps																											
	Wt																											
	Sets																											
	Reps																											
	Wt																											
	Sets																											
	Reps																											
	Wt																											
	Sets																											
	Reps																											
	Wt																											
	Sets																											
	Reps																											
	Wt																											
	Sets																											
	Reps																											
	Wt																											
	Sets																											
	Reps																											
	Wt																											
	Sets																											
	Reps																											
	Wt																											
	Sets																											
	Reps																											

5

Flexibility

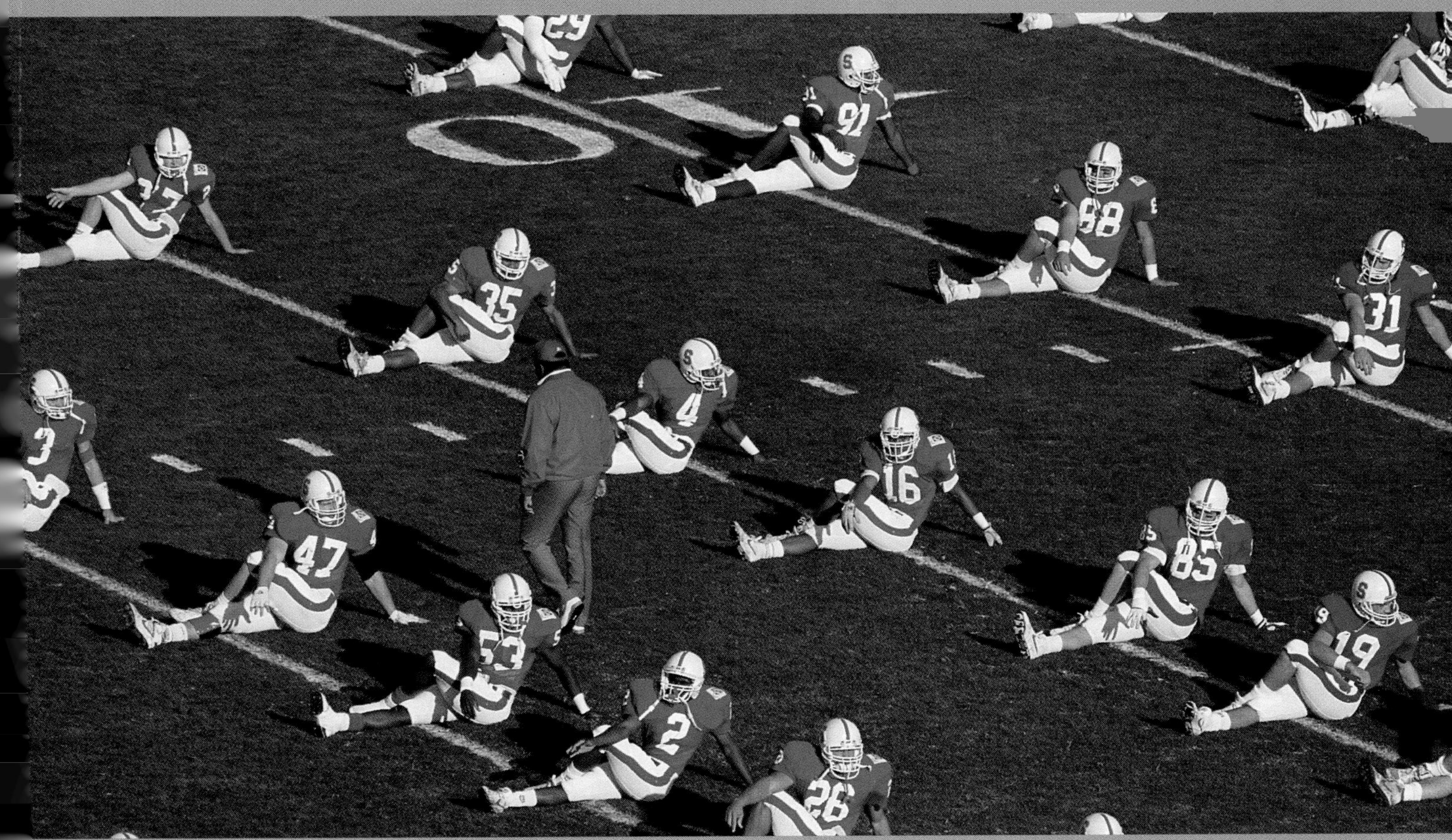

LOOKING AHEAD

After reading this chapter, you should be able to answer these questions about flexibility and stretching exercises:

- What are the benefits of flexibility and stretching exercises?
- What determines the amount of flexibility in each joint?
- What are the different types of stretching exercises, and how do they affect muscles?
- What type, intensity, duration, and frequency of stretching exercises will develop the greatest amount of flexibility with the lowest risk of injury?
- What are some common stretching exercises for major joints?
- How can low-back pain be prevented and managed?

Flexibility is the ability of a joint to move through its **range of motion.** The amount of movement is largely determined by the tightness of muscles, tendons, and ligaments that are attached to the joint. The more a muscle can stretch, the better the flexibility of the joint. Good flexibility is important for joint health and for the prevention of injuries. Leg, back, and hip muscles must be strong *and* flexible to prevent pain in the lower back. The smooth and easy performance of everyday and recreational activities is impossible if flexibility is poor.

Flexibility is a highly adaptable physical fitness component. It increases with regular activity and decreases with inactivity. Flexibility is also specific: Good flexibility in one joint doesn't necessarily mean good flexibility in another. Flexibility can be increased through stretching exercises for all major joints.

This chapter describes the factors that affect flexibility and the benefits of maintaining good flexibility. It provides guidelines for assessing your current level of flexibility and putting together a successful stretching program.

BENEFITS OF FLEXIBILITY AND STRETCHING EXERCISES

Good flexibility provides benefits for the entire muscular and skeletal system, prevents injuries and soreness, and improves performance in sports and other activities.

Maintaining Joint Health

Good flexibility is essential to good joint health. Joints that are supported by tight muscles and soft tissues are subject to abnormal stresses that can cause joint deterioration. For example, tight thigh muscles cause excessive pressure on the kneecap, leading to pain in the knee joint. Tight shoulder muscles can compress sensitive soft tissues in the shoulder, leading to pain and disability in the joint. Poor joint flexibility can also cause abnormalities in joint lubrication, leading to deterioration of the sensitive cartilage cells lining the joint; pain and further joint injury can result.

Improved flexibility can greatly improve your quality of life, particularly as you get older. Aging decreases the natural elasticity of muscles, tendons, and joints, resulting in stiffness. The problem is compounded if you have arthritis. Flexibility exercises improve the elasticity in your tissues, making it easier to move your body. When you're flexible, everything from tying your shoes to reaching for a jar on an upper shelf becomes easier.

Preventing Low-Back Pain

Low-back pain is often related to poor spinal alignment, which puts pressure on the nerves leading out from the spinal column. Poor flexibility (and weak muscles) in the back, pelvis, and thighs can increase the curve of the lower back and cause the pelvis to tilt too far forward. Good flexibility in these areas, along with good muscle strength and good posture, helps prevent abnormal pressures on sensitive spinal nerves.

Preventing Injuries

The full range of motion associated with flexibility means that muscles will not be stretched more than they can tolerate in the course of everyday activities, sports, or occasional emergencies that require physical effort. Flexible people are less likely to be injured if, for example, they slip in the shower, or extend themselves when making a difficult shot in tennis.

Additional Benefits

- *Reduction of postexercise muscle soreness.* **Delayed-onset muscle soreness,** occurring one to two days after exercise, is thought to be caused by damage to the muscle fibers and supporting connective tissue. Stretching after exercise has been shown to decrease the degree of muscle soreness after exercise.
- *Relief of aches and pains.* Flexibility exercises help relieve pain that develops from stress or prolonged sitting. Studying or working in one place for a long time can cause your muscles to become tense. Stretching helps relieve tension, so you can go back to work refreshed and effective.
- *Improved body position for sports.* Good flexibility lets a person assume the most efficient body positions and exert force through a greater range of motion. For example, swimmers with more flexible shoulders have stronger strokes because they can pull their arms through the water in the optimal position. Flexible joints and muscles let you move more fluidly without constraint. When you're flexible, you will be amazed

TERMS

range of motion The full motion possible in a joint.

delayed-onset muscle soreness Soreness that occurs 1–2 days after exercising, probably caused by tissue damage that stimulates the release of calcium and enzymes that break down muscle fibers.

joint capsules Semielastic structures, composed primarily of connective tissue, that surround major joints.

soft tissues Tissues of the human body that include skin, fat, linings of internal organs and blood vessels, connective tissues, tendons, ligaments, muscles, and nerves.

collagen White fibers that provide structure and support in collagenous tissue.

elastin Yellow fibers that make collagenous tissue flexible.

stretch receptors Sense organs in skeletal muscles that initiate a nerve signal to the spinal cord in response to a stretch; a contraction follows.

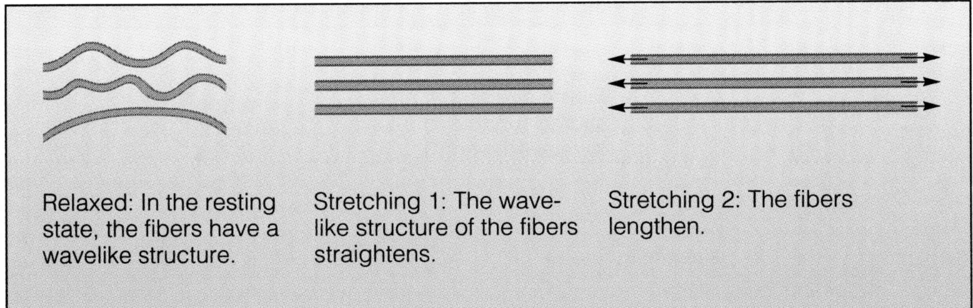

Relaxed: In the resting state, the fibers have a wavelike structure.
Stretching 1: The wave-like structure of the fibers straightens.
Stretching 2: The fibers lengthen.

Figure 5-1 ***Relaxed versus stretched elastin muscle fibers.***

at how much better you will be able to run, jump, and throw.

- *Facilitation of strength development.* Poor flexibility inhibits the ability to increase strength. Tight muscles interfere with the way the nervous system regulates muscular function.
- *Relaxation.* Flexibility exercises are a great way to relax. Studies have shown that doing flexibility exercises reduces mental tension, slows your breathing rate, and reduces blood pressure.

Flexibility and Lifetime Wellness

Part of wellness is being able to move without pain or hindrance. Flexibility exercises are an important part of this process. Sedentary people often effectively lose their mobility at an early age. Even relatively young people are often handicapped by back, shoulder, knee, and ankle pain. As they age, the pain can become debilitating, leading to injuries and a lower quality of life. Good flexibility helps keep your joints and muscles moving without pain so that you can do all the things you enjoy.

WHAT DETERMINES FLEXIBILITY?

The flexibility of a joint is affected by its structure and the nature of surrounding tissue, by muscle elasticity and length, and by nervous system activity. Some factors—joint structure, for example—can't be changed. Other factors, such as the length of resting muscle fibers, can be changed through exercise; these factors should be the focus of a program to develop flexibility.

Joint Structure and Surrounding Tissues

The amount of flexibility in a joint is determined in part by the nature and structure of the joint. Hinge joints such as those in your fingers and knees allow only limited forward and backward movement; they lock when fully extended. Ball-and-socket joints like the hip enable movement in many different directions and have a greater range of motion. Major joints are surrounded by **joint capsules,** semielastic structures that give joints strength and stability but limit movement. Flexibility can also be limited by **soft tissues**—fat, skin, or large muscles—that can prevent a joint from moving through its full range of motion. Heredity also plays a part in joint structure and flexibility.

Muscle Elasticity and Length

Muscle tissue is the key to developing flexibility because it can be lengthened if it is regularly stretched. In addition to the proteins within muscles that create movement, muscles contain collagenous tissues that provide structure, elasticity, and bulk. The two principal types of collagenous tissue are **collagen,** white fibers that provide structure and support, and **elastin,** yellow fibers that are elastic and flexible. When a muscle is stretched, the wavelike elastin fibers straighten; when the stretch is relieved, they rapidly snap back to their resting position. But elastin fibers that are gently and regularly stretched will lengthen, and flexibility will improve (Figure 5-1). Inactive, rarely stretched elastin fibers and other muscle tissues will shorten, resulting in decreased flexibility.

The stretch characteristics of elastic tissue in muscle are important considerations for a stretching program. The amount of stretch a muscle will tolerate is limited, and as the limits of its flexibility are reached, collagenous tissue becomes more brittle and may rupture if overstretched. If collagenous tissue doesn't return to its resting shape, injury results. A safe and effective program stresses muscles enough to slightly elongate elastin fibers but not so much that they cannot return to their normal shape. The effect of stretch on elastic tissue is shown in Figure 5-2.

Nervous System Activity

Muscles contain **stretch receptors** that control their length. If a muscle is stretched suddenly, stretch receptors send signals to the spinal cord, which then sends a signal back to the same muscle, causing it to contract. These reflexes occur frequently in active muscle. They help the body know what the muscles are doing and allow for fine control of muscle length.

Small movements that only slightly stimulate these receptors cause small reflex actions. Rapid, powerful, and sudden movements that strongly stimulate the receptors cause large, powerful reflex muscle contractions. Stretches that involve rapid, bouncy movements are considered dangerous because they may stimulate a reflex muscle

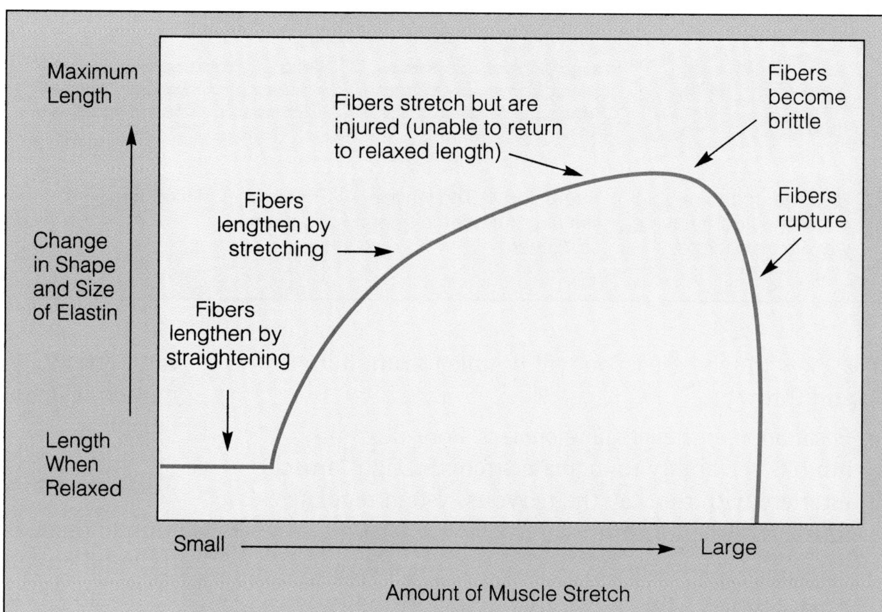

Figure 5-2 ***The effect of stretch on elastic tissue.***

contraction during a stretch. A muscle that contracts at the same time it's being stretched can be easily injured, so slow, gradual stretches are always safest.

Strong muscle contractions produce a reflex of the opposite type—one that causes muscles to relax and keeps them from contracting too hard. This inverse stretch reflex has recently been introduced as an aid to improving flexibility: Contracting a muscle prior to stretching it causes it to relax, allowing it to stretch farther. The contraction-stretch technique for developing flexibility is called **proprioceptive neuromuscular facilitation (PNF).** More research needs to be done, however, to determine precisely the degree to which PNF techniques cause muscle relaxation and help develop flexibility.

Doing each stretching exercise several times in a row can "reset" the sensitivity of muscle stretch receptors. Stretching a muscle, relaxing, and then stretching it again cause the stretch receptors to become slightly less sensitive, thereby enabling the muscle to stretch farther. It is not known if stretch receptor sensitivity continues to change following prolonged flexibility training, but it's likely that neural changes do occur to help increase flexibility.

ASSESSING FLEXIBILITY

Because flexibility is specific to each joint, there are no tests of general flexibility. The most commonly used flexibility test is the sit-and-reach test. This test rates the flexibility of the muscles in the lower back and hamstrings; flexibility in these muscles is especially important in preventing low-back pain. To assess your flexibility and identify inflexible joints, complete Lab 5-1.

CREATING A SUCCESSFUL PROGRAM TO DEVELOP FLEXIBILITY

A successful program for developing flexibility contains safe exercises executed with the most effective techniques.

Types of Stretching Techniques

Stretching techniques vary from simply stretching the muscles during the course of normal activities to sophisticated methods based on patterns of muscle reflexes. Improper stretching techniques can do more harm than good, so it's important to understand the different types of stretching exercises and how they affect the muscles. Three common techniques are static stretches, ballistic stretches, and PNF.

Static Stretching In **static stretching,** each muscle is gradually stretched, and the stretch is held for 15–30 seconds. (Holding the stretch longer than 30 seconds will not further improve flexibility, while stretching for less than 15 seconds will provide little benefit.) A slow stretch prompts less reaction from stretch receptors, and the muscles can safely stretch farther than usual. Static stretching is the type most often recommended by fitness experts because it's safe and effective. The key to this technique is to stretch the muscles and joints to the point where a pull is felt, but not to the point of pain.

Ballistic Stretching The technique of **ballistic stretching** involves dynamic muscle action whereby the muscles are stretched suddenly in a bouncing movement. For example, touching the toes repeatedly in rapid succession is

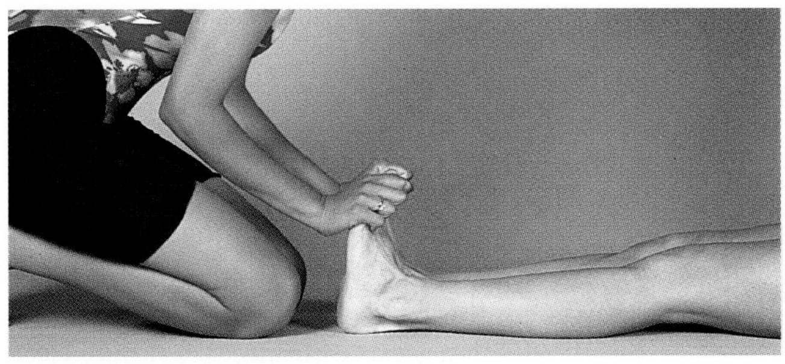

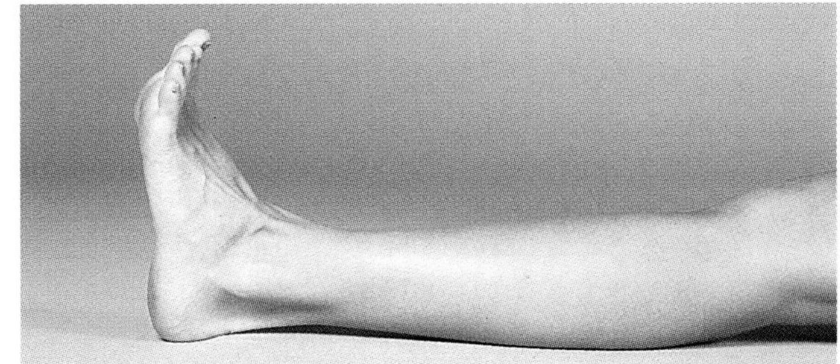

In passive stretching (left), an outside force—such as pressure exerted by another person—helps move the joint and stretch the muscles. In active stretching (right), the force to move the joint and stretch the muscles is provided by a contraction of the opposing muscles.

a ballistic stretch for the hamstrings. The problem with this technique is that the heightened activity of stretch receptors caused by the rapid stretches can continue for some time, possibly causing injuries during any physical activities that follow. For this reason, ballistic stretching is not recommended.

Proprioceptive Neuromuscular Facilitation As mentioned earlier, PNF techniques use reflexes initiated by muscle and joint receptors to cause greater training effects. The most popular PNF stretching technique is the contract-relax stretching method (usually requiring a partner), in which a muscle is contracted before it is stretched. For example, in a seated stretch of calf muscles, the first step in PNF is to contract the calf muscles: A partner can provide resistance for an isometric contraction. The second step is to stretch the calf muscles by pulling the tops of the feet toward the body. Although the contraction may cause a muscle to relax more so it can be stretched more effectively, PNF seems to cause more muscle stiffness and soreness than other stretching techniques; furthermore, it usually requires a partner and takes more time.

Passive and Active Stretching

Stretches can be done either passively or actively.

Passive Stretching In **passive stretching,** an outside force or resistance provided by yourself, a partner, gravity, or a weight helps your joints move through their range of motion. For example, a seated stretch of the hamstring and back muscles can be done by reaching the hands toward the feet until a "pull" is felt in those muscles. You can achieve a greater range of motion (a more intense stretch) using passive stretching. However, because the stretch is not controlled by the muscles themselves, there is a greater risk of injury. Communication between partners in passive stretching is very important so joints aren't forced outside their normal functional range of motion.

Active Stretching In **active stretching,** a muscle is stretched by a contraction of the opposing muscle (the muscle on the opposite side of the limb). For example, an active seated stretch of the calf muscles occurs when a person actively contracts the muscles on the top of the shin. The contraction of this opposing muscle produces a reflex that relaxes the muscles to be stretched. The muscle can be stretched farther with a low risk of injury.

The only disadvantage of active stretching is that a person may not be able to produce enough stress (enough stretch) to increase flexibility using only the contraction of opposing muscle groups. The safest and most convenient technique is active static stretching, with an occasional passive assist. For example, you might stretch your calves both by contracting the muscles on the top of your shin and by pulling your feet toward you. This way you combine the advantages of active stretching—safety and the relaxation reflex—with those of passive stretching—greater range of motion.

Intensity and Duration

For each exercise, slowly apply stretch to your muscles to the point of slight tension or mild discomfort. Hold the stretch for 15–30 seconds. As you hold the stretch, the feeling of slight tension should slowly subside; at that point, try to stretch a bit farther. Throughout the stretch, try to relax and breathe easily. Rest for about 30–60 seconds between each stretch, and do three to five repetitions of each stretch. A complete flexibility workout usually takes about 15–30 minutes.

TERMS

proprioceptive neuromuscular facilitation (PNF) A technique in which the inverse stretch reflex induces relaxation in a muscle prior to its being stretched, allowing for more stretch and more rapid development of joint flexibility.

static stretching A technique in which a muscle is slowly and gently stretched and then held in the stretched position.

ballistic stretching A technique in which muscles are stretched by the force generated as a body part is repeatedly bounced, swung, or jerked.

passive stretching A technique in which muscles are stretched by force applied by an outside source.

active stretching A technique in which muscles are stretched by the contraction of the opposing muscles.

Frequency

Do stretching exercises at least 3–5 days per week. It's best to stretch when your muscles are warm, so try incorporating stretching into your cool-down after cardiorespiratory endurance exercise or weight training. Stretching can also be a part of your warm-up, but it's best to increase the temperature of your muscles first by doing the active part of the warm-up (for example, walking or slow jogging).

Refer to the box "Safe Stretching" on p. 113 for additional tips on creating a safe and successful stretching program, and complete Lab 5-2 when you're ready to start your own program.

Exercises to Improve Flexibility

There are literally hundreds of exercises that can improve flexibility. Your program should include exercises that work all the major joints of the body by stretching their associated muscles. The exercises illustrated here are simple to do and pose a minimum risk of injury. Use these exercises, or substitute your favorite stretches, to create a well-rounded program for developing flexibility. Be sure to perform each stretch using the proper technique. Hold each position for 15–30 seconds, and repeat each exercise three to five times.

FLEXIBILITY EXERCISES

EXERCISE 1

Head Turns and Tilts

Areas stretched: Neck, upper back

Instructions:

Head turns: Turn your head to the right and hold the stretch. Repeat to the left.

Head tilts: Tilt your head to the left and hold the stretch. Repeat to the right.

Variation: Place your right palm on your right cheek; try to turn your head to the right as you resist with your hand. Repeat on the left side.

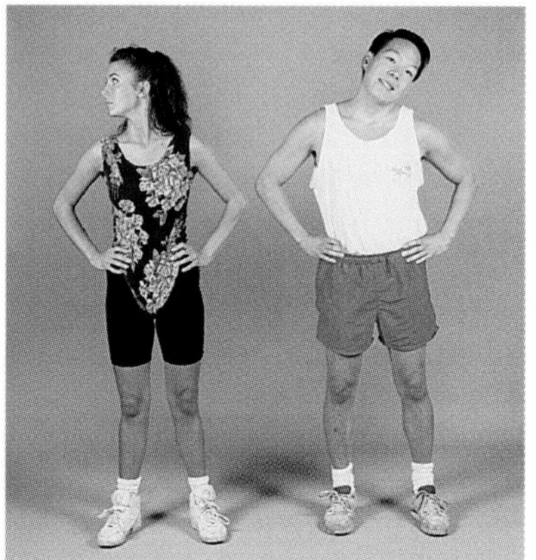

EXERCISE 2

Towel Stretch

Areas stretched: Triceps, shoulders, chest

Instructions: Roll up a towel and grasp it with both hands, palms down. With your arms straight, slowly lift it back over your head as far as possible. The closer together your hands are, the greater the stretch.

Variation: Repeat the stretch with your arms down and the towel behind your back. Grasp the towel with your palms forward and thumbs pointing out. Gently raise your arms behind your back.

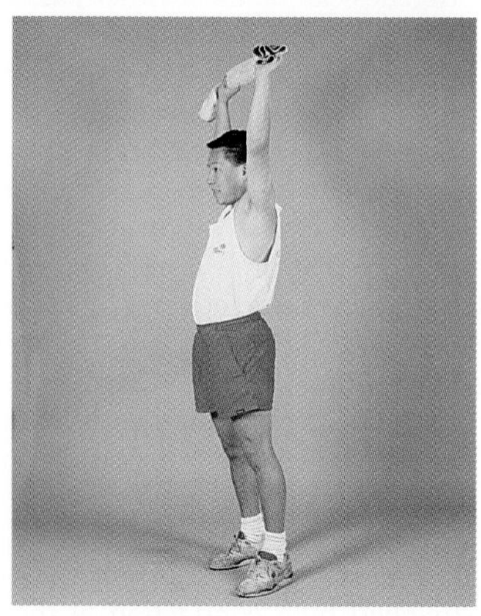

EXERCISE 3

Across-the-Body Stretch

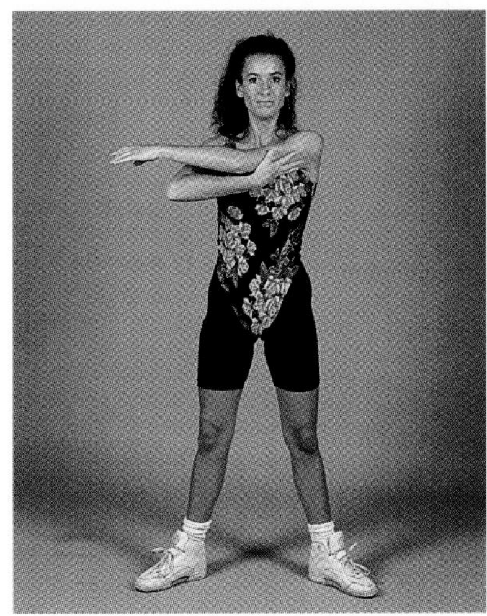

Areas stretched: Shoulders, upper back

Instructions: Keeping your back straight, cross your left arm in front of your body and grasp it with your right hand. Stretch your arm, shoulders, and back by gently pulling your arm as close to your body as possible. Repeat the stretch with your right arm.

Variation: Bend your right arm over and behind your head. Grasp your right hand with your left, and gently pull your arm until you feel the stretch. Repeat for your left arm.

EXERCISE 4

Upper-Back Stretch

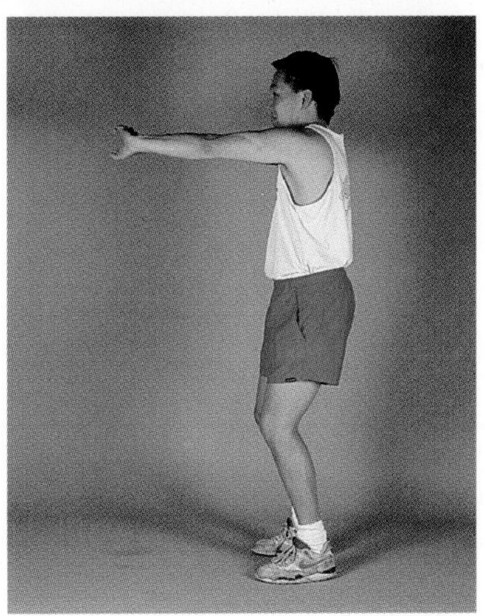

Areas stretched: Upper back

Instructions: Stand with your feet shoulder width apart, knees slightly bent, and pelvis tucked under. Clasp your hands in front of your body, and press your palms forward.

Variation: In the same position, wrap your arms around your body as if you were giving yourself a hug.

EXERCISE 5

Lateral Stretch

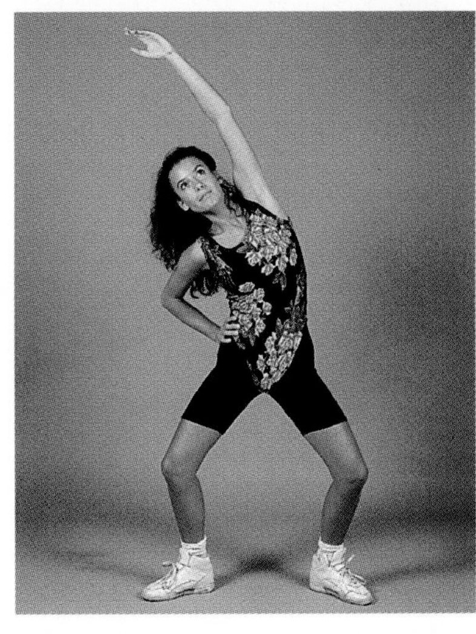

Areas stretched: Trunk muscles

Instructions: Stand with your feet shoulder width apart, knees slightly bent, and pelvis tucked under. Raise one arm over your head and bend sideways from the waist. Support your trunk by placing the hand or forearm of your other arm on your thigh or hip for support. Be sure you bend directly sideways, and don't move your body below the waist. Repeat on the other side.

Variation: Perform the same exercise in a seated position.

EXERCISE 6

Step Stretch

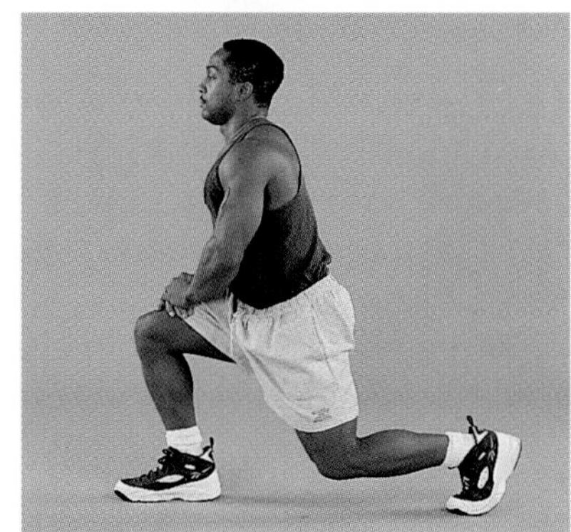

Areas stretched: Hip, front of thigh (quadriceps)

Instructions: Step forward and flex your forward knee, keeping your knee directly above your ankle. Stretch your other leg back so that it is parallel to the floor. Press your hips forward and down to stretch. Your arms can be at your sides, on top of your knee, or on the ground for balance. Repeat on the other side.

EXERCISE 7

Side Lunge

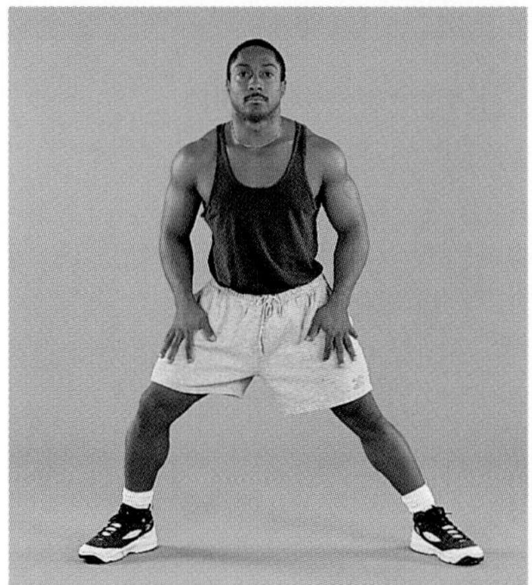

Areas stretched: Inner thigh, hip, calf

Instructions: Stand in a wide straddle with your legs turned out from your hip joints and your hands on your thighs. Lunge to one side by bending one knee and keeping the other leg straight. Keep your knee directly over your ankle; do not bend it more than 90 degrees. Repeat on the other side.

Variation: In the same position, lift the heel of the bent knee to provide additional stretch. The exercise may also be performed with your hands on the floor for balance.

EXERCISE 8

Sole Stretch

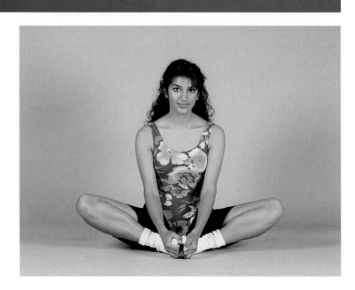

Areas stretched: Inner thigh, hip

Instructions: Sit with the soles of your feet together. Push your knees toward the floor using your hands or forearms.

Variation: When you first begin to push your knees toward the floor, use your legs to resist the movement. Then relax and press your knees down as far as they will go.

EXERCISE 9

Trunk Rotation

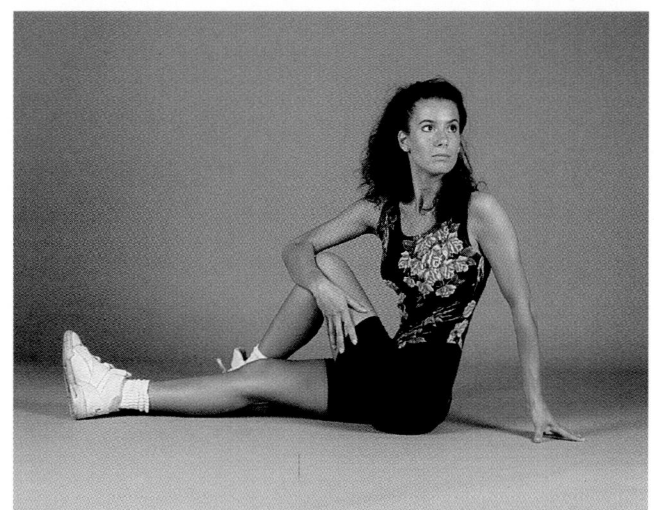

Areas stretched: Trunk, outer thigh and hip, lower back

Instructions: Sit with your right leg straight, left leg bent and crossed over the right knee, and left hand on the floor next to your left hip. Turn your trunk as far as possible to the left by pushing against your left leg with your right forearm or elbow. Keep your left foot on the floor. Repeat on the other side.

EXERCISE 10

Alternate Leg Stretcher

Areas stretched: Back of the thigh (hamstring), hip, knee, ankle, buttocks

Instructions: Lie flat on your back with both legs straight. **(a)** Grasp your left leg behind the thigh, and pull in to your chest. **(b)** Hold this position, then extend your left leg toward the ceiling. **(c)** Hold this position, then bring your left knee back to your chest and pull your toes toward your shin with your left hand. Stretch the back of the leg by attempting to straighten your knee. Repeat for the other leg.

Variation: Perform the stretch on both legs at the same time.

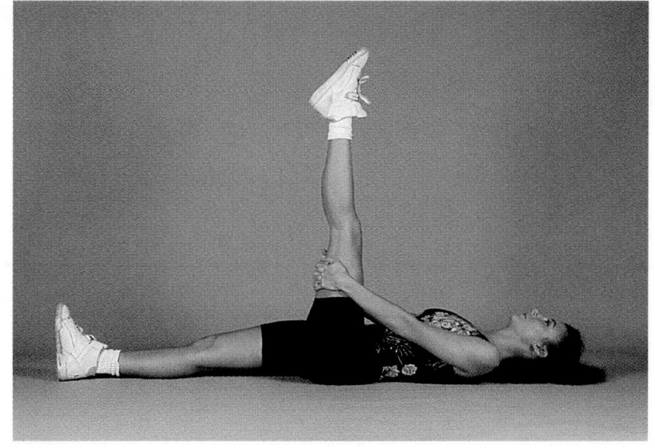

(b)

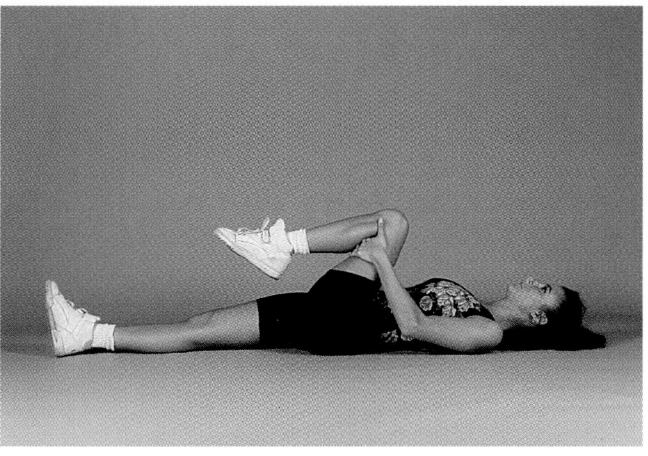

(a)

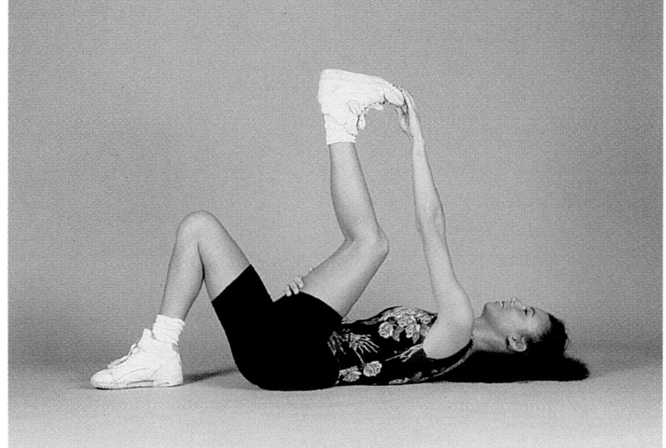

(c)

EXERCISE 11

Modified Hurdler Stretch (Seated Single-Toe Touch)

Areas stretched: Back of the thigh (hamstring), lower back

Instructions: Sit with your right leg straight and your left leg tucked close to your body. Reach toward your right foot as far as possible. Repeat for the other leg.

Variation: As you stretch forward, alternately flex and point the foot of your extended leg.

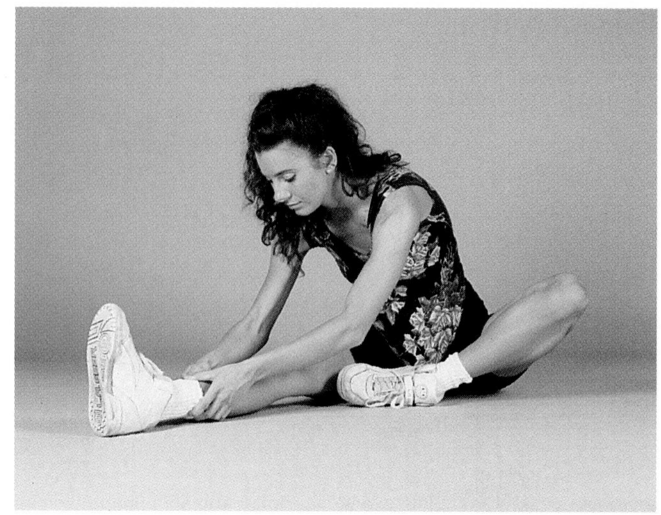

EXERCISE 12

Lower Leg Stretch

Areas stretched: Back of the lower leg (calf, soleus, Achilles tendon)

Instructions: Stand with one foot about 1–2 feet in front of the other, with both feet pointing forward.
(a) Keeping your back leg straight, lunge forward by bending your front knee and pushing your rear heel backward. Hold this position. **(b)** Then pull your back foot in slightly, and bend your back knee. Shift your weight to your back leg. Hold. Repeat on the other side.

Variation: Place your hands on a wall and extend one foot back, pressing your heel down to stretch; or stand with the balls of your feet on a step or bench and allow your heels to drop below the level of your toes.

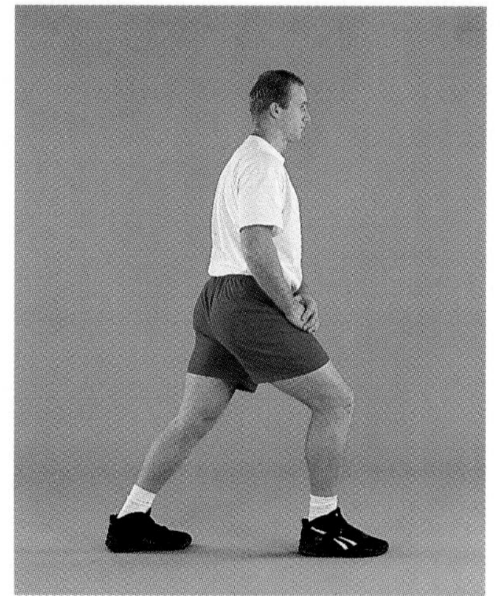

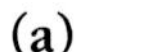

(a)

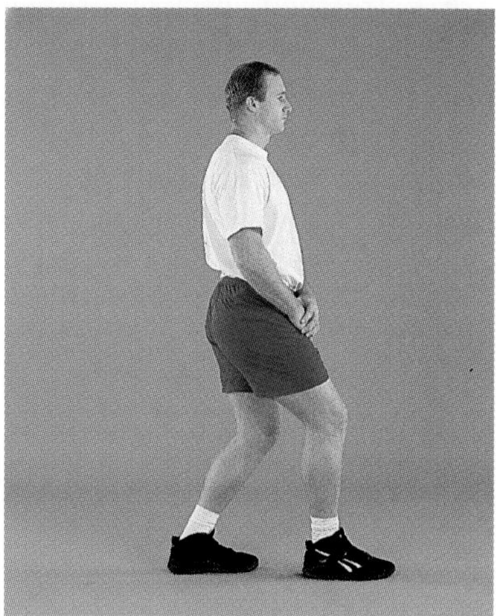

(b)

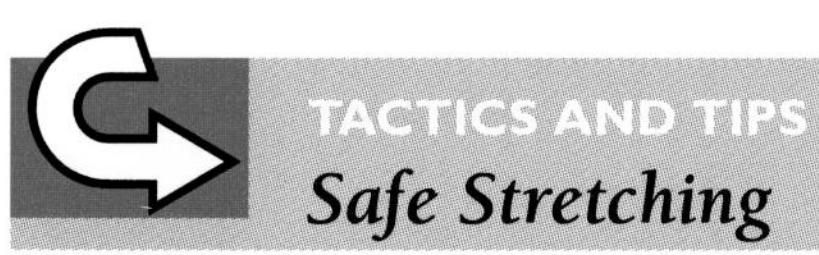

TACTICS AND TIPS

Safe Stretching

- Do stretching exercises statically. Stretch to the point of mild discomfort, and hold the position for 15–30 seconds, rest for 30–60 seconds, and repeat, trying to stretch a bit farther.
- Do not stretch until the point of pain.
- Relax and breathe easily as you stretch. Try to relax the muscles being stretched.
- Perform all exercises on both sides of your body.
- Increase your intensity and duration gradually over time. Improved flexibility takes many months to develop.
- Stretch when your muscles are warm. Do gentle warm-up exercises such as easy jogging or calisthenics before doing your pre-exercise stretching routine.
- There are large individual differences in joint flexibility. Don't feel you have to compete with others during stretching workouts.

PREVENTING AND MANAGING LOW-BACK PAIN

Over 85% of Americans will experience back pain at some time in their lives. Low-back pain is the second most common ailment in the United States—headache tops the list—and the second most common reason for absences from work. Low-back pain is estimated to cost as much as $50 billion per year in lost productivity, medical and legal fees, and disability insurance and compensation.

Back pain can result from sudden traumatic injuries, but it is more often the long-term result of weak and inflexible muscles, poor posture, or poor body mechanics during activities like lifting and carrying. Any abnormal strain on the back can result in pain. Most cases of low-back pain clear up on their own within a few weeks, but some people have recurrences or suffer from chronic pain.

Function and Structure of the Spine

The spinal column performs many important functions in the body:

- It provides structural support for the body, especially the thorax (upper-body cavity).
- It surrounds and protects the spinal cord.
- It supports much of the body's weight and transmits it to the lower body.
- It serves as an attachment site for a large number of muscles, tendons, and ligaments.
- It allows movement of the neck and back in all directions.

The spinal column is made up of bones called **vertebrae** (Figure 5-3). The spine consists of 7 cervical vertebrae in the neck, 12 thoracic vertebrae in the upper back, and 5 lumbar vertebrae in the lower back. The 9 vertebrae at the base of the spine are fused into two sections and form the sacrum and the coccyx (tailbone). The spine has four curves: the cervical, thoracic, lumbar, and sacral curves. These curves help bring the body weight supported by the spine in line with the axis of the body.

Although the structure of vertebrae depend on their location on the spine, the different types of vertebrae do share common characteristics. Each consists of a body, an arch, and several bony processes (Figure 5-4). The vertebral body is cylindrical, with flattened surfaces where **intervertebral disks** are attached. The vertebral body is designed to carry the stress of body weight and physical activity. The vertebral arch surrounds and protects the spinal cord. The bony processes serve as joints for adjacent vertebrae and attachment sites for muscles and ligaments. **Nerve roots** from the spinal cord pass through notches in the vertebral arch.

Intervertebral disks, which absorb and disperse the stresses placed on the spine, separate vertebrae from each other. Disks are made up of a gel- and water-filled nucleus surrounded by a series of fibrous rings. The liquid nucleus can change shape when it is compressed, allowing the disk to absorb shock. The intervertebral disks also help maintain the spaces between vertebrae where the spinal nerve roots are located.

TERMS

vertebrae Bony segments composing the spinal column that provide structural support for the body and protect the spinal cord.

intervertebral disk A tough, elastic disk located between adjoining vertebrae consisting of a gel- and water-filled nucleus surrounded by fibrous rings; it serves as a shock absorber for the spinal column.

nerve root The base of one of the 31 pairs of spinal nerves that branch off the spinal cord through spaces between vertebrae.

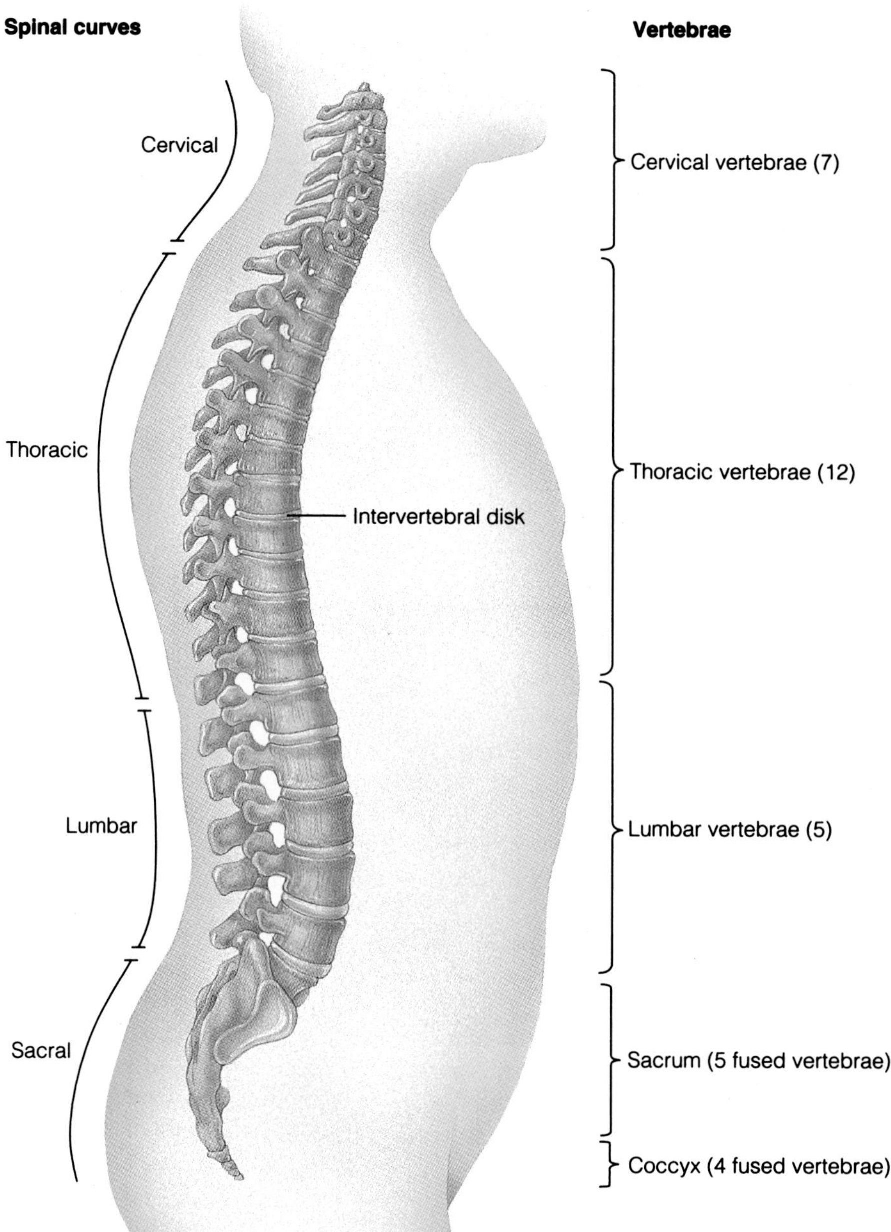

Figure 5-3 ***The spinal column.*** The spine is made up of five separate regions and has four distinct curves. An intervertebral disk is located between each vertebrae.

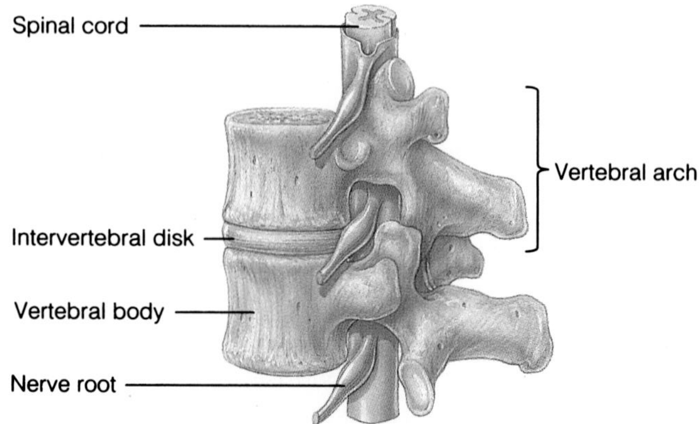

Figure 5-4 ***Vertebrae and an intervertebral disk.***

Causes of Back Pain

Back pain can occur at any point along your spine; the lumbar area, because it bears the majority of your weight, is the most common site. Any movement that causes excessive stress on the spinal column can cause injury and pain. The spine is well-equipped to bear body weight and the force or stress of body movements along its long axis. However, it is less capable of bearing loads at an angle to its long axis. You do not have to carry a heavy load or participate in a vigorous contact sport to injure your back. Picking a pencil up from the floor using poor body mechanics—reaching too far out in front of you or bending over with your knees straight, for example—can also result in back pain.

Underlying causes of back pain include weak or inflexible muscles in the back, hips, abdomen, and legs; excess body weight; poor posture when standing, sitting, or sleeping; and poor body mechanics when performing actions like lifting and carrying, or sports movements. Abnormal spinal loading resulting from any of these causes can have short-term or long-term direct and indirect effects on the spine. Strained muscles, tendons, or ligaments can cause pain and can, over time, lead to injuries to vertebrae or the intervertebral disks.

Stress can cause disks to break down and lose some of their ability to absorb shock. A damaged disk may bulge out between vertebrae and put pressure on a nerve root, a condition commonly referred to as a slipped disk. Painful pressure on nerves can also occur if damage to a disk narrows the space between two vertebrae. Depending on the amount of pressure on a nerve, symptoms may include numbness in the back, hip, leg, or foot; radiating pain; loss of muscle function; depressed reflexes; and muscle spasm. If the pressure is severe enough, loss of function can be permanent.

Preventing Low-Back Pain

Incorrect posture when standing, sitting, lying, and lifting is responsible for many back injuries. In general, think about moving your spine as a unit, with the force directed through its long axis. Strategies for maintaining good posture during daily activities are presented in the box "Avoiding Low-Back Pain" (p. 119). Follow the same guidelines for posture and movement when you engage in sports or recreational activities. Maintain control over your body movements, and warm up thoroughly before you exercise. Take special care when lifting weights as part of a strength training program. (Refer to Chapter 4 for more information on proper weight-lifting technique.)

To help maintain a healthy back, you should regularly perform exercises that stretch and strengthen the major muscle groups that affect your back. The following exercises focus on the key areas: the abdominal muscles, the muscles along your spine and sides, and the muscles of your hips and thighs. If you have back problems, check with your physician before beginning any exercise program. Perform the exercises slowly, and progress very gradually. Stop and consult your physician if any exercise causes back pain.

LOW-BACK EXERCISES

EXERCISE 1

Wall Stretch

Areas stretched: Back of thigh (hamstring), calf

Instructions: Sit on the floor with one leg extended and your foot flat against a wall or other immovable object. Bend the other leg and place your foot flat on the floor next to the knee of the straight leg. Clasp your hands behind your back or rest them loosely on the floor behind you. Bend forward from your hips, keeping your lower back flat and straight. Your bent knee can be moved slightly to the side to make room for your upper body as you lean forward. Repeat with the other leg.

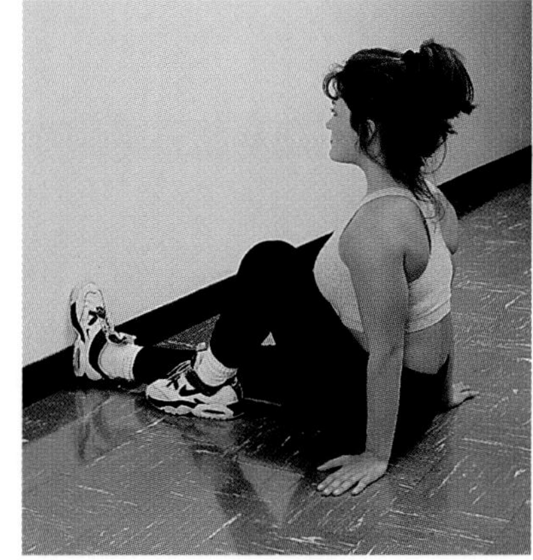

EXERCISE 2

Step Stretch (see Exercise 6 in the flexibility program)

EXERCISE 3

Alternate Leg Stretcher (see Exercise 10 in the flexibility program)

EXERCISE 4

Double Knee-to-Chest

Areas stretched: Lower back, hips

Instructions: Lie on your back with both knees bent and feet flat on the floor. **(a)** With one hand on the back of each thigh, slowly pull both knees to your chest; hold the stretch.

(b) Then straighten your knees so that both legs are extended toward the ceiling. Return to the starting position by drawing your legs back to your chest and then placing your feet on the floor.

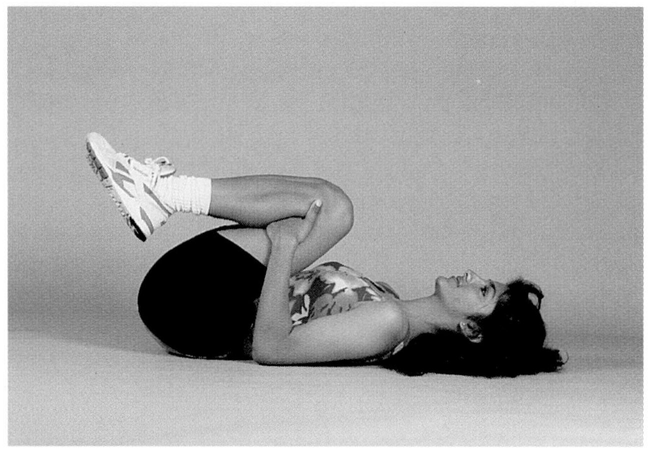

(a)

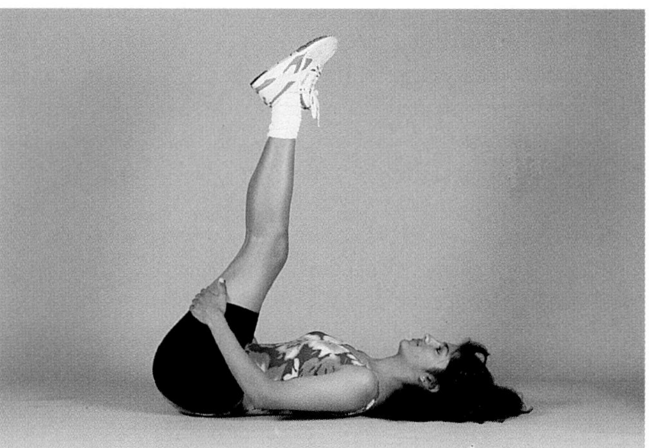

(b)

EXERCISE 5

Trunk Twist

Areas stretched: Lower back, sides

Instructions: Lie on your side with top knee bent, lower leg straight, lower arm extended out in front of you on the floor, and upper arm at your side. Push down with your upper knee while you twist your trunk backward. Try to get your shoulders and upper body flat on the floor, turning your head as well. Return to the starting position, then repeat on the other side.

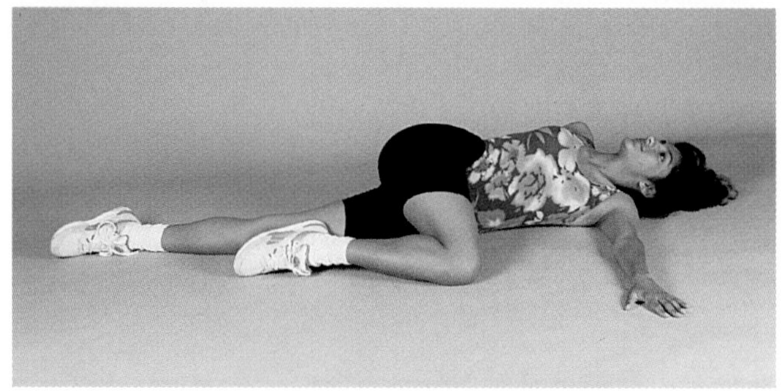

EXERCISE 6

Back Bridge

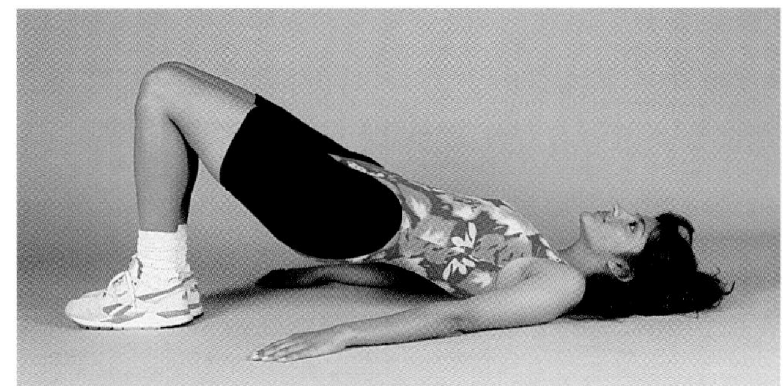

Areas strengthened: Hips, buttocks

Instructions: Lie on your back with knees bent and arms extended to the side. Tuck your pelvis under, then lift your tailbone, buttocks, and lower back from the floor. Hold this position for 5–10 seconds with your weight resting on your feet, arms, and shoulders, then return to the starting position. Work up to 10 repetitions of the exercise.

EXERCISE 7

Pelvic Tilt

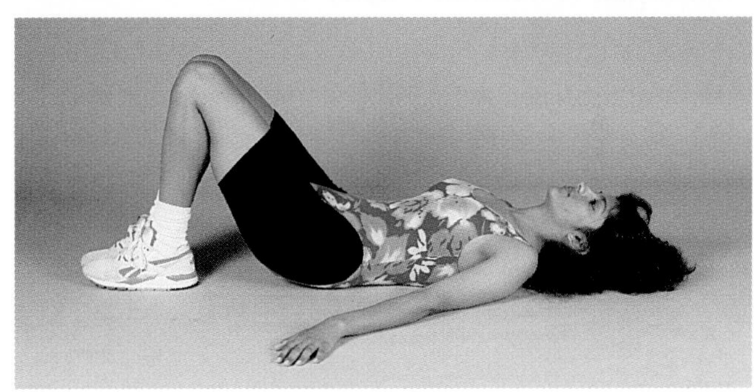

Areas strengthened: Abdomen, buttocks

Instructions: Lie on your back with knees bent and arms extended to the side. Tilt your pelvis under, and try to flatten your lower back against the floor. Tighten your buttock and abdominal muscles while you hold this position for 5–10 seconds. Don't hold your breath. Work up to 10 repetitions of the exercise. Pelvic tilts can also be done standing or leaning against a wall.

EXERCISE 8

Modified Sit-Up

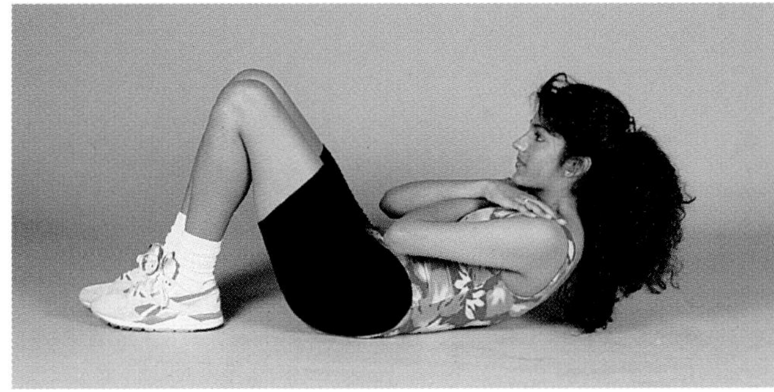

Areas strengthened: Abdomen

Instructions: Lie on your back with knees bent and arms crossed on your chest. Tilt your pelvis under, flattening your back. Tuck your chin in and slowly curl up, one vertebra at a time as you lift your head first and then your shoulders. Stop when you can see your heels, and hold for 5–10 seconds before returning to the starting position. Do 10 repetitions.

Variation: Add a twist to develop other abdominal muscles. When you have curled up so that your shoulder blades are off the floor, twist your upper body so that one shoulder is higher than the other; reach past your knee with your upper arm. Hold, then return to the starting position. Repeat on the opposite side.

EXERCISE 9

Press-Up

Areas stretched: Lower back, abdomen

Instructions: Lie face down with your hands under your face. Slowly push yourself up until your upper body is resting on your forearms. Relax and hold for 5–10 seconds. Gradually progress to straightening your elbows while keeping your pubic bone on the floor. (Stop if this exercise produces any pain.)

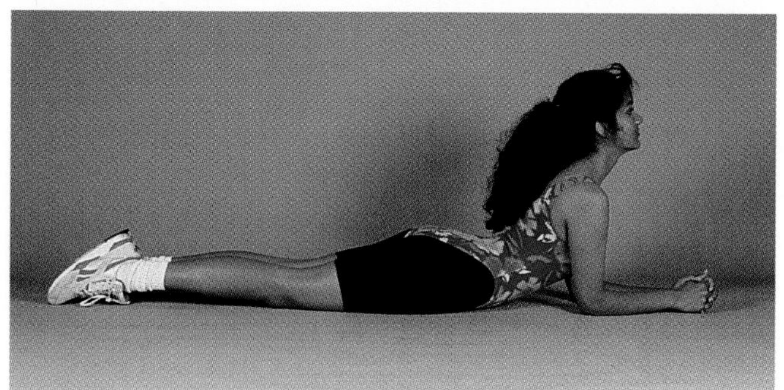

EXERCISE 10

Wall Squat (Phantom Chair)

Areas strengthened: Lower back, thighs, abdomen

Instructions: Lean against a wall and bend your knees as though you are sitting in a chair. Support your weight with your legs. Begin by holding the position for 5–10 seconds. Build up to 1 minute or more.

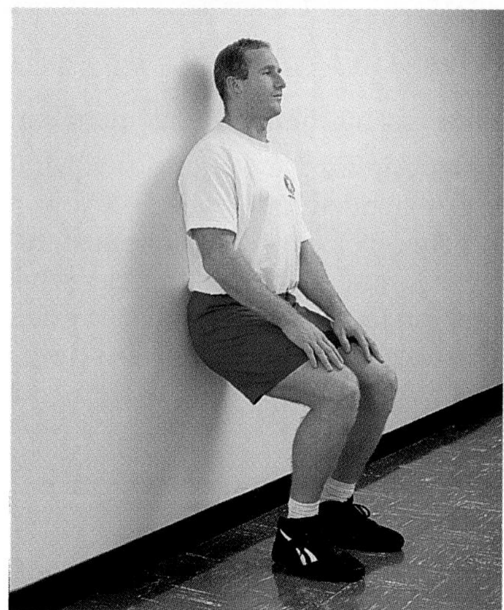

? COMMON QUESTIONS ANSWERED

Are there any stretching exercises I shouldn't do? Yes. Avoid exercises that put excessive pressure on your joints, particularly your spine and knees. Previous injuries and poor flexibility may make certain exercises dangerous for some people. Exercises that may cause problems are described in the box "Stretches to Avoid" (pp. 120–121).

Is stretching the same as warming up? People often confuse stretching and pre-exercise warm-up. While they are complementary, they're two distinct activities. A warm-up involves light exercise that increases body temperature so that your metabolism works better when you're exercising at high intensity. Stretching increases the movement capability of your joints, so you can move more easily, with less risk of injury.

Whenever you stretch, you should ideally first spend 5–10 minutes engaged in some form of low-intensity exercise, such as walking, jogging, or low-intensity calisthenics. When your muscles are warmed, then begin your stretching routine. Warmed muscles stretch better than cold ones and are less prone to injury.

Can I stretch too far? Yes. As muscle tissue is progressively stretched, it reaches a point where it becomes damaged and may rupture. The greatest danger occurs during passive stretching when a partner is doing the stretching for you. It is critical that your stretching partner not force your joint outside its normal functional range of motion.

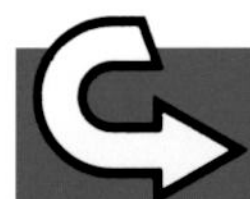

TACTICS AND TIPS

Avoiding Low-Back Pain

Changes in everyday behavior can help prevent and alleviate low-back pain.

- *Lying down.* When resting or sleeping, lie on your side with your knees and hips bent. If you lie on your back, place a pillow under your knees. Don't lie on your stomach. Sleep on a firm mattress, or place a plywood board under it.

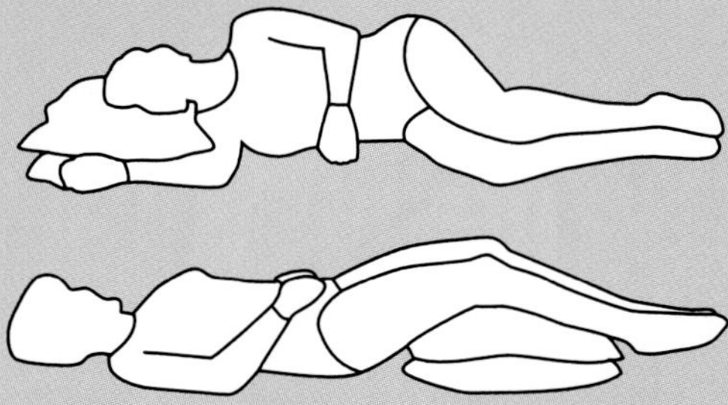

- *Sitting.* Sit with your lower back slightly rounded, knees bent, and feet flat on the floor. Alternate crossing your legs, or use a foot rest to keep your knees higher than your hips. If this position is uncomfortable or if your back flattens when you sit, try using a lumbar roll pillow behind your lower back.

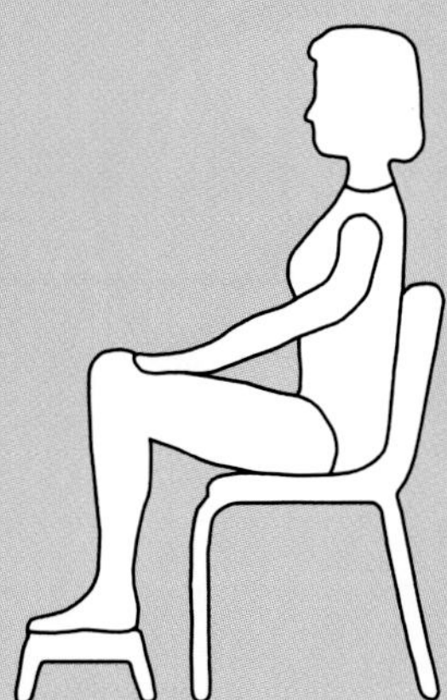

- *Lifting.* If you need to lower yourself to grasp an object, bend at the knees and hips rather than at the waist. Your feet should be shoulder width apart. Lift gradually, keeping your arms straight, by standing up or by pushing with your leg muscles. Keep the object close to your body. Don't twist; if you have to turn with the object, change the position of your feet.

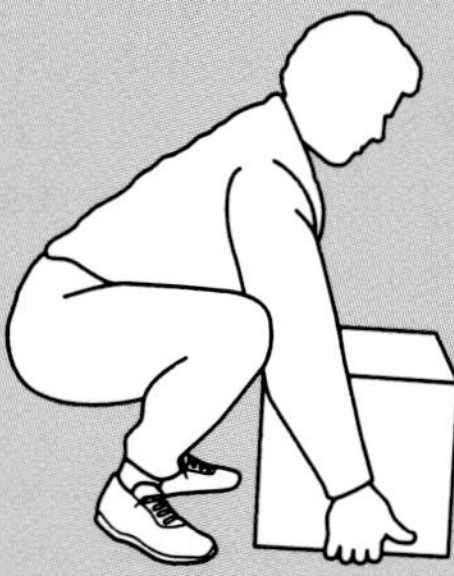

- *Standing.* When you are standing, a straight line should run from the top of your ear through the center of your shoulder, the center of your hip, the back of your kneecap, and the front of your ankle bone. Support your weight mainly on your heels, with one or both knees slightly bent. Try to keep your lower back flat by placing one foot on a stool. Don't let your pelvis tip forward or your back arch. Shift your weight back and forth from foot to foot. Avoid prolonged standing. (To check your posture, stand in a normal way with your back to a wall. Your upper back and buttocks should touch the wall; your heels may be a few inches away. Slide one hand into the space between your lower back and the wall. It should slide in easily but should almost touch both your back and the wall. Adjust your posture as needed, and try to hold this position as you walk away from the wall.)

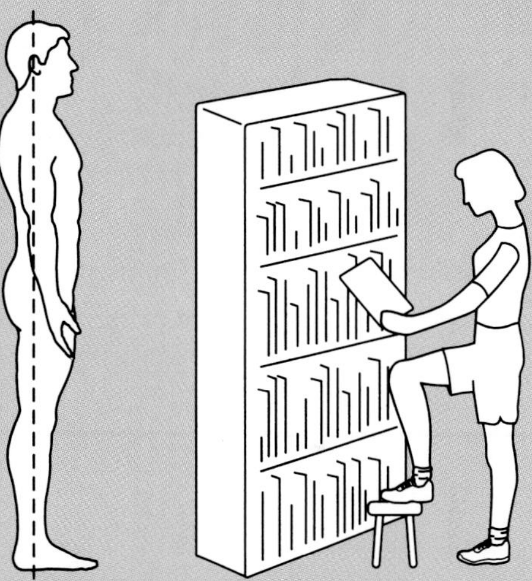

- *Walking.* Walk with your toes pointed straight ahead. Keep your back flat, head up, and chin in. Don't wear high-heeled shoes.

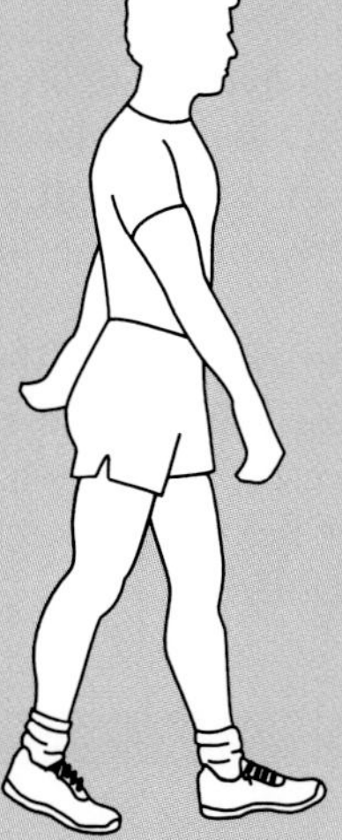

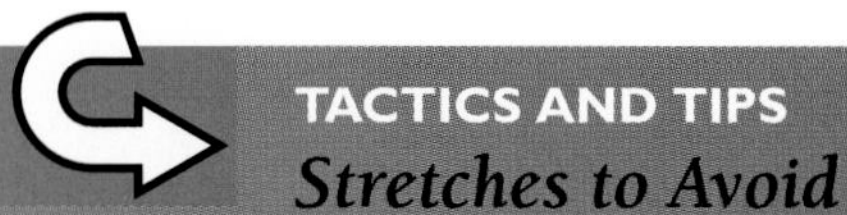

TACTICS AND TIPS
Stretches to Avoid

The safe alternatives listed here are described and illustrated on pp. 108–112 as part of the complete program of safe flexibility exercises presented in this chapter.

Standing Toe Touch

Problem: Puts excessive strain on the spine

Alternatives: Alternate leg stretcher (Exercise 10), modified hurdler stretch (Exercise 11), and lower leg stretch (Exercise 12)

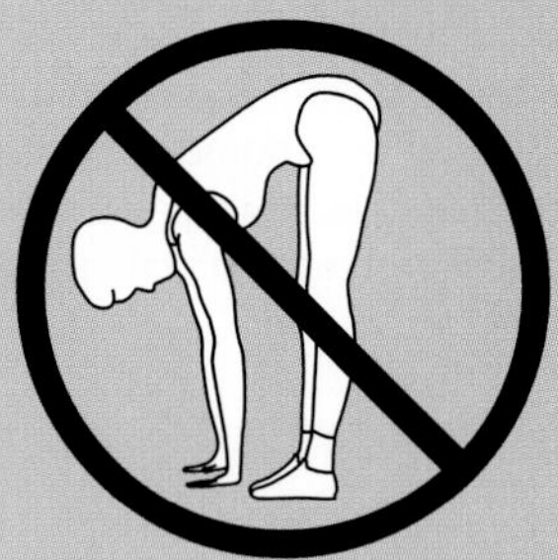

Standing Hamstring Stretch

Problem: Puts excessive strain on the knee and lower back

Alternatives: Alternate leg stretcher (Exercise 10) and modified hurdler stretch (Exercise 11)

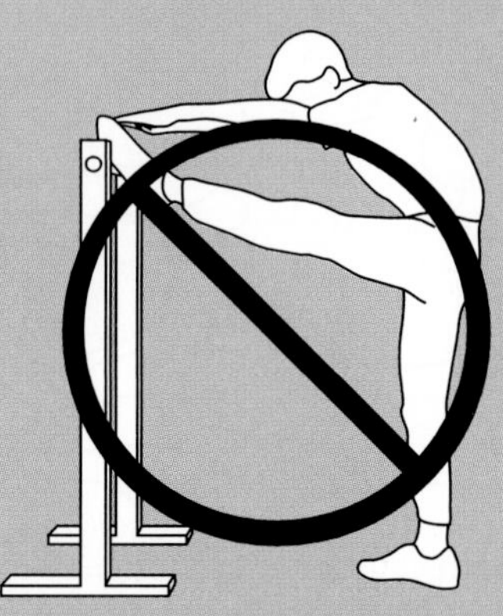

Standing Ankle-to-Buttocks Quadriceps Stretch ▶

Problem: Puts excessive strain on the ligaments of the knee

Alternative: Step stretch (Exercise 6)

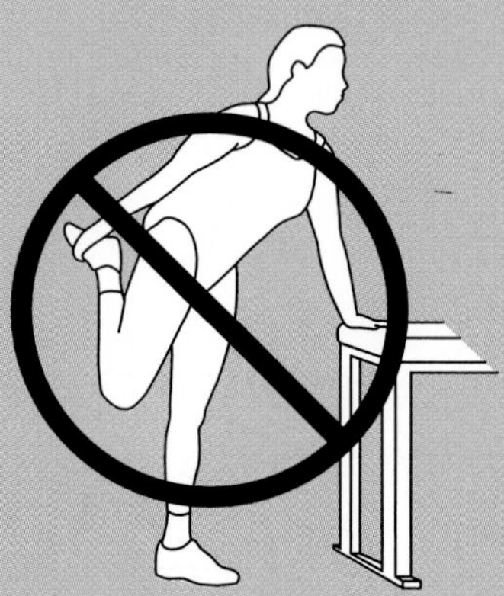

Does weight training limit flexibility? Weight training, or any physical activity, will decrease flexibility if the exercises are not performed through a full range of motion. When done properly, weight training increases flexibility.

Does jogging impair flexibility? Because of the limited range of motion used during the running stride, jogging tends to compromise flexibility. It is very important for runners to practice flexibility exercises for the hamstrings and quadriceps regularly.

SUMMARY

- Flexibility, the ability of joints to move through their full range of motion, is highly adaptable and specific to each joint.
- The benefits of flexibility include preventing abnormal stresses that lead to joint deterioration, helping maintain the correct curve of the lower back, keeping muscles from being overstretched, reducing delayed-onset muscle soreness, improving body position and therefore performance in sports, and facilitating strength development.
- Range of motion can be limited by joint structure and soft tissue obstructions, by limited muscle elasticity, and by stretch receptor activity.
- Developing flexibility depends on stretching the elastin within muscle regularly and gently until it lengthens. Overstretching can make collagenous tissue brittle and lead to rupture.
- Signals sent between stretch receptors and the spinal cord can enhance flexibility because contracting a

TACTICS AND TIPS
Stretches to Avoid (continued)

Hurdler Stretch

Problem: Turning out the bent leg can put excessive strain on the ligaments of the knee

Alternative: Modified hurdler stretch (Exercise 11)

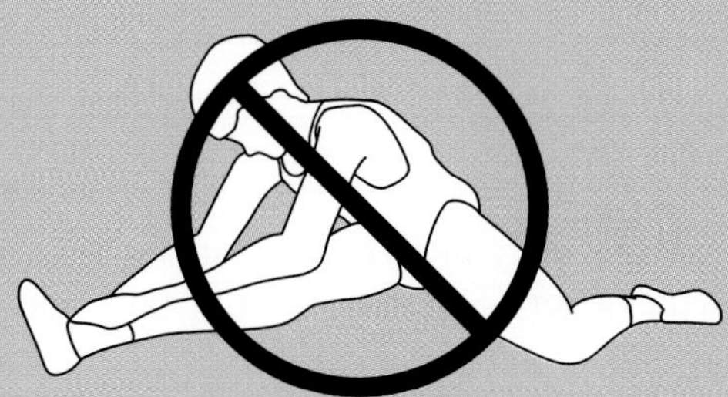

Prone Arch

Problem: Puts excessive strain on the spine, knees, and shoulders

Alternatives: Towel stretch (Exercise 2) and step stretch (Exercise 6)

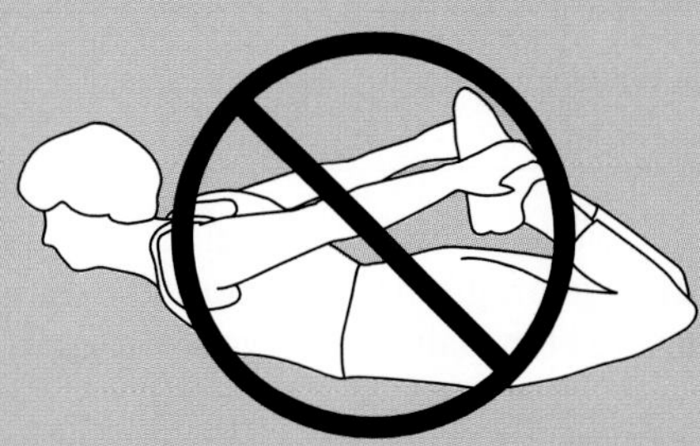

Full Squat

Problem: Puts excessive strain on the ankles, knees, and spine

Alternatives: Alternate leg stretcher (Exercise 10) and lower leg stretch (Exercise 12)

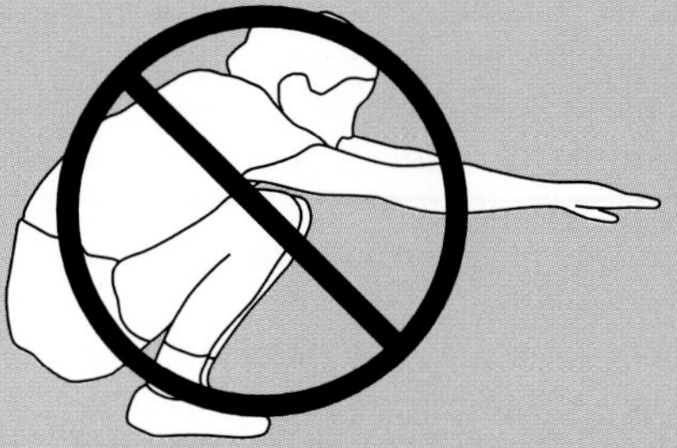

Yoga Plow

Problem: Puts excessive strain on the neck, shoulders, and back

Alternatives: Head turns and tilts (Exercise 1), across-the-body stretch (Exercise 3), and upper-back stretch (Exercise 4)

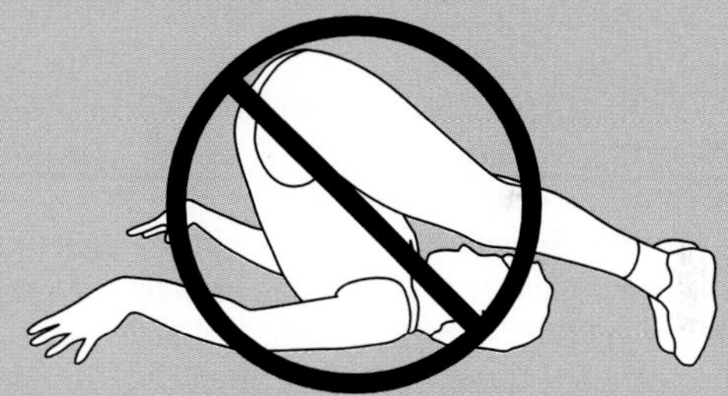

muscle stimulates a relaxation response, thereby allowing a longer muscle stretch, and because stretch receptors become less sensitive after repeated stretches, initiating fewer contractions.

- The sit-and-reach test is most often used to assess flexibility; comparisons can also be made to a chart showing normal range of motion for major joints.
- Static stretching is done slowly and held to the point of mild tension; ballistic stretching consists of bouncing stretches and can lead to injury. Proprioceptive neuromuscular facilitation uses muscle receptors in contracting and relaxing a muscle.
- Passive stretching, using an outside force in moving muscles and joints, achieves a greater range of motion (and has a higher injury risk) than active stretching, which uses opposing muscles to initiate a stretch.
- Stretches should be held for 15–30 seconds once the point of slight tension has been reached; the stretch can be increased if tension subsides. Three to five repetitions are best.
- Flexibility training should be done 3–5 days a week, preferably as part of the cool-down after cardiorespiratory endurance or weight training exercise.
- The spinal column consists of vertebrae separated by intervertebral disks. It provides structure and support for the body and protects the spinal cord.
- In addition to good posture and proper body mechanics, a program for preventing low-back pain includes exercises that stretch and strengthen major muscle groups that affect the lower back.

BEHAVIOR CHANGE ACTIVITY

Choosing Rewards

Make a list of objects, activities, and events you can use as rewards for achieving the goals of your behavior change program. Rewards should be special, relatively inexpensive, and preferably unrelated to food or alcohol; for example, a ball game, a CD, or a long-distance phone call to a family member or friend—whatever is meaningful for you. Write down a variety of rewards you can use when you reach milestones in your program and your final goal.

________________	________________
________________	________________
________________	________________
________________	________________

Many people also find it helpful to give themselves small, real rewards daily or weekly for sticking with their behavior change program. These could be things like a study break, a movie, or a Saturday morning bike ride. Make a list of rewards for maintaining your program in the short-term.

________________	________________
________________	________________
________________	________________
________________	________________

And don't forget to congratulate yourself with a pat on the back regularly during your behavior change program. Notice how much better you feel, and savor how far you've come and how you've gained control of your behavior.

FOR MORE INFORMATION

Alter, M. J. 1988. *The Science of Stretching.* Champaign, Ill.: Human Kinetics. *Includes a complete discussion of the scientific basis and correct techniques of stretching.*

Anderson, B. 1980. *Stretching.* Bolinas, Calif.: Shelter Publications. *A complete guide to stretching that includes stretching programs for general fitness, specific sports, and back care.*

Lycholat, T. 1995. *The Complete Book of Stretching,* 2d ed. Wiltshire, Eng.: Crowood. *A comprehensive guide to stretching exercises for the whole body.*

Sobel, D., and A. C. Klein. 1994. *Backache: What Exercises Work.* New York: St. Martin's. *A complete program of exercises for different conditions, along with help for living with back pain.*

Tobias, M., and J. P. Sullivan. 1994. *Complete Stretching.* New York: Knopf. *An excellent introduction to stretching exercises.*

SELECTED BIBLIOGRAPHY

American College of Sports Medicine. 1995. *Guidelines for Exercise Testing and Prescription,* 5th ed. Baltimore: Williams & Wilkins.

American Medical Association. 1995. *The AMA Pocket Guide to Back Pain.* New York: Random House.

Bandy, W. D., and J. M. Irion. 1994. The effect of time on static stretch on the flexibility of the hamstring muscles. *Physical Therapy* 74:845–852.

Brooks, G. A., T. D. Fahey, and T. White. 1996. *Exercise Physiology: Human Bioenergetics and Its Applications,* 2d ed. Mountain View, Calif.: Mayfield.

Hutton, R. S. 1992. Neuromuscular basis of stretching exercises. In *Strength and Power in Sport,* ed. P. V. Komi. London: Blackwell Scientific Publications.

Jonhagen, S., G. Nemeth, and E. Eriksson. 1994. Hamstring injuries in sprinters: The role of concentric and eccentric hamstring muscle strength and flexibility. *American Journal of Sports Medicine* 22:262–266.

Knapik, J. J., et al. 1992. Strength, flexibility and athletic injuries. *Sports Medicine* 14:277–288.

Kraines, M. G., and E. Pryor. 1997. *Jump into Jazz,* 3d ed. Mountain View, Calif.: Mayfield.

MacDougall, J. D. 1992. *Physiological Testing of the High-Performance Athlete,* 2d ed. Champaign, Ill.: Human Kinetics.

Mills, E. M. 1994. The effect of low-intensity aerobic exercise on muscle strength, flexibility, and balance among sedentary elderly persons. *Nursing Research* 43:207–211.

Osternig, L. R., et al. 1990. Differential responses to proprioceptive neuromuscular facilitation (PNF) stretch techniques. *Medicine and Science in Sports and Exercise* 22:106–111.

Smith, C. A. 1994. The warm-up procedure: To stretch or not to stretch. A brief review. *Journal of Orthopedic and Sports Physical Therapy* 19:12–17.

Sutarno, C. G., and S. M. McGill. 1995. Isovelocity investigation of the lengthening behaviour of the erector spinae muscles. *European Journal of Applied Physiology* 70:146–153.

Voigt, M., E. B. Simonsen, P. Dyhre-Poulsen, and K. Klausen. 1995. Mechanical and muscular factors influencing the performance in maximal vertical jumping after different prestretch loads. *Journal of Biomechanics* 28:293–307.

Vujnovich, A. L., and N. J. Dawson. 1994. The effect of therapeutic muscle stretch on neural processing. *Journal of Orthopedic and Sports Physical Therapy* 20:145–153.

Name ____________________ Section ____________ Date 

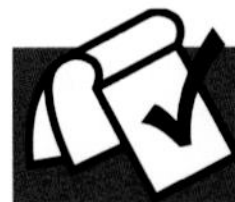

LAB 5-1 *Assessing Your Current Level of Flexibility*

Part 1. Sit-and-Reach Test

Equipment

A flexibility box or measuring device (see photograph). If you make your own measuring device, use two pieces of wood 12 inches high attached at right angles to each other. Use a ruler or yardstick to measure the extent of reach. Set the footline at 6 inches.

Preparation

Warm up your muscles with some low-intensity activity such as walking or easy jogging.

Instructions

1. Remove your shoes, and sit facing the flexibility box with your knees fully extended and your feet about 4 inches apart. Your feet should be flat against the box.
2. Reach as far forward as you can, with palms down and one hand placed on top of the other. Hold the position of maximum reach for 1–2 seconds. Keep your knees locked at all times.
3. Repeat the stretch two times. Your score is the most distant point reached with the fingertips of both hands on the third trial, measured to the nearest quarter of an inch.

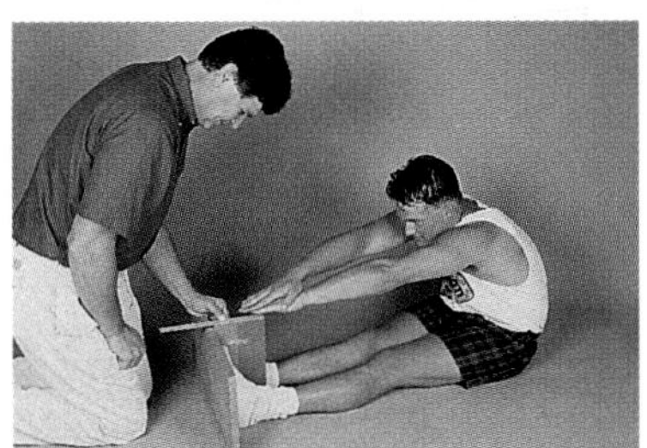

The sit-and-reach test.

Footline of your box: ____________ in.   Score of third trial: ____________ in.

Rating Your Flexibility

Find your score in the table below to determine your flexibility rating.

Rating: ____________

Ratings for Sit-and-Reach Test

	Rating/Score (in.)*				
Men	*Very Poor*	*Poor*	*Moderate*	*High*	*Very High*
Age: 15–19	Below 5.25	5.25–6.75	7.00–8.75	9.00–10.75	Above 10.75
20–29	Below 5.50	5.50–7.00	7.25–8.75	9.00–11.00	Above 11.00
30–39	Below 4.75	4.75–6.50	6.75–8.50	8.75–10.25	Above 10.25
40–49	Below 2.75	2.75–5.00	5.25–6.75	7.00–9.25	Above 9.25
50–59	Below 2.00	2.00–5.00	5.25–6.50	6.75–9.25	Above 9.25
60 and over	Below 1.75	1.75–3.25	3.50–5.25	5.50–8.50	Above 8.50
Women					
Age: 15–19	Below 7.25	7.25–8.75	9.00–10.50	10.75–12.25	Above 12.25
20–29	Below 6.75	6.75–8.50	8.75–10.00	10.25–11.50	Above 11.50
30–39	Below 6.50	6.50–8.00	8.25–9.50	9.75–11.50	Above 11.50
40–49	Below 5.50	5.50–7.25	7.50–8.75	9.00–10.50	Above 10.50
50–59	Below 5.50	5.50–7.25	7.50–8.50	8.75–10.75	Above 10.75
60 and over	Below 4.75	4.75–6.00	6.25–7.75	8.00–9.25	Above 9.25

*Footline is set at 6 inches.

Source: Adapted from Fitness Canada. 1986. *CSTF Operations Manual,* 3d ed. Ottowa: Fitness and Amateur Sport. The Canadian Standardized Test of Fitness was developed by, and is reproduced with permission of, Fitness Canada, Government of Canada.

Part 2. Range-of-Motion Assessment

This portion of the lab can be completed by doing visual comparisons or by measuring joint range of motion with a goniometer or other instrument.

Equipment

1. A partner to do visual comparisons or to measure the range of motion of your joints. (You can also use a mirror to perform your own visual comparisons.)
2. For the measurement method, you need a goniometer, flexometer, or other instrument to measure range of motion.

Preparation

None

Instructions

A. *Visual comparison method:* On the following pages, the average range of motion is illustrated for some of the major joints. Compare the range of motion in your joints to that shown in the illustration. For each joint, note (with a check mark) whether your range of motion is average or greater or needs improvement.

B. *Measurement method:* Measure the appropriate range of motion with a goniometer, flexometer, or other instrument. Record your range of motion in degrees, and find your rating in the appropriate table. (Ratings are taken from several published sources.)

For both methods, record your scores on the following pages and on the chart on the final page of this lab.

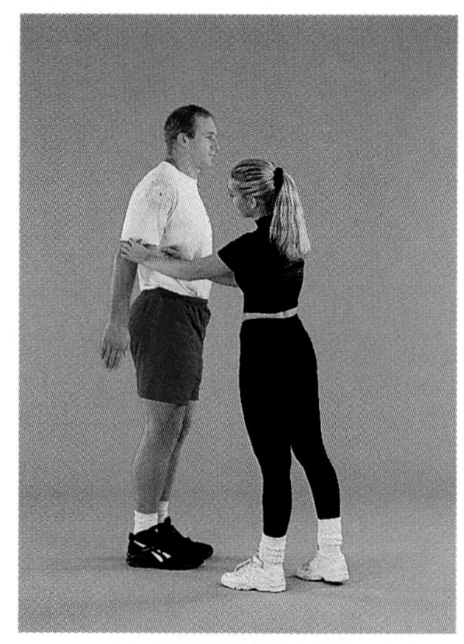

Assessment of range of motion using a goniometer.

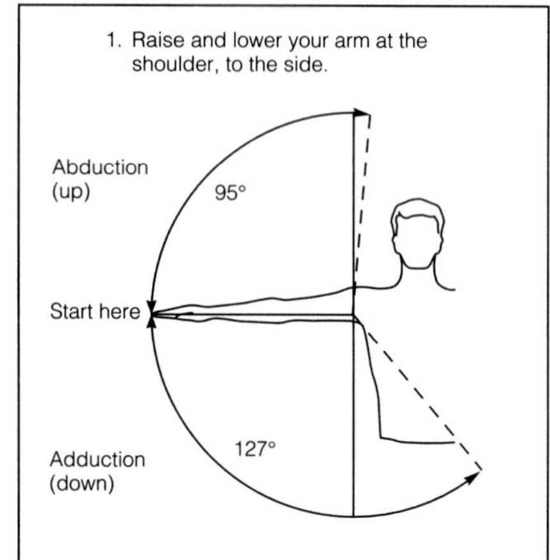
1. Raise and lower your arm at the shoulder, to the side.
Abduction (up)
95°
Start here
Adduction (down)
127°

A. Comparison Method (✓)

Abduction: Average or above ______ Needs improvement ______

Adduction: Average or above ______ Needs improvement ______

B. Measurement Method

Abduction: ______ ° Rating: ____________

Adduction: ______ ° Rating: ____________

Ratings

	Abduction	*Adduction*
Below average	<92°	<124°
Average	92°–95°	124°–127°
Above average	96°–99°	128°–130°
Excellent	>99°	>130°

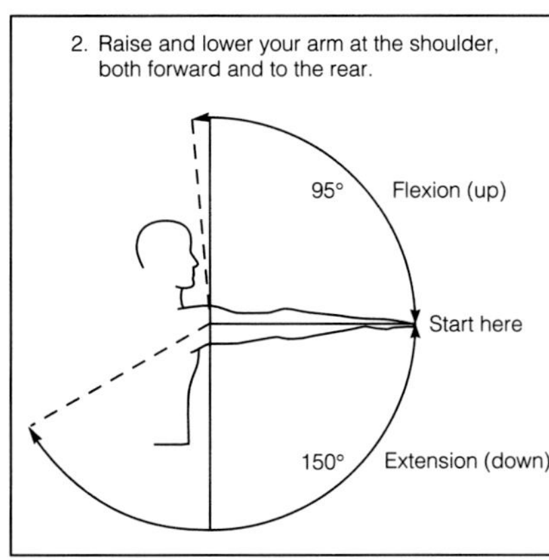
2. Raise and lower your arm at the shoulder, both forward and to the rear.
95°
Flexion (up)
Start here
150°
Extension (down)

A. Comparison Method (✓)

Flexion: Average or above ______ Needs improvement ______

Extension: Average or above ______ Needs improvement ______

B. Measurement Method

Flexion: ______ ° Rating: ____________

Extension: ______ ° Rating: ____________

Ratings

	Flexion	*Extension*
Below average	<92°	<145°
Average	92°–95°	145°–150°
Above average	96°–99°	151°–156°
Excellent	>99°	>156°

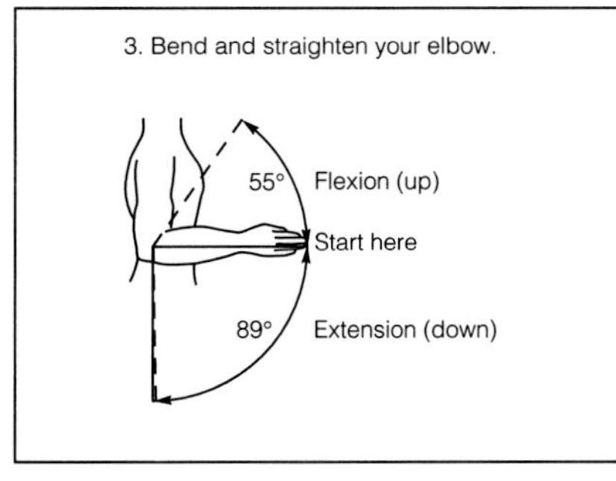
3. Bend and straighten your elbow.
55°
Flexion (up)
Start here
89°
Extension (down)

A. Comparison Method (✓)

Flexion: Average or above ______ Needs improvement ______

Extension: Average or above ______ Needs improvement ______

B. Measurement Method

Flexion: ______ ° Rating: ____________

Extension: ______ ° Rating: ____________

Ratings

	Flexion	*Extension*
Below average	<51°	<88°
Average	51°–55°	88°–89°
Above average	56°–60°	90°–91°
Excellent	>60°	>91°

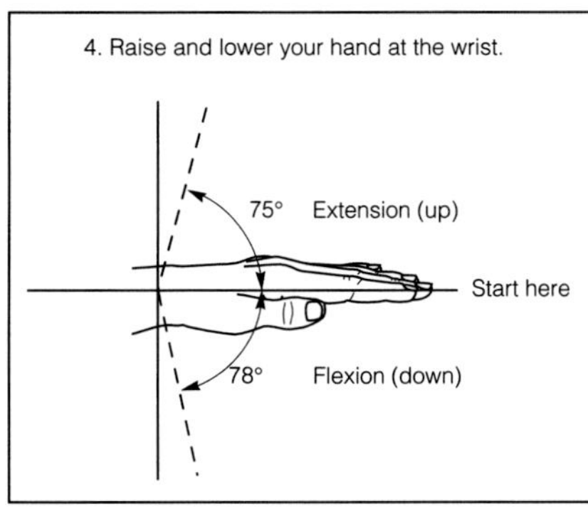
4. Raise and lower your hand at the wrist.
75°
Extension (up)
Start here
78°
Flexion (down)

A. Comparison Method (✓)

Extension: Average or above ______ Needs improvement ______

Flexion: Average or above ______ Needs improvement ______

B. Measurement Method

Extension: ______ ° Rating: ____________

Flexion: ______ ° Rating: ____________

Ratings

	Extension	*Flexion*
Below average	<70°	<73°
Average	70°–75°	73°–78°
Above average	76°–81°	79°–84°
Excellent	>81°	>84°

LABORATORY ACTIVITIES

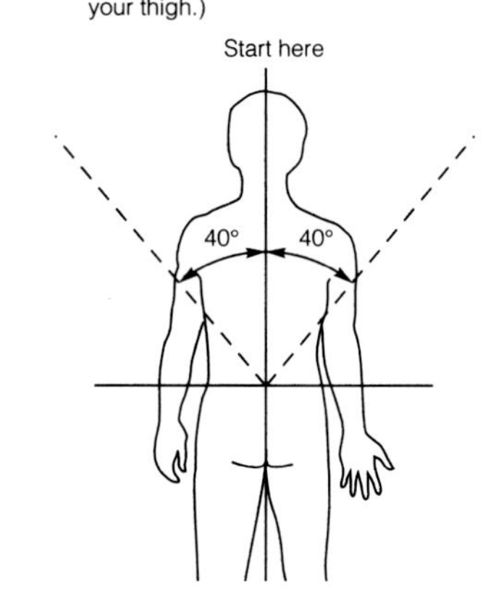

5. Bend directly sideways at your waist. (To prevent injury, keep your knees slightly bent, and support your trunk by placing your hand or forearm on your thigh.)
Start here
40°
40°

A. Comparison Method (✓)

Right lateral flexion: Average or above ______ Needs improvement ______

Left lateral flexion: Average or above ______ Needs improvement ______

B. Measurement Method:

Right lateral flexion: ______ ° Rating: ____________

Left lateral flexion: ______ ° Rating: ____________

Ratings

	Right or Left Lateral Flexion
Below average	<36°
Average	36°–40°
Above average	41°–45°
Excellent	>45

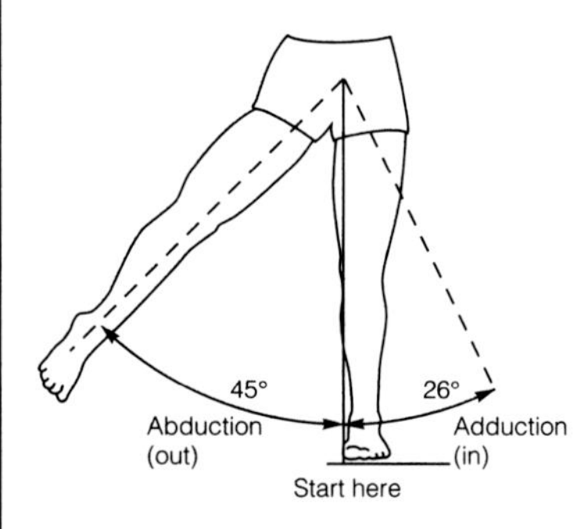

6. Raise leg to the side at the hip.

A. Comparison Method (✓)

Abduction: Average or above ______ Needs improvement ______

Adduction: Average or above ______ Needs improvement ______

B. Measurement Method

Abduction: ______ ° Rating: ____________

Adduction: ______ ° Rating: ____________

Ratings

	Abduction	*Adduction*
Below average	<40°	<23°
Average	40°–45°	23°–26°
Above average	46°–51°	27°–30°
Excellent	>51°	>30°

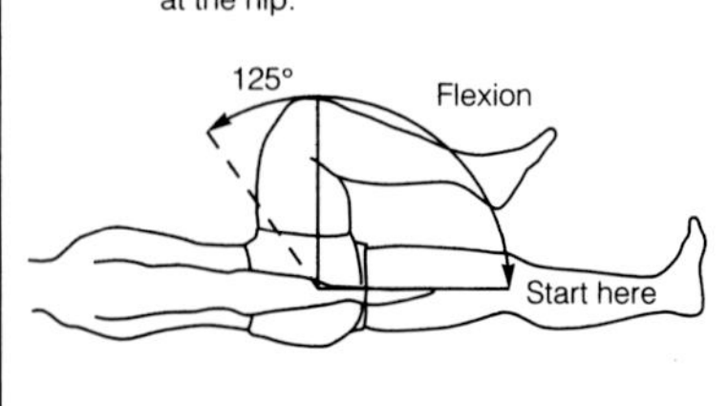

7. Raise and lower your leg forward at the hip.
125°
Flexion
Start here

A. Comparison Method (✓)

Average or above ______ Needs improvement ______

B. Measurement Method

Flexion: ______ ° Rating: ____________

Ratings

	Flexion
Below average	<121°
Average	121°–125°
Above average	126°–130°
Excellent	>130°

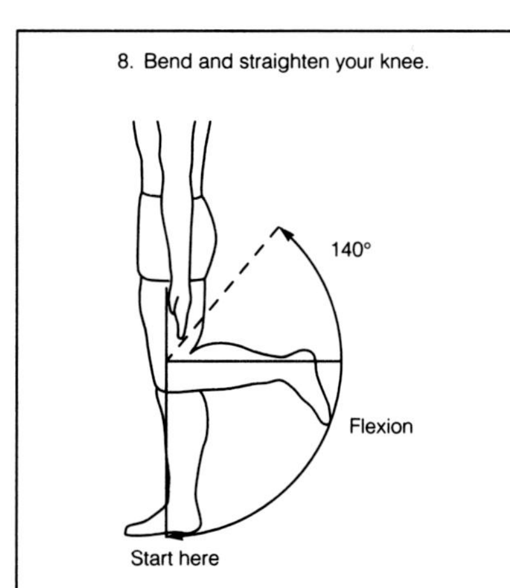

A. Comparison Method (✓)

Average or above ______ Needs improvement ______

B. Measurement Method

Flexion: ______ ° Rating: ___________

Ratings

	Flexion
Below average	<136°
Average	136°–140°
Above average	141°–145°
Excellent	>145°

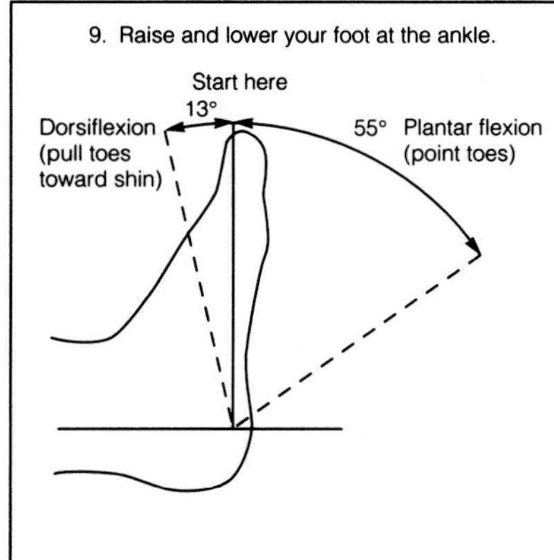

A. Comparison Method (✓)

Dorsiflexion: Average or above ______ Needs improvement ______

Plantar flexion: Average or above ______ Needs improvement ______

B. Measurement Method

Dorsiflexion: ______ ° Rating: ___________

Plantar flexion: ______ ° Rating: ___________

Ratings

	Dorsiflexion	*Plantar flexion*
Below average	<9°	<50°
Average	9°–13°	50°–55°
Above average	14°–17°	56°–60°
Excellent	>17°	>60°

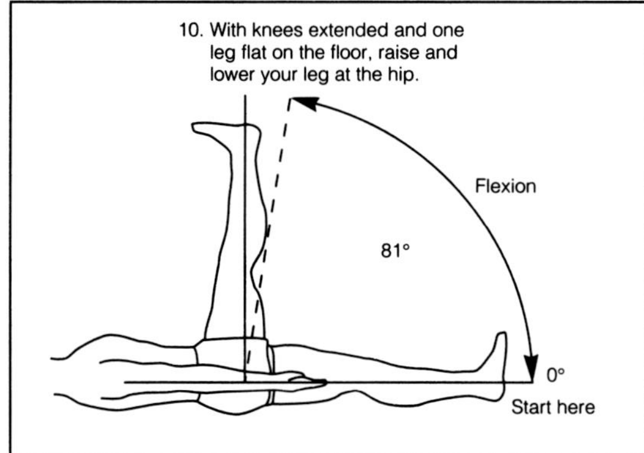

10. With knees extended and one leg flat on the floor, raise and lower your leg at the hip.
Flexion
81°
0°
Start here

A. Comparison Method (✓)

Average or above ______ Needs improvement ______

B. Measurement Method

Flexion: ______ ° Rating: ___________

Ratings

	Flexion
Below average	<79°
Average	79°–81°
Above average	82°–84°
Excellent	>84°

LABORATORY ACTIVITIES

Rating Your Flexibility

Sit-and-reach test result: ___________ in. Rating: ___________

Range of Motion Assessment

Joint		*Average ROM*	*Comparison Method (✓)* *Average or above*	*Needs improvement*	*Measurement Method* *Current range of motion (°)*	*Rating*
Shoulder (side-to-side)	Abduction	95°				
	Adduction	127°				
Shoulder (front-to-back)	Flexion	95°				
	Extension	150°				
Elbow (up-and-down)	Flexion	55°				
	Extension	89°				
Wrist (up-and-down)	Extension	75°				
	Flexion	78°				
Low back (side-to-side)	Right flexion	40°				
	Left flexion	40°				
Hip (side-to-side)	Abduction	45°				
	Adduction	26°				
Hip (bent knee)	Flexion	125°				
Knee	Flexion	140°				
Ankle	Dorsiflexion	13°				
	Plantar flexion	55°				
Hip (straight knee)	Flexion	81°				

To monitor your progress toward your goal, enter the results of this lab in the Preprogram Assessment column of Lab 15-2. After following the stretching program for several weeks, do this lab again, and enter the results in the Postprogram Assessment column of Lab 15-2. How do the results compare?

Name ______________________ Section ______________ Date ______________

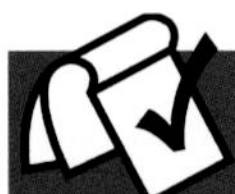

LAB 5-2 *Creating a Personalized Program for Developing Flexibility*

Complete the program plan below, and start on your flexibility program.

Exercises: The exercises contained in the program plan below are those from the general stretching program presented in Chapter 5. You can add or delete exercises depending on your needs, goals, and preferences. For any exercises you add, fill in the areas of the body affected.

Frequency: You may want to do your stretching exercises the same day you plan to do cardiorespiratory endurance exercise or weight training, because stretching is recommended after exercise and muscles stretch better when they are warm.

Intensity: All stretches should be done to the point of mild discomfort, not pain.

Duration: All stretches should be held for 15–30 seconds.

Repetitions: All stretches should be repeated 3–5 times.

Program Plan for Flexibility

Exercise	Areas Stretched	Frequency						
		M	T	W	Th	F	Sa	Su
Head turns and tilts	Neck, upper back							
Towel stretch	Triceps, shoulders, chest							
Across-the-body stretch	Shoulders, upper back							
Upper-back stretch	Upper back							
Lateral stretch	Trunk muscles							
Step stretch	Hip, front of thigh (quadriceps)							
Side lunge	Inner thigh, hip, calf							
Sole stretch	Inner thigh, hip							
Trunk rotation	Trunk, outer thigh and hip, lower back							
Alternate leg stretcher	Backs of the thigh (hamstring), hip, knee, ankle, buttocks							
Modified hurdler stretch	Back of the thigh (hamstring), lower back							
Lower leg stretch	Back of lower leg (calf, soleus, Achilles tendon)							

You can monitor your program using a chart like the one on the next page.

Flexibility Program Chart

Fill in the dates you perform each stretch, the number of seconds you hold each stretch (should be 15–30), and the number of repetitions of each (should be 3–5). For an easy check on the duration of your stretches, count "one thousand one, one thousand two," and so on. You will probably find that over time you'll be able to hold each stretch longer (in addition to being able to stretch farther).

Exercise/Date																				
	Duration																			
	Reps																			
	Duration																			
	Reps																			
	Duration																			
	Reps																			
	Duration																			
	Reps																			
	Duration																			
	Reps																			
	Duration																			
	Reps																			
	Duration																			
	Reps																			
	Duration																			
	Reps																			
	Duration																			
	Reps																			
	Duration																			
	Reps																			
	Duration																			
	Reps																			
	Duration																			
	Reps																			
	Duration																			
	Reps																			
	Duration																			
	Reps																			
	Duration																			
	Reps																			
	Duration																			
	Reps																			
	Duration																			
	Reps																			
	Duration																			
	Reps																			

6

Body Composition

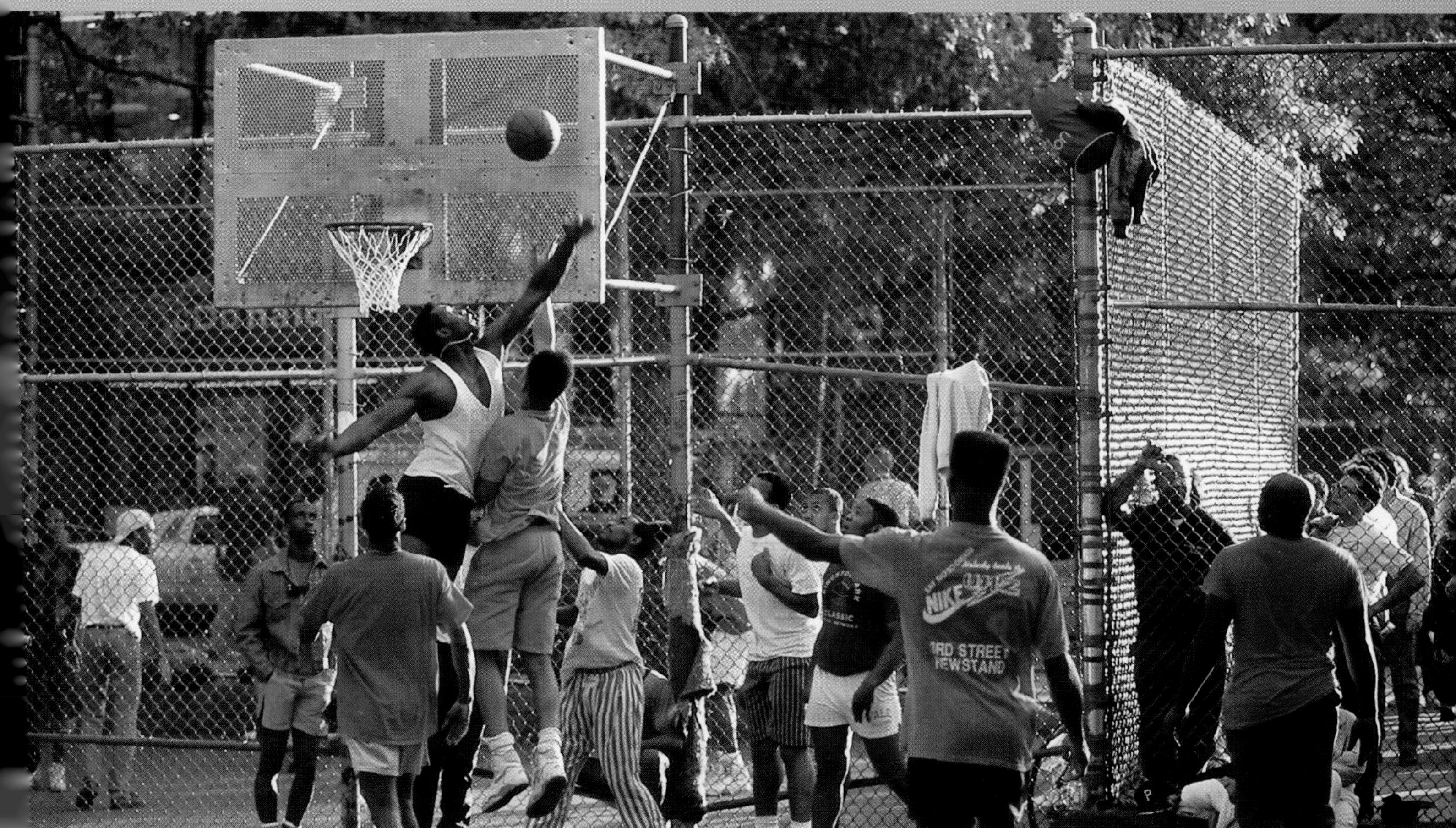

LOOKING AHEAD

After reading this chapter, you should be able to answer these questions about body composition:

- What are lean body mass, essential fat, and nonessential fat, and what are their functions in the body?
- How does body composition affect wellness?
- How are body composition and body fat distribution measured?
- What is recommended body weight, and how is it determined?

Body composition is an important component of fitness for wellness. People whose body composition is optimal tend to be healthier, to move more efficiently, and to feel better about themselves. To reach wellness, you must determine what body composition is right for you and then work to achieve it.

Although people pay lip service to the idea of exercising for health, a more immediate goal for many is to look fit and healthy. Unfortunately, many people don't succeed in their efforts to obtain a fit and healthy body because they emphasize short-term weight loss rather than the permanent changes in lifestyle that lead to fat loss and a healthy body composition. Successful management of body composition requires the coordination of many aspects of a wellness program, including proper nutrition, adequate exercise, and stress management.

This chapter focuses on defining and measuring body composition and determining recommended body weight; Chapter 9 provides specific strategies for changing your lifestyle to reach your body composition goal.

WHAT IS BODY COMPOSITION, AND WHY IS IT IMPORTANT?

The human body can be divided into lean body mass and body fat. Lean body mass is composed of all the body's nonfat tissues: bone, water, muscle, connective tissue, organ tissues, and teeth. Body fat includes both essential and nonessential body fats (Figure 6-1). **Essential fat** includes lipids incorporated into the nerves, brain, heart, lungs, liver, and mammary glands. These fat deposits, crucial for normal body functioning, make up approximately 3% of total body weight in men and 12% in women. (The larger percentage in women is due to fat deposits in the breasts, uterus, and other sites specific to females.) **Nonessential (storage) fat** exists primarily within fat cells, or **adipose tissue,** often located just below the skin and around major organs. The amount of storage fat varies from individual to individual based on many factors, including gender, age, heredity, metabolism, diet, and activity level. Excess storage fat is usually the result of consuming more energy (as food) than is expended (in metabolism and physical activity).

How much body fat is too much? In the past, many people relied on height-weight tables to answer this question. Based on insurance company statistics, these tables list a range of body weights associated with lowest mortality. People whose weight falls above the range recommended for their gender, age, height, and frame size are considered **overweight.** Unfortunately, these tables can be highly inaccurate for some people. They reflect an unrepresentative sample of data and use arbitrary **frame size** categories. At best, height-weight tables provide only an indirect measure of fatness. Because, as explained in Chapter 4, muscle tissue is denser and heavier than fat, a fit person can easily weigh more and an unfit person weigh less than recommended weights on a height-weight table.

The most important consideration when a person is looking at body composition is the proportion of the

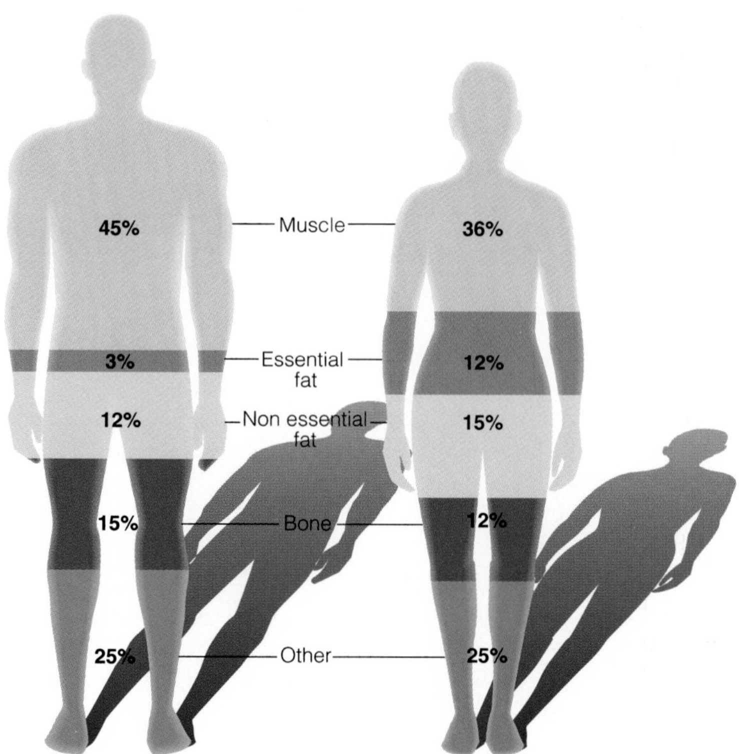

Figure 6-1 ***Body composition of a typical man and woman, 20–24 years old.*** *Source:* Adapted from Brooks, G. A., T. D. Fahey, and T. P. White. 1996. *Exercise Physiology: Human Bioenergetics and Its Applications,* 2d ed. Mountain View, Calif.: Mayfield.

body's total weight that is fat—the **percent body fat.** Too much body fat (not total weight) has a negative effect on health and well-being. Table 6-1 lists ratings of body composition based on body fat. The ratings represent approximate standards for body composition; the healthy range varies among individuals depending on health status and risk factors for disease. For example, a man with high blood pressure and high blood cholesterol levels might want to reduce his percentage of body fat even if it is within the healthy range for the general population.

Americans are getting fatter. During the last decade, the proportion of Americans having a body composition that can be categorized as **obese** has risen from one in four to one in three; many more are moderately **overfat.** The problem is particularly severe among certain groups. Almost half of African American and Mexican American women are obese. The incidence of overweight among teenagers increased from about 15% in 1985 to 21% in 1995.

The reason for increased body fat in the population is not totally clear, but it is related to increased caloric consumption and decreased physical activity. The CDC has estimated that while the fat intake of Americans (as a percent of total caloric intake) has declined during the past decade, caloric intake has increased by 100–300 calories per day. People also seem to be less active during the day. More are working in white-collar and service professions rather than jobs involving physical activity, so people are exercising less. Increased access to home computers and cable television may also contribute to more sedentary lifestyles.

Though not as prevalent a problem, having too little body fat is also dangerous. Too much or too little body fat can have negative effects on health, performance, and self-image.

Health

Obesity—the accumulation of body fat that is more than 25% of total body weight for men and 32% of total body weight for women—is associated with a wide variety of health problems, many of which are listed in the box "Negative Health Consequences of Obesity" (p. 134). Obese people have an overall mortality rate almost twice that of nonobese people. They are more than three times as likely to develop diabetes (see the box "Diabetes Mellitus," p. 135). It is estimated that if all Americans had a healthy body composition, the incidence of coronary heart disease would drop by 25%.

The distribution of fat is also an important indicator of future health. People who tend to gain weight in the abdominal area have a risk of coronary heart disease, high blood pressure, diabetes, and stroke twice as high as those who tend to gain weight in the hip area. (Fat in fat cells in the abdomen seems to be more easily mobilized and sent into the bloodstream, increasing disease-related blood lipid concentrations.) In general, men tend to gain weight in the abdominal area and women in the hip area, but women who exhibit the male pattern of fat distribution face the increased health risks associated with it. Researchers have also found ethnic differences in the relative significance of increased abdominal fat, but more studies are needed to clarify the relationship among fat distribution, ethnicity, and disease. A person doesn't have to be technically overfat to have the waist-to-hip ratio be a risk factor, nor do all overfat people face this increased risk. However, individuals in the obese range should not be complacent about their body composition regardless of their fat distribution—all obesity has serious health consequences.

Is it possible to be too lean? Health experts have generally viewed too little body fat—less than 8% for women and 5% for men—as a threat to health and well-being. Extreme leanness has been linked with reproductive, circulatory, and immune system disorders. Extremely lean people may experience muscle wasting and fatigue; they are also more likely to suffer from a dangerous eating disorder. For women, an extremely low percentage of body

TABLE 6-1 Body Fat Standards for Health and Performance

	Percent Body Fat	
Classification	*Males*	*Females*
Lean (high performance)	5–9	8–17
Healthy	10–20	18–25
Moderately overfat	21–25	26–32
Obese	Over 25	Over 32

TERMS

essential fat The fat in the body necessary for normal body functioning.

nonessential (storage) fat Extra fat or fat reserves stored in the body.

adipose tissue Connective tissue in which fat is stored.

overweight Characterized by a body weight above the recommended range according to a height-weight table based on population norms and adjusted for gender, height, and possibly frame size and age.

frame size The size of a person's bones (small, medium, or large) in relation to height.

percent body fat The percentage of total body weight that is composed of fat.

obese Characterized by an excessive accumulation of body fat: more than 25% of body weight as fat in men, and more than 32% as fat in women.

overfat Characterized by an accumulation of more body fat than is considered healthy.

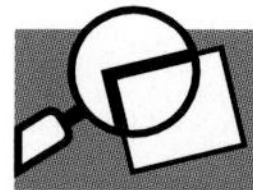

A CLOSER LOOK

Negative Health Consequences of Obesity

An obese person is at increased risk for the following:

- Early death
- Death from CVD, including sudden death
- Hypertension
- Diabetes
- Gallbladder disease
- Kidney disease
- Liver disease
- Cancer of the colon, prostate, gallbladder, ovary, endometrium, breast, and cervix
- Arthritis
- Gout
- Back pain
- Complications during pregnancy
- Menstrual abnormalities
- Shortness of breath
- Sleep apnea (intermittent cessation of breathing while sleeping)

Obesity is also associated with the following:

- Increased LDL concentration
- Decreased HDL concentration
- Impaired heart function (ventricles)
- Impaired immune function

fat is associated with **amenorrhea** and loss of bone mass. However, a recent study from Harvard Medical School found that among nonsmoking women, the leanest lived longer than women of "normal" weight. The authors of this study concluded that even mild to moderate overweight is associated with a substantial increase in the risk of premature death. Additional research is needed to determine all the effects of extremely low body fat levels on health.

Performance of Physical Activities

Too much body fat makes all types of physical activity more difficult because just moving the body through everyday activities means working harder and using more energy. In general, overfat people are less fit than others and don't have the muscular strength, endurance, and flexibility that make normal activity easy. Because exercise is more difficult, they do less of it, depriving themselves of an effective way to improve body composition.

Appearance and Self-Image

The "fashionable" body image has changed dramatically during the past 50 years, varying from slightly plump to an almost unhealthy thinness. Today a fit and healthy-looking body is the goal. And the key to this "look" is a balance of proper nutrition and exercise—in short, a lifestyle that emphasizes wellness.

The ideal body composition for appearance depends on individual preference (see the box "Exercise and Body Image," p. 136). Goals should be realistic, however; a person's ability to change body composition through diet and exercise depends not only on a wellness program, but also on heredity. Unrealistic expectations about body composition can have a negative impact on self-image and can lead to the development of eating disorders. (For more information on eating disorders, see Chapter 9.)

For most people, body fat percentage falls somewhere between ideal and a level that is significantly unhealthy. By consistently maintaining a wellness lifestyle that includes a healthy diet and regular exercise, the right body composition will naturally develop.

Wellness for Life

A healthy body composition is vital for wellness throughout life. Strong scientific evidence suggests that controlling your weight will increase your life span; reduce the risk of heart disease, cancer, diabetes, and back pain; increase your energy level; and improve your self-esteem.

ASSESSING BODY COMPOSITION

The morning weighing ritual on the bathroom scale can't reveal whether a fluctuation in weight is due to a change in muscle, body water, or fat and can't differentiate between overweight and overfat. A 260-pound football player may be overweight according to population height-weight standards yet actually have much less body fat than average. Likewise, a 40-year-old woman may weigh exactly the same as she did 20 years earlier yet have

TERMS

amenorrhea Absent or infrequent menstruation, sometimes related to low levels of body fat and excessive quantity or intensity of exercise.

body mass index (BMI) A measure of relative body weight correlating highly with more direct measures of body fat, calculated by dividing total body weight in kilograms by body height in square meters.

A CLOSER LOOK
Diabetes Mellitus

Diabetes mellitus is a disease that causes a disruption of normal metabolism. The pancreas, a long, thin organ located behind the stomach, normally secretes the hormone insulin, which stimulates cells to take up glucose to produce energy. In a person with diabetes, this process is disrupted, causing a buildup of glucose in the bloodstream. Over the long term, diabetes is associated with kidney failure, nerve damage, circulation problems, retinal damage and blindness, and increased rates of heart attack, stroke, and hypertension. It is currently the seventh leading cause of death in the United States.

Approximately 14 million Americans have one of two forms of diabetes. About 300,000 people have the more serious form, known as Type 1 or insulin-dependent diabetes. In this type of diabetes, the pancreas produces little or no insulin, so daily doses of insulin are required. (Without insulin, a person with Type 1 can lapse into a coma.) Type 1 diabetes usually strikes before age 20 and is also known as juvenile-onset diabetes.

The remaining 13.7 million Americans with diabetes have Type 2 or non–insulin-dependent diabetes. This condition can develop slowly, and about half of affected individuals are unaware of their condition. In Type 2 diabetes, the pancreas doesn't produce enough insulin, the cells don't respond to the hormone, or both. This condition is usually diagnosed in people over the age of 40 and is also called adult-onset diabetes. About one-third of people with Type 2 diabetes must inject insulin; others may take medications that increase insulin production or stimulate cells to take up glucose.

The major factors involved in the development of diabetes are age, obesity, a family history of diabetes, and lifestyle. Ethnic background also plays a role. African Americans and people of Hispanic background are 55% more likely than non-Hispanic whites to develop Type 2 diabetes. Native Americans also have a higher-than-average incidence of diabetes. Excess body fat reduces cell sensitivity to insulin, and it is a major risk factor for Type 2 diabetes. Nearly 90% of people with Type 2 diabetes are overweight.

There is no cure for diabetes, but both types can be successfully managed. Treatment involves keeping blood sugar levels within safe limits through diet, exercise, and, if necessary, medication. Blood sugar levels can be monitored using a home test. Recent research indicates that close monitoring and control of glucose levels can significantly reduce the rate of serious complications among people with diabetes. Regular exercise and a healthy diet are often sufficient to control Type 2 diabetes.

Recent studies have shown that exercise actually prevents the development of Type 2 diabetes, a benefit especially important in individuals with one or more risk factors for the disease. Exercise burns excess sugar and makes cells more sensitive to insulin. Exercise also helps keep body fat at healthy levels. A wellness lifestyle that includes a healthy diet and regular exercise is the best strategy for preventing diabetes. If you do develop diabetes, the best way to avoid complications is to recognize the symptoms and get early diagnosis and treatment. Be alert for the following warning signs:

- Frequent urination
- Extreme hunger or thirst
- Unexplained weight loss
- Extreme fatigue
- Blurred vision
- Frequent infections, especially of the bladder, gums, skin, or vagina
- Cuts and bruises that are slow to heal
- Tingling or numbness in the hands and feet
- Generalized itching, with no rash

Source: A new and better treatment for diabetes. 1994. *Consumer Reports on Health,* April. Rethinking the diabetic diet: The "rules" ease up. 1994. *Tufts University Diet and Nutrition Letter,* August. National Research Council. 1989. *Diet and Health: Implications for Reducing Chronic Disease Risk.* Washington, D.C.: National Academy Press.

a considerably different body composition. Despite these limitations, the U.S. Food and Drug Administration (FDA) and the Department of Health and Human Services recently published new height and weight recommendations, shown in Figure 6-2 (p. 137).

There are a number of simple, inexpensive ways to estimate body composition that are superior to the bathroom scale. These methods include body mass index and skinfold measurements.

Body Mass Index

Body mass index (BMI) is a rough measure of body composition that is useful if you don't have access to sophisticated equipment. Though more accurate than height-weight tables, body mass index is also based on the concept that a person's weight should be proportional to height. The measurement is fairly accurate for people who do not have an unusual amount of muscle mass. BMI is calculated by dividing your body weight (expressed in kilograms) by your height (expressed in square meters). For example, a person who weighs 130 pounds (59 kilograms) and is 5 feet, 3 inches tall (1.6 meters) would have a BMI of 59 kg $\div$ 1.6 m^2, or 23 kg/m^2. (Refer to Lab 6-1 for instructions on how to calculate your BMI.)

Optimal BMI depends on age and other health factors, but the BMI ranges for good health presented in Table 6-2 (p. 137) provide useful general guidelines.

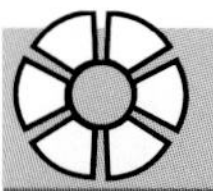

WELLNESS CONNECTION
Exercise and Body Image

If you gaze into the mirror and wish you could change the way your body looks, consider getting some exercise—not to reshape your contours but to firm up your self-image. According to a recent study from University College London, women who worked out on a regular basis rated their bodies as more attractive and healthy than women who didn't get much physical activity. Of course, the exercisers may have had particularly attractive bodies, but it should be noted that they were more satisfied than the sedentary women, even though they weighed an average of 11–12 pounds more, suggesting that active women are more comfortable bucking the Barbie-doll look that has become our cultural ideal.

One reason for the findings may be that women who exercise regularly often gain a sense of mastery and competence that enhances their self-esteem and body image. In addition, exercise contributes to a more toned look, which some women prefer. Then, too, participating in sports where size and height are advantageous, like volleyball or basketball, may help tall, relatively large women appreciate their body size and shape enough to see beyond cultural stereotypes. Finally, regular exercise and a positive family environment go hand in hand; family support provides the security to accept "sporty" body shapes even if they aren't picture-perfect by society's standards.

None of this is to say that whether a woman exercises regularly is the only factor that influences the way her body looks to her. Even the sport she prefers or engages in plays a role. In the British study, female body builders, not surprisingly, rated muscular physiques more favorably than women who chose rowing as their sport. In another study in which women were randomly assigned to weight training or brisk walking, body image improved for both groups, but more so for the weight lifters. Despite these other factors, though, the research suggests that as a group, physically active women are more comfortable with their bodies than sedentary women and are particularly tolerant of shapes that deviate from the model-thin icons.

Sources: Adapted from "Shape Up Your Body Image." 1995. *Tufts University Diet and Nutrition Letter,* May, p. 8. Tucker, L. A., and R. Mortell. 1993. Comparison of the effects of walking and weight training programs on body image in middle-aged women: An experimental study. *American Journal of Health Promotion* 8(1): 34–42.

The relative mortality rates associated with different values of BMI are shown in Figure 6-3 (p. 138). At high values of BMI, mortality rates increase rapidly. (The increased rate at very low BMI probably reflects the association between smoking and low body weight.)

BMI has its limitations, however, particularly for older people. Some people with low BMI and low muscle mass have as much fat as those with high BMI and more muscle mass. This can cause misclassification: A person with an acceptable BMI may actually be obese because he or she has less muscle mass, for example. This problem is particularly critical in older adults who have, on average, more fat than younger adults at any BMI, because of age-related loss of muscle mass. As a result, the value of BMI as a predictor of obesity decreases with age.

Skinfold Measurements

Skinfold measurement is a simple, inexpensive, and practical way to assess body composition. Skinfold measurements can be used to assess body composition because equations can link the thickness of skinfolds at various sites to percent body fat calculations from more precise laboratory techniques.

Skinfolds are measured with a device called a **caliper,** which consists of a pair of spring-loaded, calibrated jaws. High-quality calipers are made of metal, have parallel jaw surfaces, and constant spring tension. Inexpensive plastic

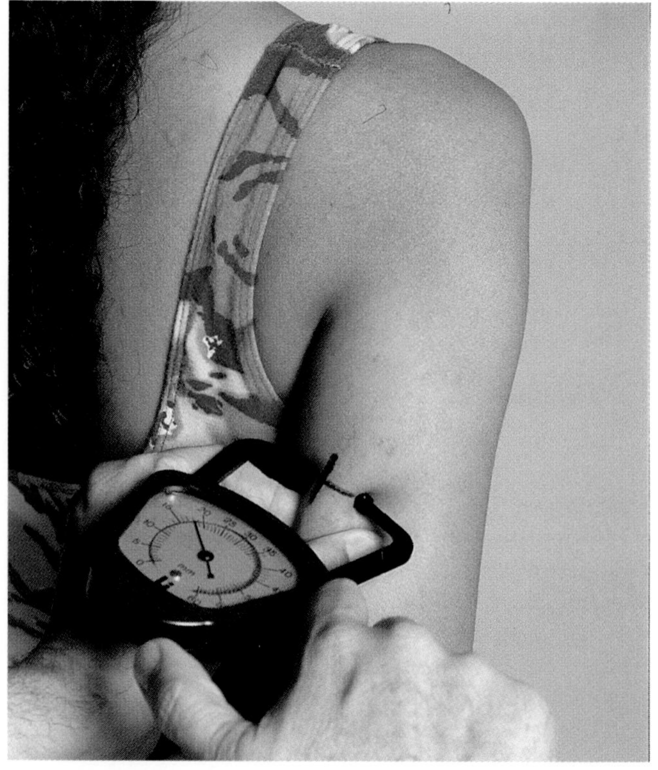

Proper technique is important in skinfold measurement. It's best to take several measurements at each site to ensure accuracy.

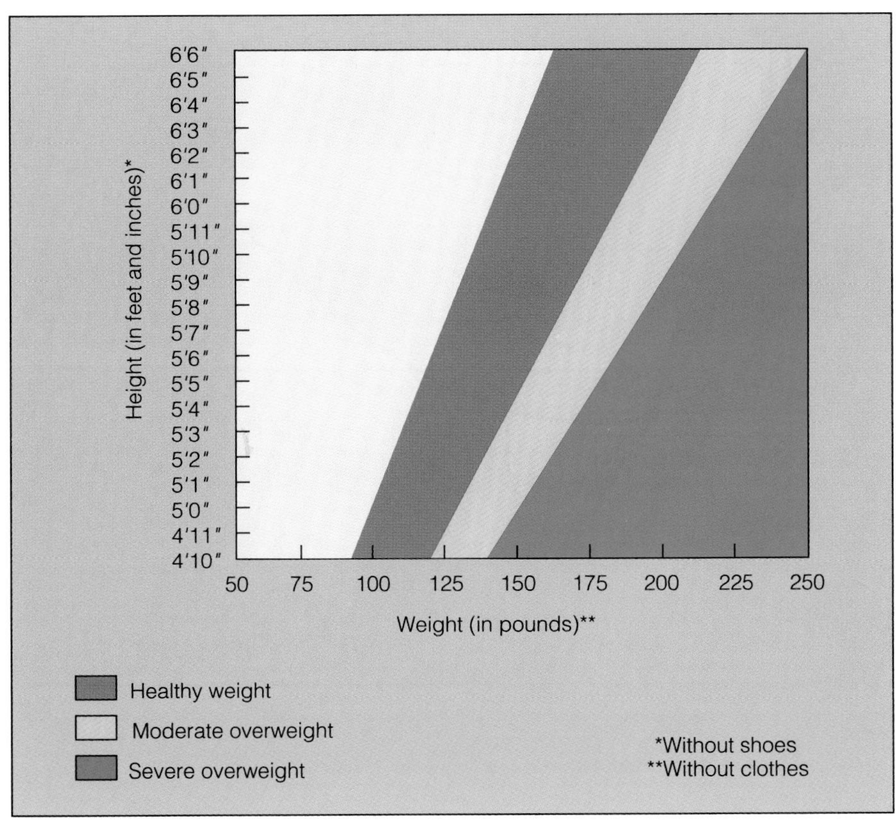

Figure 6-2 ***Suggested weights for adults.*** Weights are grouped in ranges because people of the same height may have equal amounts of body fat but different amounts of muscle and bone. The higher weights in each range apply to people with more muscle and bone, such as many men. Although weights are presented in ranges, gaining weight over time, even within the same range, is not healthy. *Source:* Adapted from U.S. Department of Agriculture. Agricultural Research Service. Dietary Guidelines Committee. 1995. *Report of the Dietary Guidelines Advisory Committee on the Dietary Guidelines for Americans.* Springfield, Va.: National Technical Information Service, pp. 23–24.

TABLE 6-2 Body Mass Index Classification

Body Mass Index	Category
20–24.9 kg/m^2	Desirable range for adult men and women
25–29.9 kg/m^2	Grade 1 obesity (moderate obesity)
30–40 kg/m^2	Grade 2 obesity (serious obesity)
>40 kg/m^2	Grade 3 obesity (morbid obesity)

Sources: Adapted from American College of Sports Medicine. 1995. *Guidelines for Exercise Testing and Prescription.* Baltimore: Williams & Wilkins. Jáequier, E. Energy, obesity, and body weight standards. 1987. *American Journal of Clinical Nutrition* 45:1035–1047.

calipers are also available, though they are less accurate than metal calipers.

Refer to Lab 6-1 for the procedure for taking skinfold measurements. Taking accurate measurements with calipers requires patience and practice. It's best to take several measurements at each site (or have several different people take each measurement) to help ensure accuracy. Be sure to take the measurements in the exact location called for in the procedure. Because the amount of water in your body changes during the day, skinfold measurements taken in the morning and evening often differ. Make sure you measure skinfolds at approximately the same time of day if you repeat the measurements in the future to track changes in your body composition.

Other Methods of Measuring Body Composition

Most of the many other methods for determining body composition are very sophisticated and require expensive equipment. Two methods available in many health clubs and sports medicine clinics are underwater weighing and bioelectrical impedance.

caliper A pressure-sensitive measuring instrument with two jaws that can be adjusted to determine thickness.

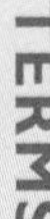

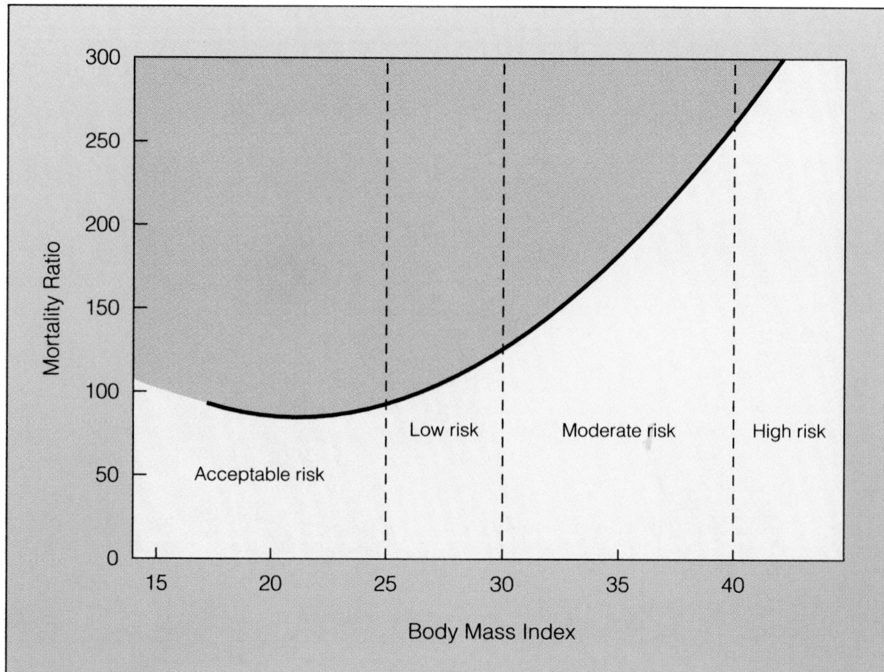

Figure 6-3 ***The relationship between BMI and mortality rates (average death rate is 100).*** *Source:* Wardlaw, G. M., and P. M. Insel. 1993. *Perspectives in Nutrition,* 2d ed. St. Louis: Mosby, p. 251.

Underwater Weighing Hydrostatic (underwater) weighing is considered the most accurate indirect way to measure body composition. It is the standard used for other techniques, including skinfold measurements. For this method, an individual is submerged and weighed underwater. The percentages of fat and fat-free weight (lean body mass) are calculated from body density. Muscle has a higher density and fat a lower density than water (1.1 grams per cubic centimeter for lean mass, 0.91 grams per cubic centimeter for fat, and 1 gram per cubic centimeter for water). Therefore, fat people tend to float and weigh less under water, and lean people tend to sink and weigh more under water.

Although somewhat cumbersome and expensive, this method is not beyond limited budgets. A harness and a spring-loaded scale can be connected to a diving board, and the school pool can be used as the underwater weighing tank. Most university exercise physiology departments or sports medicine laboratories will have an underwater weighing facility. If you want an accurate assessment of your body composition, find a place that does underwater weighing.

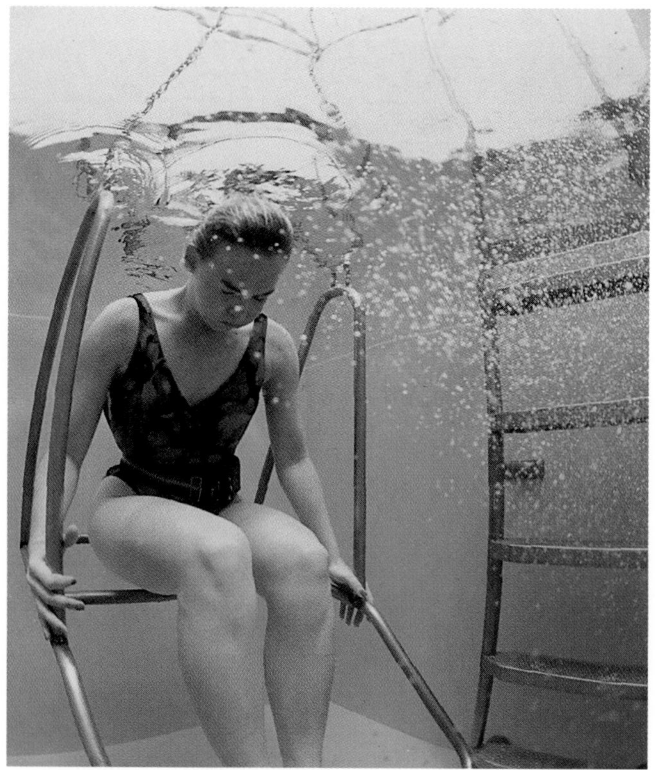

This young woman is having her body composition assessed in an underwater weighing tank. Muscle has a higher density than water, so people with more lean body mass weigh more under water.

Bioelectrical Impedance This new technique predicts body composition by estimating the amount of body water, most of which is located in lean tissue. The technique works by sending a small electrical current through the body and measuring the body's resistance to it. Although

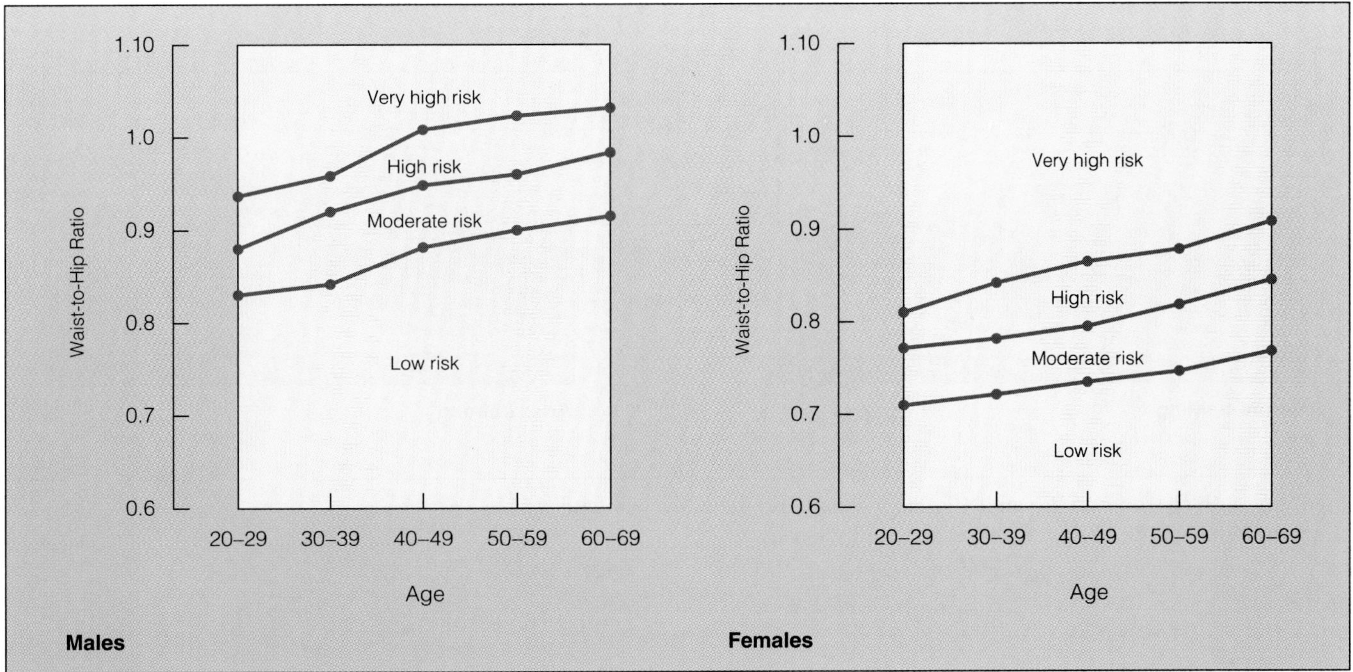

Figure 6-4 Risk of disease associated with waist-to-hip ratio. *Source:* Bray, G. A., and D. S. Gray. 1988. Obesity: Part 1—Pathogenesis. *Western Journal of Medicine* 149:429–441.

fairly accurate for most people (about the same as skinfold measurements), this method does provide very inaccurate results for some people.

Assessing Body Fat Distribution

The ratio of waist-to-hip-circumference measurements is the best available index for determining the risk associated with fat distribution. Follow the instructions in Lab 6-1 to measure and rate your body fat distribution. If your ratio is higher than that recommended for good health (Figure 6-4), it is suggested that you work on improving your body composition.

DETERMINING RECOMMENDED BODY WEIGHT

If the assessment tests indicate that fat loss would be beneficial for you, your first step is to establish a goal. Use the ratings in Table 6-1 or Table 6-2 to choose a target value for percent body fat or BMI (depending on which assessment you completed). Select a goal for percent body fat or BMI that is realistic for you and will ensure good health. If you have known risk factors for disease, such as high blood pressure or high levels of blood cholesterol, consult your physician to determine the ideal body composition for your individual risk profile.

Once you've established your goal, you can calculate a target body weight. (Though body weight is not an accurate means of assessing body composition, it's a useful method for tracking progress in a program to change body composition. If you're losing a small or moderate amount of weight and exercising, you're probably losing fat while building lean body mass.) Follow the instructions in Lab 6-2 to put the results of all the assessment tests together, get an overview of your body composition, and determine a range for recommended body weight.

Using percent body fat or BMI will generate a fairly accurate target body weight for most people. However, it's best not to stick rigidly to a recommended body weight calculated from any formula; individual genetic, cultural, and lifestyle factors are also important. Decide whether the body weight that the formulas generate for you is realistic, meets all your goals, is healthy, *and* is reasonable for you to maintain.

Track your progress toward your target body composition by checking your body weight periodically. To get a more accurate idea of your progress, especially when weight loss is large, you should directly reassess your body composition occasionally during your program: Body composition changes as weight changes. Losing a lot of weight usually includes losing some lean body mass no matter how hard a person exercises, partly because carrying less weight requires the muscular system to bear a smaller burden. (Conversely, a large gain in weight with-

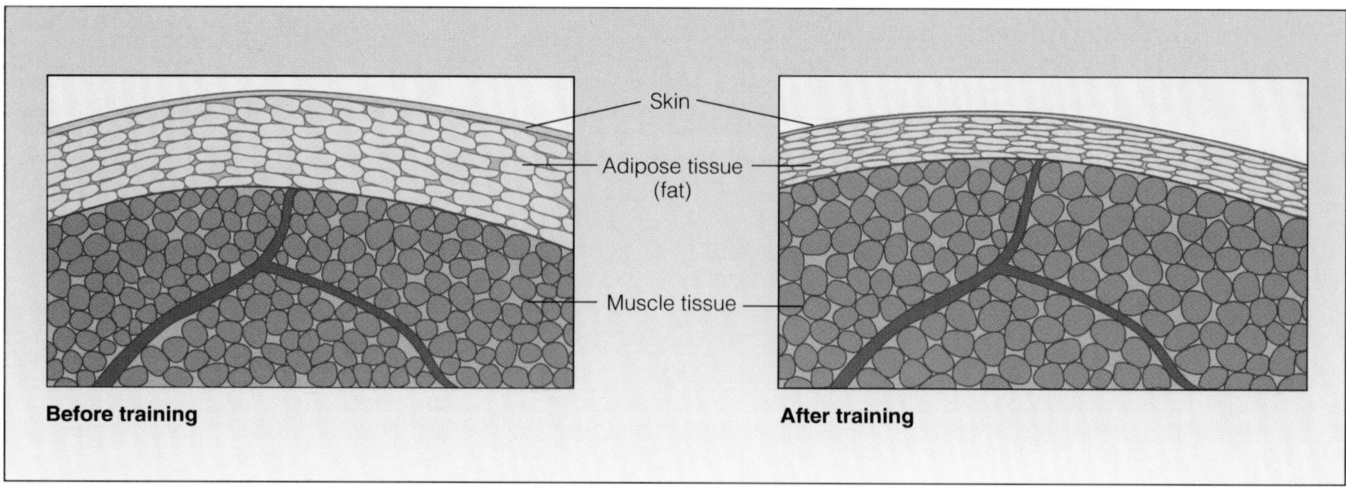

Figure 6-5 ***Effects of exercise on body composition.*** Endurance exercise and strength training reduce body fat and increase muscle mass.

out exercise still causes some gain in lean body mass, because muscles are working harder to carry the extra weight.)

? COMMON QUESTIONS ANSWERED

Is spot reducing effective? No. Spot reducing refers to attempts to lose body fat in specific parts of the body by doing exercises for those parts. For example, a person might try to spot reduce in the legs by doing leg lifts. Spot-reducing exercises contribute to fat loss only to the extent that they burn calories. The only way you can reduce fat in any specific area is to create an overall negative energy balance: Take in less energy (food) than you use up through exercise and metabolism.

How does exercise affect body composition? Cardiorespiratory endurance exercise burns calories, thereby helping create a negative energy balance. Weight training does not use very many calories and therefore is of little use in creating a negative energy balance. However, weight training increases lean body mass, which maintains a high metabolic rate (the body's energy level) and helps improve body composition. To minimize body fat and increase muscle mass, thereby improving body composition, combine cardiorespiratory endurance exercise and weight training (Figure 6-5).

How do I develop a toned, healthy-looking body? The development of a healthy-looking body requires regular exercise, proper diet, and other good health habits. However, it helps to have heredity on your side. All bodies are not created equal. Some people put on or take off fat more easily than others just as some people are taller than others. Be realistic in your goals, and be satisfied with the improvements in body composition you can make by observing the principles of a wellness lifestyle.

Are people physically fit who have a desirable body composition? Having a healthy body composition is not necessarily associated with overall fitness. For example, many body builders have very little body fat but have poor cardiorespiratory capacity and flexibility. To be fit, you must rate high on all the components of fitness.

What is liposuction, and will it help me lose body fat? Suction lipectomy, popularly known as liposuction, has become the most popular type of elective surgery in the United States. The procedure involves removing limited amounts of fat from specific areas. Typically, no more than 2.5 kg of adipose tissue is removed at a time. The procedure is usually successful if the amount of excess fat is limited and skin elasticity is good. The procedure is most effective if integrated into a program of dietary restriction and exercise. Side effects include infection, dimpling, and wavy skin contours. Although serious complications are rare, liposuction, like any surgical procedure, can lead to blood clots, shock, bleeding, impaired blood flow to vital organs, and even death. Liposuction is not an effective way to lose large amounts of fat, nor should it be a substitute for a healthy weight-management program.

What is cellulite, and how do I get rid of it? Cellulite is the name commonly given to ripply, wavy fat deposits that collect just under the skin. However, these rippling fat deposits are really the same as fat deposited anywhere else in the body. The only way to control them is to create a negative energy balance—burn up more calories than are taken in. There are no creams or lotion that will rub away surface (subcutaneous) fat deposits, and spot reducing is also ineffective. The only solution is sensible eating habits and exercise.

SUMMARY

- The human body is composed of lean body mass (which includes bone, muscle, organ tissues, and connective tissues) and body fat (essential and nonessential).
- Having too much body fat has negative health consequences, especially in terms of cardiovascular disease. Distribution of fat is also a significant factor in health.
- A fit and healthy-looking body, with the right body composition for a particular person, develops from habits of proper nutrition and exercise.
- Measuring body weight is not an accurate way to assess body composition because it does not differentiate between muscle weight and fat weight.
- Two measurements of body composition are body mass index (formulated through weight and height measurements) and percent body fat (formulated through skinfold measurements).
- Hydrostatic weighing, the most accurate indirect measure of body composition, is based on body density; muscle has a higher density and fat a lower density than water. Bioelectrical impedance estimates the amount of body water (and thereby lean tissue) by measuring the body's resistance to a small electrical current.
- Body fat distribution can be assessed through the waist-to-hip-circumference ratio.
- Recommended body weight can be determined by choosing a target BMI or target body fat percentage. Keep heredity in mind when setting a goal.

BEHAVIOR CHANGE ACTIVITY

Breaking Behavior Chains

Use the records you've collected in your health journal to trace the chain of events that lead to your target behavior. Identify points in the chain where you can make a change that will lead to your new behavior. Consider the following strategies:

- *Control or eliminate environmental stimuli that provoke the behavior.* For example, if you always end up taking a coffee break and chatting with friends when you go to the library to study, choose a different study site, such as your room. Or you may need to avoid keeping cigarettes or certain foods or drinks in your dorm room, apartment, or house.
- *Control other behaviors or habits that are linked to your target behavior.* For example, if you get the urge to eat whenever you watch television, cut back on your TV viewing, or combine it with another behavior, such as exercise.
- *Add new cues to your environment to trigger your new behavior and inspire you to continue with your program.* For example, prepare easy-to-grab healthy snacks and leave them at the front of the refrigerator, or put your walking shoes by the front door.
- *Use a system of rewards to reinforce your new behavior.* Use the rewards you listed in the Behavior Change Activity in Chapter 5, and don't forget to give yourself instant, real rewards for good behavior as your program progresses. For example, treat yourself to a phone call to a friend after you complete your workout for the day.

Review the example of a behavior chain and the potential strategies for breaking it given in Figure 6-6. Go through the same process for a typical chain of events involving your target behavior (Figure 6-7).

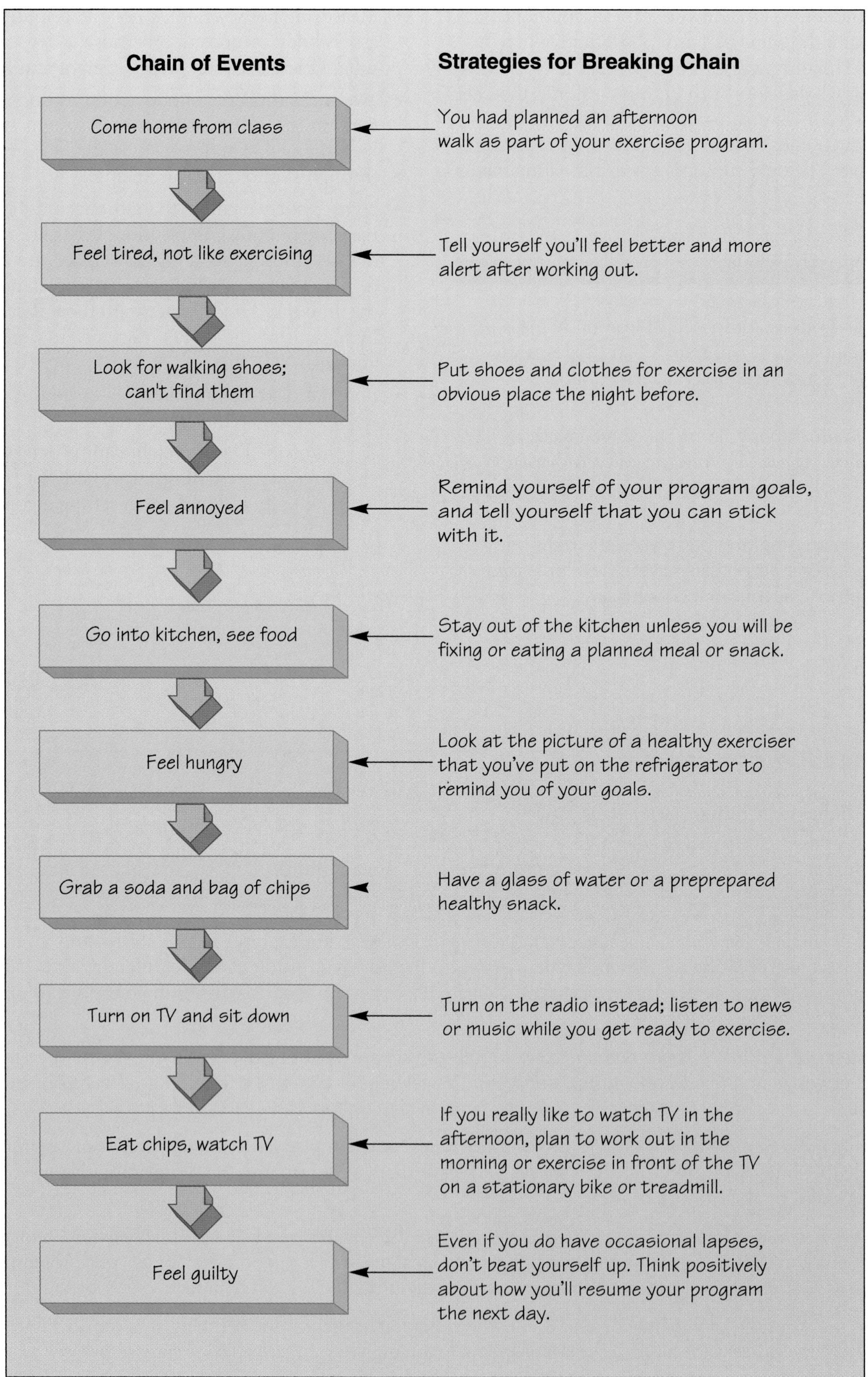

Chain of Events
Strategies for Breaking Chain
Come home from class
You had planned an afternoon walk as part of your exercise program.
Feel tired, not like exercising
Tell yourself you'll feel better and more alert after working out.
Look for walking shoes; can't find them
Put shoes and clothes for exercise in an obvious place the night before.
Feel annoyed
Remind yourself of your program goals, and tell yourself that you can stick with it.
Go into kitchen, see food
Stay out of the kitchen unless you will be fixing or eating a planned meal or snack.
Feel hungry
Look at the picture of a healthy exerciser that you've put on the refrigerator to remind you of your goals.
Grab a soda and bag of chips
Have a glass of water or a preprepared healthy snack.
Turn on TV and sit down
Turn on the radio instead; listen to news or music while you get ready to exercise.
Eat chips, watch TV
If you really like to watch TV in the afternoon, plan to work out in the morning or exercise in front of the TV on a stationary bike or treadmill.
Feel guilty
Even if you do have occasional lapses, don't beat yourself up. Think positively about how you'll resume your program the next day.

Figure 6-6 *A sample behavior chain and strategies for breaking it.*

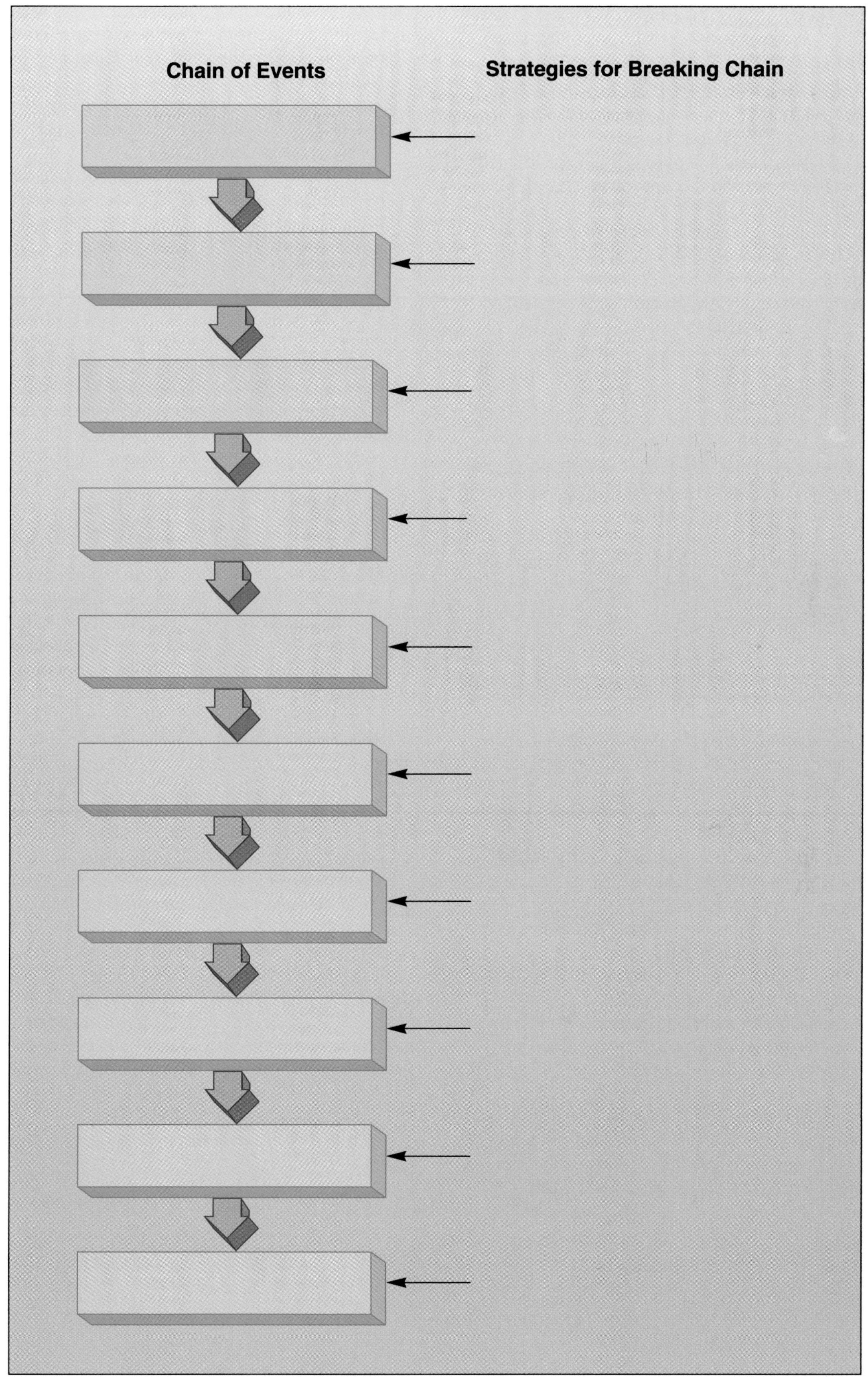

Figure 6-7 *A behavior chain for target behavior.*

FOR MORE INFORMATION

Katch, F., and W. McArdle. 1992. *Introduction to Nutrition, Exercise, and Health,* 4th ed. Baltimore: Williams & Wilkins. *A comprehensive guide, with a scientific basis, to the practice of weight control using proper diet and exercise.*

Brooks, G. A., T. D. Fahey, and T. P. White. 1996. *Exercise Physiology: Human Bioenergetics and Its Applications,* 2d ed. Mountain View, Calif.: Mayfield. *A basic exercise physiology textbook that describes principles of metabolism and body composition.*

Lohman, T. G. 1992. *Advances in Body Composition Assessment.* Champaign, Ill.: Human Kinetics. *A comprehensive guide to body composition analysis written for health and exercise professionals.*

Roche, A. F., S. T. Heymsfield, and T. G. Lohman. 1996. *Human Body Composition.* Champaign, Ill.: Human Kinetics. *This book discusses the theory and measurement of human body composition. While it is mainly directed at sports scientists, people who are seriously interested in exercise might also be interested.*

Williams, M. 1992. *Nutrition for Fitness and Sport,* 3d ed. Dubuque, Ia.: W. C. Brown. *An excellent sourcebook describing the role of nutrition in fitness and sport.*

Underwater weighing is often available through campus adult fitness programs, and health clubs may also provide tests for percent body fat.

SELECTED BIBLIOGRAPHY

American College of Sports Medicine. 1995. *Guidelines for Exercise Testing and Prescription.* Baltimore: Williams & Wilkins.

Baumgartner, R. N., S. B. Heymsfield, and A. F. Roche. 1995. Human body composition and the epidemiology of chronic disease. *Obesity Research* 3:73–95.

Blair, S. 1991. *Living With Exercise.* American Health Publishing.

Bray, G. A., and D. S. Gray. 1988. Obesity: Part I—Pathogenesis. *Western Journal of Medicine* 149:429–441.

Brodie, D. A. 1988. Techniques of measurement of body composition: part I. *Sports Medicine* 5:11–40.

Brodie, D. A. 1988. Techniques of measurement of body composition: part II. *Sports Medicine* 5:74–98.

Centers for Disease Control and Prevention. 1995. Prevalence of selected risk factors for chronic disease by education level in racial/ethnic populations, United States, 1991–1992. *Journal of the American Medical Association* 273:102.

Croft, J. B., et al. 1995. Waist-to-hip ratio in a biracial population: Measurement, implications, and cautions for using guidelines to define high risk for cardiovascular disease. *Journal of the American Dietetic Association* 95(1): 60–64.

Garrow, J. S., and C. D. Summerbell. 1995. Meta-analysis: Effect of exercise, with or without dieting, on the body composition of overweight subjects. *European Journal of Clinical Nutrition* 49:1–10.

Genest, J., and J. S. Cohn. 1995. Clustering of cardiovascular risk factors: Targeting high-risk individuals. *American Journal of Cardiology* 76:8A–20A.

Gillum, R. F. 1987. The association of body fat distribution with hypertension, hypertensive heart disease, coronary heart disease, diabetes and cardiovascular risk factors in men and women aged 18–79 years. *Journal of Chronic Disorders* 40:421–428.

Grediagin, A., M. Cody, J. Rupp, D. Benardot, and R. Shern. 1995. Exercise intensity does not affect body composition change in untrained, moderately overfat women. *Journal of the American Dietetic Association* 95:661–665.

Jackson, A. S., and M. L. Pollock. 1985. Practical assessment of body composition. *Physician and Sportsmedicine* 13:76–90.

Johnson, C. 1995. *Self-Esteem Comes in All Sizes: How to Be Happy and Healthy at Your Natural Weight.* New York: Doubleday.

Katch, F., A. R. Behnke, and V. L. Katch. 1979. Estimation of body fat from skinfolds and surface area. *Human Biology* 51:411–424.

Krotkiewski, M., et al. 1983. Impact of obesity on metabolism in men and women: Importance of regional adipose tissue distribution. *Journal of Clinical Investigation* 72:1150–1162.

Kuczmarski, R. J., K. M. Flegal, S. M. Campbell, and C. L. Johnson. 1994. Increasing prevalence of overweight among U.S. adults. The National Health and Nutrition Examination Surveys, 1960–1991. *Journal of the American Medical Association* 272:205–211.

Leutholtz, B. C., R. E. Keyser, W. W. Heusner, V. E. Wendt, and L. Rosen. 1995. Exercise training and severe caloric restriction: Effect on lean body mass in the obese. *Archives of Physical and Medical Rehabilitation* 76:65–70.

Manson, J. E., et al. 1995. Body weight and mortality among women. *New England Journal of Medicine* 333(11): 677–685.

Ng, A. V., R. Callister, D. G. Johnson, and D. R. Seals. 1994. Endurance exercise training is associated with elevated basal sympathetic nerve activity in healthy older humans. *Journal of Applied Physiology* 77:1366–1374.

Schauss, A. 1991. *Eating for A's.* New York: Pocket Books.

Stallone, D. D. 1994. The influence of obesity and its treatment on the immune system. *Nutrition Review* 52:37–50.

Stevens, J. 1995. Obesity, fat patterning and cardiovascular risk. *Advances in Experimental Medicine and Biology* 369:21–27.

Name ____________________ **Section** ____________ **Date** ____________

LAB 6-1 *Assessing Body Composition*

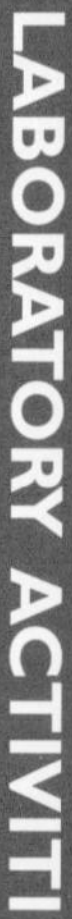

Body Mass Index

Equipment

1. Weight scale
2. Tape measure or other means of measuring height

Preparation

None

Instructions

Measure your height and weight, and record the results. Be sure to record the unit of measurement.

Height: ___________ Weight: ___________

Calculating BMI

1. Convert your body weight to kilograms by dividing your weight in pounds by 2.2.

   Body weight ___________ lb ÷ 2.2 lb/kg = body weight ___________ kg

2. Convert your height measurement to meters by multiplying your height in inches by 0.0254.

   Height ___________ in. × 0.0254 m/in. = height ___________ m

3. Square your height measurement.

   Height ___________ m × height ___________ m = height ___________ m^2

4. BMI equals body weight in kilograms divided by height in square meters (kg/m^2).

   Body weight ___________ (from step 1) kg ÷ height ___________ (from step 3) m^2 = BMI ___________ kg/m^2

Rating Your BMI

Refer to Table 6-2 (p. 137) and Figure 6-3 (p. 138) for a rating of your BMI. Record the results below and in the chart on the final page of this lab.

BMI ___________ kg/m^2

Classification (from Table 6-3) ___________

Relative risk rating (from Figure 6-2) ___________

Skinfold Measurements

Equipment

1. Skinfold calipers
2. Partner to take measurements
3. Marking pen (optional)

Preparation

None

Instructions

1. *Select and locate the correct sites for measurement.* All measurements should be taken on the right side of the body with the subject standing. Skinfolds are normally measured on the natural fold line of the skin, either vertically or at a slight angle. The skinfold measurement sites for females are triceps, suprailium, and thigh; for males, chest, abdomen, and thigh. If the person taking skinfold measurements is inexperienced, it may be helpful to mark the correct sites with a marking pen.

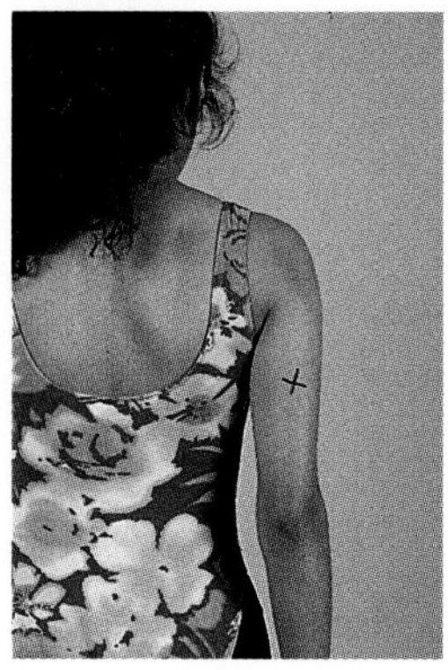
(a) Triceps

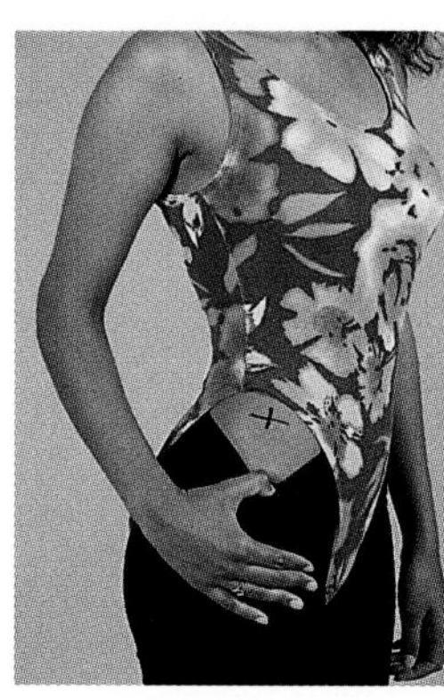
(b) Suprailium

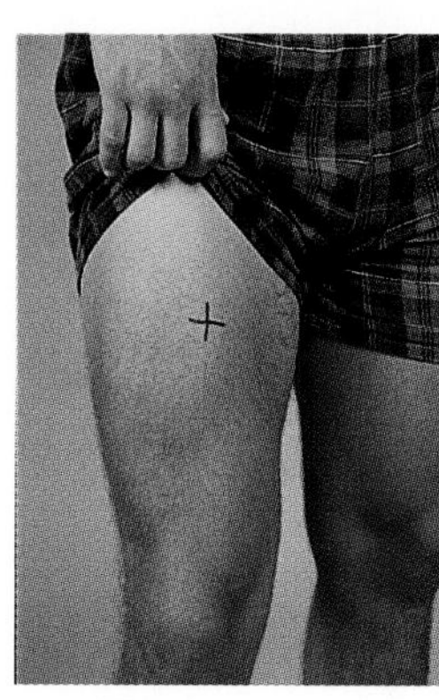
(c) Thigh

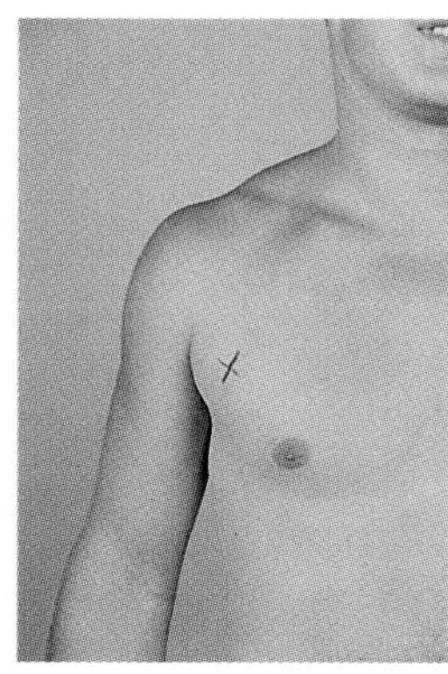
(d) Chest

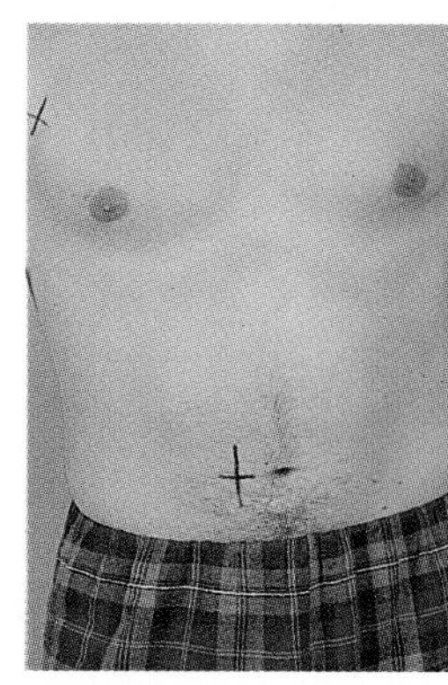
(e) Abdomen

(a) Triceps. Pinch a vertical skinfold on the back of the right arm midway between the shoulder and elbow. The elbow should be straight and should hang naturally. *(b) Suprailium.* Pinch a fold at the top front of the right hipbone. The skinfold here is taken slightly diagonally according to the natural fold tendency of the skin. *(c) Thigh.* Pinch a vertical fold midway between the top of the hipbone and the kneecap. *(d) Chest.* Pinch a diagonal fold halfway between the nipple and the shoulder crease. *(e) Abdomen.* Pinch a vertical fold about 1 inch to the right of the umbilicus (navel).

2. *Measure the appropriate skinfolds.* Pinch a fold of skin between your thumb and forefinger. Pull the fold up so that no muscular tissue is included; don't pinch the skinfold too hard. Hold the calipers perpendicular to the fold, and measure the skinfold about 0.25 inch away from your fingers. Allow the tips of the calipers to close on the skinfold, and let the reading settle before marking it down. Take readings to the nearest half millimeter. Continue to repeat the measurements until two consecutive measurements match, releasing and repinching the skinfold between each measurement. Make a note of the final measurement for each site.

   Time of day of measurements: ____________

Men		*Women*	
Chest: ______________	mm	Triceps: ______________	mm
Abdomen: ____________	mm	Suprailium: ____________	mm
Thigh: ______________	mm	Thigh: ______________	mm

Determining Percent Body Fat

Add the measurements of your three skinfolds, and then find the percent body fat that corresponds to your total in the appropriate table. For example, a 19-year-old female with measurements of 16 mm, 19 mm, and 22 mm would have a skinfold sum of 57 mm; according to the table on the next page, her percent body fat is 22.7.

Sum of three skinfolds: ____________ mm

Percent body fat: ____________ %

Rating Your Body Composition

Refer to the table on page 133 to rate your percent body fat. Record it below and on the chart on the final page of this lab.

Rating: ____________

Percent Body Fat Estimate for Men: Sum of Chest, Abdomen, and Thigh Skinfolds

Sum of Skinfolds (mm)	Age: Under 22	23–27	28–32	33–37	38–42	43–47	48–52	53–57	Over 57
8–10	1.3	1.8	2.3	2.9	3.4	3.9	4.5	5.0	5.5
11–13	2.2	2.8	3.3	3.9	4.4	4.9	5.5	6.0	6.5
14–16	3.2	3.8	4.3	4.8	5.4	5.9	6.4	7.0	7.5
17–19	4.2	4.7	5.3	5.8	6.3	6.9	7.4	8.0	8.5
20–22	5.1	5.7	6.2	6.8	7.3	7.9	8.4	8.9	9.5
23–25	6.1	6.6	7.2	7.7	8.3	8.8	9.4	9.9	10.5
26–28	7.0	7.6	8.1	8.7	9.2	9.8	10.3	10.9	11.4
29–31	8.0	8.5	9.1	9.6	10.2	10.7	11.3	11.8	12.4
32–34	8.9	9.4	10.0	10.5	11.1	11.6	12.2	12.8	13.3
35–37	9.8	10.4	10.9	11.5	12.0	12.6	13.1	13.7	14.3
38–40	10.7	11.3	11.8	12.4	12.9	13.5	14.1	14.6	15.2
41–43	11.6	12.2	12.7	13.3	13.8	14.4	15.0	15.5	16.1
44–46	12.5	13.1	13.6	14.2	14.7	15.3	15.9	16.4	17.0
47–49	13.4	13.9	14.5	15.1	15.6	16.2	16.8	17.3	17.9
50–52	14.3	14.8	15.4	15.9	16.5	17.1	17.6	18.2	18.8
53–55	15.1	15.7	16.2	16.8	17.4	17.9	18.5	19.1	19.7
56–58	16.0	16.5	17.1	17.7	18.2	18.8	19.4	20.0	20.5
59–61	16.9	17.4	17.9	18.5	19.1	19.7	20.2	20.8	21.4
62–64	17.6	18.2	18.8	19.4	19.9	20.5	21.1	21.7	22.2
65–67	18.5	19.0	19.6	20.2	20.8	21.3	21.9	22.5	23.1
68–70	19.3	19.9	20.4	21.0	21.6	22.2	22.7	23.3	23.9
71–73	20.1	20.7	21.2	21.8	22.4	23.0	23.6	24.1	24.7
74–76	20.9	21.5	22.0	22.6	23.2	23.8	24.4	25.0	25.5
77–79	21.7	22.2	22.8	23.4	24.0	24.6	25.2	25.8	26.3
80–82	22.4	23.0	23.6	24.2	24.8	25.4	25.9	26.5	27.1
83–85	23.2	23.8	24.4	25.0	25.5	26.1	26.7	27.3	27.9
86–88	24.0	24.5	25.1	25.7	26.3	26.9	27.5	28.1	28.7
89–91	24.7	25.3	25.9	26.5	27.1	27.6	28.2	28.8	29.4
92–94	25.4	26.0	26.6	27.2	27.8	28.4	29.0	29.6	30.2
95–97	26.1	26.7	27.3	27.9	28.5	29.1	29.7	30.3	30.9
98–100	26.9	27.4	28.0	28.6	29.2	29.8	30.4	31.0	31.6
101–103	27.5	28.1	28.7	29.3	29.9	30.5	31.1	31.7	32.3
104–106	28.2	28.8	29.4	30.0	30.6	31.2	31.8	32.4	33.0
107–109	28.9	29.5	30.1	30.7	31.3	31.9	32.5	33.1	33.7
110–112	29.6	30.2	30.8	31.4	32.0	32.6	33.2	33.8	34.4
113–115	30.2	30.8	31.4	32.0	32.6	33.2	33.8	34.5	35.1
116–118	30.9	31.5	32.1	32.7	33.3	33.9	34.5	35.1	35.7
119–121	31.5	32.1	32.7	33.3	33.9	34.5	35.1	35.7	36.4
122–124	32.1	32.7	33.3	33.9	34.5	35.1	35.8	36.4	37.0
125–127	32.7	33.3	33.9	34.5	35.1	35.8	36.4	37.0	37.6

Source: Jackson, A. S., and M. L. Pollock. 1985. Practical assessment of body composition. *Physician and Sportsmedicine* 13(5): 76–90. Reproduced by permission of McGraw-Hill, Inc.

Percent Body Fat Estimate for Women: Sum of Triceps, Suprailium, and Thigh Skinfolds

Sum of Skinfolds (mm)	*Age*								
	Under 22	*23–27*	*28–32*	*33–37*	*38–42*	*43–47*	*48–52*	*53–57*	*Over 57*
23–25	9.7	9.9	10.2	10.4	10.7	10.9	11.2	11.4	11.7
26–28	11.0	11.2	11.5	11.7	12.0	12.3	12.5	12.7	13.0
29–31	12.3	12.5	12.8	13.0	13.3	13.5	13.8	14.0	14.3
32–34	13.6	13.8	14.0	14.3	14.5	14.8	15.0	15.3	15.5
35–37	14.8	15.0	15.3	15.5	15.8	16.0	16.3	16.5	16.8
38–40	16.0	16.3	16.5	16.7	17.0	17.2	17.5	17.7	18.0
41–43	17.2	17.4	17.7	17.9	18.2	18.4	18.7	18.9	19.2
44–46	18.3	18.6	18.8	19.1	19.3	19.6	19.8	20.1	20.3
47–49	19.5	19.7	20.0	20.2	20.5	20.7	21.0	21.2	21.5
50–52	20.6	20.8	21.1	21.3	21.6	21.8	22.1	22.3	22.6
53–55	21.7	21.9	22.1	22.4	22.6	22.9	23.1	23.4	23.6
56–58	22.7	23.0	23.2	23.4	23.7	23.9	24.2	24.4	24.7
59–61	23.7	24.0	24.2	24.5	24.7	25.0	25.2	25.5	25.7
62–64	24.7	25.0	25.2	25.5	25.7	26.0	26.7	26.4	26.7
65–67	25.7	25.9	26.2	26.4	26.7	26.9	27.2	27.4	27.7
68–70	26.6	26.9	27.1	27.4	27.6	27.9	28.1	28.4	28.6
71–73	27.5	27.8	28.0	28.3	28.5	28.8	29.0	29.3	29.5
74–76	28.4	28.7	28.9	29.2	29.4	29.7	29.9	30.2	30.4
77–79	29.3	29.5	29.8	30.0	30.3	30.5	30.8	31.0	31.3
80–82	30.1	30.4	30.6	30.9	31.1	31.4	31.6	31.9	32.1
83–85	30.9	31.2	31.4	31.7	31.9	32.2	32.4	32.7	32.9
86–88	31.7	32.0	32.2	32.5	32.7	32.9	33.2	33.4	33.7
89–91	32.5	32.7	33.0	33.2	33.5	33.7	33.9	34.2	34.4
92–94	33.2	33.4	33.7	33.9	34.2	34.4	34.7	34.9	35.2
95–97	33.9	34.1	34.4	34.6	34.9	35.1	35.4	35.6	35.9
98–100	34.6	34.8	35.1	35.3	35.5	35.8	36.0	36.3	36.5
101–103	35.3	35.4	35.7	35.9	36.2	36.4	36.7	36.9	37.2
104–106	35.8	36.1	36.3	36.6	36.8	37.1	37.3	37.5	37.8
107–109	36.4	36.7	36.9	37.1	37.4	37.6	37.9	38.1	38.4
110–112	37.0	37.2	37.5	37.7	38.0	38.2	38.5	38.7	38.9
113–115	37.5	37.8	38.0	38.2	38.5	38.7	39.0	39.2	39.5
116–118	38.0	38.3	38.5	38.8	39.0	39.3	39.5	39.7	40.0
119–121	38.5	38.7	39.0	39.2	39.5	39.7	40.0	40.2	40.5
122–124	39.0	39.2	39.4	39.7	39.9	40.2	40.4	40.7	40.9
125–127	39.4	39.6	39.9	40.1	40.4	40.6	40.9	41.1	41.4
128–130	39.8	40.0	40.3	40.5	40.8	41.0	41.3	41.5	41.8

Source: Jackson, A. S., and M. L. Pollock. 1985. Practical assessment of body composition. *Physician and Sportsmedicine* 13(5): 76–90. Reproduced by permission of McGraw-Hill, Inc.

*Body Composition Ratings**

	Percent Body Fat					
Men	*Very Lean*	*Excellent*	*Good*	*Fair*	*Poor*	*Very Poor*
Age: 18–29	Below 5.3	5.3–9.4	9.5–14.1	14.2–17.4	17.5–22.4	Above 22.4
30–39	Below 9.2	9.2–13.9	14.0–17.5	17.6–20.5	20.6–24.2	Above 24.2
40–49	Below 11.5	11.5–16.3	16.4–19.6	19.7–22.5	22.6–26.1	Above 26.1
50–59	Below 13.0	13.0–17.9	18.0–21.3	21.4–24.1	24.2–27.5	Above 27.5
60 and over	Below 13.2	13.2–18.4	18.5–22.0	22.1–25.0	25.1–28.5	Above 28.5
Women						
Age: 18–29	Below 10.9	10.9–17.1	17.2–20.6	20.7–23.7	23.8–27.7	Above 27.7
30–39	Below 13.5	13.5–18.0	18.1–21.6	21.7–24.9	25.0–29.3	Above 29.3
40–49	Below 16.2	16.2–21.3	21.4–24.9	25.0–28.1	28.2–32.1	Above 32.1
50–59	Below 18.9	18.9–25.0	25.1–28.5	28.6–31.6	31.7–35.6	Above 35.6
60 and over	Below 16.9	16.9–25.1	25.2–29.3	29.4–32.5	32.6–36.6	Above 36.6

*These ratings are derived from norms based on the measurement of thousands of individuals. In evaluating your body composition, also consider the health-related recommendations for body fat given in Table 6-1 (p. 133). Obesity is defined as having more than 25% of body weight as fat for men and more than 32% of body weight as fat for women. Norms reflect the status of the population, while recommendations represent a more healthy and desirable status.

Source: Based on norms from the Cooper Institute for Aerobics Research, Dallas, Texas; used with permission.

Waist-to-Hip-Circumference Ratio

Equipment

1. Tape measure
2. Partner to take measurements

Preparation

Wear clothes that will not add significantly to your measurements.

Instructions

Stand with your feet together and your arms at your sides. Raise your arms only high enough to allow for taking the measurements. Your partner should make sure the tape is horizontal around the entire circumference and pulled snugly against your skin. The tape shouldn't be pulled so tight that it causes indentations in your skin. Record measurements to the nearest millimeter or one-sixteenth of an inch.

Waist. Measure at the smallest waist circumference. If you don't have a natural waist, measure at the level of your navel.

Waist measurement: ____________

Hip. Measure at the largest hip circumference.

Hip measurement: ____________

Calculating Your Ratio

You can use any unit of measurement (for example, inches or centimeters), as long as you're consistent. Waist-to-hip ratio equals waist measurement divided by hip measurement.

Waist-to-hip ratio: ____________ ÷ ____________ = ____________
waist measurement hip measurement

Determine Your Relative Risk

Find the risk category that corresponds to your ratio and age group in Figure 6-3 (p. 138). Record the risk category here and on the chart below.

Relative risk (from Figure 6-3): ___________

Rating Your Body Composition

Assessment	*Value*	*Classification/ Relative Risk*
BMI	___________ kg/m^2	___________
Skinfold measurements	___________ % body fat	___________
Waist-to-hip circumference	___________ (ratio)	___________

To monitor your progress toward your goal, enter the results of this lab in the Preprogram Assessment column of Lab 15-2. After several weeks of a program to improve body composition, do this lab again, and enter the results in the Postprogram Assessment column of Lab 15-2. How do the results compare?

Name ______________________ Section ______________ Date ______________

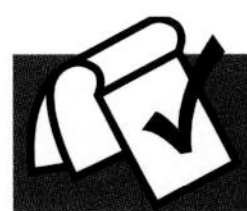

LAB 6-2 *Determining Desirable Body Weight*

Equipment

Calculator (or pencil and paper for calculations)

Preparation

Take skinfold measurements and calculate BMI as described in Lab 6-1. Keep track of height and weight as measured for these calculations.

Height: ____________

Weight: ____________

Choose a target BMI from Table 6-3. Choose a target percent body fat from Table 6-1. For example, a 190-pound male who is 5 feet, 7 inches tall and has a BMI of 29.9 and a percent body fat of 26 might set goals of 26 for BMI and 18 for percent body fat.

Instructions	*Example (see above)*
1. To calculate desirable weight from target BMI:	1. Desirable weight from target BMI:
a. Convert your height measurement to meters by multiplying your height in inches by 0.0254.	67 in. × 0.0254 m/in. = 1.70 m
b. Square your height measurement.	1.70 m × 1.70 m = 2.89 m²
c. Multiply your target BMI by your height in meters, squared, to get your target weight in kilograms.	26 kg/m² × 2.89 m² = 75.1 kg
d. Multiply your target weight in kilograms by 2.2 to get your desirable body weight in pounds.	75.1 kg × 2.2 lb/kg = 165 lb

a. Height ____________ in. × 0.0254 m/in. = height ____________ m

b. Height ____________ m × height ____________ m = height ____________ m²

c. Target BMI ____________ × height ____________ m² = target weight ____________ kg

d. Target weight ____________ kg × 2.2 lb/kg = desirable body weight ____________ lb

2. To calculate desirable body weight from actual and target body fat percentages:	2. Desirable weight from actual and target body fat percentages:
a. To determine the fat weight in your body, multiply your current weight by percent body fat (determined through skinfold measurements and expressed as a decimal).	190 lb × 0.26 = 49.4 lb
b. Subtract the fat weight from your current weight to get your current lean body weight.	190 lb − 49.4 lb = 140.6 lb
c. Subtract your target percent body fat from 1 to get target percent lean body weight.	1 − 0.18 = 0.82
d. To get your desirable body weight, divide your lean body weight by your target percent lean body weight.	140.6 lb ÷ 0.82 = 171 lb

Note: Weight can be expressed in either pounds or kilograms, as long as the unit of measurement is used consistently.

a. Current body weight ___________ × percent body fat = fat weight ___________

b. Current body weight ___________ − fat weight ___________ = lean body weight ___________

c. 1 − target percent body fat ___________ = target percent lean body weight ___________

d. Lean body weight ___________ ÷ target percent lean body weight ___________ =
desirable body weight ___________

Based on these calculations and other factors (including heredity, individual preference, and current health status), select a target weight or range of weights for yourself:

Target body weight: ___________

To monitor your progress toward your goal, enter the results of this lab in the Preprogram Assessment column of Lab 15-2. After several weeks of a program to improve body composition, do this lab again, and enter the results in the Postprogram Assessment column of Lab 15-2. How do the results compare?

7

Putting Together a Complete Fitness Program

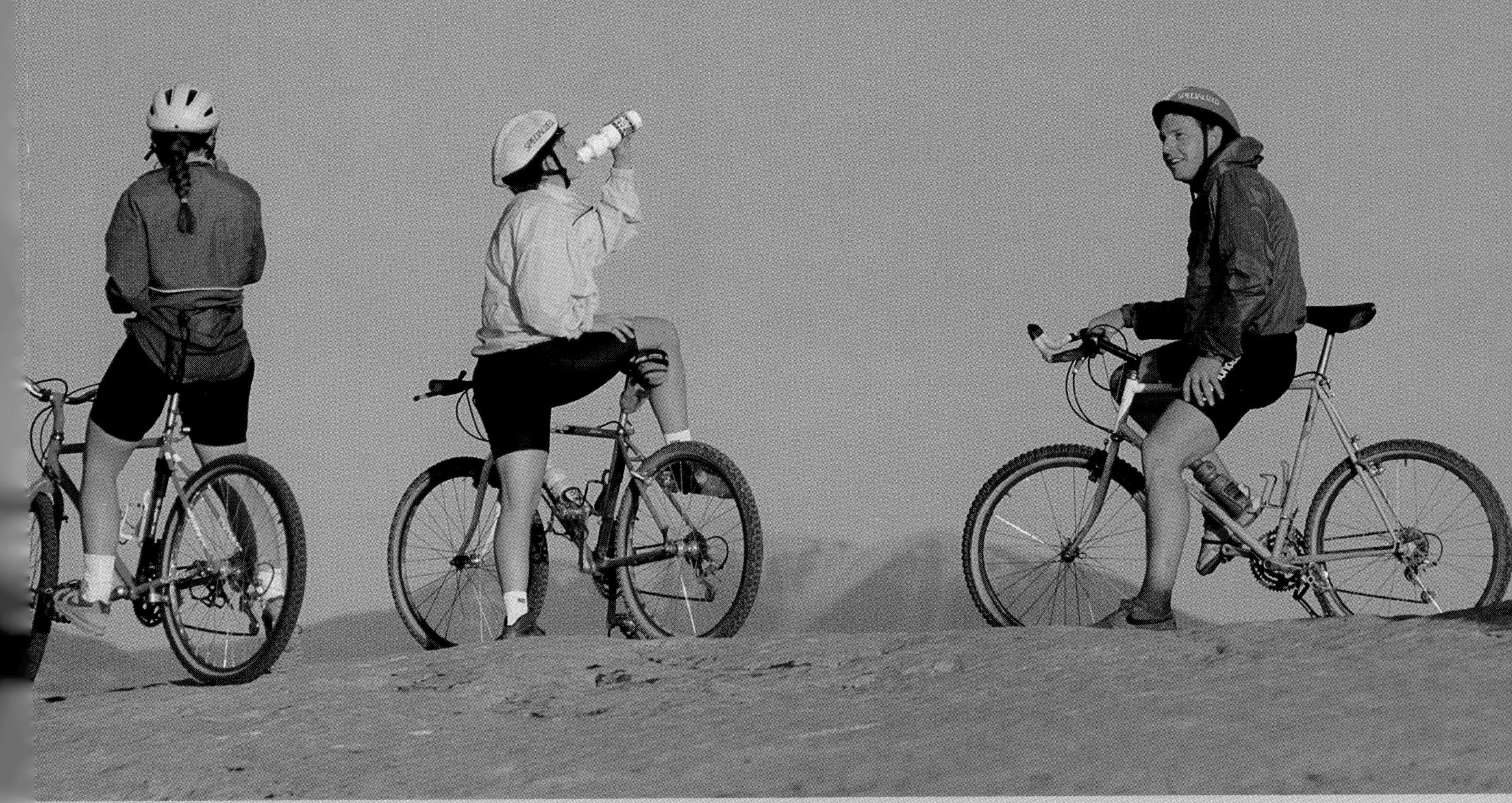

LOOKING AHEAD

After reading this chapter, you should be able to answer these questions about putting together a complete personalized exercise program:

- What are the six steps for putting together a successful personal fitness program?
- What strategies can help increase motivation and commitment to a fitness program?
- How can the sample programs presented be used to help create personalized fitness programs?

Understanding the physiological basis and wellness benefits of health-related physical fitness, as explained in Chapters 1–6, is the first step toward creating a well-rounded exercise program. The next challenge is to combine activities into a program that develops all the fitness components and maintains motivation.

This chapter presents a step-by-step procedure for creating and maintaining a well-rounded program and also provides sample programs based on popular activities. The structure these programs provide can be helpful if you're beginning an exercise program for the first time.

PUTTING TOGETHER YOUR OWN PROGRAM

If you're ready to create a complete fitness program from the activities you enjoy most, begin by preparing the program plan and contract in Lab 7-1. Refer to Figure 7-1 for a sample completed contract. A plan can help you set up a sound program and stick to it. The step-by-step procedure outlined here (adapted from *Your Guide to Getting Fit,* by Ivan Kusinitz and Morton Fine) will guide you through the steps of Lab 7-1 to the creation of an exercise program that's right for you.

1. *Set goals.* Setting specific goals to reach through exercise is a crucial first step in a successful fitness program. Refer to the general goals discussed in Chapter 2 and the results of the assessment tests you completed in Chapters 3–6. Your goals might be related to cardiovascular health, or they might relate to athletic performance or personal appearance.

   You'll find it easier to stick with your program if you choose realistic goals that are important for you. Think carefully about your reasons for exercising, and then fill in the goals portion of your program plan in Lab 7-1.

2. *Select activities.* If you have already chosen activities and created separate program plans for different fitness components in Chapters 3, 4, and 5, you can put those plans together into a single program. Cardiorespiratory endurance exercise should be the cornerstone of your fitness program; it will help you build muscular strength and endurance, maintain flexibility, and promote a healthy body composition. But more rapid gains in these other components of fitness are possible if the program includes exercises specifically designed to develop them—if weight training is included with a walking program, for example.

   To make sure all fitness components are included when you combine activities or choose new ones, refer to the activity ratings in Table 7-1 (p. 156). Choose activities based on their ability to help you reach your fitness goals. One strategy would be to select a different activity to develop each component of fitness—bicycling, weight training, and stretching, for example. Another strategy applies the principle of **cross-training,** using several different activities to develop one fitness component—aerobic dance, swimming, and volleyball, for instance.

   If you select activities that support your commitment, not activities that turn exercise into a chore, the right program will be its own incentive for continuing. Consider the following in making your choices:

   - Is this activity fun? Will it hold my interest over time?
   - Will this activity help me reach my goals?
   - Will my current fitness and skill level allow me to participate fully in this activity? (Refer to Table 7-1.)
   - Can I easily fit my participation in this activity into my daily schedule?
   - Are there any special requirements (facilities,

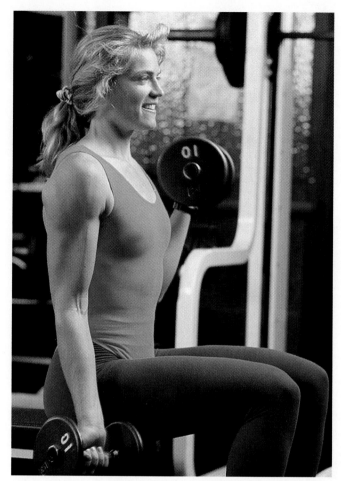

Weight training does little to develop cardiorespiratory endurance but is excellent for developing muscular strength and endurance. An overall fitness program includes exercises to develop all the components of physical fitness.

A. I Tracie Kaufman (name) am contracting with myself to follow a physical fitness program to work toward the following goals:

1. Improving cardiorespiratory fitness by raising my $\dot{V}O_{2max}$ to 37 ml/kg/min
2. Improving upper body muscular strength and endurance
3. Improving body composition (from 30% to 25% body fat)
4. Improving my tennis game
5. Developing a more positive attitude about myself

B. My program plan is as follows:

Activities	Components (Check ✓) CRE	MS	ME	F	BC	Intensity*	Duration	Frequency (Check ✓) M	Tu	W	Th	F	Sa	Su
Swimming	✓	✓	✓	✓	✓	140-150 bpm	35min	✓		✓		✓		
Tennis	✓	✓	✓	✓	✓	RPE = 14	90min						✓	
Weight Training		✓	✓	✓	✓	see Lab 4-3	30min		✓		✓		✓	
Stretching				✓		—	20min	✓		✓		✓	✓	

C. My program will begin on Sept. 21. My program includes the following schedule of mini-goals. For each step in my program, I will give myself the reward listed.

(mini-goal)	(date)	(reward)
Completing 2 full weeks of program (mini-goal 1)	Oct 5	movie with friends
$\dot{V}O_{2max}$ of 34 ml/kg/min (mini-goal 2)	Nov 2	new CD
Completing 10 full weeks of program (mini-goal 3)	Nov 30	new sweater
Percent body fat of 28% (mini-goal 4)	Dec 22	weekend away
$\dot{V}O_{2max}$ of 36 ml/kg/min (mini-goal 5)	Jan 18	new CD

D. My program will include the addition of physical activity to my daily routine (such as climbing stairs or walking to class):

1. Walking to and from campus job
2. Taking the stairs to dorm room instead of elevator
3. Bicycling to the library instead of driving
4.
5.

E. I will use the following tools to monitor my program and my progress toward my goals: I'll use a chart that lists the number of laps and minutes I swim and the charts for strength and flexibility from Labs 4-3 & 5-2.

I sign this contract as an indication of my personal commitment to reach my goal.

Tracie Kaufman (your signature) Sept 10 (date)

I have recruited a helper who will witness my contract and swim with me three days per week (list any way your helper will participate in your program)

Russell Walker (witness's signature) Sept 10 (date)

*List your target heart rate range or an RPE value if appropriate.

Figure 7-1 ***A sample personal fitness program plan and contract.***

partners, equipment, and so on) that I must plan for?

- Can I afford any special costs required for equipment or facilities?
- Does this activity conform to any special health needs I might have? Will it enhance my ability to cope with my specific health problem?

TERMS

cross-training Alternating two or more activities to improve a single component of fitness.

TABLE 7-1 Summary of Sports and Fitness Activities

This table classifies sports and activities as high (H), moderate (M), or low (L) in terms of their ability to develop each of the five components of physical fitness: cardiorespiratory endurance (CRE), muscular strength (MS), muscular endurance (ME), flexibility (F), and body composition (BC). The skill level needed to obtain fitness benefits is noted: Low (L) means little or no skill is required to obtain fitness benefits; moderate (M) means average skill is needed to obtain fitness benefits; and high (H) means much skill is required to obtain fitness benefits. The fitness prerequisite—conditioning needs of a beginner—is also noted: Low (L) means no fitness prerequisite is required; moderate (M) means some preconditioning is required; and high (H) means substantial fitness is required. The last two columns list the calorie cost of each activity when performed moderately and vigorously.

	Components							**Approximate Calorie Cost (cal/lb/min)**	
Sports and Activities	*CRE*	*MS**	*ME**	*F**	*BC*	*Skill Level*	*Fitness Prerequisite*	*Moderate*	*Vigorous*
Aerobic dance	H	M	H	H	H	L	L	.046	.062
Backpacking	H	M	H	M	H	L	M	.032	.078
Badminton, skilled, singles	H	M	M	M	H	M	M	—	.071
Ballet (floor combinations)	M	M	H	H	M	M	L	—	.058
Ballroom dancing	M	L	M	L	M	M	L	.034	.049
Baseball (pitcher and catcher)	M	M	H	M	M	H	M	.039	—
Basketball, half court	H	M	H	M	H	M	M	.045	.071
Bicycling	H	M	H	M	H	M	L	.049	.071
Bowling	L	L	L	L	L	L	L	—	—
Calisthenic circuit training	H	M	H	M	H	L	L	—	.060
Canoeing and kayaking (flat water)	M	M	H	M	M	M	M	.045	—
Cheerleading	M	M	M	M	M	M	L	.033	.049
Fencing	M	M	H	H	M	M	L	.032	.078
Field hockey	H	M	H	M	H	M	M	.052	.078
Folk and square dancing	M	L	M	L	M	L	L	.039	.049
Football, touch	M	M	M	M	M	M	M	.049	.078
Frisbee, ultimate	H	M	H	M	H	M	M	.049	.078
Golf (riding cart)	L	L	L	M	L	L	L	—	—
Handball, skilled, singles	H	M	H	M	H	M	M	—	.078
Hiking	H	M	H	L	H	L	M	.051	.073
Hockey, ice and roller	H	M	H	M	H	M	M	.052	.078
Horseback riding	M	M	M	L	M	M	M	.052	.065
Interval circuit training	H	H	H	M	H	L	L	—	.062
Jogging and running	H	M	H	L	H	L	L	.060	.104
Judo	M	H	H	M	M	M	L	.049	.090

*Ratings are for the muscle groups involved.

TABLE 7-1 Summary of Sports and Fitness Activities (continued)

	Components							Approximate Calorie Cost (cal/lb/min)	
Sports and Activities	*CR*	*MS**	*ME**	*F**	*BC*	*Skill Level*	*Fitness Prerequisite*	*Moderate*	*Vigorous*
Karate	H	M	H	H	H	L	M	.049	.090
Lacrosse	H	M	H	M	H	H	M	.052	.078
Modern dance (moving combinations)	M	M	H	H	M	L	L	—	.058
Orienteering	H	M	H	L	H	L	M	.049	.078
Outdoor fitness trails	H	M	H	M	H	L	L	—	.060
Popular dancing	M	L	M	M	M	M	L	—	.049
Racquetball, skilled, singles	H	M	M	M	H	M	M	.049	.078
Rock climbing	M	H	H	H	M	H	M	.033	.033
Rope skipping	H	M	H	L	H	M	M	.071	.095
Rowing	H	H	H	H	H	L	L	.032	.097
Rugby	H	M	H	M	H	M	M	.052	.097
Sailing	L	L	M	L	L	M	L	—	—
Skating, ice and roller	M	M	H	M	M	H	M	.049	.065
Skiing, alpine	M	H	H	M	M	H	M	.039	.078
Skiing, cross-country	H	M	H	M	H	M	M	.049	.104
Soccer	H	M	H	M	H	M	M	.052	.097
Squash, skilled, singles	H	M	M	M	H	M	M	.049	.078
Stretching	L	L	L	H	L	L	L	—	—
Surfing (including swimming)	M	M	M	M	M	H	M	—	.078
Swimming	H	M	H	M	H	M	L	.032	.088
Synchronized swimming	M	M	H	H	M	H	M	.032	.052
Table tennis	M	L	M	M	M	M	L	—	.045
Tennis, skilled, singles	H	M	M	M	H	M	M	—	.071
Volleyball	M	L	M	M	M	M	M	—	.065
Walking	H	L	M	L	H	L	L	.029	.048
Water polo	H	M	H	M	H	H	M	—	.078
Water skiing	M	M	H	M	M	H	M	.039	.055
Weight training	L	H	H	H	M	L	L	—	—
Wrestling	H	H	H	H	H	H	H	.065	.094
Yoga	L	L	M	H	L	H	L	—	—

*Ratings are for the muscle groups involved.

Source: Kusinitz, I., and M. Fine. 1995. *Your Guide to Getting Fit,* 3d ed. Mountain View, Calif.: Mayfield.

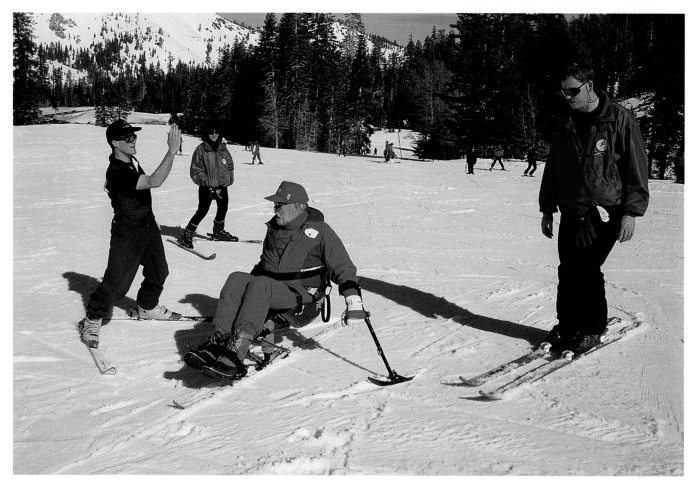

Qualified instruction can help make an exercise program both more enjoyable and more effective. This man has further increased his chance of creating a successful program by choosing an activity that he enjoys and that conforms to his special health needs.

With your goals and these guidelines in mind, select activities and add them to the program plan chart in Lab 7-1.

3. *Set a target intensity, duration, and frequency for each activity.* Refer to the calculations and plans you completed in Chapters 3, 4, and 5. For cardiorespiratory exercise, note your target heart rate zone, or RPE. To burn off the recommended 300 calories per exercise session, set a duration of 30 minutes for high-intensity activities and 60 minutes for low-intensity activities. To check that you've set the proper duration, refer to the **calorie costs** (calories per minute per pound of body weight) given in Table 7-1. For example, cycling at a moderate pace burns .045 calories per minute per pound of body weight. A 150-pound person would have to cycle for about 45 minutes to burn 300 calories.
4. *Make a commitment.* Complete your program plan in Lab 7-1 by signing your contract and having it witnessed.
5. *Begin and maintain your program.* Start out slowly to allow your body time to adjust. Be realistic and patient. In addition to the strategies presented in Chapter 1, try these to help you start and stick with your program:
   - Don't let your program become boring. Change the music you use for aerobic dance, or watch TV while stretching or riding a stationary bicycle.
   - Exercise with others who share your goals and general fitness level.
   - Vary your program. Change your activities periodically. Alter your route or distance if biking

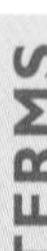

calorie cost The amount of energy used to perform a particular activity, usually expressed in calories per minute per pound of body weight.

Name Tracie Kaufman

Enter duration, distance, or other factor to track your progress.

Activity/Date	M	Tu	W	Th	F	S	S	Weekly Total	M	Tu	W	Th	F	S	S	Weekly Total
1 Swimming	800 yd		725 yd		800 yd			2325 yd	800 yd		800 yd		850 yd			2450 yd
2 Tennis						90 min		90 min						95 min		95 min
3 Weight training		✓		✓		✓				✓		✓		✓	✓	
4 Stretching	✓		✓		✓	✓			✓			✓	✓	✓	✓	
5																
6																

Figure 7-2 *A sample program log.*

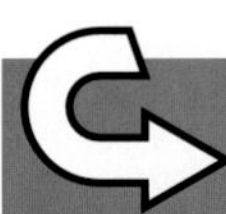

TACTICS AND TIPS

Keeping Your Fitness Program on Track

- Set realistic goals. Unrealistically high goals will only discourage you.
- Sign a contract, keep records of your activities, and track your progress.
- Start slowly, and increase intensity and duration gradually. Overzealous exercising can result in discouraging discomforts and injuries. Your program is meant to last a lifetime. The important first step is to break your established pattern of inactivity.
- Make your program fun. Participate in a variety of different activities that you enjoy. Vary the routes you take walking, running, or biking.
- Exercise with a friend. The social side of exercise is an important factor for many regular exercisers.
- Focus on the improvements you obtain from your program, how good you feel during and after exercise.
- If your program turns out to be unrealistic, revise it. Expect to make many adjustments in your program along the way.
- Expect fluctuation. On some days, your progress will be excellent, while on others, you'll barely be able to drag yourself through your scheduled activities.
- Expect lapses. Don't let them discourage you or make you feel guilty. Instead, feel a renewed commitment for your exercise program.
- Reward yourself often for sticking with your program.
- If you notice you're slacking off, try to list the negative thoughts and behaviors that are causing noncompliance. Devise a strategy to decrease the frequency of negative thoughts and behaviors. Make changes in your program plan and reward system to help renew your enthusiasm and commitment to your program.
- Review your goals. Visualize what it will be like to reach them, and keep these pictures in your mind as an incentive to stick to your program.

or jogging. Change racquetball partners, or find a new volleyball court.

6. *Record and assess your progress.* A record that tracks your daily progress will help remind you of your ongoing commitment to your program and give you a sense of accomplishment. Lab 7-2 shows you how to create a general program log (a sample is shown in Figure 7-2) and record the activity type, frequency, and duration. Or if you wish, complete specific activity logs like those in Labs 3-2, 4-3, and 5-2 in addition to, or instead of, a general log. Post your log in a place where you'll see it often as a reminder and as an incentive for improvement. You'll find additional strategies in the box "Keeping Your Fitness Program on Track."

SAMPLE PROGRAMS FOR POPULAR ACTIVITIES

Sample programs based on three different types of cardiorespiratory activities—walking/jogging/running, bicycling, and swimming—are presented below. Each sample program includes regular cardiorespiratory endurance exercise, resistance training, and stretching. To choose a sample program, first compare your fitness goals with the benefits of the different types of endurance exercise featured in the sample programs (see Table 7-1). Identify the programs that meet your fitness needs. Next, read through the descriptions of the programs you're considering and decide which will work best for you based on your present routine, the potential for enjoyment, and adaptability to your lifestyle. If you choose one of these programs, complete the personal fitness program plan in Lab 7-1, just as if you had created a program from scratch.

No program will bring about enormous changes in your fitness level in the first few weeks. Be sure to give your program a good chance. Follow the specifics of the program for 3–4 weeks. Then if the exercise program doesn't seem suitable, make adjustments to adapt it to your particular needs. But be sure to retain the basic elements of the program that make it effective for developing fitness.

General Guidelines

The following guidelines can help make the activity programs more effective for you:

- *Intensity.* To work effectively for cardiorespiratory endurance training or to improve body composition, you must raise your heart rate into its target zone. Monitor your pulse, or use rates of perceived exertion to monitor your intensity.

  If you've been sedentary, begin very slowly. Give your muscles a chance to adjust to their increased workload. It's probably best to keep your heart rate below target until your body has had time to adjust to new demands. At first you may not need to work very hard to keep your heart rate in its target zone, but as your cardiorespiratory endurance improves, you will probably need to increase intensity.
- *Duration and frequency.* To experience training effects, you should exercise for 20–60 minutes per session at least three times per week.
- *Interval training.* Some of the sample programs involve continuous activity. Others rely on **interval training,** which calls for alternating a relief interval with exercise (walking after jogging, for example, or coasting after biking uphill). Interval training is an effective way to achieve progressive overload: When your heart rate gets too high, slow down to lower your pulse rate until you're at the low end of your target zone. Interval training can also prolong the total time you spend in exercise and delay the onset of fatigue.
- *Warm-up and cool-down.* Begin each exercise session with a 10-minute warm-up. Begin your activity at a slow pace, and work up gradually to your target heart rate. Always slow down gradually at the end of your exercise session to bring your system back to its normal state. It's a good idea to do stretching exercises to increase your flexibility after cardiorespiratory exercise or strength training because your muscles will be warm and ready to stretch.
- *Record keeping.* After each exercise session, record your daily distance or time on a progress chart like the one shown in Lab 7-2.

TERMS

interval training A training technique that alternates exercise intervals with rest intervals or intense exercise intervals with low to moderate intervals.

WALKING/JOGGING/RUNNING SAMPLE PROGRAM

Walking, jogging, and running are the most popular forms of training for people who want to improve cardiorespiratory endurance; they also improve body composition and muscular endurance of the legs. It's not always easy to distinguish among these three endurance activities. For clarity and consistency, we'll consider walking to be any on-foot exercise of less than 5 miles per hour, jogging any pace between 5 and 7.5 miles per hour, and running any pace faster than that. Table 7-2 divides walking, jogging, and running into nine categories, with rates of speed (in both miles per hour and minutes per mile) and calorie costs for each. The faster your pace or the longer you exercise, the more calories you burn. The greater the number of calories burned, the higher the potential training effects of these activities.

Equipment and Technique

These activities require no special skills, expensive equipment, or unusual facilities. Comfortable clothing, well-fitted walking or running shoes, and a stopwatch or ordinary watch with a second hand are all you need. (For information on selecting appropriate shoes for walking or other activities, see the box "Choosing Exercise Footwear," p. 162.)

Developing Cardiorespiratory Endurance

The four variations of the basic walking/jogging/running sample program that follow are designed to help you regulate the intensity, duration, and frequency of

TABLE 7-2 Calorie Costs for Walking/Jogging/Running

This table gives the calorie costs of walking, jogging, and running for slow, moderate, and fast paces. Calculations for calorie costs are approximate and assume a level terrain. A hilly terrain would result in higher calorie cost. To get an estimate of the number of calories you burn, multiply your weight by the calories per minute per pound for the speed at which you're doing the activity (listed in the right-hand column), then multiply that by the number of minutes you exercise.

	Speed		
Activity	*Miles per Hour*	*Minutes: Seconds per Mile*	**Calories per Minute per Pound**
Walking			
Slow	2.0	30:00	.020
	2.5	24:00	.023
Moderate	3.0	20:00	.026
	3.5	17:08	.029
Fast	4.0	15:00	.037
	4.5	13:20	.048
Jogging			
Slow	5.0	12:00	.060
	5.5	11:00	.074
Moderate	6.0	10:00	.081
	6.5	9:00	.088
Fast	7.0	8:35	.092
	7.5	8:00	.099
Running			
Slow	8.5	7:00	.111
Moderate	9.0	6:40	.116
Fast	10.0	6:00	.129
	11.0	5:30	.141

Source: Kusinitz, I., and M. Fine. 1995. *Your Guide to Getting Fit,* 3d ed. Mountain View, Calif.: Mayfield.

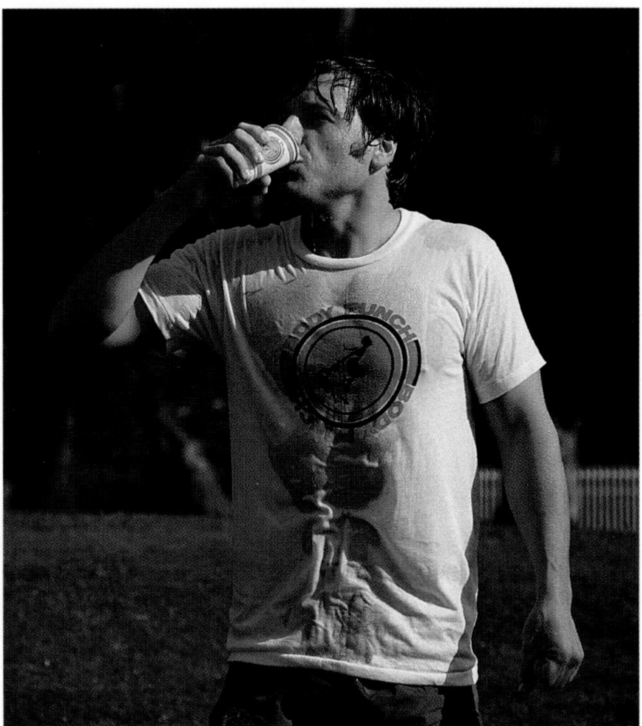

Drinking water before, during, and after exercise helps prevent dehydration from the loss of body fluids through perspiration. About 8 ounces of water or other fluid should be consumed for every 30 minutes of heavy exercise.

your program. To select the variation that's best for you at your current fitness level, consult Table 7-3, p. 164.

VARIATION 1: Walking (Starting)

Intensity, duration, and frequency: Walk at first for 15 minutes at a pace that keeps your heart rate below your target zone. Gradually increase to 30-minute sessions. The distance you travel will probably be 1–2 miles. At the beginning, walk every other day. You can gradually increase to daily walking if you want to burn more calories (helpful if you want to change body composition).

Calorie cost: Work up to using 90–135 calories in each session (see Table 7-2). To increase calorie costs to the target level, walk for a longer time or for a longer distance rather than sharply increasing speed.

At the beginning: Start at whatever level is most comfortable. Maintain a normal easy pace, and stop to rest as often as you need to. Never prolong a walk past the point of comfort. When walking with a friend (a good motivation), let a comfortable conversation be your guide to pace.

As you progress: Once your muscles have become adjusted to the exercise program, increase the duration of your sessions—but by no more than 10% each week. Increase your intensity only enough to keep your heart rate just below your target. When you're able to walk 1.5 miles in 30 minutes, using 90–135 calories per session, you should consider moving on to Variation 2 or 3. Don't be discouraged by lack of immediate progress, and don't try to speed things up by overdoing. Remember that pace and heart rate can vary with the terrain, the weather, and other factors.

CRITICAL CONSUMER

Choosing Exercise Footwear

Footwear is perhaps the most important item of equipment for almost any activity. Shoes protect and support your feet and improve your traction. When you jump or run, you place as much as six times more force on your feet than when you stand still. Shoes can help cushion against the stress that this additional force places on your lower legs and thus prevent injuries. Some athletic shoes are also designed to help prevent ankle rollover, another common source of injury.

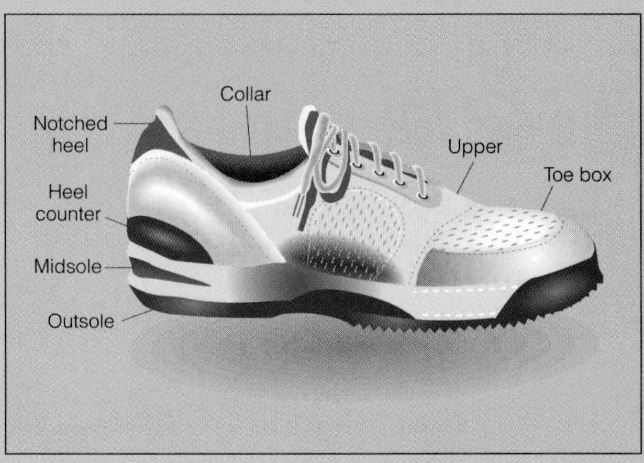

Shoe Terminology

Understanding the structural features of athletic shoes can help you make sound choices.

Outsole: The bottom of the shoe that touches the ground and provides traction. The shape and composition of an outsole depend on the activity for which the shoe is designed.

Midsole: The layer of shock-absorbing material located between the insole and the outsole; typically composed of polyurethane, ethyl vinyl acetate (EVA), rubber, or another cushioning material.

Insole: The insert or sock lining that the foot rests on inside the shoe, usually contoured to fit the foot and containing additional cushioning and arch and heel support.

Collar: The opening of the shoe where the foot goes in.

Upper: The top part of the shoe, usually made of nylon, canvas, or leather.

Toe box: The front part of the upper, which surrounds the toes.

Heel counter: The stiff cup in the back of the inside of the shoe that provides support and stability.

Notched heel: Some shoes have raised heel padding to support the Achilles tendon.

Stabilizers: Bars or strips of rubber, polyurethane, or nylon near the heel or forefoot area of some shoes; they provide additional stability.

Wedge: The thick portion of the midsole that makes the heel higher than the ball of the foot in some shoes.

General Guidelines

When choosing athletic shoes, first consider the activity you've chosen for your exercise program. Shoes appropriate for different activities have very different characteristics. For example, running shoes typically have highly cushioned midsoles, rubber outsoles with elevated heels, and a great deal of flexibility in the forefoot. The heels of walking shoes tend to be lower, less padded, and more beveled than those designed for running. For aerobic dance, shoes must be flexible in the forefoot and have straight, nonflared heels to allow for safe and easy lateral movements. Court shoes also provide substantial support for lateral movements; they typically have outsoles made from white rubber that will not damage court surfaces.

VARIATION 2: Advanced Walking

Intensity, duration, and frequency: Start at a pace at the lower end of your target heart rate zone, and begin soon afterward to increase your pace. This might boost your heart rate into the upper levels of your target zone, which is fine for brief periods. But don't overdo the intervals of fast walking. Slow down after a short time to drop your pulse rate. Vary your pattern to allow for intervals of slow, medium, and fast walking. Walk at first for 30 minutes and gradually increase your walking time until eventually you reach 60 minutes, all the while maintaining your target heart rate. The distance you walk will probably be 2–4 miles. Walk at least every other day.

Calorie cost: Work up to using about 200–350 calories in each session (see Table 7-2).

At the beginning: Begin by walking somewhat faster than you did in Variation 1. Check your pulse to make sure you keep your heart rate within your target zone. Slow down when necessary to lower your heart rate when going up hills or when extending the duration of your walks.

CRITICAL CONSUMER

Choosing Exercise Footwear (continued)

Also consider the location and intensity of your workouts. If you plan to walk or run on trails, you should choose shoes with water-resistant, highly durable uppers and more outsole traction. If you work out intensely or have a relatively high body weight, you'll need thick, firm midsoles to avoid bottoming-out the cushioning system of your shoes.

Foot type is another important consideration. If your feet tend to roll in excessively (overpronate), you may need shoes with additional stability features on the inner side of the shoe to counteract this movement. If your feet tend to roll outward excessively (oversupinate), you may need highly flexible and cushioned shoes that promote foot motion. For aerobic dancers with feet that tend to pronate or supinate, mid-cut to high-cut shoes may be more appropriate than low-cut aerobic shoes or cross-trainers (shoes designed to be worn for several different activities). If you are a woman with relatively big or wide feet, shoes designed specifically for large feet or even men's athletic shoes may fit better.

For successful shoe shopping, keep the following strategies in mind:

- Shop at an athletic shoe or specialty store that has personnel trained to fit athletic shoes and a large selection of styles and sizes.
- Shop late in the day or, ideally, following a workout. Your foot size increases over the course of the day and as a result of exercise.
- Wear socks like those you plan to wear during exercise. If you have an old pair of athletic shoes, bring them with you. The wear pattern on your old shoes can help you select a pair with extra support or cushioning in the places you need it the most.
- Ask for help. Trained salespeople know which shoes are designed for your foot type and your level of activity. They can also help fit your shoes properly.
- Don't insist on buying shoes in what you consider to be your typical shoe size. Sizes vary from shoe to shoe. In addition, foot sizes change over time, and many people have one foot that is larger or wider than the other. Try several sizes in several widths if necessary. Don't buy shoes that are too small.
- Try on both shoes, and wear them around for ten or more minutes. Try walking on a noncarpeted surface. Approximate the movements of your activity: walk, jog, run, jump, and so on.
- Check the fit and style carefully:

  Is the toe box roomy enough? Your toes will spread out when your foot hits the ground or you push off.

  Do they have enough cushioning? Do your feet feel cushioned and supported when you bounce up and down? Try bouncing on your toes and on your heels.

  Do your heels fit snugly into the shoe? Do they stay put when you walk, or do they rise up?

  Are the arches of your feet right on top of the shoes' arch supports?

  Do the shoes feel stable when you twist and turn on the balls of your feet? Try twisting from side to side while standing on one foot.

  Do you feel any pressure points?
- If the shoe isn't comfortable in the store, don't buy it. Don't expect athletic shoes to stretch over time in order to fit your feet properly.

Sources: Adapted from Choosing the right shoe. 1995. *Runner's World,* October. Gear guidelines. 1995. *Women's Sports and Fitness,* January/February. Legwold, G. 1994. Today's most comfortable walking shoes. *Consumers Digest,* January/February. Sudy, M., ed. 1991. *Personal Trainer Manual.* San Diego: American Council on Exercise.

As you progress: As your heart rate adjusts to the increased workload, gradually increase your pace and your total walking time. Gradually lengthen the periods of fast walking and shorten the relief intervals of slow walking, always maintaining target heart rate. Eventually, you will reach the fitness level you would like to maintain. And to maintain that level of fitness, continue to burn the same amount of calories in each session.

Vary your program by changing the pace and distance walked, or by walking routes with different terrains and views. Gauge your progress toward whatever calorie goal you've set by using Table 7-2.

VARIATION 3: Preparing for a Jogging Program

Intensity, duration, and frequency: Start by walking at a moderate pace (3–4 miles per hour or 15–20 minutes per mile). Staying within your target heart rate zone, begin to add brief intervals of slow jogging (5–6 miles per hour or 10–12 minutes per mile). Keep the walking intervals constant at 60 seconds or at 110 yards, but gradually increase the jogging intervals until eventually you jog 4 minutes for each minute of walking. You'll probably cover between 1.5 and 2.5 miles. Each exercise session should last 15–30 minutes. Exercise every other

TABLE 7-3 Selecting a Walking/Jogging/Running Program

Variation 1: Walking (Starting)

Choose this program if *any* of the following apply:
You have medical restrictions.
You are recovering from illness or surgery.
You tire easily after short walks.
You are obese.
You have a sedentary lifestyle.
And if you want to prepare for the advanced walking program (see below) to improve cardiorespiratory endurance, body composition, and muscular endurance.

Variation 2: Walking (Advanced)

Choose this program if:
You already can walk comfortably for 30 minutes.
And if you want to develop and maintain cardiorespiratory fitness, a lean body, and muscular endurance.

Variation 3: Walking/Jogging (Starting)

Choose this program if:
You already can walk comfortably for 30 minutes.
And if you want to prepare for the jogging/running program (see below) to improve cardiorespiratory endurance, body composition, and muscular endurance.

Variation 4: Jogging/Running

Choose this program if both of the following apply:
You already can jog comfortably without muscular discomfort.
You already can jog for 15 minutes within your target heart rate without stopping or for 30 minutes with brief walking intervals.
And if you want to develop and maintain a high level of cardiorespiratory fitness, a lean body, and muscular endurance.

Source: Kusinitz, I., and M. Fine. 1995. *Your Guide to Getting Fit,* 3d ed. Mountain View, Calif.: Mayfield.

day. If your goals include changing body composition and you want to exercise more frequently, walk on days you're not jogging.

Calorie cost: Work up to using 200–350 calories in each session (see Table 7-2).

At the beginning: Start slowly. Until your muscles adjust to jogging, you may need to exercise at less than your target heart rate. At the outset, expect to do two to four times as much walking as jogging, even more if you're relatively inexperienced. Be guided by how comfortable you feel—and by your heart rate—in setting the pace for your progress. To avoid injury, follow the guidelines for proper running technique listed in the box "Proper Running Technique."

As you progress: Adjust your ratio of walking to jogging to keep within your target heart rate zone as much as possible. When you have progressed to the point where most of your 30-minute session is spent jogging, consider moving on to Variation 4.

To find a walking/jogging progression that suits you, refer to Tables 7-4 and 7-5. (One uses time, the other distance.) Which one you choose will depend, to some extent, on where you work out. If you have access to a track or can use a measured distance with easily visible landmarks to indicate yardage covered, you may find it convenient to use distance as your organizing principle. If you'll be using parks, streets, or woods, time intervals (measured with a watch) would probably work better. The suggested progressions in Tables 7-4 and 7-5 are not meant to be rigid; they are guidelines to help you develop your own rate of progress. Let your progress be guided by your heart rate, and increase your intensity and duration only to achieve your target zone.

VARIATION 4: Jogging/Running

Intensity, duration, and frequency: The key is to exercise within your target heart rate zone. Most people who sustain a continuous jog/run program will

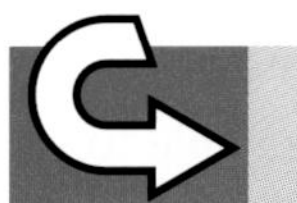

TACTICS AND TIPS

Proper Running Technique

To prevent injuries, wear an appropriate pair of running shoes. Warm up and stretch thoroughly before and after you run, and follow the guidelines presented in Chapter 3 for exercising in hot or cold weather. Drink enough liquids to stay adequately hydrated, particularly in hot weather. In addition, use the proper running technique described below:

- Run with your back straight and your head up. Look straight ahead, not at your feet. Shift your pelvis forward, and tuck your buttocks in.
- Hold your arms slightly away from your body. Your elbows should be bent so that your forearms are parallel to the ground. You may cup your hands, but do not clench your fists. Allow your arms to swing loosely and rhythmically with each stride.
- Your heel should hit the ground first in each stride. Then roll forward onto the ball of your foot and push off for the next stride. If you find this difficult, you can try a more flat-footed style; but don't land on the balls of your feet.
- Keep your steps short by allowing your foot to strike the ground just below your knee. Keep your knees bent at all times.
- Breathe deeply through your mouth. Try to use your abdominal muscles rather than just your chest muscles to take deep breaths.
- Stay relaxed.

TABLE 7-4 Sample Walking/Jogging Progression by Time

This table is based on a walking interval of 3.75 miles per hour, measured in seconds, and a jogging interval of 5.5 miles per hour, measured in minutes:seconds. The combination of the two intervals equals a single set. In the Number of Sets column, the higher figure represents the maximum number of sets to be completed.

	Walk Interval (sec)	Jog Interval (min:sec)	Number of Sets	Total Distance (mi)	Total Time (min:sec)
Stage 1	:60	:30	10–15	1.0–1.7	15:00–22:30
Stage 2	:60	:60	8–13	1.2–2.0	16:00–26:00
Stage 3	:60	2:00	5–19	1.3–2.3	15:00–27:00
Stage 4	:60	3:00	5–7	1.6–2.4	16:00–28:00
Stage 5	:60	4:00	3–6	1.5–2.7	15:00–30:00

Source: Kusinitz, I., and M. Fine. 1995. *Your Guide to Getting Fit,* 3d ed. Mountain View, Calif.: Mayfield.

TABLE 7-5 Sample Walking/Jogging Progression by Distance

This table is based on a walking interval of 3.75 miles per hour, measured in yards, and a jogging interval of 5.5 miles per hour, also measured in yards. The combination of the two intervals equals a single set.

	Walk Interval (yd)	Jog Interval (yd)	Number of Sets	Total Distance (mi)	Total Time (min:sec)
Stage 1	110	55	11–21	1.0–2.0	15:00–28:12
Stage 2	110	110	16	2.0	26:56
Stage 3	110	220	11	2.0	26:02
Stage 4	110	330	8	2.0	24:24
Stage 5	110	440	7	2.2	26:05
Stage 6	110	440	8	2.5	29:49

Source: Kusinitz, I., and M. Fine. 1995. *Your Guide to Getting Fit,* 3d ed. Mountain View, Calif.: Mayfield.

find that they can stay within their target heart rate zone with a speed of 5.5–7.5 miles per hour (8–11 minutes per mile). Start by jogging steadily for 15 minutes. Gradually increase your jog/run session to a regular 30–60 minutes (or about 2.5–7 miles). Exercise at least every other day. Increasing frequency by doing other activities on alternate days will place less stress on the weight-bearing parts of your lower body than will a daily program of jogging/running.

Calorie cost: Use about 300–750 calories in each session (see Table 7-2).

At the beginning: The greater number of calories you burn per minute makes this program less time-consuming for altering body composition than the three other variations in the walking/jogging/running program.

As you progress: If you choose this variation, you probably already have a moderate-to-high level of cardiorespiratory fitness. To stay within your target heart rate zone, increase your distance or both pace and distance as needed. Add variety to your workouts by varying your route, intensity, and duration. Alternate short runs with long ones. If you run for 60 minutes one day, try running for 30 minutes the next session. Or try doing sets that alternate hard and easy intervals—even walking, if you feel like it. You can also try a road race now and then, but be careful not to do too much too soon.

Developing Muscular Strength and Endurance

Walking, jogging, and running provide muscular endurance workouts for your lower body; they also develop muscular strength of the lower body to a lesser degree. To develop muscular strength and endurance of the upper body, and to make greater and more rapid gains in lower-body strength, you need to include resistance training in your fitness program. You can use the general wellness weight training program from Chapter 4, or tailor one to fit your personal fitness goals. If you'd like to increase your running speed and performance, you might want to focus your program on lower-body exercises. (Don't neglect upper-body strength, however; it is important for overall wellness.) Regardless of what strength training exercises you choose, follow the guidelines for successful training:

- Train 2–4 days per week.
- Perform 1–3 sets of 8–12 repetitions of 8–10 exercises.
- Include exercises that work all the major muscle groups: neck, shoulders, chest, arms, upper and lower back, abdomen, thighs, and calves.

Depending on the amount of time you are able to set aside for exercise, you may find it more convenient to alternate between your cardiorespiratory endurance workouts and your muscular strength and endurance workouts. In other words, walk or jog one day and strength train the next day.

Developing Flexibility

To round out your fitness program, you also need to include exercises that develop flexibility. The best time for a flexibility workout is when your muscles are warm, as they are immediately following cardiorespiratory endurance exercise or strength training. Perform the stretching routine presented in Chapter 5, or one that you have created to meet your own goals and preferences. Be sure to pay special attention to the hamstrings and quadriceps, which are not worked through their complete range of motion during walking or jogging. As you put your program together, remember the basic structure of a successful flexibility program:

- Stretch 3–5 days per week, preferably when muscles are warm.
- Stretch all the major muscle groups.
- Stretch to the point of mild discomfort, and hold for 15–30 seconds.
- Repeat each stretch 3–5 times.

BICYCLING SAMPLE PROGRAM

Bicycling can also lead to large gains in physical fitness. For many people, cycling is a pleasant and economical alternative to driving, and a convenient way to build fitness.

Equipment and Technique

Cycling has its own special array of equipment, including headgear, lighting, safety pennants, and special shoes. The bike is the most expensive item, ranging in cost from about $100 to well over $1000. Avoid making a large investment until you're sure you'll use your bike regularly. While investigating what the marketplace has to offer, rent or borrow a bike. Consider your intended use of the bike. Most cyclists who are interested primarily in fitness are best served by a sturdy 10-speed rather than a mountain bike or sport bike. Stationary bikes are good for rainy days and areas that have harsh winters.

Clothing for bike riding shouldn't be restrictive or binding, nor should it be so loose-fitting or so long that it might get caught in the chain. Clothing worn on the upper body should be comfortable but not so loose that it catches the wind and slows you down. Always wear a helmet (ideally equipped with a rear-view mirror) to help prevent injury in case of a fall or crash. Wearing glasses or goggles can protect the eyes from dirt, small objects, and irritation from wind.

To avoid saddle soreness and injury, choose a soft or padded saddle, and adjust it to a height that allows your legs to almost reach full extension while pedaling. Wear a pair of well-padded gloves if your hands tend to become numb while riding, or if you begin to develop blisters or calluses. To prevent backache and neck strain, warm up thoroughly, and periodically shift the position of your hands on the handlebars and your body in the saddle. Keep your arms relaxed, and don't lock your elbows. To protect your knees from strain, pedal with your feet pointed straight ahead or very slightly inward, and don't pedal in high gear for long periods.

Bike riding requires a number of precise skills that practice makes automatic. If you've never ridden before, consider taking a course. In fact, many courses are not just for beginners. They'll help you develop skills in braking, shifting, and handling emergencies, as well as teach you ways of caring for and repairing your bike.

Developing Cardiorespiratory Endurance

Cycling is an excellent way to develop and maintain cardiorespiratory endurance and a healthy body composition.

Intensity, duration, and frequency: If you've been inactive for a long time, begin your cycling program at a heart rate that is 10–20% below your target zone. Once you feel at home on your bike, try 1 mile at a comfortable speed, then stop and check your heart rate. Increase your speed gradually until you can cycle at 12–15 miles per hour (4–5 minutes per mile), a speed fast enough to bring most new cyclists' heart rate into their target zone. Allow your pulse rate to be your guide: More highly fit individuals may need to ride faster to achieve their target heart rate. Cycling for at least 20 minutes three times per week will improve your fitness.

Calorie cost: Use Table 7-6 (p. 168) to determine the number of calories you burn during each outing. You can increase the number of calories burned by cycling faster or for a longer duration (it's usually better to increase distance rather than to add speed).

At the beginning: It may require several outings to get the muscles and joints of your legs and hips adjusted to this new activity. Begin each outing with a 10-minute warm-up that includes stretches for your hamstrings and your back and neck muscles. Until you become a skilled cyclist, select routes with the fewest hazards, and avoid heavy automobile traffic. See the box "Bicycling Safety" (p. 169) for additional tips.

As you progress: Interval training is also effective with bicycling. Simply increase your speed for periods of 4–8 minutes or for specific distances, such as 1–2 miles. Then coast for 2–3 minutes. Alternate the speed intervals and slow intervals for a total of 20–60 minutes, depending on your level of fitness. Hilly terrain is also a form of interval training.

Developing Muscular Strength and Endurance

Bicycling develops a high level of endurance and a moderate level of strength in the muscles of the lower body. To develop muscular strength and endurance of the upper body—and to make greater and more rapid gains in lower-body strength—you need to include resistance training as part of your fitness program. You can use the general wellness weight training program from Chapter 4, or tailor one to fit your personal fitness goals. If one of your goals is to increase your cycling speed and performance, be sure to include exercises for the quadriceps, hamstrings, and buttocks muscles in your strength training program. No matter which exercises you include in your program, follow the general guidelines for successful and safe training:

- Train 2–4 days per week.
- Perform 1–3 sets of 8–12 repetitions of 8–10 exercises.
- Include exercises that work all the major muscle groups: neck, shoulders, chest, arms, upper and lower back, abdomen, thighs, and calves.

Depending on your schedule, you may find it more convenient to alternate between your cardiorespiratory endurance workouts and your muscular strength and endurance workouts. In other words, cycle one day and strength train the next day.

Developing Flexibility

A complete fitness program also includes exercises that develop flexibility. The best time for a flexibility workout is when your muscles are warm, as they are immediately following a session of cardiorespiratory endurance exercise or strength training. Perform the stretching routine presented in Chapter 5, or develop one that meets your own goals and preferences. Pay special attention to the hamstrings and quadriceps, which are not worked through their complete range of motion during bike riding, and to the muscles in your

TABLE 7-6 *Determining Calorie Costs for Bicycling*

This table gives the approximate calorie costs per pound of body weight for cycling from 5–60 minutes for distances of .50 mile up to 15 miles on a level terrain. To use the table, find on the horizontal line the time most closely approximating the number of minutes you cycle. Next, locate on the vertical column the approximate distance in miles you cover. The figure at the intersection represents an estimate of the calories used per minute per pound of body weight. Multiply this figure by your own body weight. Then multiply the product of these two figures by the number of minutes you cycle to get the total number of calories burned. For example, assuming you weigh 154 pounds and cycle 6 miles in 40 minutes, you would burn 260 calories: 154 × .042 (calories per pound, from table) = 6.5 × 40 (minutes) = 260 calories burned.

	Time (min)											
Distance (mi)	*5*	*10*	*15*	*20*	*25*	*30*	*35*	*40*	*45*	*50*	*55*	*60*
.50	.032											
1.00	.062	.032										
1.50		.042	.032									
2.00		.062	.039	.032								
3.00			.062	.042	.036	.032						
4.00				.062	.044	.039	.035	.032				
5.00				.097	.062	.045	.041	.037	.035	.032		
6.00					.088	.062	.047	.042	.039	.036	.034	.032
7.00						.081	.062	.049	.043	.040	.038	.036
8.00							.078	.062	.050	.044	.041	.039
9.00								.076	.062	.051	.045	.042
10.00								.097	.074	.062	.051	.045
11.00									.093	.073	.062	.052
12.00										.088	.072	.062
13.00											.084	.071
14.00												.081
15.00												.097

Source: Kusinitz, I., and M. Fine. 1995. *Your Guide to Getting Fit,* 3d ed. Mountain View, Calif.: Mayfield.

lower back, shoulders, and neck. As you put your stretching program together, remember these basic guidelines:

- Stretch 3–5 days per week, preferably when muscles are warm.
- Stretch all the major muscle groups.
- Stretch to the point of mild discomfort, and hold for 15–30 seconds.
- Repeat each stretch 3–5 times.

SWIMMING SAMPLE PROGRAM

Swimming is one of the best activities for developing all-around fitness. Because water supports the body weight of the swimmer, swimming places less stress than weight-bearing activities on joints, ligaments, and tendons and tends to cause fewer injuries.

Equipment

Aside from having access to a swimming pool, the only equipment required for a swimming program is a swimsuit and a pair of swimming goggles to protect the eyes from irritation in chlorinated pools.

Developing Cardiorespiratory Endurance

Any one or any combination of common swimming strokes—front crawl stroke, breaststroke, backstroke, butterfly stroke, sidestroke, or elementary backstroke

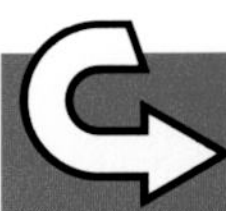

TACTICS AND TIPS

Bicycling Safety

The National Injury Information Clearinghouse classifies bicycle riding as the nation's most dangerous sport. Many injuries are the result of the cyclist's carelessness. For safe cycling, follow these rules:

- Always wear a helmet.
- Keep on the correct side of the road. Bicycling against traffic is usually illegal and always dangerous.
- Obey all traffic signs and signals.
- On public roads, ride in single file, except in low-traffic areas (if the law permits). Ride in a straight line; don't swerve or weave in traffic.
- Be alert; anticipate the movements of other traffic and pedestrians. Listen for approaching traffic that is out of your line of vision.
- Slow down at street crossings. Check both ways before crossing.
- Use hand signals—the same as for automobile drivers—if you intend to stop or turn. Use audible signals to warn those in your path.
- Maintain full control. Avoid anything that interferes with your vision. Don't jeopardize your ability to steer by carrying anything (including people) on the handlebars.
- Keep your bicycle in good shape. Brakes, gears, saddle, wheels, and tires should always be in good condition.
- See and be seen. Use a headlight at night, and equip your bike with rear reflectors. Use side reflectors on pedals, front and rear. Wear light-colored clothing or use reflective tape at night and bright colors or fluorescent tape by day.
- Be courteous to other road users. Anticipate the worst, and practice preventive cycling.
- Use a rear-view mirror.

—can help develop and maintain cardiorespiratory fitness. (Swimming may not be as helpful as walking, jogging, or cycling for body fat loss.)

Intensity, duration, and frequency: Because swimming is not a weight-bearing activity and is not done in an upright position, it elicits a lower heart rate per minute. Therefore, you need to adjust your target heart rate zone. To calculate your target heart rate for swimming, use this formula:

Maximum swimming heart rate (MSHR) = 205 − age

Heart rate reserve (HRR) = MSHR − resting heart rate (RHR)

Target heart rate zone = 50–85% of HRR + RHR

For example, a 19-year-old with a resting heart rate of 67 bpm would calculate her target heart rate zone for swimming as follows:

MSHR = 205 − 19 = 186 bpm

HRR = 186 − 67 = 119 bpm

Target heart rate zone for swimming:

at 50% intensity: (.50 × 119) + 67 = 127 bpm

at 85% intensity: (.85 × 119) + 67 = 168 bpm

Base your duration of swimming on your intensity and target calorie costs. Swim at least three times per week.

Calorie cost: Calories burned while swimming are the result of the pace: how far you swim and how fast (see Table 7-7, p. 170). Work up to using at least 300 calories per session.

At the beginning: If you don't have much experience swimming, invest the time and money for instruction. You'll make more rapid gains in fitness if you learn correct swimming technique. If you've been sedentary and haven't done any swimming for a long time, begin your program with 2–3 weeks, three times per week, of leisurely swimming at a pace that keeps your heart rate 10–20% below your target zone. Start swimming **laps** of the width of the pool if you can't swim the length. To keep your heart rate below target, take rest intervals as needed. Swim one lap, then rest 15–90 seconds as needed.

TERMS

lap In swimming, one width or one length of a pool, regardless of pool size.

TABLE 7-7 Determining Calorie Costs for Swimming

To use this table, find on the horizontal line the distance in yards that most closely approximates the distance you swim. Next, locate on the appropriate vertical column (below the distance in yards) the time it takes you to swim the distance. Then locate in the first column on the left the approximate number of calories burned per minute per pound for the time and distance. To find the total number of calories burned, multiply your weight by the calories per minute per pound. Then multiply the product of these two numbers by the time it takes you to swim the distance (minutes:seconds). For example, assuming you weigh 130 pounds and swim 500 yards in 20 minutes, you would burn 106 calories: 130 × .041 (calories per pound, from table) = 5.33 × 20 (minutes) = 106 calories burned.

Calories per Minute per Pound	Distance (yd) 25	100	150	250	500	750
.033	1:15	5:00	7:30	12:30	25:00	30:30
.041	1:00	4:00	6:00	10:00	20:00	30:00
.049	0:50	3:20	5:00	8:20	18:40	25:00
.057	0:43	2:52	4:18	7:10	17:20	21:30
.065	0:37.5	2:30	3:45	6:15	10:00	
.073	0:33	2:13	3:20	5:30	8:50	
.081	0:30	2:00	3:00	5:00	8:00	
.090	0:27	1:48	2:42	4:30	7:12	
.097	0:25	1:40	2:30	4:10	6:30	

Source: Kusinitz, I., and M. Fine. 1995. *Your Guide to Getting Fit,* 3d ed. Mountain View, Calif.: Mayfield.

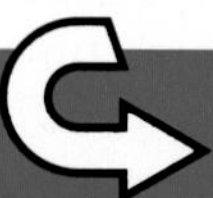

TACTICS AND TIPS

Health and Safety for Swimming

Following these few simple rules can help keep you safe and healthy during your swimming sessions:

- Swim only in a pool with a qualified lifeguard on duty.
- Always walk carefully on wet surfaces.
- Wear goggles to prevent eye irritation.
- Dry your ears well after swimming. If you experience the symptoms of swimmer's ear (itching, discharge, or even a partial hearing loss), consult your physician. If you swim while recovering from swimmer's ear, protect your ears with a few drops of lanolin on a wad of lamb's wool.
- To avoid back pain, try not to arch your back excessively when you swim.
- Be courteous to others in the pool.

If you swim in a setting other than a pool with a lifeguard, remember the following important rules:

- Don't swim beyond your skill and endurance limits.
- Avoid being chilled by water colder than 70°F.
- Never drink alcohol before going swimming.
- Never swim alone.

Start with 10 minutes of swim/rest intervals and work up to 20 minutes. How long it takes will depend on your swimming skills and muscular fitness. Be sure to follow the tips listed in the box "Health and Safety for Swimming."

As you progress: Gradually increase either the duration, the intensity, or both duration and intensity of your swimming to raise your heart rate to a comfortable level within your target zone. Gradually increase your swimming intervals and decrease your rest intervals as you progress. Once you can swim the length of the pool at a pace that keeps your heart rate on target, continue swim/rest intervals for 20 minutes. Your rest intervals should be 30–45 seconds. You may find it helpful to get out of the pool during your rest intervals and walk until you've lowered your heart rate. Next, swim two laps of the pool length per swim interval and continue swim/rest intervals for 30 minutes. For the 30-second rest interval, walk (or rest) until you've lowered your heart rate. Gradually increase the number of laps you swim consecutively and the total duration of your session until you reach your target calorie expenditure and fitness level. But take care not to swim at too fast a pace: It can raise your heart rate too high and limit your ability to sustain your swimming. Alternating strokes can rest your muscles and help prolong your swimming time. A variety of strokes will also let you work more muscle groups.

Developing Muscular Strength and Endurance

The swimming program outlined in this section will result in moderate gains in strength and large gains in endurance in the muscles used during the strokes you've chosen. To develop strength and endurance in all the muscles of the body, you need to include resistance training as part of your fitness program. You can use the general wellness weight training program from Chapter 4, or tailor one to fit your personal fitness goals. To improve your swimming performance, include exercises that work key muscles. For example, if you swim primarily front crawl, include exercises to increase strength in your shoulders, arms, and upper back. (Training the muscles you use during swimming can also help prevent injuries.) Regardless of which strength training exercise you include in your program, follow the general guidelines for successful training:

- Train 2–4 days per week.
- Perform 1–3 sets of 8–12 repetitions of 8–10 exercises.
- Include exercises that work all the major muscle groups: neck, shoulders, chest, arms, upper and lower back, abdomen, thighs, and calves.

Depending on the amount of time you have for exercise, you might want to schedule your cardiorespiratory endurance workouts and your muscular strength and endurance workouts on alternate days. In other words, swim one day and strength train the next day.

Developing Flexibility

For a complete fitness program, you also need to include exercises that develop flexibility. The best time for a flexibility workout is when your muscles are warm, as they are immediately following cardiorespiratory endurance exercise or strength training. Perform the stretching routine presented in Chapter 5 or one you have created to meet your own goals and preferences. Be sure to pay special attention to the muscles you use during swimming, particularly the shoulders and back. As you put your program together, remember the basic structure of a successful flexibility program:

- Stretch 3–5 days per week, preferably when muscles are warm.
- Stretch all the major muscle groups.
- Stretch to the point of mild discomfort, and hold for 15–30 seconds.
- Repeat each stretch 3–5 times.

? COMMON QUESTIONS ANSWERED

Should I exercise every day? Some daily exercise is beneficial, and many health experts recommend that you engage in at least 30 minutes of moderate physical activity over the course of every day. However, if you train intensely every day without giving yourself a rest, you will likely get injured or become overtrained. When strength training, for example, rest at least one day between workouts before exercising the same muscle group. For cardiorespiratory endurance exercise, rest or exercise lightly the day after an intense or long-duration workout. Balancing the proper amount of rest and exercise will help you feel better and improve your fitness faster.

When is the best time of day to exercise? Exercise physiologists have determined that your performance and body temperature are highest during the afternoon and early evening. Training during those times will feel better, and you will tend to run, swim, and cycle slightly faster than during other times of the day. However, other studies have shown that people who exercise in the morning are much more faithful to their programs.

I'm just starting an exercise program; how much activity should I do at first? Be conservative. Walking is a good way to begin almost any fitness program. At first, walk for approximately 10 minutes, and then increase the distance and pace. After several weeks, you can progress to something more vigorous. Let your body be your guide. If the intensity and duration of a workout seem easy, increase them a little next time. The key is to be progressive; don't try to achieve physical fitness in one or two workouts. Build your fitness gradually.

I'm concerned about my safety when I go for a jog or walk. What can I do to make sure that my training sessions are safe and enjoyable? A person exercising alone in the park can be a tempting target for criminals. Don't exercise alone. You are much less likely to be a crime victim if you are training in a group or with a partner. Another alternative is to take an exercise class. Classes are fun and much more safe than exercising by yourself. If you must train alone, try to exercise where there are plenty of people. A good bet is the local high school or college track.

Make sure you're wearing proper safety equipment. If you're riding a bike, wear a helmet. If you're playing racquetball or handball, wear eye protectors. Don't go in-line skating unless you're wearing the proper pads and protective equipment. If jogging at night, wear reflective clothing that can be seen easily.

Refer to Appendix A for more information on personal safety.

SUMMARY

- The six steps involved in putting together a successful fitness program are (1) setting realistic goals, (2) selecting appropriate activities, (3) setting targets for intensity, duration, and frequency, (4) making a commitment, (5) beginning the program and maintaining motivation, and (6) recording and assessing progress.
- Interval training is an important way to maintain target heart rate as exercise becomes more intense.
- The walking/jogging/running programs build to a high level of intensity with an increase in calorie cost. Running can cause great stress on weight-bearing parts of the body, so frequency should be limited to every other day.
- Bicycling requires more equipment than foot exercise and swimming do, as well as some precise skills and safety precautions.
- Swimming is not a weight-bearing activity and therefore places less stress on joints, ligaments, and tendons, resulting in fewer injuries. It also elicits a lower heart rate per minute.

BEHAVIOR CHANGE ACTIVITY

Making a Contract for Behavior Change

We are all familiar with the power of signed contracts. Documentation that commits our word, money, and/or property carries a strong impact and results in a higher chance of follow-through than casual, offhand promises. Contracts can be used to try to change a health behavior if they include the time, date, and the details of the behavior change program. A witness may be asked to sign the contract; this helps set in motion the support and encouragement of a social network. Contracts help prevent procrastination by specifying the dates and other details of the behavioral tasks and goals. They also act as reminders of a personal commitment to change.

A blank program plan and contract for exercise is included in Lab 7-1; a blank, generic contract is also included in Lab 1-2. You can use the principles embodied in these contracts to tailor one to fit any type of behavior change program. Let's take the example of Michael, who wants to break a long-standing habit of eating candy and chips every afternoon and evening. Setting up a formal contract and program for giving up these snacks will help him succeed in changing his behavior. He begins by keeping track of his snacking in his health journal. Based on this information, he can set goals for his program and develop strategies for breaking the behavior chains that typically lead to his snacking. He sets intermediate milestones for the program and allows himself plenty of time to achieve each goal. He also chooses appropriate rewards. Finally, he enlists the help of one of his housemates as a witness to his contract; she will also offer encouragement and check on his progress. Michael's contract is shown in Figure 7-3. Once he has signed it, he's ready to begin his efforts to change his behavior.

FOR MORE INFORMATION

Many popular activities like bike riding and running have monthly magazines devoted to them—check your local library. Some books about common fitness activities are listed below.

American Association of Retired Persons (AARP). 1995. *Pep Up Your Life: A Fitness Book for Mid-Life and Older Persons.* Washington, D.C.: AARP. *A basic guide to fitness for people over 40.*

American College of Sports Medicine. 1993. *The American College of Sports Medicine's Fitness Book.* Champaign, Ill.: Human Kinetics. *A comprehensive fitness guide compiled by the foremost sports science organization.*

Arnot, R. 1995. *Dr. Bob Arnot's Guide to Turning Back the Clock.* Boston: Little, Brown. *A sensible exercise guide by a popular TV personality and physician.*

Carmichael, C., and E. Burke. 1994. *Fitness Cycling.* Champaign, Ill.: Human Kinetics. *A guide for people interested in cycling as their primary form of exercise.*

My Personal Contract for Giving Up Snacking on Candy and Chips

I agree to stop snacking on candy and chips twice every day. I will begin my program on 10/4 and plan to reach my final goal by 11/15. I have divided my program into two parts, with two separate goals. For each step in my program, I will give myself the reward listed.

1. I will stop having candy or chips for an afternoon snack on 10/4.
(Reward: new CD)

2. I will stop having candy or chips for an evening snack on 10/25.
(Reward: Concert)

My plan for stopping my snacking includes the following strategies:

1. Avoid snack bar by taking a walk or reading at student union.
2. Eating healthy snacks instead of candy and chips.
3. Studying at the library instead of at home.

I understand that it is important for me to make a strong personal effort to make this change in my behavior. I sign this contract as an indication of my personal commitment to reach my goal.

Michael Cook 9/28

Witness: Katie Lim 9/28

Figure 7-3 ***A sample completed contract.***

Huey, L., and R. Forster. 1993. *The Complete Waterpower Workout Book.* New York: Random House. *An introduction to a popular new form of exercise.*

Maglischo, E. W., and C. F. Brennan. 1984. *Swim for the Health of It.* Mountain View, Calif.: Mayfield. *Conditioning and stroke techniques for people who want to use swimming to improve their health and physical fitness.*

Myers, C. 1992. *Walking: A Complete Guide to the Complete Exercise.* New York: Random House. *Strategies for putting together individualized walking programs for weight management and cardiovascular fitness.*

Nokes, T. D. 1991. *Lore of Running,* 3d ed. Champaign, Ill.: Leisure Press. *A comprehensive guide that includes discussions of the physiology of running; training for running; and recognizing, avoiding, and treating running injuries.*

Pryor, E., and M. Kraines. 1997. *Keep Moving! It's Aerobic Dance.* 3d ed. Mountain View, Calif.: Mayfield. *The fitness principles and techniques every aerobic dancer should know.*

Rippe, J. M., and A. Ward. 1989. *Rockport's Complete Book of Fitness Walking.* New York: Prentice-Hall. *An excellent, easy-to-read guide for people interested in walking for exercise.*

Sloane, E. A. 1995. *Sloane's Complete Book of Bicycling.* 5th ed. New York: Simon & Schuster. *A comprehensive guide for beginning and expert cyclists that includes information on equipment selection and maintenance and cycling health and safety.*

Stutz, D. R., and the editors of Consumer Reports Books. 1994. *40+ Guide to Fitness.* Yonkers, N.Y.: Consumers Union of the United States. *A book on fitness for older adults.*

Yanker, G.1995. *Walkshaping: Indoors or Out, 6 Weeks to a Better Body.* New York: Morrow. *A basic book on using walking to develop fitness.*

Community and campus resources for fitness programs, in addition to those mentioned in earlier chapters, include fitness trails or courses (a walking/jogging trail with stations for performing fitness activities); bike trails; community recreation programs; and public swimming pools.

SELECTED BIBLIOGRAPHY

American College of Sports Medicine. 1995. *Guidelines for Exercise Testing and Prescription,* 5th ed. Baltimore: Williams & Wilkins.

Brooks, G. A., T. D. Fahey, and T. P. White. 1996. *Exercise Physiology: Human Bioenergetics and Its Applications,* 2d ed. Mountain View, Calif.: Mayfield.

Butts, N. K., K. M. Knox, and T. S. Foley. 1995. Energy costs of walking on a dual-action treadmill in men and women. *Medicine and Science in Sports and Exercise* 27:121–125.

Dishman, R. K. 1994. Prescribing exercise intensity for healthy adults using perceived exertion. *Medicine and Science in Sports and Exercise* 26:1087–1094.

Fellingham, G. W. 1978. Caloric cost of walking and running. *Medicine and Science in Sports and Exercise* 10(2): 132–136.

Getchell, B., and P. Cleary. 1980. The caloric costs of rope skipping and running. *Physician and Sportsmedicine* 8:56.

Jones T. F., and C. B. Eaton. 1995. Exercise prescription. *American Family Physician* 52:543–550, 553–555.

Kusinitz, I., and M. Fine. 1995. *Your Guide to Getting Fit,* 3d ed. Mountain View, Calif.: Mayfield.

Lombard, D. N., T. N. Lombard, and R. A. Winett. 1995. Walking to meet health guidelines: The effect of prompting frequency and prompt structure. *Health Psychology* 14:164–170.

Maglischo, E. W. 1993. *Swimming Even Faster: A Comprehensive Guide to the Science of Swimming.* Mountain View, Calif.: Mayfield.

O'Shea, J. P., C. Novak, and F. Gaulard. 1982. Bicycle interval training for cardiovascular fitness. *Physician and Sportsmedicine* 10:156.

Pierce, E. F., S. W. Butterworth, T. D. Lynn, J. O'Shea, and W. G. Hammer. 1992. Fitness profiles and activity patterns of entering college students. *Journal of American Collegiate Health* 41:59–62.

Sallis, J. F., et al. 1989. A multivariate study of determinants of vigorous exercise in a community sample. *Preventive Medicine* 18:35–44.

Siegel, P. Z., R. M. Brackbill, and G. W. Heath. 1995. The epidemiology of walking for exercise: Implications for promoting activity among sedentary groups. *American Journal of Public Health* 85:706–710.

Name ____________________ Section ____________ Date ____________

LAB 7-1 *A Personal Fitness Program Plan and Contract*

A. I, ______________________________ (name), am contracting with myself to follow a physical fitness program to work toward the following goals:

1. ______________________________
2. ______________________________
3. ______________________________
4. ______________________________
5. ______________________________

B. My program plan is as follows:

Activities	Components (Check ✓)					*Intensity**	*Duration*	Frequency (Check ✓)						
	CRE	MS	ME	F	BC			M	Tu	W	Th	F	Sa	Su

*You should conduct activities for achieving CRE goals at your target heart rate or RPE value.

C. My program will begin on __________ (date). My program includes the following schedule of minigoals. For each step in my program, I will give myself the reward listed.

______________________________ (minigoal 1) __________ (date) __________ (reward)

______________________________ (minigoal 2) __________ (date) __________ (reward)

______________________________ (minigoal 3) __________ (date) __________ (reward)

______________________________ (minigoal 4) __________ (date) __________ (reward)

______________________________ (minigoal 5) __________ (date) __________ (reward)

LABORATORY ACTIVITIES

D. My program will include the addition of physical activity to my daily routine (such as climbing stairs or walking to class):

1. ______________________________

2. ______________________________

3. ______________________________

4. ______________________________

5. ______________________________

E. I will use the following tools to monitor my program and my progress toward my goals:

____
(list any charts, graphs, or journals you plan to use)

____

____

I sign this contract as an indication of my personal commitment to reach my goal.

______________________________ ______________
(your signature) (date)

I have recruited a helper who will witness my contract and ______________________________

____
(list any way your helper will participate in your program)

____

______________________________ ______________
(witness's signature) (date)

Name ______________________ Section ____________ Date ____________

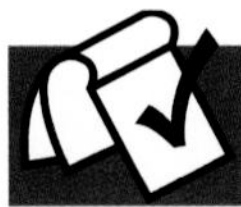

LAB 7-2 *Monitoring Your Program Progress*

Track your adherence to your program and your progress by filling out a program log. Use the one below, or make one specifically designed to match your program. If you prefer detailed program logs for each of your fitness components, use the logs in Labs 3-2, 4-3, and 5-2.

To use the log below, fill in the activities that are part of your program. Each day, note the distance and/or time for each activity. For flexibility or strength training workouts, you may prefer just to enter a check mark each time you complete a workout. At the end of each week, total your distances and/or times.

Activity/Date	M	Tu	W	Th	F	Sa	Su	Weekly Total	M	Tu	W	Th	F	Sa	Su	Weekly Total
1																
2																
3																
4																
5																
6																

Activity/Date	M	Tu	W	Th	F	Sa	Su	Weekly Total	M	Tu	W	Th	F	Sa	Su	Weekly Total
1																
2																
3																
4																
5																
6																

Activity/Date	M	Tu	W	Th	F	Sa	Su	Weekly Total	M	Tu	W	Th	F	Sa	Su	Weekly Total
1																
2																
3																
4																
5																
6																

Activity/Date	M	Tu	W	Th	F	Sa	Su	Weekly Total	M	Tu	W	Th	F	Sa	Su	Weekly Total
1																
2																
3																
4																
5																
6																

Activity/Date	M	Tu	W	Th	F	Sa	Su	Weekly Total	M	Tu	W	Th	F	Sa	Su	Weekly Total
1																
2																
3																
4																
5																
6																

8

Nutrition

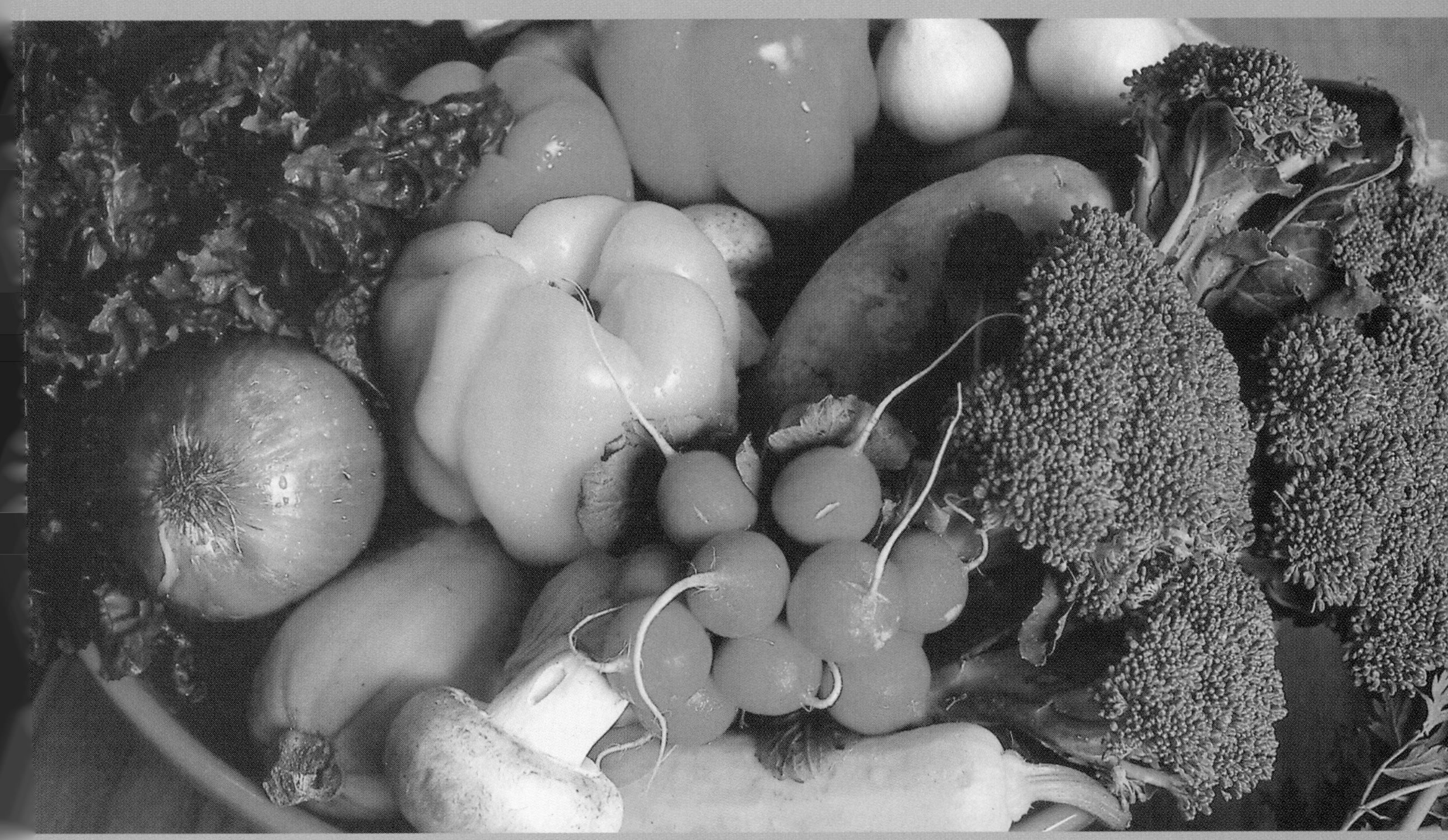

LOOKING AHEAD

After reading this chapter, you should be able to answer these questions about nutrition:

- What are the different kinds of nutrients, and what functions do they perform in the body?
- What percentages of calories come from protein, fats, and carbohydrates in the average American diet, and what percentages of these nutrients are recommended?
- What guidelines have been developed to help people choose a healthy diet, avoid nutritional deficiencies, and protect themselves from diet-related chronic diseases?
- What special nutritional guidelines apply to vegetarian diets?
- How can people adapt nutritional information to their own lives and circumstances?

Nutrition is a vitally important component of wellness. Diet affects energy levels, well-being, and overall health. Diet can also be closely linked with certain diseases, disabling conditions, and other health problems. Of particular concern is the connection between lifetime nutritional habits and the risk of the major chronic diseases, including heart disease, cancer, stroke, and diabetes. On the more positive side, however, a well-planned diet in conjunction with a fitness program can help prevent such conditions and even reverse some of them.

Creating a diet plan to support maximum fitness and protect against disease is a two-part project. First, you have to know which nutrients are necessary and in what amounts. Second, you have to translate those requirements into a diet consisting of foods you like to eat that are both available and affordable. Once you have an idea of what constitutes a healthy diet for you, you may also have to make adjustments in your current diet to bring it into line with your goals.

This chapter provides the basic principles of nutrition. It introduces the six classes of essential nutrients, explaining their role in the functioning of the body. It also provides different sets of guidelines, including guidelines for a vegetarian diet, that are available to help you design a healthy diet plan. Finally, it offers practical tools and advice to help you apply the guidelines to your own life, whether you are eating at home, at school, or in a restaurant. Diet is an area of your life in which you have almost total control. Using your knowledge and understanding of nutrition to create a healthy diet plan is a significant step toward wellness.

COMPONENTS OF A HEALTHY DIET

Most people think about their dietary patterns in terms of the food they eat—deciding, for example, on a turkey sandwich and a glass of milk or a steak and salad for a meal. But it is the nutrients contained in these foods—the carbohydrates, proteins, fats, vitamins, minerals, and water—that should determine daily food choices. Nutritional scientists have identified approximately 45 different **essential nutrients**—that is, nutrients that are necessary to but not manufactured by the human body, at least not in sufficient amounts. The six classes of nutrients, along with their functions and major sources, are listed in Table 8-1.

Nutrients are released into the body by the process of **digestion,** which breaks them down into compounds that the gastrointestinal tract can absorb and the body can use (Figure 8-1). In this form, the essential nutrients provide energy, build and maintain body tissues, and regulate body functions.

Providing energy is the most immediate function of nutrients. The energy in foods is measured in **kilocalories** (abbreviated **kcalories**). One kcalorie represents the amount of heat it takes to raise the temperature of 1 kilogram of water 1°C. The average adult requires about 2000 kcalories per day to meet energy needs. Kilocalories consumed in excess of energy needs are stored as body fat. In common usage, the term *kilocalorie* is generally shortened to **calorie,** although a calorie is actually a very small energy unit—a kilocalorie contains 1000 calories. For convenience, this chapter will use the more familiar term, *calorie,* to stand for the larger energy unit.

Three of the six classes of nutrients supply energy: proteins, carbohydrates, and fats. Fats provide the most energy—9 calories per gram; protein and carbohydrates each provide 4 calories per gram. (Alcohol, although it is not an essential nutrient, also supplies energy, providing 7 calories per gram.) Experts advise against high fat consumption, in part because fats provide so many calories. Given the typical American diet, most Americans simply do not need the extra calories to meet energy needs.

Meeting our energy needs is only one of the functions of food. All the nutrients perform numerous other vital functions. In terms of quantity, water is the most significant nutrient: The body is approximately 60% water and can survive only a few days without it. Vitamins and minerals are needed in much smaller quantities, but they are still vital.

Practically all foods are mixtures of nutrients, although foods are commonly classified according to their predominant nutrients. For example, spaghetti is considered a carbohydrate food although it contains small amounts of other nutrients. The following is a closer look at the functions and sources of the six classes of nutrients.

Proteins

Protein is an important component of muscle, bone, blood, enzymes, cell membranes, and some hormones. As mentioned above, protein can also provide energy at 4 calories per gram of protein weight. Proteins are composed of **amino acids.** Twenty common amino acids are found in food, but only nine of these are essential to an adult diet: histidine, isoleucine, leucine, lysine, methionine, phenylalanine, threonine, tryptophan, and valine.

TERMS

essential nutrients Vitamins, minerals, some amino acids, linoleic acid, water, and other substances the body must obtain from food because it can't manufacture them in sufficient quantity for its physiological needs.

digestion The process of breaking down foods in the gastrointestinal tract into nutrients the body can absorb.

kilocalorie (kcalorie) The unit of fuel potential in a food. One kcalorie represents the amount of heat required to raise the temperature of 1 kilogram of water 1°C.

calorie The amount of heat required to raise the temperature of 1 gram of water 1°C; the word commonly used when kilocalorie is meant.

amino acids The components of proteins used to build muscle and other tissue.

TABLE 8-1 The Six Classes of Essential Nutrients

Nutrient	Function	Major Sources
Proteins	Form important parts of muscles, bone, blood, enzymes, some hormones, and cell membranes; repair tissue; regulate water and acid-base balance; help in growth; supply energy	Meat, fish, poultry, eggs, milk products, legumes, nuts
Carbohydrates	Supply energy to cells in brain, nervous system, and blood; supply energy to muscles during exercise	Grains (breads and cereals), fruits, vegetables
Fats	Supply energy; insulate, support, and cushion organs; provide medium for absorption of fat-soluble vitamins	Saturated fats primarily from animal sources, palm and coconut oils, and hydrogenated vegetable fats; unsaturated fats from grains, fish, vegetables
Vitamins	Promote (initiate or speed up) specific chemical reactions within cells	Abundant in fruits, vegetables, and grains; also found in meat and dairy products
Minerals	Help regulate body functions; aid in the growth and maintenance of body tissues; act as catalysts for the release of energy	Found in most food groups
Water	Makes up 50–70% of body weight; provides a medium for chemical reactions; transports chemicals; regulates temperature; removes waste products	Fruits, vegetables, and other liquids

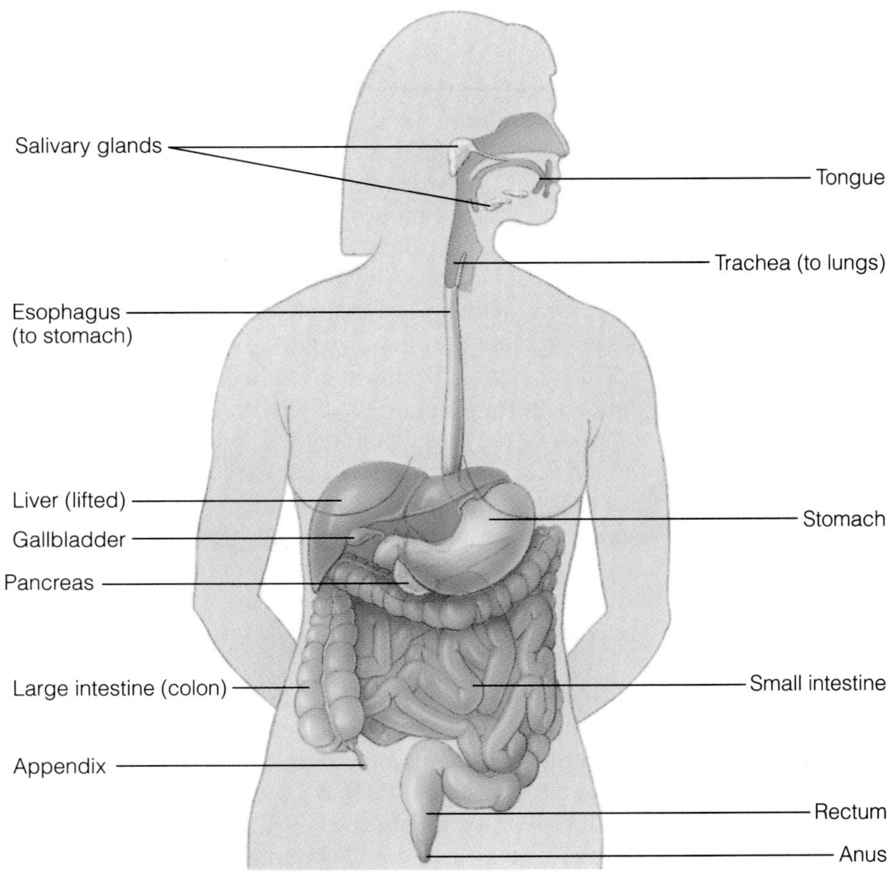

Figure 8-1 ***The digestive tract.*** Digestion begins in the mouth, but most digestion takes place in the small intestine and stomach.

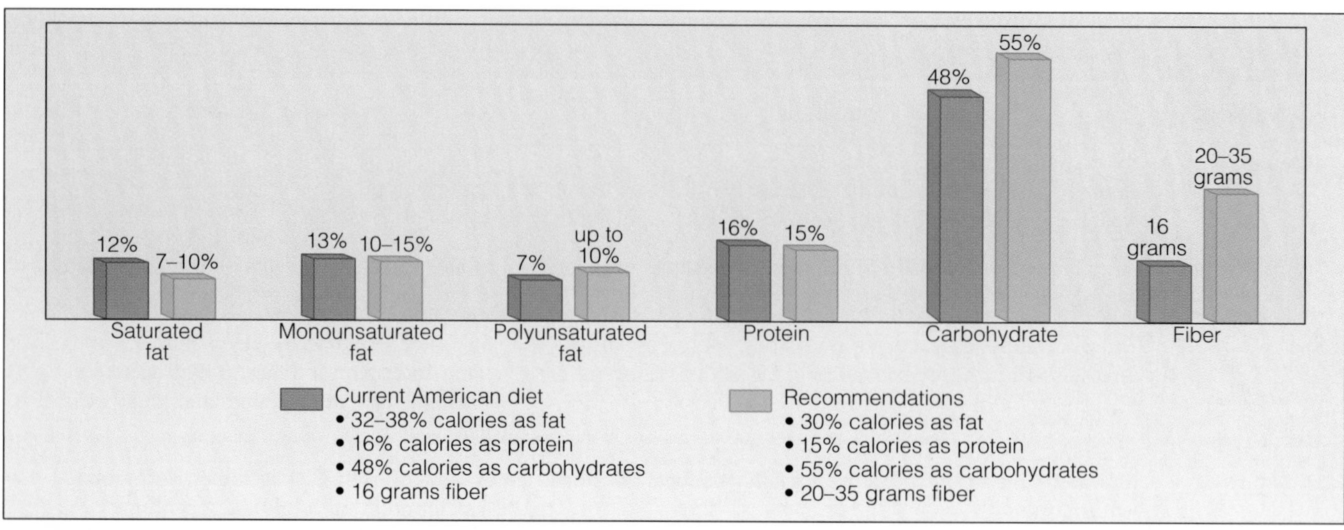

VITAL STATISTICS

Figure 8-2 *What Americans eat, compared to what they should eat, as recommended by major health authorities.*

"Essential," again, means that they are required for normal health and growth but must be provided in the diet because the body manufactures them in insufficient quantities, if at all. The other eleven amino acids can be produced by the body as long as the necessary ingredients are supplied by foods.

Foods are rated as "complete" or "high-quality" protein sources if they supply all nine essential amino acids in adequate amounts; they are classified as "incomplete" or "low-quality" protein sources if they supply only some. Meat, fish, poultry, eggs, milk, cheese, and other foods from animal sources provide complete proteins. Incomplete proteins come from plant sources such as beans, peas, and nuts; these are good sources of most essential amino acids but are usually low in one or two. Different vegetable proteins are low in different amino acids, so combinations can provide complete proteins. Vegetarians who eat no foods from animal sources can obtain all essential amino acids by eating a wide variety of foods each day.

The leading sources of protein in the American diet are (1) beef, steaks, and roasts; (2) hamburgers and meatloaf; (3) white bread, rolls, and crackers; (4) milk; and (5) pork. About two-thirds of the protein in the American diet comes from animal sources, which means the nation's diet is rich in amino acids. About 10–15% of the total calories in a well-balanced diet should come from protein (Figure 8-2). However, many Americans consume more than that amount every day. This excess protein is synthesized into fat for energy storage or burned for energy. For most people, extra protein in the diet is not harmful, but it does contribute fat to the diet because protein-rich foods are often fat-rich as well. Nutritionists recommend that daily protein intake not exceed twice what is needed.

Fats

At 9 calories per gram, fats (also known as lipids) are the most concentrated source of energy. The fats stored in the body insulate the body, cushion the organs, and provide usable energy. Fats in the diet absorb fat-soluble vitamins and add important flavor and texture to foods. During periods of rest and light activity, fats are the major body fuel. The nervous system, brain, and red blood cells are fueled by carbohydrates, but most of the rest of the body's organs are fueled by fats. Two fats—linoleic acid and alpha-linolenic acid—are essential to the diet; they are key regulators of such body functions as the maintenance of blood pressure and the progress of a healthy pregnancy.

Fats are categorized according to their structure. The three most important fats are glycerides, phospholipids, and sterols, the most common of which is **cholesterol.** Of these three, **glycerides** are the most common. They consist of a glycerol molecule to which one, two, or three fatty acids are attached. Based on the number of fatty acids, glycerides are called monoglycerides, diglycerides, or triglycerides. About 95% of the fat in food and 99% of the fat stored in the body are in the form of **triglycerides.**

Saturated and Unsaturated Fats Fatty acids differ in the length of their carbon atom chains and in their degree of saturation—the number of double bonds between the carbon atoms (Figure 8-3). If no double bonds exist between the carbon atoms, the fatty acid is called **saturated.** Fatty acids with one double bond are called **monounsat-**

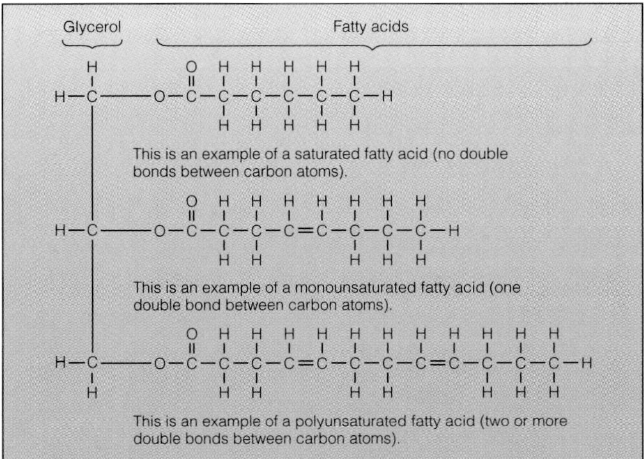

Figure 8-3 ***Chemical structures of saturated and unsaturated fatty acids.*** This example of a triglyceride consists of a molecule of glycerol with three fatty acids attached. Fatty acids can differ in the length of their carbon chains and their degree of saturation.

urated, and those with two or more double bonds are called **polyunsaturated.**

Food fats are often composed of both saturated and unsaturated fatty acids, but the dominant type of fatty acid determines the fat's characteristics. "Saturated fats" are those food fats that contain large amounts of saturated fatty acids. They are generally found in animal products and are usually solid at room temperature. The leading sources of saturated fat in the American diet are unprocessed animal flesh (hamburger, steak, roasts) and whole milk, cheese, and hot dogs or lunch meats. Other significant sources include poultry skin, ice cream, and many baked products. In familiar terms, it is the fats high in saturated fatty acids we generally mean when we use the term *fats*. For the relative amounts of fatty acids in common dietary fats, see Figure 8-4 (p. 184).

Food fats that contain large amounts of monounsaturated and polyunsaturated fatty acids usually come from plant sources and are liquid at room temperature. These fats are generally referred to as "oils." Olive, canola, and peanut oils contain mostly monounsaturated fatty acids. Sunflower, corn, soybean, and safflower oils contain mostly polyunsaturated fatty acids. Notable exceptions are palm oil and coconut oil, used in some processed foods. Although derived from plants, these oils are highly saturated, as are hydrogenated vegetable oils. The process of **hydrogenation,** used by food manufacturers to improve the texture of foods and extend shelf life, turns a liquid oil into a more solid fat.

Dietary Fats and Health Human beings need only a single tablespoon of vegetable oil per day, but the average American diet supplies a great deal more. In fact, fats constitute about 32–38% of most Americans' caloric intake (see Figure 8-2). Health experts recommend that fat intake be held to less than 30% of total calories, with no more than 7–10% of total calories from saturated fat.

Controlling the amount of saturated fat in the diet is the most important diet-related action an individual can take to limit the levels of cholesterol in the blood. Elevated total and LDL ("bad") cholesterol levels are associated with an increased risk for premature heart disease (discussed in more detail in Chapter 11). As a preventive strategy, all adults should minimize their saturated fat intake. This is especially true for those with high blood cholesterol levels—over 200 milligrams of cholesterol per 100 milliliters of blood serum. Consuming hydrogenated and partially hydrogenated vegetable oils, including stick margarine and shortening, also poses a risk to health because the process of hydrogenation produces **trans fatty acids,** which increase serum cholesterol levels.

Controlling total fat intake and shifting from saturated fats to unsaturated fats can benefit health. And consuming foods rich in monounsaturated fats, such as olive oil, may raise the levels of HDL ("good") cholesterol in the blood. Certain forms of polyunsaturated fatty acids, referred to as **omega-3** polyunsaturates and found in many kinds of fish, may also have a positive effect on cardiovascular health. Most polyunsaturated fats consumed by Americans are omega-6 forms and come primarily from corn and soybean oil. Omega-3 fatty acids, on the other hand, have been shown to reduce the tendency of blood to clot, to decrease inflammatory responses in the body, and to increase levels of HDL cholesterol in women; they even appear to lower the risk of heart disease in some people. Because of these benefits, nutritionists now recommend that Americans increase the proportion of omega-3 polyunsaturated fats in their diet by increasing

TERMS

cholesterol A type of sterol, or fat, that is manufactured in the body and also found in animal-derived foods; elevated levels in the blood can lead to cardiovascular disease (CVD).

glycerides The most common type of lipid, consisting of a glycerol molecule attached to one or more fatty acids.

triglyceride The most common lipid found in fatty tissues; high levels increase the risk of CVD.

saturated fatty acid A fatty acid that has no double bonds between carbon atoms.

monounsaturated fatty acid A fatty acid that has one double bond between carbon atoms.

polyunsaturated fatty acid A fatty acid that has two or more double bonds between carbon atoms.

hydrogenation A process by which liquid oils are turned into solid fats; used to extend the shelf life of certain foods.

trans fatty acid A type of unsaturated fatty acid produced during the process of hydrogenation; high levels of trans fatty acids in the diet increase serum cholesterol levels.

omega-3 fatty acids Polyunsaturated fatty acids commonly found in fish oils that are beneficial to cardiovascular health.

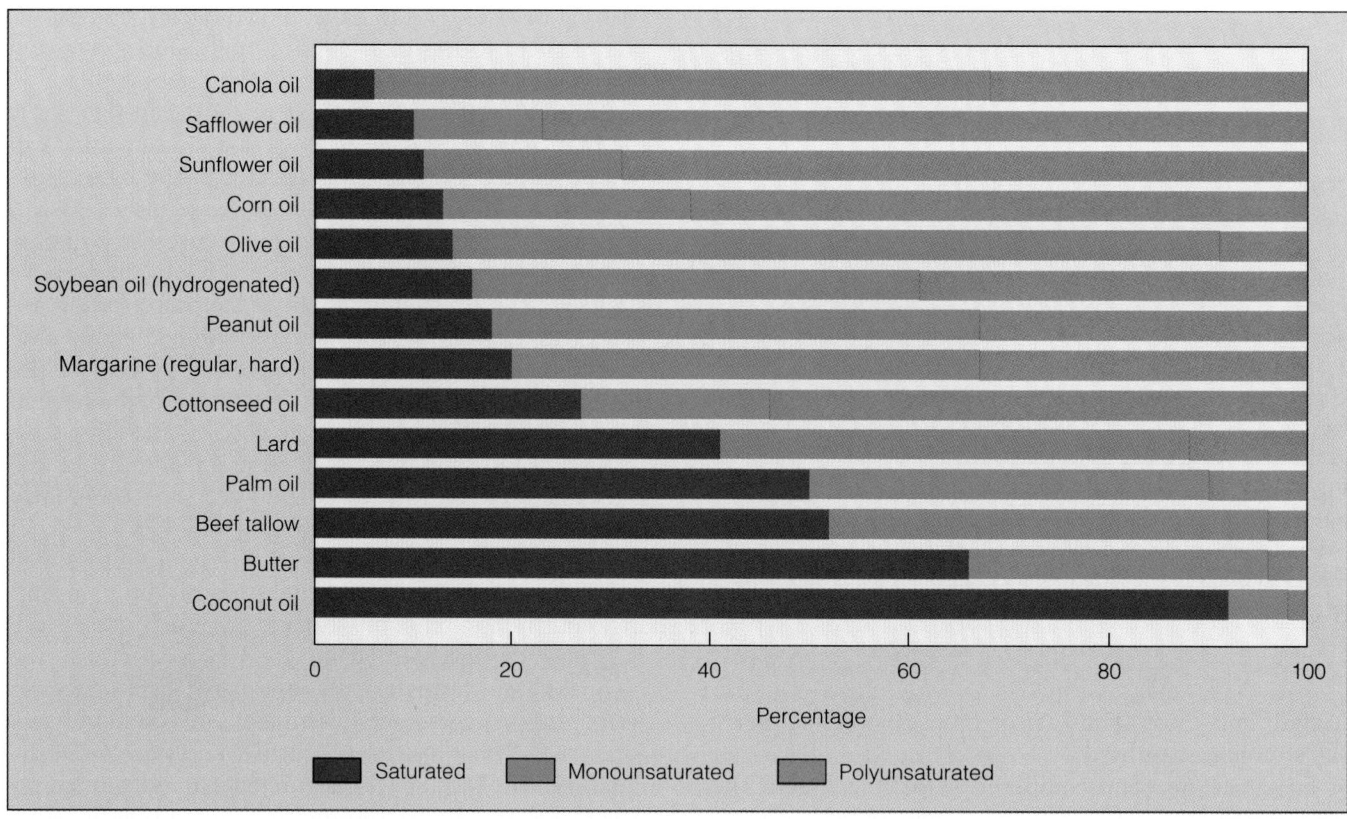

Figure 8-4 *Comparisons of dietary fats.*

their consumption of fish to two or more times a week. Mackerel, whitefish, herring, salmon, and lake trout are all good sources of omega-3 fatty acids.

Monitoring Fat Intake To calculate how much fat a food contains, you first need to know the total number of calories and grams of fat it contains. For prepared foods, food labels provide this information. (For fat and calorie information on many common foods, see Appendix B.) Multiply the grams of fat by 9 (because there are 9 calories in a gram of fat). Then divide that number by the total calories. For example, a tablespoon of peanut butter has 8 grams of fat and 95 calories. So 8 × 9 = 72, divided by the number of calories (95) equals 0.76, or about 76% of calories from fat.

To monitor the fat percentage in your diet, multiply the grams of fat in any individual food by 9. If the result is more than a third of the total calories, the food is relatively high in fat. You can still eat it, but make sure you limit the amount you eat—especially if it's also high in saturated fat. And make sure to balance it with low-fat foods.

Your goal is to end up with fewer than 30% of your total daily calories from fat. This can be accomplished by setting a goal for fat consumption and then keeping track of the amount of fat you consume during the day. To set a goal for your daily fat consumption, first determine approximately how many calories you consume per day. Depending on your activity level, daily caloric needs range from about 2200–3500 calories for men and about 1700–2500 for women. Multiply your chosen daily calorie intake by 30% (0.3) to get the maximum fat calories allowed per day. Divide this figure by 9 to get the maximum number of grams of fat you can consume per day and still stay within the 30% guideline at your level of caloric intake. For example, if you consume about 1800 calories per day, your maximum fat intake would be 1800 × 0.3 = 540 calories from fat, or 60 grams of fat. Food labels calculate this for a 2000-calorie and sometimes a 2500-calorie diet. By checking food labels, you can keep a running total of the grams of fat you consume and make food choices that keep you within the limit you've set for yourself.

Carbohydrates

Carbohydrates function primarily to supply energy to body cells. Some cells, such as those in the brain and other parts of the nervous system and in the blood, use only carbohydrates for fuel. During high-intensity exercise, muscles also get most of their energy from carbohydrates. When the diet contains insufficient amounts of carbohydrates to satisfy the needs of the brain and red blood cells, the body makes its own carbohydrates from proteins. This synthesizing process is costly, in terms of both energy used for metabolism and money spent on protein foods, compared with carbohydrate foods. (Compare the price of a 1-pound loaf of whole wheat bread with the price of 3/4 of a pound of lean beef, both of which yield about 1100 calories.)

In situations of extreme deprivation, when the diet lacks sufficient amounts of both carbohydrates and proteins, the body turns to its own proteins, resulting in severe muscle wasting. But since the body's daily carbohydrate requirement is filled by just three or four slices of bread, the average American would have to struggle to consume a diet so low in carbohydrates that the body would have to synthesize them from dietary or body proteins. The only common situations in which this might occur are crash diets or medically supervised very-low-carbohydrate diets, sometimes used in weight-reduction programs.

Simple and Complex Carbohydrates Carbohydrates are classified into two groups: simple and complex. Simple carbohydrates contain only one or two sugar units in each molecule. A one-sugar carbohydrate is called a **monosaccharide;** a two-sugar carbohydrate, a **disaccharide.** They include sucrose (table sugar), fructose (fruit sugar, honey), maltose (malt sugar), and lactose (milk sugar). Simple carbohydrates provide much of the sweetness in foods. Starches and most types of dietary fiber are complex carbohydrates; they consist of chains of many sugar molecules and are called **polysaccharides.** Starches are found in a variety of plants, especially grains, **legumes,** tubers, and nuts. Dietary fiber includes pectins, found in fruits, especially apples, and some vegetables; gums and mucilages; and cellulose, the indigestible, insoluble material concentrated in the outer layers of grains, seeds, skins, and peels.

During digestion in the mouth and small intestine, the body breaks down starches and disaccharides into monosaccharides, such as **glucose,** for absorption into the bloodstream. Once the glucose is absorbed, cells take it up and use it for energy. The liver and muscles also take up glucose and store it in the form of a starch called **glycogen.** The muscles use glycogen as fuel during endurance events or long workouts. Carbohydrates consumed in excess of the body's energy needs are changed into fat and stored. Whenever calorie intake exceeds calorie expenditure, fat storage can lead to weight gain. This is true whether the excess calories come from carbohydrates, proteins, fat, or alcohol.

Carbohydrates are found primarily in plant foods; the only significant animal source of carbohydrates is milk. The average American adult consumes more than 200 grams of carbohydrates a day (about 48% of total caloric intake), well above the minimum requirement of 50–100 grams. However, health experts recommend that Americans increase their consumption of carbohydrates, particularly complex carbohydrates, to 55% of total daily calories, reducing their fat intake by the same measure (see Figure 8-2). Potatoes, rice, pasta, bread, vegetables, and beans are all good sources of complex carbohydrates.

Athletes who are in training can benefit from a high-carbohydrate diet to increase the amount of carbohydrates stored in their muscles as glycogen. Athletes who consume carbohydrates while they are actually engaged in prolonged athletic events (usually as a high-carbohydrate drink) can help fuel muscles and prevent the depletion of glycogen.

Dietary Fiber Commonly known as "bulk" or "roughage," **dietary fiber** consists of carbohydrate plant substances that are difficult or impossible for humans to digest. Instead, fiber passes through the intestinal tract and provides bulk for feces in the large intestine, which in turn facilitates elimination. In the large intestine, some types of fiber are broken down by bacteria into acids and gases, which explains why consuming too much fiber can lead to intestinal gas.

Nutritionists classify dietary fiber as soluble or insoluble. **Soluble fiber** slows the body's absorption of glucose and binds cholesterol-containing compounds in the intestine, lowering blood cholesterol levels and reducing the risk of cardiovascular disease. **Insoluble fiber** binds water, making the feces bulkier and softer so they pass more quickly and easily through the intestines.

Both kinds of fiber contribute to disease prevention. A diet high in soluble fiber can help people manage diabetes and high blood cholesterol levels. A diet high in insoluble

TERMS

monosaccharide A simple carbohydrate consisting of one sugar molecule.

disaccharide A simple carbohydrate consisting of two single-sugar molecules (monosaccharides) linked together.

polysaccharide A complex carbohydrate composed of many sugar molecules (monosaccharides) linked together.

legumes Vegetables such as peas and beans that are high in fiber and are also important sources of protein.

glucose A simple sugar that is the body's basic fuel.

glycogen A complex carbohydrate stored principally in the liver and skeletal muscles; the major fuel source during most forms of exercise.

dietary fiber Carbohydrates and other substances in plants that are difficult or impossible for humans to digest.

soluble fiber Dietary fiber that dissolves in water or is broken down by bacteria in the large intestine. It tends to absorb cholesterol-containing compounds in the intestine.

insoluble fiber Fiber that does not dissolve in water and is not broken down by bacteria in the large intestine; it binds water and increases bulk in the stool.

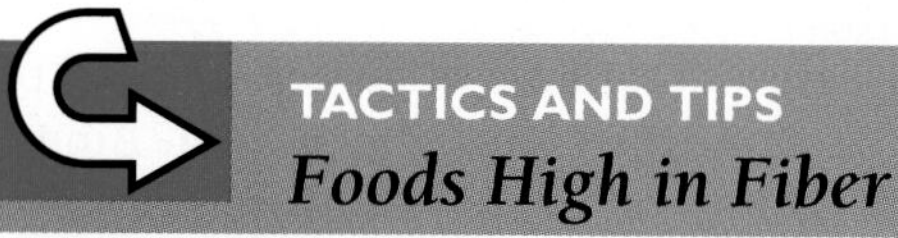

TACTICS AND TIPS

Foods High in Fiber

Fiber is found only in plant foods. To meet the recommended daily intake of 20–35 grams of fiber, choose fiber-rich fruits, vegetables, grains and cereals, and legumes.

Food Item	Serving Size	Fiber (g)
Fruits		
Apple, with skin	1	4.0
Apricot, with skin	3	2.0
Avocado	1/4 cup	2.5
Banana	1	2.3
Cantaloupe	1/2	2.0
Nectarine	1	3.3
Orange	1	3.8
Pear	1	4.8
Prunes, uncooked	5	3.9
Raisins	1/4 cup	2.5
Raspberries	1/2 cup	3.0
*Grains and Cereals**		
Bread, whole wheat	1 slice	2.5
Bread, mixed grain	1 slice	1.4
Oatmeal, cooked	2/3 cup	3.0
Legumes		
Kidney beans, cooked	1/2 cup	4.6
Lima beans, cooked	1/2 cup	4.3
Pinto beans, cooked	1/2 cup	4.3
Vegetables		
Artichoke, cooked	1	4.0
Beans, green, cooked	1/2 cup	2.0
Broccoli, cooked	1/2 cup	2.1
Brussels sprouts, cooked	1/2 cup	2.2
Carrot, raw	1	1.8
Corn, cooked	1/2 cup	4.6
Eggplant, cooked	1 cup	2.0
Peas, green, cooked	1/2 cup	3.5
Potato, baked with skin	1	5.0
Spinach, cooked	1/2 cup	3.5
Squash, winter, cooked	1/2 cup	3.0
Tomato, medium	1	1.8

*Many breakfast cereals contain significant amounts of dietary fiber (2–5 grams per serving). Check the labels for exact amounts.

fiber can help prevent a variety of health problems, including constipation, hemorrhoids, and diverticulitis (a painful condition in which abnormal pouches form and become inflamed in the wall of the large intestine). Some studies have linked high levels of insoluble fiber in the diet with a decreased incidence of colon and rectal cancer; conversely, a low-fiber diet may increase the risk of colon cancer. There is even some evidence that high levels of insoluble fiber can suppress and reverse precancerous changes that can lead to colon and rectal cancer.

All plant foods contain some dietary fiber, but fruits, legumes, oats (especially oat bran), barley, and psyllium (found in some laxatives) are particularly rich in it. Wheat (especially wheat bran), cereals, grains, and vegetables are all good sources of insoluble fiber (see the box "Foods High in Fiber"). However, the processing of packaged foods can remove fiber, so it's important to depend on fresh fruits and vegetables and foods made from whole grains as sources of dietary fiber.

Although it is not yet clear precisely how much and what types of fiber are ideal, most experts believe the average American would benefit from an increase in daily fiber intake. Currently, most Americans consume about 16 grams of fiber a day, whereas the recommended daily amount is 20–35 grams of food fiber—not from supplements, which should be taken only under medical supervision. However, too much fiber—more than 40–60 grams a day—can cause health problems, such as overlarge stools or the malabsorption of important minerals. In fiber intake, as in all aspects of nutrition, balance and moderation are key principles.

Water

Water is the major component of both foods and the human body. As mentioned earlier, the human body is about 60% water. In terms of weight, the need for water is much greater than for other nutrients. Human beings can live for up to 50 days without food, but they can survive only a few days without water.

Water is distributed throughout the body, in tissues as well as in body fluids. Water is used in the digestion and absorption of food and is the medium in which most of the chemical reactions take place within the body. Water-based fluids, such as blood and lymph, transport substances around the body, and other fluids, such as the synovial fluid in joints, serve as lubricants or cushions. Water also helps regulate body temperature.

Water is found in almost all foods, particularly liquids, fruits, and vegetables. Consumption accounts for 80–90% of the average person's daily water intake; the rest is generated through the metabolism of energy nutrients. Water is lost each day in urine, feces, sweat, and evaporation in the lungs. To maintain a balance between water consumed and water lost, people need to take in about 1 milliliter of water for each calorie burned—a total of about 2 liters, or 8 cups, of fluid a day. People who live in hot climates or engage in vigorous exercise need to take in more.

Thirst is the body's first sign of dehydration, a signal that it needs more water. If this thirst mechanism is faulty, as it may be during illness or vigorous exercise, hormonal mechanisms can help conserve water by reducing the output of urine. Severe dehydration causes weakness and can lead to death. Drinking enough water is a simple and essential action everyone can take to promote physical well-being.

Vitamins

Vitamins are organic (carbon-containing) substances required in very small amounts to promote specific chemical reactions within living cells. Humans need 13 vitamins. Four of these—vitamins A, D, E, and K—are fat-soluble, meaning they can be absorbed only in the presence of fat. The other nine are water-soluble—vitamin C and the eight B-complex vitamins: thiamin, riboflavin, niacin, vitamin B-6, folate, vitamin B-12, biotin, and pantothenic acid. A summary of facts about vitamins is presented in Table 8-2 (p. 188).

Vitamins provide no energy to the body directly; they unleash the energy stored in carbohydrates, proteins, and fats by acting with catalysts to initiate or speed up chemical reactions. In addition, some vitamins act as **antioxidants,** aiding in the preservation of the body's healthy cells. When the body uses oxygen or breaks down certain fats, it gives rise to substances called free radicals (see Chapter 3). In their search for electrons, free radicals react with fats, proteins, and DNA, damaging cell membranes and causing gene mutations. Antioxidants react with free radicals and donate electrons, rendering them harmless. Key vitamin antioxidants in our diet are vitamin E, vitamin C, and the vitamin A derivative beta-carotene. Obtaining a regular intake of these nutrients is vital for maintaining the health of the body.

The human body does not manufacture most of the vitamins it requires and must obtain them from foods. (A few vitamins are made in certain parts of the body, however. The skin makes vitamin D when it is exposed to sunlight, and intestinal bacteria make biotin and vitamin K.) When the intake of a particular vitamin is insufficient, the deficiency results in characteristic symptoms. For example, vitamin A deficiency can cause night blindness, niacin deficiency can lead to mental illness, vitamin B-6 deficiency can cause seizures, vitamin B-12 deficiency can cause a severe type of anemia, and vitamin D deficiency can result in bone deformities. Although everyone who eats poorly is at risk for vitamin deficiency, risk is particularly high in people with alcoholism.

Vitamins are abundant in fruits, vegetables, and grains. In addition, many processed foods, such as flour and breakfast cereals, are enriched with certain vitamins during the manufacturing process. On the other hand, both vitamins and minerals can be lost or destroyed as a result of certain food-preparation and food-storage techniques. For tips on minimizing such losses, see the box "Keeping the Nutrient Value in Food" (p. 190).

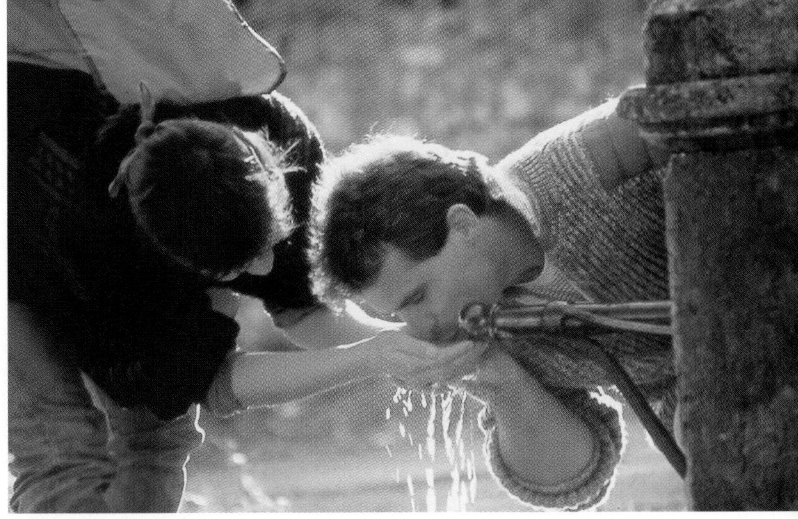

Often overlooked but absolutely crucial to life, water is an essential part of our diet.

Minerals

Minerals are inorganic (non–carbon-containing) compounds needed by the body in relatively small amounts to help regulate body functions, aid in growth and tissue maintenance, and act as catalysts to release energy. There are at least 17 essential minerals. The major minerals are those the body needs in amounts exceeding 100 milligrams: calcium, chloride, magnesium, phosphorus, potassium, sodium, and sulfur. Essential trace minerals are those needed in only minute amounts; these include fluoride, iron, selenium, zinc, arsenic, boron, chromium, cobalt, copper, iodine, manganese, molybdenum, nickel, silicon, and vanadium.

If an essential mineral is consumed in a quantity either too small or too large, characteristic symptoms develop. The minerals most commonly lacking in the human diet are iron and calcium, with zinc and magnesium sometimes lacking as well. People of all ages suffer from iron-deficiency **anemia,** a blood disorder, and researchers believe that poor calcium intake leads to **osteoporosis,** a condition in which the bones become weak and brittle (see the box "Osteoporosis," p. 191). Any health-promoting diet must include good food choices for

TERMS

antioxidant A substance that inhibits reactions promoted by oxygen, usually by reacting with it itself, thereby providing protection against the damaging effects of oxidation.

anemia A deficiency in the oxygen-carrying material in the red blood cells.

osteoporosis A condition in which the bones become extremely thin and brittle; fractures of the wrist, spine, and hip commonly result.

TABLE 8-2 Facts About Vitamins

Vitamin	Major Functions	Signs of Prolonged Deficiency	Toxic Effects of Megadoses	Important Dietary Sources
Fat-Soluble				
Vitamin A	Maintenance of eyes, vision, skin, linings of the nose, mouth, digestive and urinary tracts, immune function	Night blindness; dry, scaling skin; increased susceptibility to infection; loss of appetite; anemia; kidney stones	Headache, vomiting and diarrhea, dryness of mucous membranes, vertigo, double vision, bone abnormalities, liver damage, miscarriage and birth defects, convulsions, coma, respiratory failure	Liver, milk, butter, cheese, and fortified margarine; carrots, spinach, cantaloupe, and other orange and deep-green vegetables and fruits contain carotenes that the body converts to vitamin A
Vitamin D	Aid in calcium and phosphorus metabolism, promotion of calcium absorption, development and maintenance of bones and teeth	Rickets (bone deformities) in children; bone softening, loss, and fractures in adults	Calcium deposits in kidneys and blood vessels, causing irreversible kidney and cardiovascular damage	Fortified milk and margarine, fish liver oils, butter, egg yolks (sunlight on skin also produces vitamin D)
Vitamin E	Protection and maintenance of cellular membranes	Red blood cell breakage and anemia, weakness, neurological problems, muscle cramps	Relatively nontoxic, but may cause excess bleeding or formation of blood clots	Vegetable oils, whole grains, nuts and seeds, green leafy vegetables, asparagus, peaches; smaller amounts widespread in other foods
Vitamin K	Production of factors essential for blood clotting	Hemorrhaging	None observed	Green leafy vegetables; smaller amounts widespread in other foods
Water-Soluble				
Vitamin C	Maintenance and repair of connective tissue, bones, teeth, and cartilage; promotion of healing; aid in iron absorption	Scurvy (weakening of collagenous structures resulting in widespread capillary hemorrhaging), anemia, reduced resistance to infection, bleeding gums, weakness, loosened teeth, rough skin, joint pain, poor wound healing, hair loss, poor iron absorption	Urinary stones in some people, acid stomach from ingesting supplements in pill form, nausea, diarrhea, headache, fatigue	Peppers, broccoli, spinach, brussels sprouts, citrus fruits, strawberries, tomatoes, potatoes, cabbage, other fruits and vegetables
Thiamin	Conversion of carbohydrates into usable forms of energy, maintenance of appetite and nervous system function	Beriberi (symptoms include edema or muscle wasting, mental confusion, anorexia, enlarged heart, abnormal heart rhythm, muscle degeneration and weakness, nerve changes)	None reported	Yeast, whole-grain and enriched breads and cereals, organ meats, liver, pork, lean meats, poultry, eggs, fish, beans, nuts, legumes

TABLE 8-2 *Facts About Vitamins (continued)*

Vitamin	Major Functions	Signs of Prolonged Deficiency	Toxic Effects of Megadoses	Important Dietary Sources
Riboflavin	Energy metabolism; maintenance of skin, mucous membranes, and nervous system structures	Cracks at corners of mouth, sore throat, skin rash, hypersensitivity to light, purple tongue	None reported	Dairy products, whole-grain and enriched breads and cereals, lean meats, poultry, green vegetables, liver
Niacin	Conversion of carbohydrates, fats, and protein into usable forms of energy; essential for growth, synthesis of hormones	Pellagra (symptoms include weakness, diarrhea, dermatitis, inflammation of mucous membranes, mental illness)	Flushing of the skin, nausea, vomiting, diarrhea, changes in metabolism of glycogen and fatty acids	Eggs, chicken, turkey, fish, milk, whole grains, nuts, enriched breads and cereals, lean meats, legumes*
Vitamin B-6	Enzyme reactions involving amino acids and the metabolism of carbohydrates, lipids, and nucleic acids	Anemia, convulsions, cracks at corners of mouth, dermatitis, nausea, confusion	Neurological abnormalities and damage	Eggs, poultry, whole grains, nuts, legumes, liver, kidney, pork
Folate	Amino acid metabolism, synthesis of RNA and DNA, new cell synthesis	Anemia, gastrointestinal disturbances, decreased resistance to infection, depression	Diarrhea, reduction of zinc absorption, possible kidney enlargement and damage	Green leafy vegetables, yeast, oranges, whole grains, legumes, liver
Vitamin B-12	Synthesis of red and white blood cells; other metabolic reactions	Anemia, fatigue, nervous system damage, sore tongue	None reported	Eggs, milk, meat, liver
Biotin	Metabolism of fats, carbohydrates, and proteins	Rash, nausea, vomiting, weight loss, depression, fatigue, hair loss; not known under natural circumstances	None reported	Cereals, yeast, nuts, cheese, egg yolks, soy flour, liver; widespread in foods
Pantothenic acid	Metabolism of fats, carbohydrates, and proteins	Fatigue, numbness and tingling of hands and feet, gastrointestinal disturbances; not known under natural circumstances	Diarrhea, water retention	Peanuts, whole grains, legumes, fish, eggs, liver, kidney; smaller amounts found in milk, vegetables, and fruits

*Niacin can be made in the body from tryptophan, so this list includes foods containing niacin and/or tryptophan.

Sources: National Research Council. 1989. *Recommended Dietary Allowances,* 10th ed. Washington, D.C.: National Academy Press. Shils, M. E., and V. R. Young, eds. 1993. *Modern Nutrition in Health and Disease,* 8th ed. Baltimore: Williams & Wilkins.

minerals. Table 8-3 (p. 192) provides a summary of basic facts about selected minerals.

Should You Take Supplements?

Nutrition scientists generally agree that most Americans can obtain the vitamins and minerals they need to prevent deficiencies by consuming a varied, nutritionally balanced diet. However, controversy currently exists among scientists about whether supplements of particular vitamins and minerals should be recommended for their potential disease-fighting properties, as for the antioxidant vitamins C and E. At this time, the FDA and the National Academy of Sciences take the position that recommend-

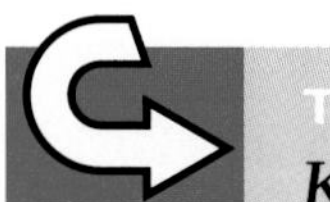

TACTICS AND TIPS

Keeping the Nutrient Value in Food

1. *Consume or process vegetables immediately after purchasing (or harvesting).* The longer vegetables are kept before they are eaten or processed, the more vitamins are lost, especially vitamin C and folate.
2. *Store vegetables and fruits properly.* If you can't eat fruits and vegetables immediately after purchasing (or harvesting) but plan to do so within a few days, keep them in the refrigerator. Place them in covered containers or plastic bags to lessen moisture loss. The best method for longer-term preservation is to freeze fruits and vegetables when possible. Canning fruits and vegetables preserves them, but it's a lot of work and causes a greater nutrient loss.
3. *Minimize the preparation and cooking of vegetables and other foods.* The more preparation and cooking of foods that is done before eating, the greater the nutrient loss. To reduce the losses:
    - Avoid soaking vegetables in water.
    - When possible, cook vegetables, like potatoes, whole and in their skins.
    - Don't soak and rinse rice before cooking; you'll wash off the B vitamins.
    - Cook in as little water as possible.
    - Don't add baking soda to vegetables to enhance the green color.
    - Bake, steam, broil, or microwave vegetables.
    - If you stew meats, consume the broth, too.
    - When boiling, use tight-fitting lids to minimize the evaporation of water.
    - Cook vegetables as little as possible. Develop a taste for a more crunchy texture.
    - Don't thaw frozen vegetables before cooking.
    - Prepare lettuce salads right before eating.

ing such supplements to the general public is premature. It's possible that in the future recommendations for vitamins and minerals may be broadened to include both a minimum amount to prevent a deficiency and a higher value to optimize chronic disease prevention.

The question of whether or not to take supplements is a serious one because some vitamins and minerals are dangerous when ingested in excess, as shown in Tables 8-2 and 8-3. For example, high doses of vitamin A are toxic and increase the risk of birth defects. Vitamin D toxicity causes calcium deposits to form in the kidneys. And vitamin B-6 can cause irreversible nerve damage when taken in large doses. Large doses of particular nutrients can also cause health problems by affecting the absorption of other vitamins and minerals. For instance, a high amount of copper in a supplement can inhibit the body's absorption of zinc.

Relying on supplements for vitamins and minerals can also be a problem because of what they do *not* contain. Foods contain many substances other than vitamins and minerals, some of which have been linked to disease prevention. These **phytochemicals** (*phyto* means plant) are discussed in more detail in Chapters 11 and 12.

For all of these reasons, people need to think carefully about whether or not to take supplements. Although vitamins are sold over the counter, the decision to take supplements should be made in consultation with a physician or a registered dietitian. Supplements may be prescribed in certain cases, including the following:

- Women with heavy menstrual flows may need extra iron to compensate for the monthly loss.
- Pregnant or nursing women may need extra iron, folate, and calcium.
- People who are unable to consume adequate calories may need a range of vitamin and mineral supplements.
- Some vegetarians may need extra calcium, iron, zinc, and vitamin B-12.
- Newborns need a single dose of vitamin K, which must be administered under the direction of a physician.
- People who have certain diseases or who take certain medications may need specific vitamin and mineral supplements. For example, people who use thiazide diuretics may require extra potassium, and people with osteoporosis may require extra vitamin D. Such supplement decisions must be made by a physician because some vitamins and minerals counteract the actions of certain medications.

If you do decide to take a vitamin and mineral supplement, the Council on Scientific Affairs of the American Medical Association recommends a supplement containing 50–150% of the adult Daily Value for vitamins. We suggest the same guidelines for minerals. Choose a balanced formulation to avoid developing a vitamin or

TERMS

phytochemical A naturally occurring substance found in plant foods that is not an essential nutrient but does have health benefits (such as preventing cancer and heart disease).

A CLOSER LOOK
Osteoporosis

Osteoporosis is a condition in which the bones become dangerously thin and fragile over time. It currently afflicts some 25 million Americans, 80% of them women, and results in 1.5 million bone fractures each year. The incidence of osteoporosis may double in the next 25 years as the population ages.

The bones in your body are continually being broken down and rebuilt in order to adapt to mechanical strain. About 20% of your body's bone mass is replaced each year. In the first few decades of life, bones become thicker and stronger as they are rebuilt. Most of your bone mass (95%) is built by age 18. After bone mass peaks between the ages of 25 and 35, the rate of bone loss exceeds the rate of replacement, and bones become thinner. In osteoporosis, this thinning becomes so severe that bones become very fragile.

Fractures are the most serious consequences of osteoporosis; up to 25% of all people who suffer a hip fracture die within a year. Other problems associated with osteoporosis are loss of height and a stooped posture caused by vertebral fractures, severe back and hip pain, and breathing problems caused by changes in the shape of the skeleton.

Who Is at Risk?

Women are at greater risk than men for osteoporosis because they have 10–25% less bone in their skeleton. As they lose bone mass with age, women's bones become dangerously thin sooner than men's bones. More men will probably develop osteoporosis in the future as they live into their 80s and 90s. Bone loss accelerates in women during the first 5–10 years after the onset of menopause because of a drop in estrogen production. (Estrogen improves calcium absorption and reduces the amount of calcium the body excretes.)

Other risk factors for osteoporosis include a family history of osteoporosis, early menopause (before age 45), abnormal menstruation, a history of anorexia, a thin small frame, and European or Asian background. Certain medications can also have a negative impact on bone mass, including thyroid medication and high doses of cortisonelike drugs for asthma or arthritis.

What Can You Do?

To prevent osteoporosis, the best strategy is to build as much bone as possible during your young years and then do everything you can to maintain it as you age. After age 35 there's not much you can do to add to bone mass, but up to 50% of bone loss is determined by controllable lifestyle factors.

- *Ensure an adequate intake of calcium.* Consuming an adequate amount of calcium is important throughout life to build and maintain bone mass. Americans average 400–600 mg of calcium per day, only about half of what is currently recommended (and many scientists would like to see the recommendations increased). Milk, yogurt, and fortified orange juice, bread, and cereals are all good sources of calcium. Nutritionists suggest that you obtain calcium from foods first and then take supplements only if needed to make up the difference. Supplements containing calcium carbonate are usually the least expensive.
- *Ensure an adequate intake of vitamin D.* Vitamin D is necessary for bones to absorb calcium. It can be obtained from foods (milk and fortified cereals, for example) and is manufactured by the skin when exposed to sunlight. Obtaining enough vitamin D can be a problem for housebound older adults and for people who live in northern latitudes where the sun is weaker, especially during the winter. Candidates for vitamin D supplements include people who don't eat many foods rich in vitamin D; those who don't expose their face, arms, and hands to the sun (without sunscreen) for 5–15 minutes a few times each week; and people who live north of an imaginary line roughly between Boston and the Oregon-California border. Many calcium supplements also contain vitamin D.
- *Exercise.* Weight-bearing aerobic activities help build and maintain bone mass throughout life, but they must be performed regularly in order to have lasting effects. Strength training is also helpful: It improves bone density, muscle mass, strength, and balance, protecting against both bone loss and falls, a major cause of fractures.
- *Don't smoke.* Smoking reduces the body's estrogen levels and is linked to earlier menopause and more rapid postmenopausal bone loss.
- *Drink alcohol only in moderation.* Alcohol reduces the body's ability to absorb calcium and may interfere with estrogen's bone-protecting effects. Follow the Dietary Guidelines, and consume no more than one alcoholic beverage per day.
- *Monitor your consumption of caffeine.* The association between caffeine-containing beverages and osteoporosis isn't clear, but researchers recommend that caffeine consumers take special care to include calcium-rich foods in their diet because calcium may counterbalance any caffeine-linked drop in bone mass.
- *After menopause, consider estrogen replacement therapy (ERT) or another drug treatment.* ERT combats bone loss as well as menopausal symptoms and heart disease. However, it is not without side effects and risks, including a possible increase in breast cancer risk. A physician can review your risk factors and test your bone density to help you decide whether ERT is a wise choice for you. Other new drug treatments include alendronate (Fosamez) and calcitonin (Miacalcin), which slow the resorption of bone by the body, and fluoride, which helps build bone in women who already have osteoporosis.

Scientists recently discovered a gene linked to bone density, so a test to identify people at high risk for osteoporosis may become available in the future. Although not helpful in treating the condition, such a test could alert those at greater risk.

TABLE 8-3 Facts About Selected Minerals

Mineral	Major Functions	Signs of Prolonged Deficiency	Toxic Effects of Megadoses	Important Dietary Sources
Calcium	Maintenance of bones and teeth, blood clotting, maintenance of cell membranes, control of nerve impulses and muscle contraction	Stunted growth in children, bone mineral loss in adults	Nausea, vomiting, hypertension, constipation, urinary stones, calcium deposits in soft tissues, inhibition of absorption of certain minerals	Milk and milk products, tofu, fortified orange juice and bread, green leafy vegetables, bones in fish
Fluoride	Maintenance of tooth (and possibly bone) structure	Higher frequency of tooth decay	Increased bone density, mottling of teeth, impaired kidney function, neurological disturbances	Fluoride-containing drinking water, tea, marine fish eaten with bones
Iron	Component of hemoglobin (carries oxygen to tissues), myoglobin (in muscle fibers), and enzymes	Iron-deficiency anemia, weakness, impaired immune function, cold hands and feet, gastrointestinal distress	Iron deposits in soft tissues, causing liver and kidney damage, joint pains, sterility, and disruption of cardiac function	Lean meats, legumes, enriched flour, green vegetables, dried fruit, liver; absorption is enhanced by the presence of vitamin C
Iodine	Essential part of thyroid hormones, regulation of body metabolism	Goiter (enlarged thyroid), cretinism (birth defect)	Depression of thyroid activity, hyperthyroidism in susceptible individuals	Iodized salt, seafood
Magnesium	Transmission of nerve impulses, bone and tooth structure, energy transfer, composition of many enzyme systems	Neurological disturbances, impaired immune function, kidney disorders, nausea, weight loss, growth failure in children	Nausea, vomiting, central nervous system depression, coma; death in people with impaired kidney function	Widespread in foods and water (except soft water); especially found in wheat bran, milk products, legumes, nuts, seeds, leafy vegetables

mineral imbalance. In making a decision about supplements, consider whether you consume a fortified breakfast cereal, which may contain up to 100% of the adult Daily Values for vitamins and minerals.

NUTRITIONAL GUIDELINES

The second part of putting together a healthy food plan—after you've learned about necessary nutrients—is choosing foods that satisfy nutritional requirements and that meet your personal criteria. Various tools have been created by scientific and government groups to help people design healthy diets. These tools are presented in some detail here so that you can learn to use them in conjunction with the information already provided on essential nutrients. The **Recommended Dietary Allowances (RDAs),** Estimated Safe and Adequate Daily Intakes (ESADDIs), and Estimated Minimum Requirements are standards that protect against nutritional deficiencies (Table 8-4, p. 194). The **Food Guide Pyramid** translates these nutrient recommendations into a balanced plan that includes all essential nutrients. A second set of guidelines, **Dietary Guidelines for Americans,** provides further guidance for choosing a healthy diet. Together, these items make up a complete set of resources for dietary planning.

Recommended Dietary Allowances (RDAs)

The Food and Nutrition Board of the National Academy of Sciences meets approximately every 5 years to set RDAs and related guidelines. The most recent version was published in 1989 (see Table 8-4). The board sets recommendations for individual nutrients in one of three categories:

1. *Recommended Dietary Allowances (RDAs).* These are specific recommended intakes of nutrients that are

TABLE 8-3 Facts About Selected Minerals (continued)

Mineral	Major Functions	Signs of Prolonged Deficiency	Toxic Effects of Megadoses	Important Dietary Sources
Phosphorus	Bone growth and maintenance (combined with calcium), energy transfer in cells	Weakness, bone loss, kidney disorders, cardiorespiratory failure	Drop in blood calcium levels	Present in nearly all foods, especially milk, cheese, cereal, legumes, meats
Potassium	Nerve function and body water balance	Muscular weakness, nausea, drowsiness, paralysis, confusion, disruption of cardiac rhythm	Cardiac arrest	Meats, milk, fruits, vegetables, grains, legumes
Sodium	Body water balance, acid-base balance, nerve function	Muscle weakness, loss of appetite, nausea, vomiting; sodium deficiency is rarely seen	Edema, hypertension in sensitive people	Salt, soy sauce, salted foods
Zinc	Enzyme reactions, including synthesis of proteins, RNA, and DNA; wound healing; immune response; ability to taste	Growth failure, reproductive failure, loss of appetite, impaired taste acuity, skin rash, impaired immune function, poor wound healing, night blindness	Vomiting, impaired immune function, decline in serum HDL levels, impaired magnesium absorption	Whole grains, meat, eggs, liver, seafood (especially oysters)

Sources: National Research Council. 1989. *Recommended Dietary Allowances,* 10th ed. Washington, D.C.: National Academy Press. Shils, M. E., and V. R. Young, eds. 1993. *Modern Nutrition in Health and Disease,* 8th ed. Baltimore: Williams & Wilkins.

well known and well researched: calories, protein, eleven vitamins, and seven minerals.

2. *Estimated Safe and Adequate Daily Dietary Intakes (ESADDIs).* These are ranges of values for nutrients about which knowledge is still sketchy: two vitamins and five minerals.
3. *Estimated Minimum Requirements.* These are minimum values for three minerals: sodium, potassium, and chloride.

The RDAs are intended as guidelines for meeting nutritional needs with food rather than vitamin and mineral supplements. This aim is important, because the board has not yet set recommendations for some essential nutrients about which too little is still known. Because many supplements contain only nutrients for which RDAs have been established, those who rely on them can become deficient in other nutrients, which are available in foods. (Supplements also lack potentially beneficial phytochemicals that are found only in foods.)

None of the essential nutrients is needed daily. For example, a person can survive for about a year without vitamin A. But diets that meet only half the recommended intake levels are likely to be insufficient to replace daily losses, so over the long run they can lead to deficiencies. Nutritional deficiencies can develop slowly, and symptoms can be subtle. There may be a decrease in the effectiveness of the immune system, for example, reduced organ function, a diminished ability to carry oxygen in the

TERMS

Recommended Dietary Allowances (RDAs) Amounts of certain nutrients considered adequate to meet the needs of most healthy people.

Food Guide Pyramid A food group plan that provides practical advice to ensure a balanced intake of the essential nutrients.

Dietary Guidelines for Americans General principles of good nutrition provided by the USDA and the U.S. Department of Health and Human Services.

TABLE 8-4 *Recommended Dietary Allowances, Revised 1989*[a, b, c]

Category	Age (years) or Condition	Weight[d] (kg)	Weight[d] (lb)	Height[d] (cm)	Height[d] (in.)	Protein (g)	Fat-Soluble Vitamins: *Vitamin A* (μg RE)[e]	Fat-Soluble Vitamins: *Vitamin D* (μg)	Fat-Soluble Vitamins: *Vitamin E* (mg α-TE)[f]	Fat-Soluble Vitamins: *Vitamin K* (μg)
Infants	0.0–0.5	6	13	60	24	13	375	7.5	3	5
	0.5–1.0	9	20	71	28	14	375	10	4	10
Children	1–3	13	29	90	35	16	400	10	6	15
	4–6	20	44	112	44	24	500	10	7	20
	7–10	28	62	132	52	28	700	10	7	30
Males	11–14	45	99	157	62	45	1000	10	10	45
	15–18	66	145	176	69	59	1000	10	10	65
	19–24	72	160	177	70	58	1000	10	10	70
	25–50	79	174	176	70	63	1000	5	10	80
	51+	77	170	173	68	63	1000	5	10	80
Females	11–14	46	101	157	62	46	800	10	8	45
	15–18	55	120	163	64	44	800	10	8	55
	19–24	58	128	164	65	46	800	10	8	60
	25–50	63	138	163	64	50	800	5	8	65
	51+	65	143	160	63	50	800	5	8	65
Pregnant						60	800	10	10	65
Lactating	1st 6 Months					65	1300	10	12	65
	2nd 6 Months					62	1200	10	11	65

[a]The allowances, expressed as average daily intakes over time, are intended to provide for individual variations among most normal people as they live in the United States under usual environmental stresses. Diet should be based on a variety of common foods in order to provide other nutrients for which human requirements have been less well defined.
[b]Estimated Safe and Adequate Daily Dietary Intakes (ESADDIs) for adults: 30–100 μg biotin; 4.0–7.0 mg pantothenic acid; 1.5–3.0 mg copper; 2.0–5.0 mg manganese; 1.0–4.0 mg fluoride; 50–200 μg chromium; 75–250 mg molybdenum. (For information on other age groups, see National Research Council. 1989. *Recommended Dietary Allowances,* 10th ed. Washington, D.C.: National Academy Press.)
[c]Estimated Minimum Requirements of healthy adults: 500 mg sodium; 750 mg chloride; 2000 mg potassium. (For information on other age groups, see *Recommended Dietary Allowances,* 10th ed.)
[d]Weights and heights are medians for the U.S. population of the designated age. The use of these figures does not imply that the height-to-weight ratios are ideal.
[e]Retinol equivalents: 1 retinol equivalent = 1μg retinol or 6μg β-carotene.
[f]α-Tocopherol equivalents: 1 mg d-α tocopherol = 1 α-TE.

bloodstream, or general ongoing cell damage. Signs of these problems may not be apparent for a long time; instead, a person may simply become ill more often without knowing why. Designing a nutritionally sound diet around the RDAs is a way of preventing hard-to-detect deficiencies.

A variant of the RDAs is the **Daily Values,** which have been set by the FDA as a means of expressing nutrient content on food labels. The Daily Values are based on two dietary standards: the RDAs, used for vitamins and minerals; and current scientific consensus, used for nutrients for which there is no RDA per se, such as protein, saturated fat, and dietary fiber. Nutrient content is expressed as a percentage of the Daily Values.

The Food Guide Pyramid

Most Americans know the three important principles of a healthy diet—variety, balance, and moderation. Many also know that a good diet is composed of items from a number of distinct food groups. Although the principles have remained constant over the years, the food groups themselves have changed as new information has become available. The latest food group plan is the Food Guide

TABLE 8-4 Recommended Dietary Allowances, Revised 1989[a, b, c] (continued)

Water-Soluble Vitamins							Minerals						
Vitamin C (mg)	*Thiamin (mg)*	*Riboflavin (mg)*	*Niacin (mg)*	*Vitamin B-6 (mg)*	*Folate (μg)*	*Vitamin B-12 (μg)*	*Calcium (mg)*	*Phosphorus (mg)*	*Magnesium (mg)*	*Iron (mg)*	*Zinc (mg)*	*Iodine (μg)*	*Selenium (μg)*
30	0.3	0.4	5	0.3	25	0.3	400	300	40	6	5	40	10
35	0.4	0.5	6	0.6	35	0.5	600	500	60	10	5	50	15
40	0.7	0.8	9	1.0	50	0.7	800	800	80	10	10	70	20
45	0.9	1.1	12	1.1	75	1.0	800	800	120	10	10	90	20
45	1.0	1.2	13	1.4	100	1.4	800	800	170	10	10	120	30
50	1.3	1.5	17	1.7	150	2.0	1200	1200	270	12	15	150	40
60	1.5	1.8	20	2.0	200	2.0	1200	1200	400	12	15	150	50
60	1.5	1.7	19	2.0	200	2.0	1200	1200	350	10	15	150	70
60	1.5	1.7	19	2.0	200	2.0	800	800	350	10	15	150	70
60	1.2	1.4	15	2.0	200	2.0	800	800	350	10	15	150	70
50	1.1	1.3	15	1.4	150	2.0	1200	1200	280	15	12	150	45
60	1.1	1.3	15	1.5	180	2.0	1200	1200	300	15	12	150	50
60	1.1	1.3	15	1.6	180	2.0	1200	1200	280	15	12	150	55
60	1.1	1.3	15	1.6	180	2.0	800	800	280	15	12	150	55
60	1.0	1.2	13	1.6	180	2.0	800	800	280	10	12	150	55
70	1.5	1.6	17	2.2	400	2.2	1200	1200	320	30	15	175	65
95	1.6	1.8	20	2.1	280	2.6	1200	1200	355	15	19	200	75
90	1.6	1.7	20	2.1	260	2.6	1200	1200	340	15	16	200	75

Pyramid, provided by the United States Department of Agriculture (USDA) and shown in Figure 8-5 (p. 196).

The Food Guide Pyramid is based on a recommended number of servings from six food groups:

1. Bread, cereals, rice, and pasta group: 6–11 servings
2. Vegetable group: 3–5 servings
3. Fruit group: 2–4 servings
4. Meat, poultry, fish, dry beans, eggs, and nuts group: 2–3 servings
5. Milk, yogurt, and cheese group: 2–3 servings
6. Fats, oils, and sweets group: No recommended servings

The Food Guide Pyramid is a general guide to what you should eat every day. You can get all essential nutrients by eating a balanced variety of foods from each of the six food groups. Serving sizes and examples of foods are included in Table 8-5 (p. 197). If you choose some plant proteins (from the meat, poultry, fish, dry beans, eggs, and nuts group) and follow the other suggestions listed in the table, your daily diet will be adequate in all nutrients, except possibly iron for women with heavy menstrual flows. To maximize the nutrient value of this diet, include a source of vitamin C in the fruit group; a dark-green or orange vegetable in the vegetable group; mostly whole grains in the bread, cereal, rice, and pasta group; and a tablespoon of vegetable oil if it is not already present in other foods. A diet based on these choices will yield about 1600–1800 calories.

Dietary Guidelines for Americans

To provide further guidance, the USDA and the U.S. Department of Health and Human Services have issued Dietary Guidelines for Americans, most recently in 1995. Following is a summary of these guidelines, with addi-

TERMS

Daily Values A simplified version of the RDAs used on food labels; also included are values for nutrients with no RDA per se.

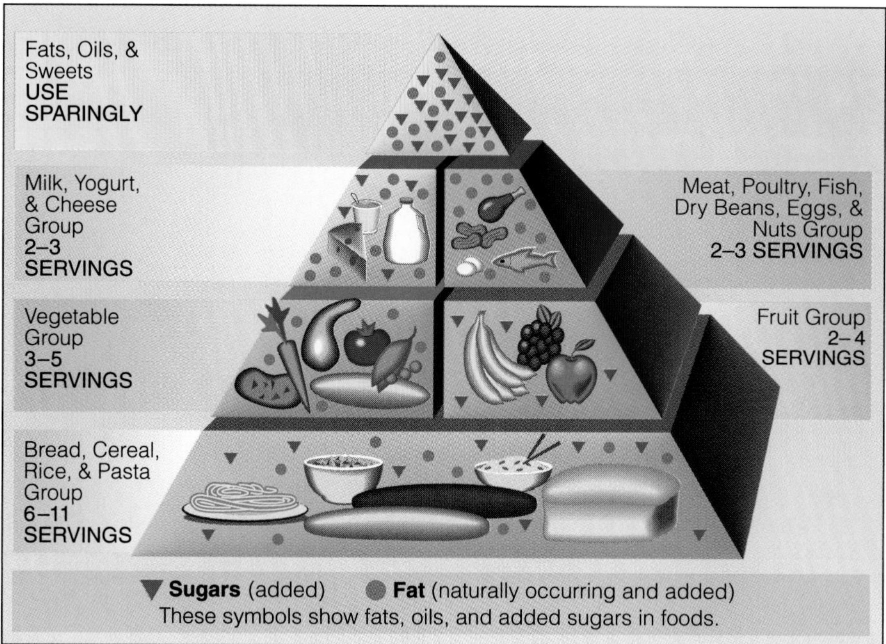

Figure 8-5 ***The Food Guide Pyramid.*** *Source:* U.S. Department of Agriculture. 1992. Human Nutrition Information Service, *Food Guide Pyramid,* Home and Garden Bulletin No. 249.

tional comments from the U.S. Surgeon General, the American Heart Association, the National Cancer Institute, and the National Academy of Sciences.

1. *Eat a variety of foods.* Focus on the six food groups shown on the Food Guide Pyramid, and choose an appropriate number of servings from each group. Choose a variety of foods from within each group to take advantage of the fact that some foods are better sources of certain nutrients than other foods. Everyone, but especially adolescent girls and women, should take special care to meet their RDAs for calcium and iron. Protein intake should be limited to no more than 150% of the Daily Value.
2. *Balance the food you eat with physical activity—maintain or improve your weight.* Many Americans gain weight in adulthood, increasing their risk of diabetes, heart disease, cancer, and other diseases. Therefore, most adults should not gain weight once they achieve a healthy adult weight. In order to stay at the same weight, balance the amount of calories in the foods you eat with the amount of calories your body uses.

   Overweight people, especially those who already have obesity-related health problems, should try to lose weight or, at the very least, not gain weight. Weight loss, however, should be gradual—no more than ½–1 pound per week. Healthy weight loss is the result of a balance of two efforts: eating low-calorie, nutrient-rich foods and increasing calorie-burning physical activity. Drastic calorie restriction can be dangerous and is recommended only under strict medical supervision.
3. *Choose a diet with plenty of grain products, vegetables, and fruits.* A healthy diet emphasizes grain products, vegetables, and fruits because they tend to be low in fat and high in complex carbohydrates, dietary fiber, vitamins, minerals, and other beneficial phytochemicals. Five or more servings of vegetables or fruits per day are recommended, plus six or more servings of bread, cereals, and legumes. This goal will dovetail with that of consuming 20–35 grams of dietary fiber.
4. *Choose a diet that is low in fat, saturated fat, and cholesterol.* Fat intake should be limited to 30% or less of total daily calorie intake. Saturated fat should be no more than one-third of total daily fat intake (10% of total daily calories), and dietary cholesterol should be limited to 300 milligrams a day. These levels are below current typical levels: The average American consumes 12% of the total daily number of calories as saturated fat and 230 mg for women and 370 mg for men of dietary cholesterol a day.

   To reduce the intake of fat and saturated fat, experts recommend choosing lean meat, fish, poultry, and dry beans and peas as protein sources; using nonfat or low-fat milk and milk products; limiting the intake of fats and oils high in saturated fat; trimming fat off meats; broiling, baking, or boiling instead of frying, deep-frying, and breading; and strictly limiting fast-food meals, in which fat tends to make up 40% or more of the total calorie count. For more ideas, see the box "Reducing the Fat in Your Diet" (p. 198).

   Although less dangerous for heart health than saturated fat, high cholesterol intake can be a problem for some people. Cholesterol is found only in animal foods. If you want to cut back on your cholesterol intake, follow the Food Guide Pyramid's recommendations for consumption of animal foods;

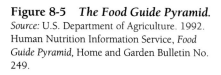

TABLE 8-5 Using the Food Guide Pyramid

Food Group	Number of Servings	Major Contributions	Foods and Serving Sizes[a]
Milk, yogurt, and cheese	2–3[b]	Carbohydrate, protein, calcium, riboflavin, potassium, zinc	1 cup milk 1½ oz cheese 2 oz processed cheese 1 cup yogurt 2 cups cottage cheese
Meat, poultry, fish, dry beans, eggs, and nuts	2–3	Protein, niacin, iron, vitamin B-6, zinc, thiamin, vitamin B-12[c]	2–3 oz cooked meat, poultry, fish 1–1½ cups cooked dry beans 4 tbsp peanut butter 2 eggs ½–1 cup nuts
Fruits	2–4	Carbohydrate, vitamin C, dietary fiber	1 whole piece of fruit 1 melon wedge ½ cup berries ½ grapefruit ¼ cup dried fruit ½ cup cooked or canned fruit ¾ cup juice
Vegetables	3–5	Carbohydrate, vitamin A, vitamin C, folate, magnesium, dietary fiber	½ cup raw or cooked vegetables 1 cup raw leafy vegetables ¾ cup juice
Bread, cereals, rice, and pasta	6–11	Carbohydrate, thiamin, riboflavin[d], iron, niacin, folate, magnesium[e], dietary fiber[e], zinc[e]	1 slice of bread ½ hamburger bun, English muffin, or bagel (depending on size) 1 small roll, biscuit, or muffin 1 oz ready-to-eat cereal ½–¾ cup cooked cereal, rice, or pasta 3–4 small or 2 large crackers
Fats, oils, and sweets		Foods from this group should not replace any from the other groups. Amounts consumed should be determined by individual energy needs.	

[a]May be reduced for child servings.
[b]Two servings for adults age 25 or over; 3 servings for children, teens, young adults, and pregnant or lactating women.
[c]Only in animal food choices.
[d]If enriched.
[e]Whole grains especially.

pay particular attention to serving sizes. In addition, limit your intake of foods that are particularly high in cholesterol content, including egg yolks and liver. The cholesterol content of many common foods is listed in Appendix B; nutrition labels on prepared foods also include cholesterol information.

5. *Choose a diet moderate in sugars.* Diets high in sugars do not cause hyperactivity or diabetes, but they do promote tooth decay. In addition, some foods that contain a lot of sugars supply calories but few or no nutrients. For people who are very active and have high calorie needs, sugars can be an additional source of energy. However, because eating a nutritious diet and maintaining a healthy body weight are very important, healthy people should use sugars in moderation, and people with low calorie needs should use sugars sparingly. Reducing sugar consumption means cutting back on items with added sugar, such as baked goods, candies, sweet desserts, sweetened beverages, canned fruits, and presweetened breakfast cereals.
6. *Choose a diet moderate in salt and sodium.* Sodium is an essential nutrient, but it is required only in small amounts—500 milligrams, or ¼ teaspoon, per day. Most Americans consume 8–12 times this amount. It is recommended that people limit their salt intake to

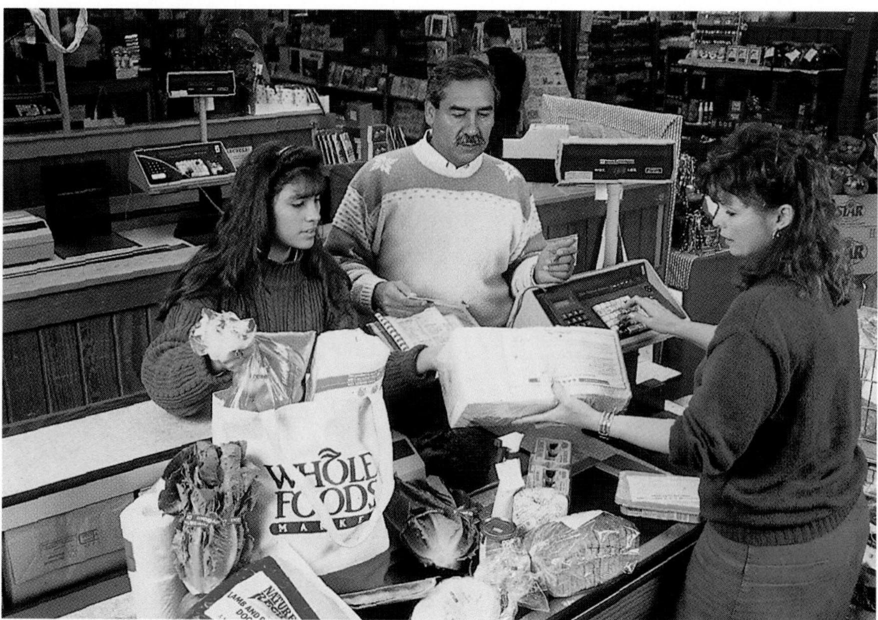

Our bodies need adequate amounts of all essential nutrients to grow and function properly. Guidelines like the Food Guide Pyramid can help people translate nutritional requirements into food choices when they're planning meals and shopping.

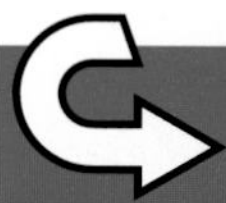

TACTICS AND TIPS

Reducing the Fat in Your Diet

- Steam, boil, bake, or microwave vegetables, or stir-fry them in a small amount of vegetable oil.
- Season vegetables with herbs and spices rather than with sauces, butter, or margarine.
- Try lemon juice or a fat-free dressing on salad, or use a yogurt-based dressing instead of mayonnaise or sour cream dressing.
- To reduce saturated fat, use vegetable oil or tub margarine instead of butter or stick margarine when possible.
- Replace whole milk with skim or low-fat milk in puddings, soups, and baked products. Substitute plain nonfat yogurt, blender-whipped cottage cheese, low-fat sour cream, or buttermilk in recipes that call for sour cream.
- Choose lean cuts of meat, and trim any visible fat from meat before and after cooking. Remove skin from poultry before or after cooking. Monitor portion sizes.
- Roast, bake, or broil meat, poultry, or fish so that fat drains away as the food cooks.
- Use a nonstick pan for cooking so added fat will be unnecessary; use a vegetable spray for frying.
- Chill broths from meat or poultry until the fat becomes solid. Spoon off the fat before using the broth.
- Eat a low-fat vegetarian main dish at least once a week.

2400 milligrams, or about 1 teaspoon, per day. Strategies for reducing salt intake include cutting back on salty foods, such as lunch meats, salted snack foods, canned soups, regular cheese, and many tomato-based products; choosing low sodium versions of high sodium foods; adding only small amounts of salt during cooking and at the table; and using lemon juice, herbs, and spices, rather than salt, to enhance the flavor of food.

7. *If you drink alcoholic beverages, do so in moderation.* Alcoholic beverages supply calories but few or no nutrients. Current evidence suggests that moderate drinking—no more than one drink daily for women and two drinks daily for men—is associated with a lower risk for cardiovascular disease in some people. However, higher levels of alcohol intake are associated with an increased risk for a variety of diseases and with higher overall mortality rates. Adults who drink alcoholic beverages should do so in moderation, with meals, and when its consumption does not put themselves or others at risk. (Alcohol is discussed in more detail in Chapter 13.)

One further recommendation, geared specifically for cancer prevention, is to eat salt-cured, smoked, and nitrate-cured foods such as bacon and sausage only in moderation. These foods may increase the risk of colon cancer.

Reading Food Labels

Consumers can get help in applying the principles of the Food Guide Pyramid and the Dietary Guidelines for Americans from food labels. Beginning in 1994, all processed foods regulated by either the FDA or the USDA have included standardized nutrition information on their labels. Every food label shows serving sizes and the amount of fat, saturated fat, cholesterol, protein, dietary fiber, and sodium in each serving. To make intelligent choices about food, learn to read and understand food labels (see the box "Using Food Labels to Make Dietary Choices," p. 200).

The Typical American Diet

Although much has been made in the press about recent decreases in the consumption of fat and saturated fat, the average American diet still does not comply with the Dietary Guidelines. Reports of a shift to low-fat and nonfat milk seem to have been exaggerated, since whole milk and whole-milk beverages are among the five major contributors of calories to the American diet. The other four are white bread, rolls, and crackers; doughnuts, cakes, and cookies; alcoholic beverages; and hamburgers, cheeseburgers, and meatloaf. Some of these foods have a certain degree of nutritional value, but they certainly do not reflect a trend toward whole grains and fiber and away from saturated fat, alcohol, and sugar. Low consumption of fruits and vegetables also continues to be a problem. Recent surveys indicate that only 20% of Americans consume the recommended five or more servings of fruits and vegetables per day.

On a list of ideal, health-enhancing foods, the top five calorie contributors would be replaced by low-fat and nonfat milk; whole-wheat bread and whole-grain cereals; and lean meat, tuna, beans, and other vegetable proteins; additional nutrients would come from oranges, Romaine lettuce, carrots, and broccoli.

The Vegetarian Alternative

Some people choose a diet with one essential difference from the diets we've already described: Foods of animal origin (meat, poultry, fish, eggs, milk) are eliminated or restricted. Today, about 12 million Americans follow a vegetarian diet. Most do so because they think foods of plant origin are a more natural way to nourish the body. Some do so for religious, health, ethical, or philosophical reasons. If you choose to be a vegetarian, you can be confident of meeting your nutritional needs by following a few basic rules. (Vegetarian diets for children and pregnant women warrant individual professional guidance.)

There is a variety of vegetarian styles; the wider the variety of the diet eaten, the easier to meet nutritional needs. **Vegans** eat only plant foods. **Lacto-vegetarians** eat plant foods and dairy products. **Lacto-ovo-vegetarians** eat plant foods, dairy products, and eggs. Finally, **partial** or **semivegetarians** eat plant foods, dairy products, eggs, and usually a small selection of poultry, fish, and other seafood. Including some animal protein in a diet makes planning much easier.

A food-group plan has been developed for lacto-vegetarians; it includes 6–11 servings from grains and 2–4 servings from legumes, nuts, and seeds. Add to this 3–5 servings from the vegetable group, 2–4 servings from the fruit group, and two or more servings from the milk, yogurt, and cheese group to complete the plan. By following this plan, lacto-vegetarians should have no problem obtaining an adequate diet. Consuming fruits with most meals is especially helpful, because any vitamin C present will improve iron absorption (the iron in plants is more difficult to absorb than the iron in animal sources).

In contrast to those who eat dairy products, vegans must do much more special diet planning to obtain all essential nutrients. A vegan must take special care to consume adequate amounts of protein, riboflavin, vitamin D, vitamin B-12, calcium, iron, and zinc; good strategies for obtaining these nutrients include the following:

- Eat proteins from a wide variety of sources, and include a couple of protein sources at each meal. A good rule of thumb is 11 servings of grains and 4 servings of legumes, nuts, and seeds. Soy milk and tofu (soybean curd) make important nutrient contributions to this diet plan.
- Eat green leafy vegetables, whole grains, yeast, and legumes to obtain riboflavin.
- Obtain vitamin D by spending at least a half-hour a day out in the sun or, if not possible on a regular basis, by taking a supplement.
- Obtain vitamin B-12 (found only in animal foods) from a supplement or by consuming foods fortified with vitamin B-12, such as special yeast products, soy milk, and breakfast cereals. (Vitamin B-12 deficiency takes a long time to develop, but it can cause irreversible nerve damage.)

TERMS

vegan A vegetarian who eats no animal products.

lacto-vegetarian A vegetarian who includes dairy products in the diet.

lacto-ovo-vegetarian A vegetarian who includes dairy products and eggs in the diet.

partial or **semivegetarian** A person who eats plant foods, dairy products, eggs, and small amounts of poultry, fish, and seafood.

CRITICAL CONSUMER

Using Food Labels to Make Dietary Choices

Food labels are designed to help consumers make food choices based on the nutrients that are most important to good health. A food label states how much fat, saturated fat, cholesterol, protein, dietary fiber, and sodium the food contains. In addition to listing nutrient content by weight, the label puts the information in the context of a daily diet of 2000 calories that includes no more than 65 grams of fat (approximately 30% of total calories). For example, if a serving of a particular product has 13 grams of fat, the label will show that the serving represents 20% of the daily fat allowance. If your daily diet contains fewer or more than 2000 calories, you need to adjust these calculations accordingly. Refer to p. 184 for instructions on setting an appropriate limit on your fat intake.

Food labels contain uniform serving sizes. This means that if you look at different brands of salad dressing, for example, you can compare calories and fat content based on the serving amount. Regulations also require that foods meet strict definitions if their packaging includes the terms "light," "low-fat," or "high-fiber." Health claims such as "good source of dietary fiber" or "low in saturated fat" on packages are signals that those products can wisely be included in your diet. Overall, the food label is an important tool to help you choose a diet that conforms to the Food Guide Pyramid and the Dietary Guidelines.

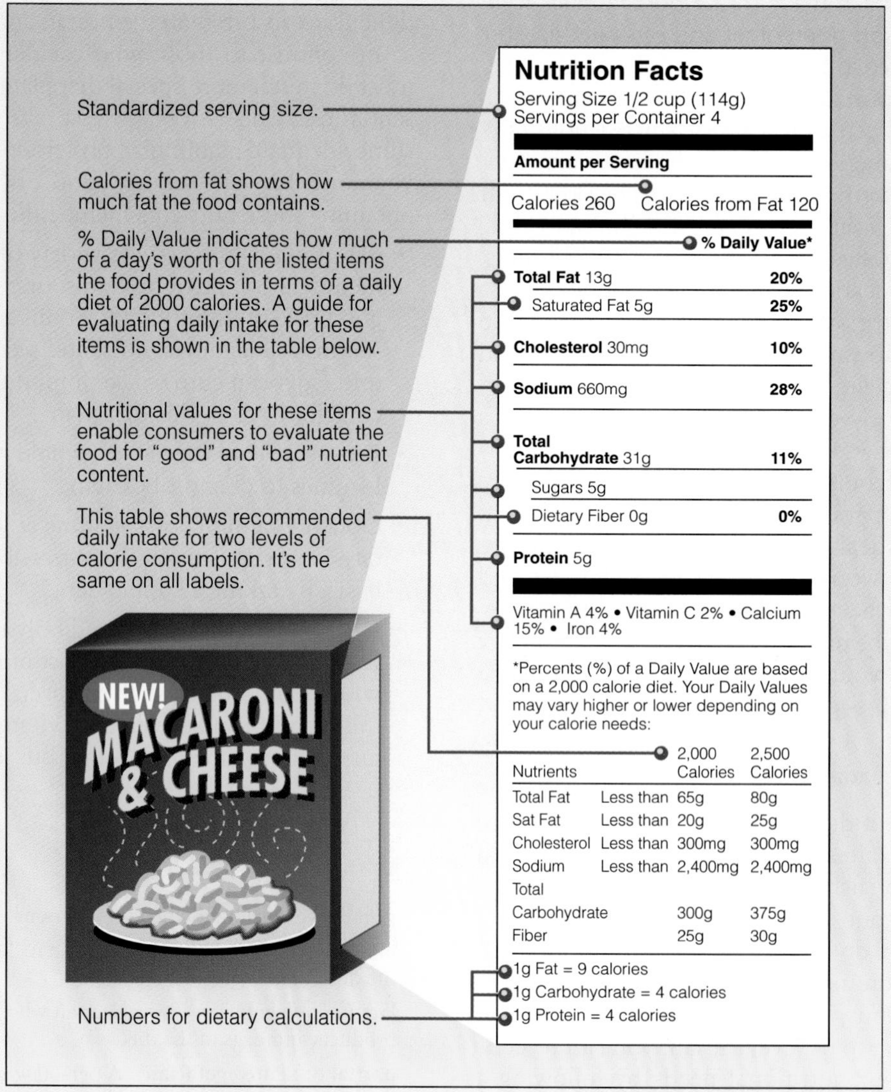

Standardized serving size.
Calories from fat shows how much fat the food contains.
% Daily Value indicates how much of a day's worth of the listed items the food provides in terms of a daily diet of 2000 calories. A guide for evaluating daily intake for these items is shown in the table below.
Nutritional values for these items enable consumers to evaluate the food for "good" and "bad" nutrient content.
This table shows recommended daily intake for two levels of calorie consumption. It's the same on all labels.
Numbers for dietary calculations.
NEW!
MACARONI & CHEESE
Nutrition Facts
Serving Size 1/2 cup (114g)
Servings per Container 4
Amount per Serving
Calories 260 Calories from Fat 120
% Daily Value*
Total Fat 13g 20%
Saturated Fat 5g 25%
Cholesterol 30mg 10%
Sodium 660mg 28%
Total Carbohydrate 31g 11%
Sugars 5g
Dietary Fiber 0g 0%
Protein 5g
Vitamin A 4% • Vitamin C 2% • Calcium 15% • Iron 4%
*Percents (%) of a Daily Value are based on a 2,000 calorie diet. Your Daily Values may vary higher or lower depending on your calorie needs:
Nutrients 2,000 Calories 2,500 Calories
Total Fat Less than 65g 80g
Sat Fat Less than 20g 25g
Cholesterol Less than 300mg 300mg
Sodium Less than 2,400mg 2,400mg
Total Carbohydrate 300g 375g
Fiber 25g 30g
1g Fat = 9 calories
1g Carbohydrate = 4 calories
1g Protein = 4 calories

- Consume fortified tofu, green leafy vegetables, nuts, and fortified orange juice, bread, and soy milk to obtain calcium. Supplements may be necessary.
- Consume whole grains, fortified breakfast cereals, dried fruits, nuts, and legumes to obtain iron.
- Obtain zinc from whole grains and legumes.

It takes a little planning and common sense to put together a good vegetarian diet. If you are a vegetarian or are considering becoming one, devote some extra time and thought to your diet. It's especially important that you eat as wide a variety of foods as possible to ensure that all of your nutritional needs are satisfied.

A PERSONAL PLAN: APPLYING NUTRITIONAL PRINCIPLES

Now that you understand the basics of good nutrition, you can put together a diet that works for you. The basic principles of a healthy diet are simple—variety, balance, and moderation. But within this framework, no single diet is optimal for everyone. Many different diets can meet people's nutritional requirements. Every individual needs to customize a food plan based on age, gender, height, weight, activity level, medical risk factors—and, of course, personal tastes.

Assessing and Changing Your Diet

The first step in planning a healthy diet is to examine what you currently eat. Labs 8-1 and 8-2 are designed to help you analyze your current diet and compare it to optimal dietary goals. (This analysis can be completed using either Appendix B or the nutritional software that accompanies the text.)

Next, experiment with additions and substitutions to your current diet to bring it closer to your goals. If you are consuming too much fat, for example, try substituting fruit for a calorie-rich dessert. If you aren't getting enough iron, try adding some raisins to your cereal or garbanzo beans to your salad. If you need to plan your diet from the ground up, use the Food Guide Pyramid and the Dietary Guidelines. To see a sample diet for one day for a 20-year-old male that meets the RDAs and follows the Dietary Guidelines, refer to the box "A Sample Diet for One Day" (p. 202).

To put your plan into action, use the behavioral self-management techniques and tips described in Chapter 1. If you identify several changes you want to make, be sure to focus on one at a time. You might start, for example, by substituting nonfat or low-fat milk for whole milk. When you become used to that, you can try substituting whole-wheat bread for white bread. The information on eating behavior in Lab 8-1 will help you identify and change problem behaviors.

Staying Committed to a Healthy Diet

Beyond knowledge and information, you also need support in difficult situations. The final section of this chapter offers some practical tips for maintaining your commitment to a healthy diet in a variety of circumstances.

Keeping to your plan is easiest when you choose and prepare your own food at home. There, advance planning is the key: mapping out meals and shopping appropriately, cooking in advance when possible, and preparing enough food for leftovers later in the week. A tight budget does not necessarily make it more difficult to eat healthy meals. It makes good health sense and good budget sense to use only small amounts of meat and to have a few meatless meals each week.

In restaurants, keeping to food plan goals becomes somewhat more difficult. Portion sizes in restaurants tend to be larger than serving sizes of the Food Guide Pyramid, but by remaining focused on your goals, you can eat only part of your meal and take the rest home for lunch later in the week.

Don't hesitate to ask questions when you're eating in a restaurant. Most restaurant personnel are glad to explain how menu selections are prepared and to make small adjustments, such as serving salad dressings and sauces on the side so they can be avoided or used sparingly. To limit your fat intake, order meat or fish broiled or grilled rather than fried or sauteed, choose rice or a plain baked potato over french fries, and select a clear soup rather than a creamy one. Desserts that are irresistible can, at least, be shared.

Strategies like these can be helpful, but small changes cannot change a fundamentally high-fat, high-calorie meal into a moderate, healthful one. Often, the best advice is to bypass a steak with potatoes au gratin for a flavorful but low-fat entree. Many of the selections offered in ethnic restaurants are healthy choices (see the box "Ethnic Diets and Cuisines," p. 203).

Fast-food restaurants offer the biggest challenge to a healthy diet. Surveys show that about 70% of 18- to 24-year-olds and 64% of 25- to 34-year-olds visit a fast-food restaurant at least once a week. Fast-food meals are often high in calories, total fat, saturated fat, sodium, and sugar; they may be low in fiber and in some vitamins and minerals (see Appendix C). Although not all fast food is bad, the best strategy is to limit the number of times you eat in fast-food restaurants. If you do eat at a fast-food restaurant, make sure the rest of your meals that day are low-fat meals. For more ideas, see the box "Eating at Fast-Food Restaurants" (p. 204).

For young people, another challenge is eating in a college dining hall or cafeteria. In general, institutional food is known for its large portions and particularly high fat content. For ideas about how to manage a diet centered on the dining hall or cafeteria, see the box "College Eating" (p. 204).

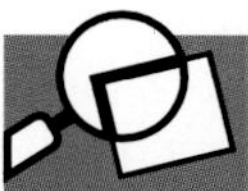

A CLOSER LOOK

A Sample Diet for One Day

This sample diet meets or exceeds the RDAs for a 20-year-old male and follows the suggestions provided by the Dietary Guidelines for Americans.

Breakfast

Cereal, wheat flakes, 1 cup
Raisins, 1/4 cup
Cantaloupe, 1/2
Orange juice, 6 oz
Nonfat milk, 12 oz

Snack

Pear, 1

Lunch

Turkey sandwich
- Wheat bread, 2 slices
- Sliced turkey, 1 1/2 oz
- Lettuce, green leaf, 2 leaves
- Tomato, 1/2
- Mayonnaise, 2 tsp
- Mustard, 1 tsp

Vegetable soup, 6 oz
Banana, 1
Nonfat milk, 8 oz

Snack

Crackers, whole grain rye, 4
Peanut butter, 2 tbsp
Apple juice, 6 oz

Dinner

Meat loaf, 1 slice
Potato, boiled, 1
Carrots, cooked, 1/2 cup
Spinach, cooked, 1/2 cup
Margarine, 2 tsp
Strawberries, 1 cup
Water, 12 oz

Snack

Popcorn, plain, 1 cup
Cranberry-apple juice, 6 oz

Approximate Nutrition Totals

Calories: 2200
- 15% from protein
- 65% from carbohydrates
- 20% from fat
  - 5.5% from saturated fat
  - 8.6% from monounsaturated fat
  - 5.9% from polyunsaturated fat
- 167 mg of cholesterol
- 38 g of dietary fiber
- 2.4 g of sodium

Knowledge of food and nutrition is essential to the success of your program. The information provided in this chapter should give you the tools you need to design and implement a diet that promotes long-term health and well-being. If you need additional information or have questions about nutrition, be sure the source you consult is a reliable one.

? COMMON QUESTIONS ANSWERED

How can I tell what a serving of a particular food is? Food labels on prepared food list serving sizes; Table 8-5 gives serving sizes used in the Food Guide Pyramid. Sometimes it's difficult to translate these serving sizes into the amount of food you put on your plate, however. Studies have shown that most people underestimate serving sizes—in many cases by as much as 50%. If you need to retrain your eye, try using measuring cups and spoons and an inexpensive kitchen scale when you eat at home. With a little practice, you'll learn the difference between 3 and 8 ounces of chicken or meat, and what a half-cup of rice really looks like. For quick estimates, use the following equivalents:

1 teaspoon of margarine: the tip of your thumb
1 ounce of cheese: your thumb or a one-inch cube
3 ounces of chicken or meat: a deck of cards
1 cup of pasta: your fist

DIMENSIONS OF DIVERSITY
Ethnic Diets and Cuisines

Every cultural group has its own eating practices—its own habitually eaten foods (its diet) and its own manner of preparing foods (its cuisine). Culture-based eating practices are influenced by many factors, including the availability of food items, cultural and religious beliefs and values about what people can and can't eat, and even the symbolic meaning of various foods.

There is no one ethnic diet that clearly surpasses all others in providing people with healthful foods. However, every diet has its advantages and disadvantages, and within each cuisine, some foods are better choices. It is in this area of personal choice that individuals can make a difference in their own health.

The dietary guidelines described in this chapter can be applied to any ethnic cuisine. For additional guidance, refer to the table below, which lists some of the more and less healthful choices you can make when you eat out at various ethnic restaurants or cook ethnic meals at home.

	Choose Often	Choose Less Often
Chinese	Chinese greens Rice, brown or white Steamed beef with pea pods Stir-fry dishes Wonton soup	Crispy duck Egg rolls Fried rice Kung pao (fried chicken) Pork spare ribs Sweet-and-sour dishes
Japanese	Chiri nabe (fish stew) Sushi Yakitori (grilled chicken) Shabu-shabu (foods in boiling broth)	Age tofu (fried tofu) Tonkatsu (fried pork) Tempura (fried chicken, shrimp, or vegetables) Sukiyaki
Thai	Forest salad Larb (minty chicken salad) Po tak (seafood soup) Yum neua (broiled beef with onions)	Fried fish, duck, or chicken Curries with coconut milk Yum koon chaing (sausage with peppers) Peanut sauce
Italian	Cioppino (seafood stew) Minestrone soup (vegetarian) Pasta with marinara sauce Pasta primavera (pasta with vegetables) Red clam sauce	Antipasto Cannelloni, ravioli Fettucine alfredo Garlic bread Veal or eggplant parmigiana Fried calamari
Mexican	Beans and rice Black bean/vegetable soup Burritos, bean Enchiladas, bean Gazpacho Tortillas, steamed Tostadas, bean or chicken Refried beans (nonfat or low-fat)	Chiles relleños Chimichangas Enchiladas, beef or cheese Flautas Guacamole Nachos or fried tortillas Quesadillas Refried beans (made with lard)
Indian	Chapati (tortillalike bread) Dal (lentils) Karhi (chick-pea soup) Khur (milk/rice dessert) Tandoori, chicken or fish	Bhatura (fried bread) Coconut milk Ghee (clarified butter) Korma (rich meat dish) Samosa (fried meat and vegetables in dough)

Sources: Adapted from The best of Asian cuisines. 1993. *University of California at Berkeley Wellness Letter,* January. Hurley, J., and B. Liebman. 1994. When in Rome . . . *Nutrition Action,* January/February. Eating in ethnic restaurants. 1990. *Runner's World,* January.

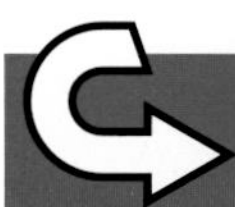

TACTICS AND TIPS
Eating at Fast-Food Restaurants

- *Skip the croissants at breakfast.* Croissants are usually fatty, especially when stuffed with eggs or bacon. For breakfast, choose plain scrambled eggs, a bagel, an English muffin, or plain hotcakes.
- *Choose plain burgers.* A bacon cheeseburger has twice the fat of a plain hamburger.
- *Hold the mayonnaise and the tartar sauce.* Tartar sauce accounts for about one-third of the fat in a fish sandwich.
- *Choose chicken items made from chicken breast, not processed chicken.* Processed chicken, whether in sandwiches or bite-size pieces, is higher in fat. Chicken filet sandwiches are usually lower in fat than bite-size chicken pieces.
- *Avoid rich salads and salad dressings.* Heavily dressed potato or pasta salads are usually high in fat. Choose a plain or low-calorie dressing, and don't add croutons or bacon to vegetable salads.
- *Avoid french fries and onion rings.* As currently prepared, french fries and onion rings usually get about 50% of their calories from fat. If you can't give them up entirely, order the smallest portion size available and eat them plain (no additional salt or ketchup). When available, choose mashed potatoes, a baked potato, or corn.
- *Choose vegetable pizza.* Avoid double-cheese and fatty meat (sausage and pepperoni) toppings. Choose vegetable toppings to limit fat and increase your intake of vitamins and minerals.
- *Drink water, mineral water, sugar-free soft drinks, or low-fat milk.* Milkshakes and regular soft drinks are high in calories and sugar.
- *Skip dessert.* Unless a low-fat, low-sugar dessert is available, save your dessert calories for another meal.

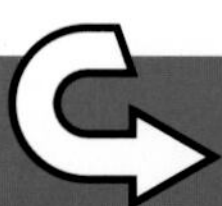

TACTICS AND TIPS
College Eating

- If menus are posted or distributed, decide what you want to eat before you get in the food-service or cafeteria line, and then stick to your choices. Consider what you plan to do and eat for the rest of the day before making your choices.
- Choose a meal plan that includes breakfast, and don't skip it. Even if you have just a slice of bread or a piece of fruit, a small breakfast can help keep you from snacking later in the morning.
- Avoid high-fat breakfast food choices, like cheese omelets and sausage. Choose cereals, plain bagels or whole-grain toast, fruit, yogurt, nonfat milk, and juice.
- Avoid fried foods and heavy sauces at lunch and dinner. Rice and potatoes are excellent choices if you limit the amount of butter or sour cream you add. If necessary, build your meal around soup, salad, and bread.
- Do some research about the foods and preparation methods used in your dining hall or cafeteria. Find out what oils are used in frying foods and what goes into creamy sauces. Many food services offer a limited number of food choices, so a little research can provide a lot of nutrition information. Discuss any food and nutrition suggestions you have with your food service manager.

Which is the healthier choice—butter or margarine? Both butter and margarine are concentrated sources of fat, containing about 11 grams of fat and 100 calories per tablespoon. However, butter is richer in saturated fat, the type of fat most closely associated with elevated levels of artery-clogging LDLs ("bad" cholesterol). Each tablespoon of butter has about 8 grams of saturated fat; margarine averages only 2 grams of saturated fat per tablespoon, regardless of the type of vegetable oil it contains. In addition, butter contains cholesterol; margarine does not.

Based on this information, margarine is clearly the best choice. However, recent research has turned up a potential health problem with margarine, too. The process of hydrogenation, which is used to turn vegetable oil into a more solid form of fat like shortening or margarine, produces trans fatty acids. Although not as well-studied as saturated fat, trans fatty acids have also been shown to raise blood cholesterol levels. The most concentrated sources of trans fatty acids in the American diet are commercially prepared foods and deep-fried fast foods, which are typically fried in vegetable shortening. (Trans fatty acids are not listed separately on food labels; to check for them, look for "hydrogenated vegetable oils" on the list of ingredients.)

So what should you choose? Most scientists agree that consumption of saturated fat is a more serious problem than consumption of trans fatty acids. Americans currently consume about 12% of their calories as saturated fat and 2% as trans fatty acids. Your best strategy is to consume a diet that is low in all kinds of fat; that way, you can control your intake of both saturated fat and trans fatty acids. When you do incorporate fats, favor vegetable oils over margarine, tub or squeeze margarines over stick margarines (they are less hydrogenized), and any type of vegetable oil or margarine over butter.

How common is food poisoning? Food poisoning—or foodborne illness, as scientists call it—is very common. Tens of millions of cases occur each year; it is likely that your last case of "stomach flu" was actually a case of foodborne illness. The most common symptoms are diarrhea, abdominal cramps, vomiting, fever, and weakness. Most cases clear up in a few days, as long as people consume enough fluids to prevent dehydration. Foodborne illness poses a greater risk for young children, the elderly, and people with underlying chronic illnesses. And in cases where a particularly dangerous organism is involved, even a healthy adult can become seriously ill. Foodborne illness is believed to kill 6000–9000 Americans each year.

Bacteria and the toxins they produce cause most cases of foodborne illness; parasites and viruses are less common causes. *Salmonella* bacteria are responsible for almost 60% of all cases of foodborne illness; they are most often found in eggs, poultry, meat, milk, and inadequately refrigerated and reheated leftovers. The bacteria *Staphylococcus aureus* is responsible for 20–40% of cases. It is usually transferred to food when people handle or sneeze or cough over food; it is most common on meat, prepared salads, cream sauces, and cream-filled pastries. Illness from *Clostridium botulinum* and *Escherichia coli* are rare, but both can be deadly. Botulism results primarily from improperly canned foods; *E. coli* is spread mainly by undercooked ground beef.

Virtually all foods contain some bacteria. The key to protecting yourself from foodborne illness is to handle, cook, and store foods in ways that prevent the bacteria from spreading and multiplying. Keep the following tips in mind:

- Don't buy food in containers that leak, bulge, or are severely dented.
- Use or freeze fresh meats within 3–5 days after purchase; use or freeze fresh poultry, fish, and ground meat within 1–2 days.
- Thoroughly wash your hands with hot soapy water before and after handling food, especially raw meat, fish, poultry, or eggs.
- Make sure counters, cutting boards, dishes, and other equipment are thoroughly cleaned before and after use. If possible, use separate cutting boards for meat and for foods that will be eaten raw, such as fruits or vegetables. Wash dishcloths and kitchen towels frequently.
- Thoroughly rinse and scrub fruits and vegetables, with a brush, if possible; or peel off the skin.
- Cook foods thoroughly, especially beef, poultry, fish, pork, and eggs. Cooking kills most microbes. When eating out, order red meat prepared "well-done."
- Cook stuffing separately from poultry; or wash poultry thoroughly, stuff immediately before cooking, and then transfer the stuffing to a clean bowl immediately after cooking.
- Store foods below 40°F or above 140°F. Do not leave cooked or refrigerated foods, such as meats or salads, at room temperature for more than 2 hours.
- Don't eat raw animal products. Use only pasteurized milk.

SUMMARY

- The six classes of nutrients are carbohydrates, proteins, fats, vitamins, minerals, and water.
- The 45 nutrients essential to humans are released into the body through digestion. Nutrients in foods provide energy, measured in kilocalories (commonly called calories); build and maintain body tissues; and regulate body functions.
- Protein, an important component of body tissue, is composed of amino acids, nine of which are essential to a diet. Animal proteins are complete; vegetable proteins can be made complete through combination.
- Fat, the major body fuel at times of rest and light activity, also insulates the body and cushions the organs.
- Saturated fats most often come from animal sources and unsaturated fats from plant sources. Limiting saturated fat in the diet can limit blood cholesterol levels and reduce the risk of CVD; monounsaturated and omega-3 unsaturated fats may promote cardiovascular health.
- Carbohydrates provide energy to the brain, nervous system, and blood and to muscles during high-intensity exercise. Digestion breaks down complex carbohydrates into glucose, which is absorbed into the bloodstream; some is stored as glycogen. Dietary fiber cannot be broken down; it helps reduce cholesterol levels (soluble fiber) and promotes the passage of wastes through the intestines (insoluble fiber).

- Water, distributed in body tissues and fluids, aids in digestion and food absorption, allows chemical reactions to take place, serves as a lubricant or cushion, and helps regulate body temperature.
- The 13 essential vitamins are either water- or fat-soluble; they help unleash energy in food sources and act as antioxidants. The 17 known essential minerals regulate body functions, aid in growth and tissue maintenance, and act as catalysts to release energy. Deficiencies in vitamins and minerals can cause severe symptoms over time, but excess doses are also dangerous. Supplements are required in certain cases, especially for iron and calcium.
- The Recommended Dietary Allowances, Food Guide Pyramid, and Dietary Guidelines for Americans provide standards and recommendations for getting all essential nutrients from a varied, balanced diet and for eating in ways that protect against chronic disease.
- Basic recommendations for a healthy diet include eating a variety of foods; reducing all fat, especially saturated fat; increasing complex carbohydrates; and limiting sugar, salt, alcohol, and smoked and nitrate-cured foods.
- A vegetarian diet requires special planning to meet all nutrient requirements; grains, legumes, and a variety of fruits and vegetables are central. Supplements and professional advice may be necessary.
- Using behavioral self-management techniques and specific strategies (for fast-food restaurants and college dining halls, for example), it's possible to change to or maintain a diet plan for wellness that is customized according to age, gender, height, weight, activity level, medical risk factors, and personal tastes.

BEHAVIOR CHANGE ACTIVITY

Building Motivation and Commitment

Complete the following checklist to determine whether you are motivated and committed to changing your behavior. Check the statements that are true for you.

_______ I feel responsible for my own behavior and capable of managing it.

_______ I am not easily discouraged.

_______ I enjoy setting goals and then working to achieve them.

_______ I am good at keeping promises to myself.

_______ I like having a structure and schedule for my activities.

_______ I view my new behavior as a necessity, not an optional activity.

_______ Compared with previous attempts to change my behavior, I am more motivated now.

_______ My goals are realistic.

_______ I have a positive mental picture of the new behavior.

_______ Considering the outside stresses in my life, I feel confident that I can stick to my program.

_______ I feel prepared for lapses and ups-and-downs in my behavior change program.

_______ I feel that my plan for behavior change is enjoyable.

_______ I feel comfortable telling other people about the change I am making in my behavior.

Did you check most of these statements? If not, you need to boost your motivation and commitment. Try the following strategies:

- Review the potential benefits of changing your behavior and the costs of not changing it. Pay special attention to the short-term benefits of changing your behavior, including feelings of accomplishment and self-confidence.
- Visualize yourself achieving your goal and enjoying its benefits. For example, if you want to manage time more effectively, picture yourself as a confident, organized person who systematically tackles important tasks and sets aside time each day for relaxation, exercise, and friends.

- Put aside obstacles and objections to change. Counter thoughts such as "I'll never have time to exercise" with thoughts like "Lots of other people do it and so can I."
- Bombard yourself with propaganda. Take a class dealing with the change you want to make. Read books and watch television shows on the subject. Post motivational phrases or pictures on your refrigerator or over your desk. Talk to people who have already made the change.
- Build up your confidence. Remind yourself of other goals you've achieved. At the end of each day, mentally review your good decision and actions. See yourself as a capable person, one who is in charge of her or his health.

FOR MORE INFORMATION

For reliable nutrition advice, talk to one of the following:

- A faculty member in the nutrition department on your campus.
- A registered dietitian (R.D.).
- Your physician. (Individuals who have high blood cholesterol levels, high blood pressure, or diabetes; who suffer from food allergies or digestive problems; or who are beginning to develop osteoporosis should have a careful evaluation by a physician.)

In addition, many large communities have a telephone service called Dial a Dietitian. By calling this number, people can receive nutrition information from an R.D. free of charge.

Experts on quackery suggest that you steer clear of anyone who puts forth any of the following false statements:

- Most diseases are caused by faulty nutrition.
- Large doses of vitamins are effective against many diseases.
- Hair analysis can be used to determine a person's nutritional state.
- A computer-scored nutritional deficiency test is a basis for prescribing vitamins.

Any practitioner—licensed or not—who sells vitamins in his or her office should be thoroughly scrutinized.

Written resources on nutrition for wellness include the following:

Consumers Guide Editors. 1994. *Complete Book of Vitamins and Minerals.* New York: NAL/Dutton. *A comprehensive review of vitamins and minerals.*

Editors of Vegetarian Times Magazine. 1995. *Vegetarian Times Complete Cookbook.* New York: Macmillan. *Contains introductory chapters on the health benefits of vegetarianism and on meal planning, along with over 600 recipes.*

Finn, S. C., and L. Stern. 1992. *The Real Life Nutrition Book.* New York: Penguin. *A nice review of nutrition for the consumer, written by a past president of the American Dietetic Association.*

Herbert, V., and G. J. Subak-Sharpe, eds. 1994. *Total Nutrition: The Only Guide You Will Ever Need—From the Mount Sinai School of Medicine.* New York: St. Martin's Press. *An excellent review of current nutrition topics.*

Nutrition Action Health Letter. 1875 Connecticut Ave., N.W., Suite 300, Washington, DC 20009-5728. *The most widely read monthly newsletter focusing on nutrition and health.*

Tufts University Diet and Nutrition Letter. P.O. Box 57857, Boulder, CO 80322-7857. *A monthly newsletter that covers a variety of nutrition and weight-management concerns.*

Wardlaw, G. M., and P. M. Insel. 1996. *Perspectives in Nutrition,* 3d ed. St. Louis: Mosby-Yearbook. *An easy-to-understand review of major concepts in nutrition—from infancy to elderly years.*

Woteki, C. E., and P. R. Thomas. 1992. *Eat for Life.* Washington, D.C.: National Academy Press. *A summary for general readers of* Improving America's Diet and Health *by the same authors (see Selected Bibliography); up-to-date and useful information on the relationship between diet and health status.*

In addition, the Human Nutrition Information Service (HNIS) publishes a wide variety of resources. Topics of HNIS booklets and pamphlets include meeting the RDAs for vitamins and minerals and following the Dietary Guidelines in a variety of circumstances. Contact the HNIS at 6506 Belcrest Road, Hyattsville, MD 20782.

SELECTED BIBLIOGRAPHY

Achterberg, C., et al. 1994. How to put the Food Guide Pyramid into practice. *Journal of the American Dietetic Association* 94:1030.

ADA Reports: Position of the American Dietetic Association: Vegetarian diets. 1993. *Journal of the American Dietetic Association* 93:1317.

Alaimo, K., et al. 1994. Dietary intake of vitamins, minerals, and fiber of persons ages 2 months and over in the United States. *Third National Health and Nutrition Examination Survey,* Phase 1, 1988–91, Advance Data 258:1, November 14.

Anderson, J. W., et al. 1991. Lipid responses of hypercholesterolemic men to oat-bran and wheat-bran intakes. *American Journal of Clinical Nutrition* 54:678.

Anderson, J. W., et al. 1994. Health benefits and practical aspects of high-fiber diets. *American Journal of Clinical Nutrition* 59:1242S.

Ascherio, A., et al. 1995. Dietary intake of marine *n-3* fatty acids, fish intake, and the risk of coronary disease among men. *New England Journal of Medicine* 332:977–982.

The bare-bones facts for avoiding osteoporosis. 1994. *Tufts University Diet and Nutrition Letter* 12(4): 3–6.

Dawson-Hughes, B. 1995. For avoiding broken bones, more vitamin D. *Tufts University Diet and Nutrition Letter* 13(5): 1.

Food and Nutrition Board. 1989. *Diet and Health: Implications for Reducing Chronic Disease Risk.* Washington, D.C.: National Academy Press.

Food and Nutrition Board. 1989. *Recommended Dietary Allowances.* Revised. Washington, D.C.: National Academy of Sciences—National Research Council.

Food poisoning: When microbes are on the menu. 1994. *Harvard Health Letter,* December, 4–5.

Friedlander, A. L., H. K. Genant, S. Sadowsky, N. N. Byl, and C. C. Gluer. 1995. A two-year program of aerobics and weight training enhances bone mineral density of young women. *Journal of Bone and Mineral Research* 10:574–585.

Glore, S. R., et al. 1994. Soluble fiber and serum lipids: A literature review. *Journal of the American Dietetic Association* 94:425.

Greendale, G. A., E. Barrett-Connor, S. Edelstein, S. Ingles, and R. Haile. 1995. Lifetime leisure exercise and osteoporosis. The Rancho Bernardo study. *American Journal of Epidemiology* 141:951–959.

Haddad, E. H. 1994. Development of a vegetarian food guide. *American Journal of Clinical Nutrition* 59:1248S.

Halliwell, B. 1994. Free radicals and antioxidants: A personal view. *Nutrition Reviews* 52:253.

How much fish is enough? 1995. *University of California at Berkeley Wellness Letter,* August, 2.

Judd, J. T., et al. 1994. Dietary trans fatty acids: Effects on plasma lipids and lipoproteins of healthy men and women. *American Journal of Clinical Nutrition* 59:861.

Kurtzwell, P. 1994. Food label close-up. *FDA Consumer,* April, 15.

Lachance, P., and L. Langseth. 1994. The RDA concept: Time for a change? *Nutrition Reviews* 52:266.

Lofgren, P. A., et al. 1994. Eating in America today: A dietary pattern and intake report. *Food and Nutrition News* 66:9.

Mayfield, E. 1994. A consumer's guide to fats. *FDA Consumer,* May, 15.

McDowell, M. A., et al. 1994. Energy and macronutrient intakes of persons ages 2 months and over in the United States. *Third National Health and Nutrition Examination Survey.* Advanced Data No. 255, October 24.

Mensink, R. P., and M. B. Katan. 1989. Effect of a diet enriched with monounsaturated or polyunsaturated fatty acids on levels of low-density and high-density lipoprotein cholesterol in healthy women and men. *New England Journal of Medicine* 321:436–441.

NIH Consensus Development Panel on Optimal Calcium Intake. 1994. Optimal calcium intake. *Journal of the American Medical Association* 272:1942.

Perkin, B. B. 1990. Dietary guidelines for Americans, 1990 edition. *Journal of the American Dietetic Association* 90:1725.

Psychological conditioning. 1994. *Harvard Women's Health Watch,* January, 6.

Saltos, E., et al. 1994. The new food label as a tool for healthy eating. *Nutrition Today,* May/June, 18.

Semba, R. D., et al. 1995. Reduced seroconversion to measles in infants given vitamin A with measles vaccination. *Lancet* 345:1330–1332.

Study links excess vitamin A and birth defects. 1995. *New York Times,* October 7, 1.

U.S. Department of Agriculture, U.S. Department of Health and Human Services. 1990. *Nutrition and Your Health: Dietary Guidelines for Americans,* 3d ed. Washington, D.C.: U.S. Government Printing Office, Home and Garden Bulletin No. 232.

U.S. Department of Agriculture, U.S. Department of Health and Human Services. 1995. *Nutrition and Your Health: Dietary Guidelines for Americans,* Home and Garden Bulletin No. 232. Internet address: http://www.nalusda.gov/fnic/

Vitamin A and infants with HIV. 1995. *New York Times,* August 9, C6.

Wise up about serving sizes. 1994. *University of California at Berkeley Wellness Letter,* June.

Woteki, C. E., and P. R. Thomas. 1991. *Improving America's Diet and Health.* Washington, D.C.: National Academy Press.

Name ______________________ Section ______________ Date ______________

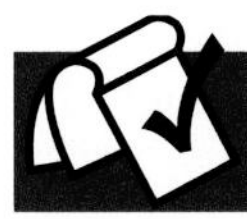

LAB 8-1 *Your Daily Diet Versus the Food Guide Pyramid*

Keep a record of everything you eat for 3 consecutive days. Record all foods and beverages you consume, breaking each food item into its component parts (for example, a turkey sandwich would be listed as 2 slices of bread, 3 oz of turkey, 1 tsp mayonnaise, and so on). Complete the first two columns of the chart during the course of the day; fill in the remaining information at the end of the day using Table 8-5.

DAY 1

Food	*Portion Size*	*Food Group*	*Number of Servings**

Daily Total

Food Group	*Number of Servings*
Milk, yogurt, cheese	
Meat, poultry, fish, dry beans, eggs, nuts	
Fruits	
Vegetables	
Breads, cereals, rice, pasta	

*Your portion sizes may be smaller or larger than the serving sizes given in the Food Guide Pyramid; list the actual number of Food Guide Pyramid servings contained in the foods you eat.

LABORATORY ACTIVITIES

DAY 2

Food	*Portion Size*	*Food Group*	*Number of Servings**

Daily Total

Food Group	*Number of Servings*
Milk, yogurt, cheese	
Meat, poultry, fish, dry beans, eggs, nuts	
Fruits	
Vegetables	
Breads, cereals, rice, pasta	

*Your portion sizes may be smaller or larger than the serving sizes given in the Food Guide Pyramid; list the actual number of Food Guide Pyramid servings contained in the foods you eat.

DAY 3

Food	*Portion Size*	*Food Group*	*Number of Servings**

Daily Total

Food Group	*Number of Servings*
Milk, yogurt, cheese	
Meat, poultry, fish, dry beans, eggs, nuts	
Fruits	
Vegetables	
Breads, cereals, rice, pasta	

*Your portion sizes may be smaller or larger than the serving sizes given in the Food Guide Pyramid; list the actual number of Food Guide Pyramid servings contained in the foods you eat.

LABORATORY ACTIVITIES

Next, average your serving totals for the 3 days, and enter them into the chart below. Fill in the recommended serving totals that apply to you from Table 8-5.

Food Group	*Recommended Number of Servings*	*Actual Number of Servings*
Milk, yogurt, cheese		
Meat, poultry, fish, dry beans, eggs, nuts		
Fruits		
Vegetables		
Breads, cereals, rice, pasta		

Are there any groups for which you need to increase your consumption? Decrease your consumption? List any areas of concern below, along with ideas for changing them. Think carefully about the reasons behind your food choices. For example, if you eat doughnuts for breakfast every morning because you feel rushed, make a list of ways to save time to allow for a more healthful breakfast.

Problem: ______________________________

Possible solutions: ______________________________

____

____

____

____

____

____

Problem: ______________________________

Possible solutions: ______________________________

____

____

____

____

____

____

Problem: ______________________________

Possible solutions: ______________________________

____

____

____

____

____

____

Name ______________________ Section ______________ Date ______________

LAB 8-2 *Dietary Analysis*

You can complete this activity using either the software that accompanies the text or Appendix B and the charts printed below.

Part 1. Analyze Your Diet for 3 Days

If you are using the software, follow the instructions to complete an analysis of your diet on 3 separate days. Otherwise, complete the charts on the first three pages of this lab. When you have completed this analysis, go on to the second part of the lab.

Date______________________ Day: M Tu W Th F Sa Su

Food	Amount	Calories	Protein (g)	Fat, total (g)	Saturated fat (g)	Carbohydrate (g)	Dietary fiber (g)	Cholesterol (mg)	Sodium (mg)	Calcium (mg)	Iron (mg)
Recommended totals*			≤15%	≤30%	7–10%	≥55%	20–35 g	≤300 mg	≤2400 mg		
Actual totals**			g / %	g / %	g / %	g / %					

*Fill in the appropriate RDA values for calcium and iron from Table 8-4.

**Total the values in each column. To calculate the percentage of total calories from protein, carbohydrate, fat, and saturated fat, use the formula on p. 184. Protein and carbohydrate provide 4 calories per gram; fat provides 9 calories per gram. For example, if you consume a total of 270 grams of carbohydrate and 2000 calories, your percentage of total calories from carbohydrate would be (270 g × 4 cal/g) ÷ 2000 cal = 54%.

Date______________________ Day: M Tu W Th F Sa Su

Food	Amount	Calories	Protein (g)	Fat, total (g)	Saturated fat (g)	Carbohydrate (g)	Dietary fiber (g)	Cholesterol (mg)	Sodium (mg)	Calcium (mg)	Iron (mg)
Recommended totals*			≤15%	≤30%	7–10%	≥55%	20–35 g	≤300 mg	≤2400 mg		
Actual totals**			g / %	g / %	g / %	g / %					

Date________________________________ Day: M Tu W Th F Sa Su

Food	Amount	Calories	Protein (g)	Fat, total (g)	Saturated fat (g)	Carbohydrate (g)	Dietary fiber (g)	Cholesterol (mg)	Sodium (mg)	Calcium (mg)	Iron (mg)
Recommended totals*			≤15%	≤30%	7–10%	≥55%	20–35 g	≤300 mg	≤2400 mg		
Actual totals**			g / %	g / %	g / %	g / %					

Part 2. Making Changes in Your Diet to Meet the Dietary Guidelines

(*Note:* If your daily diet follows all the recommended intakes, you don't need to complete this section.) Choose one of your daily diet records. Make changes, additions, and deletions from it until it conforms to all or most of the Dietary Guidelines. Or, if you prefer, start from scratch to create a day's diet that meets all guidelines. Use the chart below to experiment and record your final, healthy sample diet for one day.

Date________________________________ Day: M Tu W Th F Sa Su

Food	Amount	Calories	Protein (g)	Fat, total (g)	Saturated fat (g)	Carbohydrate (g)	Dietary fiber (g)	Cholesterol (mg)	Sodium (mg)	Calcium (mg)	Iron (mg)
Recommended totals*			≤15%	≤30%	7–10%	≥55%	20–35 g	≤300 mg	≤2400 mg		
Actual totals**			g / %	g / %	g / %	g / %					

To monitor your progress toward your goal, enter the results of this lab in the Preprogram Assessment column of Lab 15-2. After several weeks of dietary changes, do this lab again and enter the results in the Postprogram Assessment column of Lab 15-2. How do the results compare?

9

Weight Management

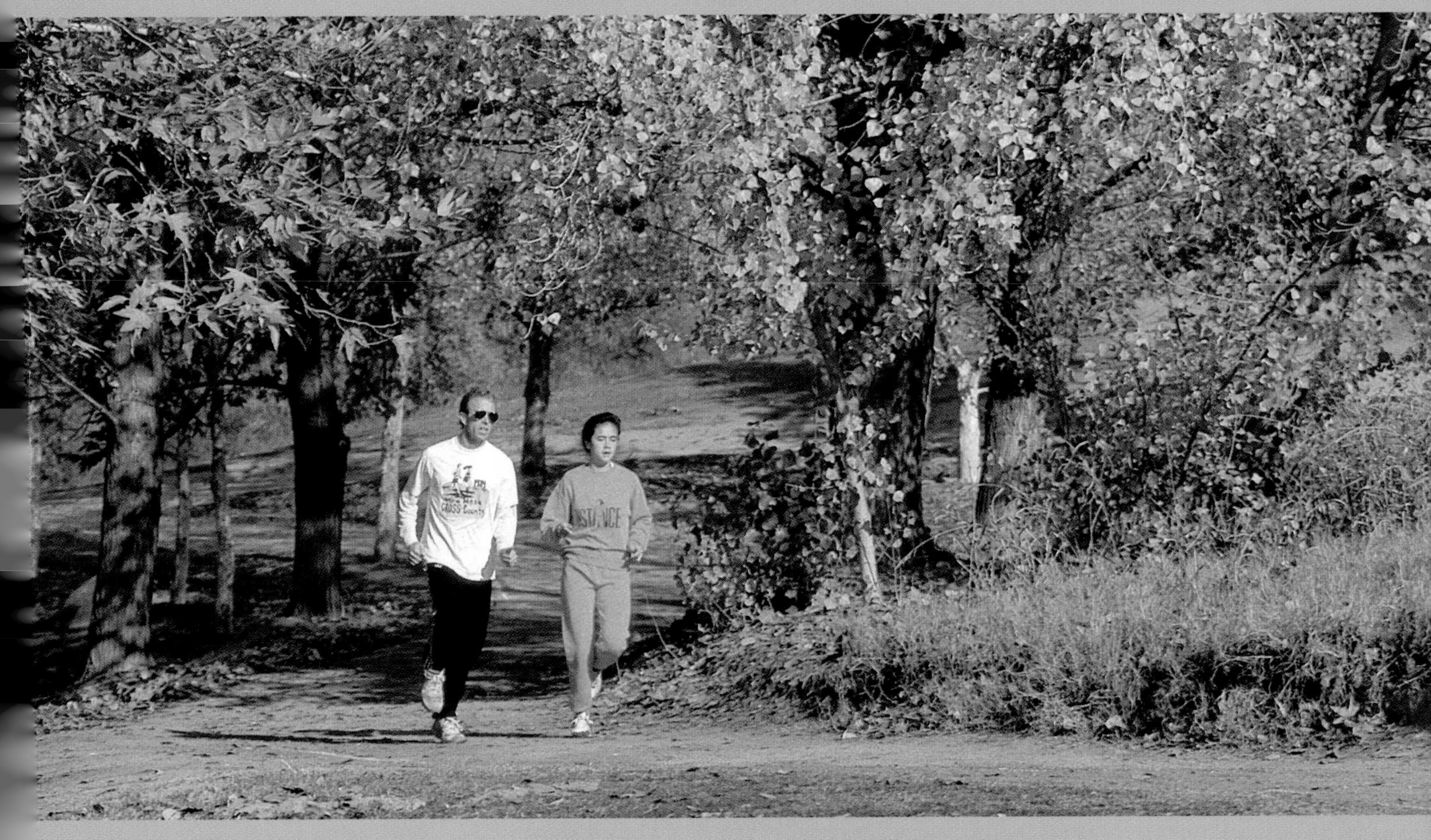

LOOKING AHEAD

After reading this chapter, you should be able to answer these questions about weight management:

- How do overweight and obesity affect health?
- How do genetic factors and metabolic rate influence a person's weight?
- What are the components of a lifestyle that leads naturally to a healthy body weight?
- Why is dieting not a successful approach to weight loss?
- What are the symptoms, possible causes, and treatments for eating disorders?
- What are the most effective strategies for losing weight?

Controlling body weight is really a matter of controlling body fat. As explained in Chapter 6, the most important consideration for health is not total weight but body composition—the proportion of body fat to lean body mass. Many people who are "overweight" are also overfat, and the health risks they face are due to the latter condition. Although this chapter uses the common terms *weight control* and *weight loss,* the goal of a wellness lifestyle is to achieve a healthy body composition, not to conform to rigid standards of total body weight.

Controlling body weight and body fat is not a mysterious process. The "secret" of weight control is simply balancing calories consumed with calories expended in daily activities—in other words, eating a moderate, low-fat diet and exercising regularly. Unfortunately, this simple formula is not as exciting as the latest fad diet or "scientific breakthrough" that promises slimness without effort. The American public is assaulted year after year by a steady stream of diet books, dietary supplements, commercial weight-loss programs, and medical procedures for weight loss. However, dieting can undermine the development of a truly healthy lifestyle that will naturally allow a person to maintain an appropriate body weight. Dieting is not part of a wellness lifestyle.

This chapter sorts out the factors that contribute to a weight problem, takes a closer look at weight management through lifestyle, and suggests specific strategies for permanent weight loss. This information is designed to provide all the tools necessary for integrating effective weight management into an overall wellness program.

HEALTH IMPLICATIONS OF OVERWEIGHT AND OBESITY

Excess body weight increases a person's risk of developing numerous diseases and unhealthy conditions, as discussed in Chapter 6. These include cardiovascular disease (CVD), hypertension, gallbladder disease, and diabetes. Obesity may also be associated with high levels of blood fats, and it is correlated with certain types of cancer, including cancer of the colon, prostate, gallbladder, ovary, endometrium, breast, and cervix. Women who are obese are more likely to suffer from menstrual abnormalities and complications during pregnancy; and in severely obese people of both genders, the rates of respiratory problems and degenerative joint disease are higher than normal.

The overall health risks of obesity were illustrated in the results of a study published in 1995 that followed over 100,000 women for more than 15 years. Among women who had never smoked, the slimmest—those with a body mass index (BMI) of 19 or less—had the lowest risk of death from all causes. The relative risk of death increased as BMI increased, and the risk doubled for women with a BMI over 29. Gaining pounds over the years was also shown to be hazardous: The women who reported gaining 22 or more pounds since they were 18 years old showed a sevenfold increase in their risk of coronary heart disease. The results of this study reinforce the compelling conclusion of many others: Obesity shortens lives.

Currently, about 34% of American adults are obese, making obesity one of the most serious and widespread challenges to health and wellness.

FACTORS THAT CONTRIBUTE TO A WEIGHT PROBLEM

Why do some people become obese and others remain thin? A variety of factors—physical, psychological, cultural, and social—play significant roles in determining body weight. Research has linked genetic factors and metabolism, in particular, to body weight problems.

Genetic Factors Versus Environmental Factors

Both genetic and environmental factors influence the development of obesity. Genes influence body size and shape, body fat distribution, and metabolic rate. It is estimated that 25–70% of the BMI variance among people is due to genetics and associated biological factors. If both parents are overweight, their children are twice as likely to be overweight as children who have only one overweight parent. In a study that compared adoptees and their biological parents, the weights of the adoptees were found to be more like those of the biological parents than the adoptive parents, again indicating a strong genetic link.

Genetic factors also affect the ease with which weight is gained as a result of overeating. In a study of the effects of overfeeding on sets of identical twin brothers, researchers found that the twins in each pair gained almost exactly the same amount of weight, in the same places. But when the sets of twins were compared to each other, it was found that some pairs gained far more weight than others. In some pairs, the weight was added as fat and in others as muscle mass. In addition, pairs of twins varied in where the new body weight was added, some gaining inches in the abdomen and others in the thighs and buttocks.

In studies of mice, scientists located a gene (named *ob*) that appears to influence the development of obesity. The gene produces a hormonelike protein called leptin that is secreted by the body's fat cells and carried to the brain. Leptin seems to let the brain know how big or small the body's fat stores are, and the brain can regulate appetite and metabolic rate accordingly. Mice with a defective or missing *ob* gene overate and gained weight. But when injected with leptin, the obese mice ate less, had higher metabolic rates, and lost weight. Even mice of normal weight lost weight when injected with leptin. Could leptin "cure" obesity in humans? As encouraging as this finding is, obesity in humans is likely to turn out to be more

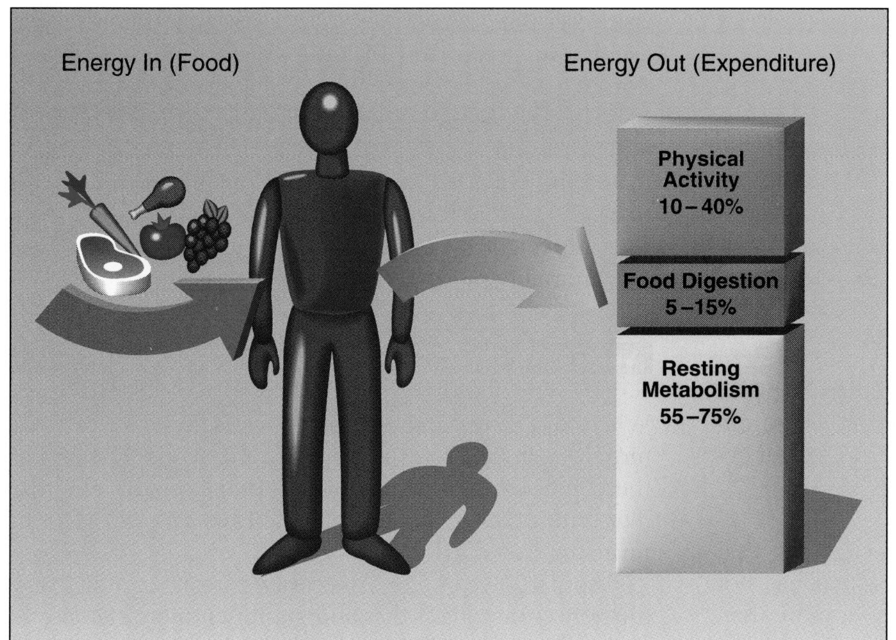

Figure 9-1 ***The energy-balance equation.*** Total energy expenditure is composed of physical activity, digestion, and resting metabolism.

complicated than a one-gene phenomenon. Many obese people have been found to have normal levels of leptin in their bloodstream; researchers hypothesize that they may have faulty leptin receptors in their brain. Working with rats, a different group of researchers identified another natural appetite suppressor (gluconlike peptide-1, or GLP-1), which may also be significant for humans. However, additional studies will be needed before a treatment can be developed based on any of these findings.

All this research points to a genetic component in the determination of body weight. However, hereditary influences must be balanced against the contribution of environmental factors. In a study comparing men born and raised in Ireland with their biological brothers who lived in the United States, the American men were found to weigh, on average, 6% more than their Irish brothers. Environmental factors like diet and exercise are likely responsible for this difference in weight. Thus, the tendency to develop obesity may be inherited, but the expression of this tendency is affected by environmental influences.

The message you should take from this research is that genes are not destiny. It is true that some people have a much harder time losing weight and maintaining weight loss than others. However, with increased exercise and attention to diet, even those with a genetic tendency toward obesity can maintain a healthy body weight. And regardless of genetic factors, lifestyle choices remain the cornerstone of successful weight management.

Metabolism and Energy Balance

Metabolism is the sum of all the vital processes by which food energy and nutrients are made available to and used by the body. The largest component of metabolism, measured as **resting metabolic rate (RMR),** is the energy required to maintain vital body functions. As Figure 9-1 shows, RMR accounts for 55–75% of the energy used by the body. The energy required to digest food accounts for an additional 5–15% of daily energy expenditure. The remaining 10–40% is expended during physical activity.

Both genetics and behavior affect metabolic rate. Men, who have a higher proportion of muscle mass than women, have higher metabolic rates (muscle tissue is more metabolically active than fat). In addition, some individuals inherit higher or lower metabolic rates than others. A higher metabolic rate means that a person burns more calories while at rest and can therefore take in more calories.

Recent evidence also suggests that people with a history of weight loss have lower metabolic rates. For example, a man who formerly weighed 165 pounds but who now weighs 150 pounds must eat about 15% fewer calories to maintain his new, lower weight than a man who has weighed 150 pounds throughout adult life. Researchers found that among individuals who had lost weight, both RMR and the energy required to perform physical tasks were lowered. The message from this research is that although weight loss can be achieved and maintained, it requires ongoing commitment.

Exercise has a positive effect on metabolism. When people exercise, they increase their RMR—which is, to reiterate, the number of calories their bodies burn *at rest.* They also increase their lean body mass, which is associated with a higher metabolic rate. The exercise itself also burns calories, raising total energy expenditure. The

TERMS

resting metabolic rate (RMR) The energy required (in calories) to maintain the body.

higher the energy expenditure, the more the person can eat without gaining weight.

The two factors in the energy-balance equation illustrated in Figure 9-1 that fall under individual control are the amount of energy intake (in food) and the number of calories expended in physical activity. For these simple reasons alone, increased physical activity is a critical component of a long-term program of weight management. (To determine your own RMR, complete Lab 9-1.)

Other Explanations for Overweight

Researchers have proposed various other explanations for overweight besides heredity and metabolism. These explanations include overeating, eating style, and weight cycling.

Overeating Although common sense suggests that overeating is involved in weight gain, research has not proved that all or even many obese people eat more than people who are not obese. However, some research has raised serious questions about the accuracy of self-reported caloric intake. Both obese and nonobese individuals have been found to underestimate their caloric intake in daily diet records, but obese subjects typically underreport their intakes by 30–35%, a much greater margin than that of nonobese subjects. Also, **binge eating**—episodes of high consumption—may account for obesity even in overweight people who do not generally overeat.

Eating Style Some researchers have compared the eating styles of obese and nonobese people in an attempt to identify a distinctive pattern that might account for overweight. No such style distinction turned up; the only factor that seemed to distinguish the two groups was that when food tasted good, obese people kept eating longer.

Another theory suggested that obese people were more sensitive to external cues to eat than people of normal weight. Researchers examined the association between eating and time of day, elapsed time between eating episodes, the sight of food, and other cues in the environment. They found that these cues are in fact intimately linked to eating behavior, but these links exist for people in every weight category.

Weight Cycling Repeated dieting resulting in cycles of weight loss and weight gain ("yo-yo dieting") may be harmful—both to weight management and to overall health. Researchers hypothesized that cycling increases the body's efficiency at extracting and storing calories from food, making weight loss more and more difficult with each successive diet. Although some studies have found support for this idea, most have not; and current thinking is that weight cycling probably does not result in increased efficiency. Other studies have shown an association between weight variability and altered body fat distribution, increased preference for dietary fat, and death from CVD. More research will be needed to clarify the effects of weight cycling on weight management and disease mortality rates.

TERMS

binge eating A pattern of eating in which normal food consumption is interrupted by episodes of high consumption.

WEIGHT MANAGEMENT AND LIFESTYLE

When all the research has been assessed, it is clear that most weight problems are lifestyle problems. Looking at these problems in a historical context reveals why fad diets and other quick-fix approaches are not effective in reversing overweight.

About 100 years ago, Americans consumed a diet very different from today's diet and got much more exercise as well. Americans now eat more fat and refined sugars and fewer complex carbohydrates. And despite an increased interest in fitness, Americans today get far less exercise than their great-grandparents did. Walking, bicycling, and farm and manual labor have all declined, resulting in a decrease in daily energy expenditure of about 200 calories.

This decline, coupled with a continuing tendency to consume processed foods instead of fresh foods and complex carbohydrates, is measurable in the number of overweight Americans: about 34 million, and rising. The solution to this problem lies in lifestyle management. Four lifestyle factors are particularly relevant to weight control: nutrition, exercise, thoughts and emotions, and coping strategies.

Nutrition

At the core of a program to maintain a healthy weight or to reverse overweight and overfat is knowledge of sound nutritional principles and the body's nutritional requirements. Here we review some of the information covered in Chapter 8 that particularly relates to overweight.

Fat Most experts agree that the basic problem in the American diet is the overconsumption of fat. Despite the ideal of 30% or less, Americans get about 34% of total daily calories from fat sources. These include oils, margarine, butter, cream, and lard, which are almost pure fat; meat and processed foods, which contain a great deal of "hidden" fat; and nuts, seeds, and avocados, which are plant sources of fats.

Some people are better fat burners than others; that is, they burn more of the fat they take in as calories and therefore have less fat to store. Low fat burners convert more dietary fat to stored body fat. This tendency to hoard fat calories may be an important part of the genetic tendency toward obesity. For low fat burners, restricting fat calories to a level even below the 30% recommended by the Dietary Guidelines may be helpful in weight management. As Chapter 8 made clear, moving toward a vegetarian diet strong in complex carbohydrates and fresh fruits and vegetables, and away from a reliance on meat and processed foods, is an effective approach to reducing fat consumption.

Sugar Although there is no evidence suggesting that fat people consume more sugar than thin people, excess sugar, a major component of the American diet, can be a problem. Sugar makes up a large proportion of our "fun" foods and, like fat, is "hidden" in the packaged convenience foods most of us rely on. Substituting fresh fruits for sugar-rich desserts is the way to end a reliance on sugar without giving up natural sweetness.

Protein Typically, Americans eat about 100–150 grams of protein every day, but an adult male needs only 70 grams and an adult female only 45. Not only is excess protein stored by the body as fat, but foods high in protein are also often high in dietary fat. Coming to rely on complex carbohydrates for a feeling of fullness and using meat as a condiment rather than the center of a meal can trim the excess protein and fat from the diet.

Complex Carbohydrates It has long been the fashion among dieters to cut back on bread, pasta, and potatoes to control weight gain. But complex carbohydrates from these sources, as well as from vegetables, legumes, and whole grains, are precisely the nutrients that can help people attain and maintain proper weight. Whereas the body can convert dietary fat to body fat with relative ease, digesting complex carbohydrates actually uses calories, and studies have shown that very little carbohydrate becomes stored as fat in the body. In addition, eating a hearty amount of complex carbohydrates results in a full, or satiated, feeling, thereby preventing overeating. For these reasons, as long as no high-fat sauces and toppings are added to these satisfying foods, a high-carbohydrate diet can actually result in weight loss without conscious calorie-cutting or exercise. However, doing without butter on bread, sour cream on baked potatoes, and cheese on pasta may require changing some eating habits.

Total Calories and Portion Sizes Although decreasing fat consumption is the most important dietary change people can make for successful weight management, the total number of calories consumed should not be overlooked. According to the Centers for Disease Control and Prevention (CDC), fat consumption as a proportion of total calories has declined slightly over the past decade, while the average caloric intake has increased by 100–300 calories per day. Levels of physical activity did not increase during this period, so the net result was a substantial increase in the number of Americans who are obese.

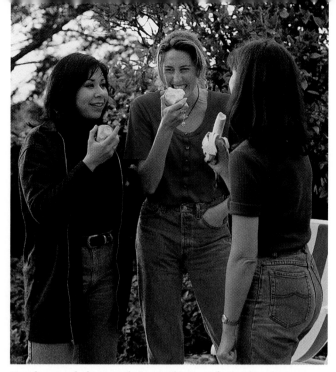

Good eating habits, such as snacking on fruit when hungry, are an important part of successful weight management.

Counting calories, even with the help of food labels, can be a time-consuming activity. For permanent weight management, you need to adopt a strategy that you can maintain over the long term. Many people find that concentrating on portion sizes rather than calories is an easier way to monitor and manage total food intake. Refer to Chapter 8 for a discussion of the serving sizes recommended in the Food Guide Pyramid.

Hunger and Satiety Most people decide they're hungry when their stomach growls or when they get the "shakes" from not eating. But research suggests that many people are unable to recognize stomach contractions as a signal of hunger, and that some might even confuse anxiety or physiological arousal with hunger. Telling such people to "eat only when you're hungry" is poor advice. More practical advice is to "stop eating when you feel full" because people are much more accurate at noticing satiety—sense of fullness—than hunger. Unfortunately, many people who know they're full continue to eat because the food tastes good. Everyone needs to monitor feelings of fullness and stop eating when physically satisfied.

Eating Habits Equally important to weight control is eating small, frequent meals—three or more a day plus snacks—on a dependable, regular schedule. This pattern, along with some personal "decision rules" governing food choices, is a way of thinking about and then internalizing the many details that go into a healthy, low-fat diet. Decision rules governing breakfast might be these, for example: Choose a sugar-free, high-fiber cereal with nonfat milk most of the time; once in a while (no more than once a week), a poached or soft-boiled egg is okay; save pancakes and waffles for special occasions.

A CLOSER LOOK
Exercise and Weight Management

Exercise is a critical component of a weight-management program. In order to achieve long-term success, you must be able to stick with your program for a lifetime. Cutting food intake in order to lose weight is a difficult strategy to maintain; increasing your physical activity is a much better approach. A 45-minute exercise session burns a significant number of calories—in addition to its many other health benefits. And exercise has weight-management benefits beyond the increased energy expenditure that occurs during each exercise session.

Both strength training and endurance exercise can raise your metabolic rate. Resistance training builds muscle mass, and more muscle translates into a higher metabolic rate. Resistance training can also help you maintain your muscle mass during a period of weight loss, helping you to avoid the significant drop in RMR associated with weight loss.

Endurance training increases the rate at which your body uses calories after your exercise session is over. One study found that a 30-minute session of endurance exercise increased RMR by an extra 150 calories over the 12-hour period following the workout. The number of excess calories burned during the recovery period can equal up to 50% of the calories burned during the exercise itself. That's like getting the weight-management benefits of an extra 15 minutes of walking, jogging, or stair climbing.

The body's fuel-use patterns vary with exercise intensity and change during recovery. During exercise, a higher proportion of energy comes from fat during low-intensity exercise (50%) compared with high-intensity exercise (40%). However, high-intensity exercise burns more calories overall, so even though a lower proportion of those calories comes from fat, high-intensity exercise tends to burn more fat than low-intensity exercise.

Intense exercise also causes your body to use more fat as fuel during the recovery period. When you haven't eaten in 3–4 hours and are at rest, your body normally breaks down some of its fat for energy. Following vigorous exercise, the body can increase its use of fat by 300%. Intense training also turns on wasteful metabolic energy pathways known as futile cycling, causing the body to burn still more calories during the postexercise period. In addition, exercise increases metabolism by increasing muscle temperature, thereby causing the body to use calories at a faster rate than normal. The harder and longer you exercise, the greater the muscle temperature and the more calories you burn after exercise.

But high-intensity exercise is not necessarily the best strategy for controlling weight. All exercise will help you manage your weight, and many people find that a program of moderate-intensity exercise is easier to maintain over the long term. However, you might want to consider gradually increasing the intensity of exercise in one or two of your training sessions each week to maximize postexercise fat burning.

Sources: Adapted from Fahey, T. D. 1995. Exercise burns more calories. *Healthline*, March. Ask the experts. 1994. *University of California at Berkeley Wellness Letter*, November.

Decreeing some foods "off limits" generally sets up a rule to be broken. The better principle is "everything in moderation." If a particular food becomes troublesome, it might be placed off limits temporarily until control can be regained.

Exercise and Physical Activity

Exercise is the second important component of weight control through lifestyle management. Exercise and physical activity burn calories and keep the metabolism geared to using food for energy instead of storing it as fat. See the box "Exercise and Weight Management" for more information on how physical activity affects metabolism.

A well-rounded exercise program geared for wellness and weight control includes endurance exercise, weight training, and activities to promote flexibility, relaxation, and enjoyment. Moderate endurance exercise, sustained for 45 minutes to 1 hour, can help trim body fat permanently. Weight training helps increase or maintain lean body mass during diet-induced weight loss, which results in more calorie burning even outside of exercise periods. (Chapter 7 explains how to put together a customized exercise program.)

Thoughts and Emotions

The third component of a lifestyle for weight management is thoughts and emotions. A healthy psychological adjustment can result from *and* encourage weight control for fitness. Psychological distress, on the other hand, can discourage and undermine a healthy program. Someone who is having difficulty making a commitment to weight management may be motivated by knowing that a low-fat diet based on solid nutritional principles can yield psychological as well as physical well-being.

Research on people who have a weight problem indicates that low self-esteem and the accompanying negative emotions are a significant part of the picture. These emotions, interacting with beliefs and attitudes about the "ideal self," give rise to negative **self-talk**—self-deprecating or self-blaming internal comments—that can undermine weight control and contribute to anxiety and depression. Realistic self-talk, on the other hand—internal

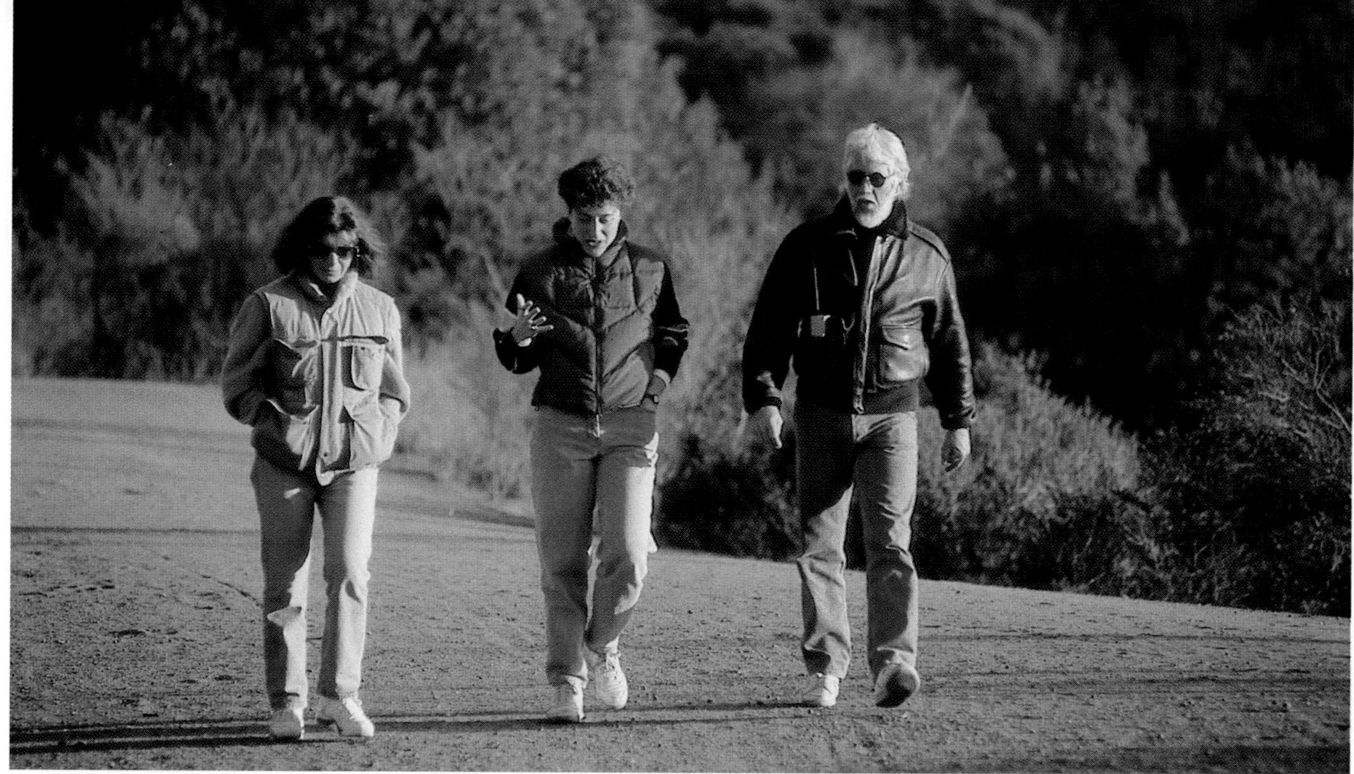

An active lifestyle is one of the keys to lifelong weight management. A vigorous walk is not just a pleasant way to start the day; it also burns calories, raises the metabolic rate, and builds lean body mass.

dialogue that leads step by step toward a goal and then offers praise for success—can be an important component in sustaining the commitment to a weight-management program over time. (The Behavior Change Activity at the end of this chapter includes strategies for developing realistic self-talk.)

Coping Strategies

The fourth component of a healthy lifestyle for weight control is appropriate strategies for handling the stresses and challenges of life. Many people use eating as a means of coping, just as many use drugs, alcohol, smoking, spending, or gambling. They might use food to alleviate loneliness, as a pickup for fatigue, as an antidote to boredom, or as a distraction from problems. Some people even overeat as a means of punishing themselves for real or imagined transgressions.

Those who recognize that they are using food in these ways can analyze their eating habits with fresh eyes. At that point, they can consciously attempt to find new coping strategies and begin to use food appropriately—to fuel life's activities, to foster growth, and to bring pleasure, *not* to manage stress. For a summary of the components of weight management through healthy lifestyle choices, see the box "A Lifestyle for Weight Management."

THE DANGEROUS SEARCH FOR THE "PERFECT" BODY

Many Americans attempt to control their weight by means other than a healthy lifestyle. Decade by decade, the American obsession with slimness has become more intense. Dieting has become an American way of life. In one recent survey, nearly 25% of the adult men and 50% of the adult women reported being on a diet. The rates are even higher among younger people. A national survey found that 61% of adolescent girls and 28% of adolescent boys had dieted during the previous year. Another study identified a small but alarming segment of young "chronic dieters"—girls and boys who reported that they always dieted or had been on a diet more than ten times in the past year.

These are dangerous findings, because chronic dieting among teenagers can lead to growth retardation, menstrual irregularities, and the development of eating disorders. The cultural pressure to be thin is so strong, especially for female adolescents, that it may well predispose weight-conscious young people to abnormal eating patterns (see the box "Eating Disorders," p. 225).

Striving for an ultraslender body can lead not only to diet failure but also to serious psychological distress. Dieters who fail to attain unrealistic goals may consider themselves failures and, discouraged, give up all attempts to manage their weight and other health and fitness behaviors. On the other hand, small, reasonable weight-loss goals can benefit health and fitness significantly. For an

self-talk A person's internal comments and discussion; instrumental in shaping self-image.

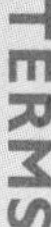

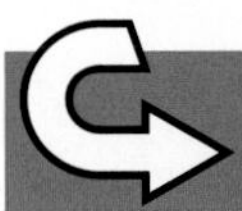

TACTICS AND TIPS
A Lifestyle for Weight Management

- Eat a moderate number of calories every day.
- Limit your intake of dietary fat and refined sugars.
- Increase your intake of complex carbohydrates.
- Limit your protein intake to recommended levels.
- Eat small, frequent meals.
- Maintain a structured pattern of eating.
- Engage in moderate cardiorespiratory endurance exercise of medium to long duration as part of a program of regular exercise.
- Include weight training as part of your exercise program.
- Develop realistic goals for yourself and your behavior.
- Think positively about yourself, and praise yourself for your accomplishments.
- Develop healthy ways of dealing with stress, boredom, fatigue, and loneliness that don't involve food.

obese person, for example, losing as little as 10 pounds can reduce blood pressure as much as antihypertensive medication. And people who participate in behavioral weight-loss programs tend to experience improvement in mood, sometimes after losing just a few pounds.

Obesity is a serious health risk, but people can manage their weight only if they set realistic goals—goals that take into account their particular weight history, social circumstances, metabolic profile, and psychological condition. Setting goals to conform to the current ideals of ultrathin and ultrafit can result only in discouragement and failure. But people who commit themselves to a program that balances exercise, nutritional needs, and healthy weight goals look better, feel better, and have more control of their lives.

STRATEGIES FOR LOSING WEIGHT

In cases in which weight loss is clearly desirable, the next step is assessing the various options and the available resources for support and guidance. No single weight-reduction approach is appropriate for all people. For example, most people who are less than 20% over their healthy goal weight can safely cut back on their fat intake and increase their exercise on their own. People who are 20–40% overweight, however, will be better served with some professional guidance and support—perhaps in a commercial weight-loss program (carefully researched to protect against dangerous or fraudulent claims) or a behavioral program supervised by a health professional. More serious degrees of overweight, in the range 40–100%, require a more aggressive approach under strict medical supervision.

People who are more than 100% overweight or who have 100 pounds to lose should consider a medically supervised **very-low-calorie diet.** Good judgment is important here. Consumers should choose from only those programs with careful pretreatment assessment criteria, open-ended programs that include guidance in weight maintenance, and a full staff that includes physicians, psychologists, and registered dietitians. In programs that withstand strict scrutiny, the success rate is about 65% of all participants. After this, the most extreme option is surgery, a serious medical alternative to be considered with the advice of a physician.

Do-It-Yourself Approaches

People who aren't dangerously obese might find it most convenient to set up an individual program.

Doing It Alone Current research regarding long-term success in weight management is optimistic. About 64% of the people in one study achieved long-term success without joining a formal program, while public health records put the success record at about 50%. In another study, subjects who maintained their desired weight for 2 years or more had made exercise a permanent part of their lifestyle and kept records of their weight and eating habits.

On the other hand, people who give up on weight control generally do so after their initial rapid weight loss (of body water) slows down. They may be unaware that slower, more gradual losses are the ones that matter because mostly fat is being lost, even if fewer pounds are be-

TERMS

very-low-calorie diet A medically supervised, usually liquid, diet designed for dangerously obese people, usually consisting of no more than 800 calories per day.

anorexia nervosa An eating disorder characterized by an intense fear of weight gain leading to self-starvation and excessive weight loss.

bulimia nervosa An eating disorder characterized by alternating binge eating and purging through vomiting or using laxatives or diuretics. Bulimics can be at normal weight or overweight.

A CLOSER LOOK

Eating Disorders

Overweight is not the only kind of weight and body image problem that occurs in our society. A growing number of people, especially young women, suffer from what are called eating disorders. Western society's emphasis on extreme thinness as the ideal for females places many women in conflict about their weight. The gap between reality and ideal for most women is reflected in high rates of body dissatisfaction (50–80% say they feel "fat") and in the widespread use of low-calorie diets (used by as many as 50% of college students). A preoccupation with body shape and weight, along with extreme dieting, can contribute to the development of an eating disorder in an individual with poor self-image or underlying emotional problems.

Anorexia Nervosa

Anorexia nervosa is a serious medical and psychiatric disorder that afflicts 1–3 million Americans, mostly women. A person suffering from anorexia nervosa doesn't eat enough food to maintain a healthy body weight. Anorexics are often females of average or slightly above-average weight who start dieting to lose weight and then never stop. People suffering from anorexia starve themselves and exercise excessively to burn a high number of calories. They develop a distorted body image, so that even when they're dangerously thin, they think they're still "fat."

The symptoms of anorexia include continual extreme dieting, weight loss of 15–25% of total body weight, amenorrhea, hyperactivity, intense fear of weight gain, and unusual behavior toward food. Anorexics are often obsessed with diet, cooking, and food, even though they eat very little. Anorexia nervosa causes life-threatening chemical imbalances and organ damage; it ends in death 15–20% of the time.

Anorexia nervosa often begins during adolescence and is believed to be related to the stresses of puberty. Anorexia is more prevalent in the middle and upper social classes in families that stress high achievement; genetic factors may also play a role. Anorexics tend to be introverted, emotionally reserved, socially insecure, self-critical, self-denying, and overly rigid in their thinking. Psychological control is often an important issue for the anorexic: Taking charge of their eating habits, though it's in an unhealthy way, may be a way anorexics can exercise control over their lives or their families.

Anorexics are usually treated with a combination of behavioral and drug therapies. Hospitalization is often required to restore body weight to a normal level. Because family behavior and interpersonal relations often play a role, entire families must sometimes enter therapy in order for the anorexic individual to recover.

Bulimia Nervosa

Bulimia nervosa is often less visible than anorexia because people suffering from bulimia usually maintain a normal weight. But like anorexics, bulimics have an intense fear of becoming fat and a distorted body image. Bulimia is characterized by cycles of uncontrollable binge eating followed by self-induced vomiting to prevent food from being absorbed. Bulimics also use laxatives and diuretics to purge themselves. A bulimic may binge and purge more than 20 times a day, consuming over 6000 calories in a 24-hour period.

Symptoms of bulimia include uncontrollable urges to eat, cycles of binge eating and self-induced vomiting, frequent use of laxatives and diuretics, menstrual irregularities, large fluctuations in weight, dental decay (caused by contact with vomited stomach acids), and feelings of guilt and depression. Bulimics usually know that their eating habits are abnormal, so they conceal them. The bulimic eating pattern can cause kidney failure, mineral depletion, abnormalities of heart rhythm, and infection.

The majority of people who suffer from bulimia are women in their late teens and early twenties of high socioeconomic status. Bulimia may begin after a period of restrictive dieting or a traumatic event, such as the loss of or separation from a significant person, or during a stressful life stage that might elicit discomfort with sexuality. Bulimia is more common among individuals who have difficulty handling emotions like depression, loneliness, boredom, and anger. Bulimics tend to be moody and impulsive, to have low self-esteem, and to be very critical of themselves. Like anorexics, people with bulimia often come from families that stress high achievement; their eating behavior may be an attempt to take control of their lives and achieve perfection.

Treatments for bulimia include drug therapy and psychotherapy to help treat depression and underlying emotional problems, and behavioral therapy to help break the bulimic eating patterns.

Although anorexia nervosa and bulimia nervosa are both characterized by underlying emotional and psychological problems, in a sense they are an extension of the concern with weight that pervades our society. Most people don't succumb to irrational or distorted ideas about their bodies, but many do become obsessed with dieting. Many people experiment with the unhealthy behaviors associated with eating disorders—fasting, purging, very-low-calorie diets—without developing a specific disorder. These people are suffering the consequences of being overly concerned with weight. The challenge facing Americans today is to achieve and maintain a healthy body weight without excessive dieting.

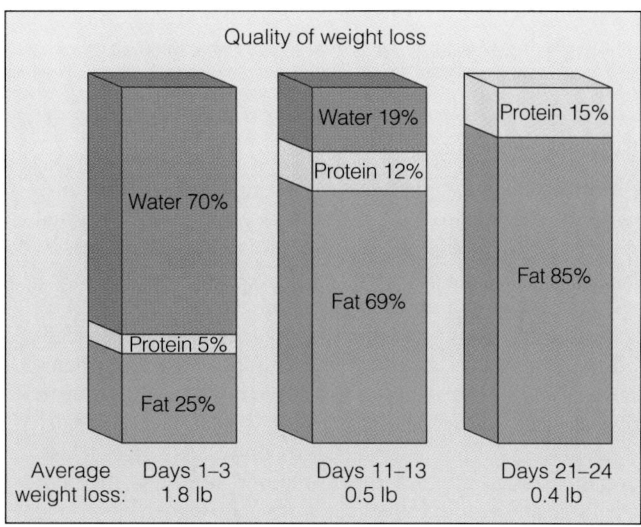

Figure 9-2 ***The quality of weight loss.*** *Source:* Grande, F. 1961. Nutrition and energy balance in body composition studies. In *Techniques for Measuring Body Composition.* Washington, D.C.: National Academy Press.

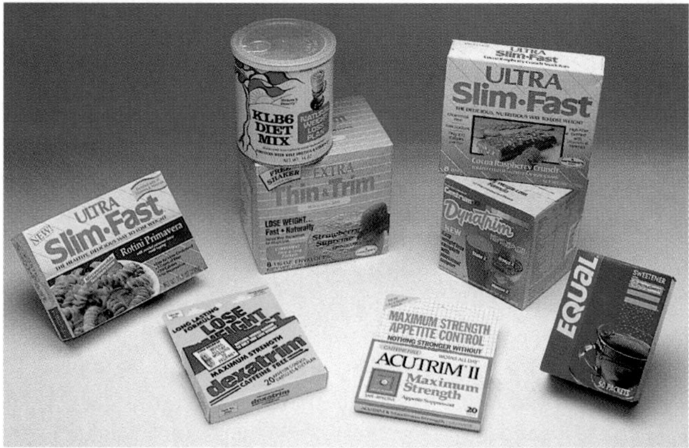

Over-the-counter diet aids such as those shown here are not part of a healthy lifestyle. Although they can help control hunger and weight in the short term, they encourage dependence on commercial products rather than the development of healthy eating and exercise habits.

ing shed (Figure 9-2). If you decide to lose weight on your own, refer to the section that follows on creating an individual weight-loss plan.

Using a Diet Book New diet books are published regularly, many of them making exciting but empty promises, and it can be dangerous or discouraging to rely on them too heavily. In assessing diet books, reject those that do the following:

- Advocate unbalanced meal plans—for example, those that advocate a high-carbohydrate–only diet or a low-carbohydrate/high-protein diet.
- Claim to be based on a "scientific breakthrough" or a "secret."
- Use gimmicks, such as combining foods in certain ways or claiming that weight problems are due to food allergies, food sensitivities, or yeast infections.
- Promise fast weight loss or limit the food selection. Responsible diet books advocate a balanced approach to diet that includes exercise and sound nutritional principles.

Using Diet Aids Diet aids are widely available without prescription, and many people are tempted to rely on them for quick-and-easy weight loss. However, the promises associated with these products are advertising gimmicks, and overreliance on them can be dangerous. Among the more common of these aids are dietary supplements for modified fasting. These supplements, in the forms of food bars and powder for shakes, provide far less than the daily nutritional and caloric requirements and should be used only under the guidance of a physician. They also teach dependence on products, not on sound, lifelong eating habits, and weight lost as a result of them is often regained.

Diet pills are another common diet aid. There are numerous brands of over-the-counter pills and diet aids, containing many ineffective ingredients. The most common ingredient of diet pills sold in drugstores is phenylpropanolamine hydrochloride (PPA), which has been deemed a safe and effective mild appetite suppressant by the FDA. Nevertheless, studies on PPA's effectiveness are contradictory at best, and some reports suggest that it can cause dizziness, headaches, rapid pulse, palpitations, sleeplessness, and hypertension. The use of PPA is approved by the FDA for periods of no more than 12 weeks.

Fiber is the second most common ingredient in diet aids sold in drugstores. Despite manufacturers' claims, the amount generally provided is inconsequential, and the FDA has found no data to suggest that fiber aids in weight control.

Getting Help

Some people are helped by the support and experience of others as well as by professional guidance.

Participating in a Weight-Loss Program Commercial weight-loss programs can be helpful for providing a food-and-exercise plan and reinforcing motivation. However, if you are considering enrolling in such a program, be sure to use your most acute consumer skills in assessing the available options (see the box "Evaluating Commercial Weight-Loss Programs"). Any weight-loss program should include medical supervision, counseling, nutrition education, and maintenance training.

Prescription Medications Several prescription drugs have been found to be safe and effective for helping some people lose weight. The most widely prescribed regimen

CRITICAL CONSUMER
Evaluating Commercial Weight-Loss Programs

Almost 8 million Americans enroll in some kind of structured weight-loss program each year. Unfortunately, many of these people fail to lose weight permanently. Before you join a commercial program, look for these six criteria:

1. *Proof that it works.* Most programs have data on quick weight loss, but ask for long-term results of all clients who have completed the program.
2. *Qualified staff.* A registered dietitian and specialists in behavior modification and exercise should design and supervise the program.
3. *A nutritionally balanced diet.* You should be allowed to eat reasonable portions from all the basic food groups and flexibility based on needs and preferences. You should not be required to buy special products.
4. *Exercise.* At a minimum, you should receive instructions for starting a safe, moderate exercise program. Trained staff should be available to tailor the program and answer your questions.
5. *Lifestyle change.* Ask to see materials used for helping you identify and change behaviors. Find out how they reward and monitor your progress.
6. *Follow-up and support.* After you complete the formal part of the program, be sure you can obtain ongoing support easily and inexpensively.

Source: Weight control: What works and why. 1994. *Supplement to Mayo Clinic Health Letter,* June.

is a combination of two drugs, phentermine and fenfluramine. The antidepressant fluoxetine (Prozac) is also sometimes prescribed. These drugs don't work for everyone, however, and are used primarily for people who are at least 30% overweight. They have side effects and may have as-yet-undetermined long-term risks. These drugs are not a quick fix, but they may help people maintain the lifestyle choices—a healthy diet and regular exercise—required for successful long-term weight management.

Professional Counseling It is not clear whether psychotherapy alone can help with weight loss. People often choose this option out of a sense of failure. Although there is no empirical evidence that it contributes to success rates, professional counseling may ease the emotional distress associated with frustrated weight-loss efforts and poor body image.

CREATING AN INDIVIDUAL WEIGHT-MANAGEMENT PLAN

Would you like to lose weight on your own? Here are some strategies for creating a program of weight management that will last a lifetime.

Assess Your Motivation and Commitment

Before embarking on your chosen weight-management program, it's important that you take a fresh look within and assess your motivation and commitment. The point is not only to achieve success but also to guard against frustration, negative changes in self-esteem, and the sense of failure that attends broken resolves or "yo-yo dieting." Think about the reasons you want to lose weight. Self-focused reasons, such as to feel good about yourself or to have a greater sense of well-being, can often lead to success. Trying to lose weight for others or out of concern for how others view you is a poor foundation for a weight-management program. Make a list of your reasons for wanting to manage your weight, and post it in a prominent place.

Set Reasonable Goals

Choose a goal weight or body fat percentage that is both healthy and reasonable. Refer to the calculations you completed in Lab 6-2. Subdivide your long-term goal into a series of short-term goals. Be willing to renegotiate your final goal as your program moves along.

Assess Your Current Energy Balance

Your energy balance is the balance between calories consumed and calories used in physical activity. When your weight is constant, you are burning approximately the same number of calories as you are taking in. To tip your energy balance toward weight loss, you must either consume fewer calories or burn more through physical activity. To lose the recommended ½–1 pound per week, you'll need to create a negative energy balance of between 1750 and 3500 calories a week, or 250–500 calories a day. Complete Labs 9-1 and 9-2 to assess your current energy balance and set negative calorie balance goals.

Increase Your Level of Physical Activity

To generate a negative energy balance, it's usually best to increase your activity level rather than decrease your calorie consumption. As discussed earlier, dieting reduces RMR; exercise raises it. Furthermore, a diet with fewer than 1600 calories per day will probably not meet the RDAs for all essential nutrients. (No diet should reduce

*TABLE 9-1 Calorie Costs of Selected Physical Activities**

To determine how many calories you burn when you engage in a particular activity, multiply the calorie multiplier given below by your body weight in pounds and then by the number of minutes you exercise.

Activity	Cal/lb/min	×	Body weight	×	Min	=	Activity cal
Cycling (13 mph)	.071		______		______		______
Digging	.062		______		______		______
Driving a car	.020		______		______		______
Housework	.029		______		______		______
Painting a house	.034		______		______		______
Shoveling snow	.052		______		______		______
Sitting quietly	.009		______		______		______
Sleeping and resting	.008		______		______		______
Standing quietly	.012		______		______		______
Typing or writing	.013		______		______		______
Walking, briskly (4.5 mph)	.048		______		______		______

*For the calorie costs of various fitness activities, see Chapter 7.

Source: Adapted from Kusinitz, I., and M. Fine. 1995. *Your Guide to Getting Fit,* 3d ed. Mountain View, Calif.: Mayfield.

calorie intake below 1500 for men or 1200 for women.) Increasing energy output by adopting a program of regular exercise and by incorporating more physical activity into your daily routine is a better strategy. Table 9-1 lists the calorie costs of selected physical activities; refer to Table 7-1 for the calorie costs of different types of sports and fitness activities.

Make Changes in Your Diet and Eating Habits

If you can't generate a large enough negative calorie balance solely by increasing physical activity, you may want to supplement exercise with small cuts in your calorie intake. Don't think of this as "going on a diet"; your goal is to make small changes in your diet that you can maintain for a lifetime. Focus on cutting your fat intake and on eating a variety of nutritious foods in moderation. Don't try skipping meals, fasting, or a very-low-calorie diet. These strategies seldom work, and they can have negative effects on your ability to manage your weight and on your overall health.

Making changes in eating habits is another important strategy for weight management. If your program centers on conscious restriction of certain food items, you're likely to spend all your time thinking about the forbidden foods. Focus on *how* to eat rather than *what* to eat. Try adopting some of the behaviors listed in the box "Strategies for Managing Your Weight." You may find that your new eating habits make it much easier for you to achieve and maintain a healthy weight.

Put Your Plan into Action

Be systematic in your effort to change your behavior. Keeping written records of food intake and dietary changes seems to increase the likelihood of success, so devise a food journal similar to the one in Lab 8-1 or Figure 2-3. Write down what you plan to eat, in what quantity, before you eat it. Many people find that just having to record a food they know they should avoid helps stop them from eating it. Also, keep track of your daily activities and your formal exercise program so you can monitor increases in physical activity.

Other strategies for putting a successful plan into action include the following:

- Examine the environmental cues that trigger poor eating and exercise habits, and devise strategies for dealing with them. Anticipate problem situations, and plan ways to handle them more effectively.
- Get others to help. Talk to friends and family members about what they can do to support your efforts.
- Give yourself lots of praise and rewards. Avoid self-criticism, even when you slip.
- Don't get discouraged. Be aware that although weight loss is bound to slow down after the first loss of body

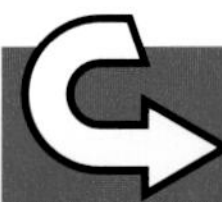

TACTICS AND TIPS
Strategies for Managing Your Weight

- When shopping for food, take along a list, and stick to it. Don't shop when you're hungry. Avoid aisles that contain problem foods.
- When serving food, use a small food scale to measure out portions before putting them on your plate. Serve meals on small plates and in small bowls to help you eat smaller portions without feeling deprived.
- Eat three meals a day; replace impulse snacking with planned, healthy snacks. Drink plenty of water to help fill you up.
- Eat only in specifically designated places. Remove food from other areas of your house or apartment. When you eat, just eat—don't do anything else, such as read or watch TV.
- Eat more slowly. Pay attention to every bite, and enjoy your food. Try putting your fork or spoon down between bites.
- For problem foods, try eating small amounts under controlled conditions. Go out for a scoop of ice cream, for example, rather than buying half a gallon for your freezer.
- When you eat out, choose a restaurant where you can make healthy food choices. Ask that bread and butter not be put on the table before the meal and that sauces and salad dressings be served on the side.
- If you're eating at a friend's, eat a little and leave the rest. Don't eat to be polite; if someone offers you food you don't want, thank the person and decline firmly.

Source: Adapted from Nash, J. D. 1986. *Maximize Your Body Potential.* Palo Alto, Calif.: Bull Publishing.

fluid, the weight loss at this slower rate is more permanent than earlier, more dramatic losses.

- Remember that weight management is a lifelong project. You need to adopt reasonable goals and strategies that you can maintain over the long term.

? COMMON QUESTIONS ANSWERED

How can I safely gain weight? Although for most of us the focus of a weight-management program is losing weight, some people face the opposite challenge. Just as for losing weight, a program for weight gain should be gradual and should include both exercise and dietary changes. The foundation of a successful and healthy program for weight gain is a combination of strength training and a high-carbohydrate, high-calorie diet. Strength training is critical because it will help you add weight as muscle rather than fat.

Energy balance is also important in a program for gaining weight. You need to consume more calories than your body needs in order to gain weight, but you need to choose those extra calories wisely. Fatty, high-calorie foods may seem like an obvious choice, but consuming additional calories as fat can jeopardize your health and your weight-management program. A diet high in fat carries health risks, and your body is more likely to convert dietary fat into fat tissue than into lean body tissue. A better strategy is to consume additional calories as complex carbohydrates—from grains, fruits, and vegetables. Experts recommend that a diet for weight gain should contain about 60–65% of total daily calories from carbohydrates. You do not need to be concerned with protein: Although protein requirements increase when you exercise, most Americans already consume protein in far greater amounts than the RDA minimum recommendation.

In order to gain primarily muscle weight instead of fat, a gradual program of weight gain is your best bet. Try the following strategies for consuming extra calories:

- Don't skip any meals.
- Add two or three snacks to your daily eating routine.
- Try a sports drink or supplement that has at least 60% of calories from carbohydrates, as well as significant amounts of protein, vitamins, and minerals. (But don't use such supplements to replace meals, because they don't contain all food components.)

Can reduced-fat foods and snacks help me lose weight? Reduced-fat foods can be a part of a weight-management program, but they must be used carefully. Consider both what the food is and how much of it you eat. A reduced-fat food contains at least 25% less fat than the "regular" version of the food. But the total amount of fat depends on the type of food. For example, a serving of regular peanut butter has 17 grams of fat; the same serving of reduced-fat peanut butter has about 12—a lower amount, but still a substantial amount of fat. In addition, reduced-fat foods often contain the same number of calories as their regular versions. Studies indicate that many of us actually take in more calories when we consume low-fat foods by rationalizing that we can eat more if we decrease our fat intake. To be part of a successful weight-management program, reduced-fat foods cannot be considered as a license to eat more.

You also need to consider nutrients. Fruits and vegetables are still likely to be lower in fat and calories and higher in vitamins and minerals than reduced-fat cookies or muffins. Nutrients may also be a concern if you eat foods made with olestra (trade name, Olean), a fat substitute approved by the FDA in 1996 for use in deep-fried foods. While olestra does significantly lower the fat content of popular foods like potato and tortilla chips, it also binds with certain nutrients, causing them to be carried through the digestive tract without being absorbed by the body. Foods made with olestra are fortified with some of these nutrients, including vitamins A and E, but not all of them. Some scientists are concerned that consumption of significant amounts of olestra could lead to nutrient deficiencies. (In addition, olestra can cause gastrointestinal problems.)

Overall, reduced-fat desserts and snacks should be considered as occasional treats rather than as a regular part of a healthy diet.

How can I achieve a "perfect" body? The current ideal of an ultrathin, ultrafit body is impossible for most people to achieve. A reasonable goal for body weight and body shape must take into account an individual's heredity, weight history, social circumstances, metabolic rate, and psychological well-being. Don't set goals based on movie stars or fashion models. Modern photographic techniques can make people look much better on film or in magazines than they look in person. Many of these people are also genetically endowed with body shapes that are impossible for most of us to emulate. The best approach is to work with what you've got. Adopting a wellness lifestyle that includes regular exercise and a healthy diet will naturally result in the best possible body shape for you. Obsessively trying to achieve unreasonable goals can lead to problems such as eating disorders, overtraining, and injuries.

SUMMARY

- Excess body weight increases the risk of numerous diseases, particularly cardiovascular disease, cancer, gallbladder disease, and diabetes.
- Although genetic factors help determine a person's weight, the influence of heredity can be overcome.
- Resting metabolic rate, the amount of energy needed to maintain body functions, is partly determined by heredity; it can be increased through exercise and an increase in lean body mass.
- Weight factors that an individual can control are calories taken in and calories expended in physical activity. Americans today expend fewer calories than in the past and rely too heavily on high-calorie processed foods.
- Nutritional guidelines for weight control and wellness include reducing consumption of fat, sugar, and protein; increasing consumption of complex carbohydrates (which require energy for digestion); monitoring portion sizes; learning to stop eating when full; and developing an eating schedule based on decision rules.
- Activity guidelines for weight control emphasize regular, prolonged endurance exercise and weight training.
- The sense of well-being that results from a well-balanced, low-fat diet can reinforce commitment to weight control, improve self-esteem, and lead to realistic, as opposed to negative, self-talk. Successful weight-management results in not using food as a way to cope with stress.
- The dieting that results from an obsession with thinness can lead to physical problems and serious eating disorders, especially among adolescents, including anorexia nervosa and bulimia nervosa. Reasonable goals lead to success and enhanced physical well-being.
- In cases of extreme obesity, weight loss requires medical supervision; otherwise, people can set up individual nutritional programs, perhaps getting guidance from reliable books, or they can get help by joining a commercial weight-loss program.
- A successful personal plan assesses motivation, sets reasonable and healthy goals, and emphasizes increased activity rather than decreased calories.

BEHAVIOR CHANGE ACTIVITY

Developing Realistic Self-Talk

Self-talk is the ongoing internal dialogue we have with ourselves throughout much of the day. Our thoughts can be accurate, positive, and supportive, or they can be exaggerated and negative. Self-talk is closely related to self-esteem and self-concept. Realistic self-talk can help maintain positive self-esteem, the belief that one is a good and competent person, worthy of friendship and love. A negative internal dialogue can reinforce negative self-esteem and can make behavior change very difficult. Substituting realistic self-talk for negative self-talk can help you build and maintain self-esteem and cope better with the challenges in your life.

First, take a closer look at your current pattern of self-talk. Use your health journal to track self-talk, especially as it relates to your target behavior. Does any of your self-talk fall into the common patterns of distorted negative self-talk shown in Table 9-2? If so, use the examples of realistic self-talk from the table to develop more accurate and rational responses. Write your current negative thoughts in the left-hand column, then record more realistic responses in the right-hand column.

Current Self-Talk	More Realistic Self-Talk
____________________	____________________
____________________	____________________
____________________	____________________
____________________	____________________
____________________	____________________
____________________	____________________

TABLE 9-2 Developing More Realistic Self-Talk

Cognitive Distortion	Negative Self-Talk	Realistic Self-Talk
Focusing on negatives	School is so discouraging—nothing but one hassle after another.	School is pretty challenging and has its difficulties, but there certainly are rewards. It's really a mixture of good and bad.
Expecting the worst	Why would my boss want to meet with me this afternoon if not to fire me?	I wonder why my boss wants to meet with me. I guess I'll just have to wait and see.
Overgeneralizing	(After getting a poor grade on a paper) Just as I thought—I'm incompetent at everything.	I'll start working on the next paper earlier. That way, if I run into problems, I'll have time to consult with the TA.
Minimizing	I won the speech contest, but none of the other speakers was very good. I wouldn't have done as well against stiffer competition.	It may not have been the best speech I'll ever give, but it was good enough to win the contest. I'm really improving as a speaker.
Blaming others	I wouldn't have eaten so much last night if my friends hadn't insisted on going to that restaurant.	I overdid it last night. Next time I'll make different choices.
Expecting perfection	I should have scored 100% on this test. I can't believe I missed that one problem through a careless mistake.	Too bad I missed one problem through carelessness, but overall I did very well on this test. Next time I'll be more careful.
Believing you're the cause of everything	Sarah seems so depressed today. I wish I hadn't had that argument with her yesterday; it must have really upset her.	I wish I had handled the argument better, and in the future I'll try to. But I don't know if Sarah's behavior is related to what I said, or even if she's depressed. In any case, I'm not responsible for how Sarah feels or acts; only she can take responsibility for that.
Thinking in black and white	I've got to score 10 points in the game today. Otherwise, I don't belong on the team.	I'm a good player or else I wouldn't be on the team. I'll play my best—that's all I can do.
Magnifying events	They went to a movie without me. I thought we were friends, but I guess I was wrong.	I'm disappointed they didn't ask me to the movie, but it doesn't mean our friendship is over. It's not that big a deal.

Source: Adapted from Schafer, W. 1992. *Stress Management for Wellness,* 2d ed. Fort Worth: Harcourt Brace Jovanovich.

FOR MORE INFORMATION

If you have questions about your body composition or about the right program of weight control for you, consult your physician. The books listed below may also be useful.

Bailey, C. 1991. *The New Fit or Fat,* rev. ed. Boston: Houghton Mifflin. *Originally published in 1977, an entertaining description of ways to become healthy by developing better diet and exercise habits.*

Finn, S., and L. S. Kass. 1992. *The Real Life Nutrition Book.* New York: Penguin. *Nutrition basics, with the philosophy that your lifestyle should dictate your nutrition and fitness regimen.*

Goldberg, L. 1991. *The New Controlled ChEATing Weight-Loss and Fitness Program.* Kansas City: Andrews and McMeel. *How to eat your favorite foods without guilt, with responsible diet and exercise advice.*

Nash, J. D. 1986. *Maximize Your Body Potential.* Palo Alto, Calif.: Bull Publishing. *A comprehensive book on nutrition, exercise, behavior, and the psychological aspects of weight management.*

Nash, J. D. 1992. *Now That You've Lost It: How to Maintain Your Best Weight.* Palo Alto, Calif.: Bull Publishing. *The psychological and motivational factors that can produce long-lasting success at weight management.*

Roth, G. 1991. *When Food Is Love.* New York: Dutton. *The connection between eating disorders and close relationships, including early family experiences.*

If you are concerned about anorexia nervosa or bulimia nervosa, you can get information and support from the American Anorexia/Bulimia Association, 133 Cedar Lane, Teaneck, NJ 07666.

SELECTED BIBLIOGRAPHY

Bouchard, C., et al. 1990. The response to long-term overfeeding in identical twins. *New England Journal of Medicine* 322(21): 1477–1482.

Brownell, K. D. 1991. Dieting and the search for the perfect body: Where physiology and culture collide. *Behavior Therapy* 22:1–12.

Brownell, K. D., and J. Rodin. 1994. The dieting maelstrom: Is it possible and advisable to lose weight? *American Psychologist* 49:781–791.

Burgess, N. S. 1991. Effect of a very-low-calorie diet on body composition and resting metabolic rate in obese men and women. *Journal of the American Dietetic Association* 91(4): 430–434.

Collier, S. N., et al. 1990. Assessment of attitudes about weight and dieting among college-aged individuals. *Journal of the American Dietetic Association* 90(2): 276–278.

Flynn, M. E. 1995. Fat-free food: A dieter's downfall? Studies show calories do count. *Environmental Nutrition* 18(4): 1, 6.

Gillette, C. A., R. C. Bullough, and C. L. Melby. 1994. Post-exercise energy expenditure in response to acute aerobic or resistive exercise. *International Journal of Sport Nutrition* 4:347–360.

Gortmaker, S. L., W. H. Dietz, and L. W. Y. Cheung. 1990. Inactivity, diet, and the fattening of America. *Journal of the American Dietetic Association* 90:1247–1252.

Halaas, J. L. 1995. Weight-reducing effects of the plasma protein encoded by the obese gene. *Science* 269:543–546.

Jeffery, R. W., R. R. Wing, and S. A. French. 1992. Weight cycling and cardiovascular risk factors in obese men and women. *American Journal of Clinical Nutrition* 55:641–644.

Kleiner, S. M. 1995. Healthy muscle gain. *Physician and Sportsmedicine* 23(4): 21–22.

Kuczmarski, R. J. 1992. Prevalence of overweight and weight gain in the United States. *American Journal of Clinical Nutrition* 55:495S–502S.

Lissner, L., et al. 1991. Variability of body weight and health outcomes in the Framingham population. *New England Journal of Medicine* 324(26): 1839–1844.

Low-fat mind games. 1995. *Tufts University Diet and Nutrition Letter* 13(9): 1.

Manson, J. E. 1995. Body weight and mortality among women. *New England Journal of Medicine* 333(11): 677–685.

Miles, D. S. 1991. Weight control and exercise. *Clinics in Sports Medicine* 10(1): 157–169.

Nash, J. D. 1987. Eating behavior and body weight: Physiological influences. *American Journal of Health Promotion* 1(3): 5–15.

Nash, J. D. 1987. Eating behavior and body weight: Psychological influences. *American Journal of Health Promotion* 2(1): 5–14.

Obesity insights. 1995. *Harvard Women's Health Watch,* October.

Pelleymounter, M. A., et al. 1995. Effects of the *obese* gene product on body weight regulation in *ob/ob* mice. *Science* 269: 540–543.

Peterkin, B. B. 1990. Dietary guidelines for Americans, 1990 edition. *Journal of the American Dietetic Association* 90: 1725–1727.

Pi-Sunyer, F. X. 1991. Health implications of obesity. *American Journal of Clinical Nutrition* 53:1595S–1603S.

Rand, C. S. W., and J. M. Kuldau. 1992. Epidemiology of bulimia and symptoms in a general population: Sex, age, race, and socioeconomic status. *International Journal of Eating Disorders* 11:37–44.

Sale, J. E., L. J. McCargar, S. M. Crawford, and J. E. Taunton. 1995. Effects of exercise modality on metabolic rate and body composition. *Clinical Journal of Sport Medicine* 5: 100–107.

Sichieri, R., J. E. Everhart, and V. S. Hubbard. 1992. Relative weight classifications in the assessment of underweight and overweight in the United States. *International Journal of Obesity* 16:303–312.

Simoes, E. J., T. Byers, R. J. Coates, M. K. Serdula, A. H. Mokdad, and G. W. Heath. 1995. The association between leisure-time physical activity and dietary fat in American adults. *American Journal of Public Health* 85(2): 240–244.

Stunkard, A. J., et al. 1990. The body-mass index of twins who have been reared apart. *New England Journal of Medicine* 322(21): 1483–1487.

U.S. Department of Health and Human Services. 1990. *Healthy People 2000: National Health Promotion and Disease Prevention Objectives.* Washington, D.C.: U.S. Government Printing Office, DHHS Pub. (PHS) 91-50212.

"Why Lost Weight Finds Its Way Back." 1995. *San Francisco Chronicle.* 9 March, pp. A1, A13.

Zhang, Y., et al. 1994. Positional cloning of the mouse *obese* gene and its human homologue. *Nature* 372:425–431.

Name ______________________ Section ______________ Date ______________

LAB 9-1 *Calculating Daily Energy Balance*

I. Resting Metabolic Rate

Resting metabolic rate varies depending on age, gender, and weight. Use the equations below to calculate your approximate RMR.

World Health Organization Equations

1. Convert body weight to kilograms:

   ___________ lb ÷ 2.2 lb/kg = ___________ kg

2. Find the appropriate formula in the table below, and calculate your RMR. (For example, a 19-year-old male weighing 80 kg would have an RMR of approximately [15.3 × 80] + 679 = 1224 + 679 = 1903 calories per day.)

Males	*Age Range (years)*	*Equation to Derive RMR in cal/day*
	10–18	(17.5 × wt) + 651
	18–30	(15.3 × wt) + 679
	30–60	(11.6 × wt) + 879
	Over 60	(13.5 × wt) + 487
Females		
	10–18	(12.2 × wt) + 746
	18–30	(14.7 × wt) + 496
	30–60	(8.7 × wt) + 829
	Over 60	(10.5 × wt) + 596

RMR = (___________ × ___________ kg) + ___________ = ___________ **cal/day**
(factor from table) (body weight) (factor from table)

Harris Benedict Equations

1. Convert body weight to kilograms:

   ___________ lb ÷ 2.2 lb/kg = ___________ kg

2. Convert height to centimeters:

   ___________ in. × 2.54 cm/in. = ___________ cm

3. Use the appropriate equation to calculate RMR. (For example, a 20-year-old female 160 tall, weighing 60 kg, would have an RMR of approximately 655 + [9.56 × 60] + [1.85 × 160] − [4.68 × 20] = 1431 calories per day.)

   Women: RMR = 655 + (9.56 × weight ________ kg) + (1.85 × height ________ cm) −
   (4.68 × age ________ yr) = ________ **cal/day**

   Men: RMR = 66.5 + (13.8 × weight ________ kg) + (5 × height ________ cm) −
   (6.76 × age ________ yr) = ________ **cal/day**

Approximate Resting Metabolic Rate

Average the values you obtained from these equations to determine your approximate RMR.

World Health Organization Equation: ____________ cal/day

Harris Benedict Equation: ____________ cal/day

Average value for RMR: ____________ cal/day

II. Daily Energy Expenditures

List all of your activities for a 3-day period, and classify them according to the categories listed in the table below. (Representative values of the calorie costs of different types of activities are presented below as multiples of resting metabolic rate.) Table 7-1 provides general guidelines for how to classify the sports and fitness activities you participate in: Activities with high cardiorespiratory endurance ratings probably fall in the heavy category, those with medium CRE ratings in the moderate category, and those with low CRE ratings in the light category. Take your intensity into account when classifying fitness activities; basketball, for example, can be played at an easy pace or very intensely.

Your total daily energy expenditure can be estimated by calculating a daily activity factor based on the amount of time you engage in activities in each category of intensity. By adding up weighted activity factors and finding the average, you can calculate total daily energy requirements. Since your activity levels probably vary widely from day to day, it's more accurate to calculate energy output for several different days to come up with an average daily range of calorie output.

Activity Category	*Representative Value for Activity Factor per Unit Time of Activity*
Resting	
Sleeping, lying down	RMR × 1.0
Very light	
Seated and standing activities such as driving, lab work, writing, typing, cooking, playing cards or a musical instrument	RMR × 1.5
Light	
Walking on a level surface 2.5–3.0 mph, house cleaning, child care, carpentry, restaurant trades, and sports/activities with low fitness ratings such as golf, bowling, and sailing	RMR × 2.5
Moderate	
Walking 3.5–4.0 mph, gardening, carrying a load, and sports/activities with medium fitness ratings such as baseball and volleyball	RMR × 5.0
Heavy	
Walking with a load uphill, heavy manual labor, sports/activities with high fitness ratings such as aerobic dance and cross-country skiing	RMR × 7.0

For each day's activities, add up the total number of hours for each activity category. Then multiply the total duration for each category by the category's activity factor. Add the weighted activity factors, then divide the total weighted activity factor by 24 to get an average daily activity factor. A sample of completed calculations for one day is shown on the next page.

SAMPLE

Activity	Duration	Category
sleeping	8 hours	resting
eating in dorm	1-1/2	very light
class	5	very light
bicycling to class, lab...	1	moderate
job in library	2-1/2	very light
cleaning room/laundry	1	light
basketball	1	heavy
studying in library	4	very light

Category	Activity Factor	Duration	Weighted Activity Factor
Resting	1.0	8	8.0
Very light	1.5	13	19.5
Light	2.5	1	2.5
Moderate	5.0	1	5.0
Heavy	7.0	1	7.0
Total		24 hours	42.0
Average daily activity factor (Total of weighted factors ÷ 24)			1.75

RECORDS FOR THREE DAYS

Day 1

Activity	Duration	Category

Day 1

Category	Activity Factor	Duration	Weighted Activity Factor
Resting	1.0		
Very light	1.5		
Light	2.5		
Moderate	5.0		
Heavy	7.0		
Total		24 hours	
Average daily activity factor (Total of weighted factors ÷ 24)			

Day 2

Activity	Duration	Category

Day 2

Category	Activity Factor	Duration	Weighted Activity Factor
Resting	1.0		
Very light	1.5		
Light	2.5		
Moderate	5.0		
Heavy	7.0		
Total		24 hours	
Average daily activity factor (Total of weighted factors ÷ 24)			

Day 3

Activity	*Duration*	*Category*

Day 3

Category	*Activity Factor*	*Duration*	*Weighted Activity Factor*
Resting	1.0		
Very light	1.5		
Light	2.5		
Moderate	5.0		
Heavy	7.0		
Total		24 hours	
Average daily activity factor (Total of weighted factors ÷ 24)			

Finally, use the middle or average of your three daily activity factors to calculate your average daily energy output. For RMR, use the value you calculated in the first part of this lab.

Average of three daily activity factors ___________ × RMR ___________ cal/day =
approximate daily energy expenditure: ___________ cal/day

How does this value compare to the average number of calories you eat each day, as determined in Lab 8-2?

To monitor your progress toward your goal, enter the results of this lab in the Preprogram Assessment column of Lab 15-2. After several weeks of a program to increase daily energy expenditure, do this lab again and enter the results in the Postprogram Assessment column of Lab 15-2. How do the results compare?

Sources: World Health Organization. 1985. *Energy and Protein Requirements: Report of a Joint FAO/WHO/UNO Expert Consultation*. Geneva: World Health Organization, Technical Report Series 724. National Research Council. 1989. *Recommended Dietary Allowances*, 10th ed. Washington, D.C.: National Academy Press.

Name ______________________ Section ______________ Date ______________

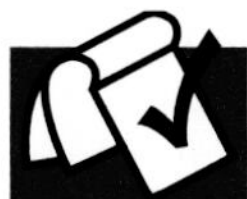

LAB 9-2 *Identifying Weight-Loss Goals and Ways to Meet Them*

Negative Calorie Balance

Complete the following calculations to determine your weekly and daily negative calorie balance goals and the number of weeks to achieve your target weight.

Current weight __________ lb − target weight (from Lab 6-1) __________ lb =
total weight to lose __________ lb

Total weight to lose __________ lb ÷ weight to lose each week __________ lb =
time to achieve target weight __________ weeks

Weight to lose each week __________ lb × 3500 cal/lb = weekly negative calorie balance __________ cal/week

Weekly negative calorie balance __________ cal/week ÷ 7 days/week = daily negative calorie balance
__________ cal/day

To keep your weight-loss program on schedule, you must achieve the daily negative calorie balance by either decreasing your calorie consumption (eating less) or increasing your calorie expenditure (being more active). A combination of the two strategies will probably be most successful.

Changes in Activity Level

Adding a few minutes of exercise every day is a good way of expending calories. Use the calorie costs for different activities listed in Table 7-1 and Table 9-1 to plan ways for raising your calorie expenditure level.

Activity	Duration	Calories Used
	Total calories expended:	

Changes in Diet

Look closely at your diet from one day, as recorded in Lab 8-2. Identify ways to cut calorie consumption by eliminating certain items or substituting lower-calorie choices. Be realistic in your cuts and substitutions; you need to develop a plan you can live with.

Food Item	Substitute Food Item	Calorie Savings
	Total calories cut:	

Total calories expended _______ + total calories cut _______ = Total negative calorie balance _______

Have you met your required negative energy balance? If not, revise your dietary and activity changes to meet your goal.

Common Problem Eating Behaviors

For each of the groups of statements that appear below, check those that are true for you. If you check several statements for a given pattern or problem, it will probably be a significant factor in your weight-control program. One possible strategy for dealing with each type of problem is given. For those eating problems you identify as important, add your own ideas to the strategies listed.

1. _____ I often skip meals.

   _____ I often eat a number of snacks in place of a meal.

   _____ I don't have a regular schedule of meal and snack times.

   _____ I make up for missed meals and snacks by eating more at the next meal.

   Problem: Irregular eating habits

   Possible solutions:

   - Write out a plan for each day's meals in advance. Carry it with you, and stick to it.
   - ______________________________
   - ______________________________

2. _____ I eat more than one sweet dessert or snack each day.

   _____ I usually snack on foods high in calories and fat (chips, cookies, ice cream).

   _____ I drink regular (not sugar-free) soft drinks.

   _____ I choose types of meat that are high in fat.

   _____ I consume more than one alcoholic beverage per day.

   Problem: Poor food choices

   Possible solutions:

   - Keep a supply of raw vegetables handy for snacks.
   - ______________________________
   - ______________________________

3. _____ I always eat everything on my plate.

   _____ I often go back for seconds and thirds.

   _____ I take larger helpings than most people.

   _____ I eat up leftovers instead of putting them away.

   Problem: Portion sizes too large

   Possible solutions:

   - Measure all portions with a scale or measuring cup.
   - ______________________________
   - ______________________________

10

Stress

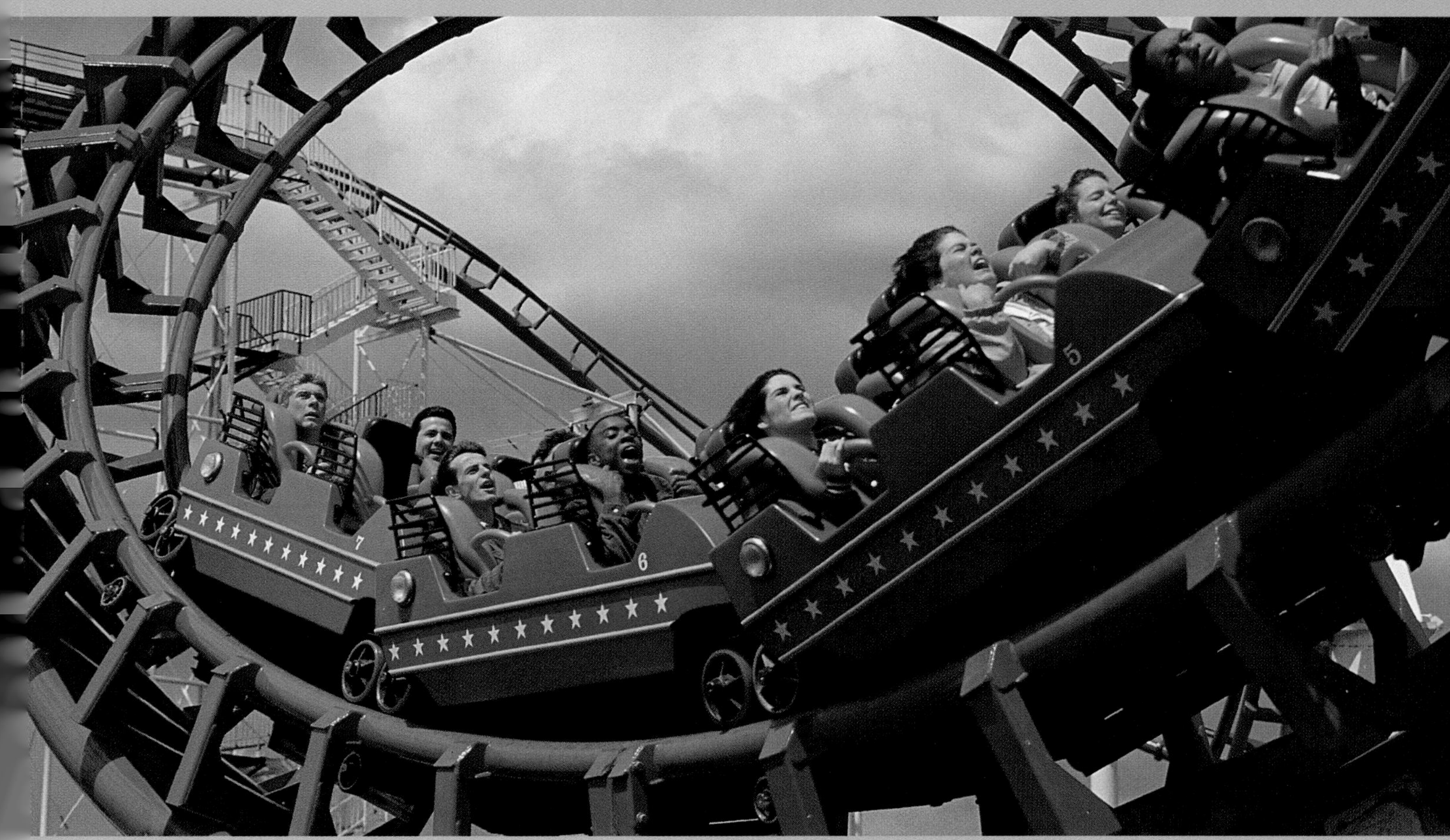

LOOKING AHEAD

After reading this chapter, you should be able to answer these questions about stress:

- What is stress, and how does it affect health and wellness?
- How does the body respond to stress?
- How do emotional and behavioral responses to stress affect the ability to manage stress?
- What is the relationship between stress and disease, and what are some possible mechanisms of this relationship?
- What are some approaches to successful stress management?

Like the term *fitness,* **stress** is a word most people use without really understanding its precise meaning. Stress is popularly viewed as an uncomfortable response to a negative event, which probably describes *nervous tension* more than the cluster of physical and psychological responses that actually constitute stress. In fact, stress is not limited to negative situations; it is also a response to pleasurable physical challenges and the achievement of personal goals. Whether stress is experienced as pleasant or unpleasant depends largely on the situation and the individual. Because learning effective responses to whatever induces stress can enhance psychological health and help prevent a number of serious diseases, it is an important component in any fitness program.

This chapter explains the physiological and psychological reactions that make up the stress response and describes how these reactions can be risks to good health. Ways of managing stress with a personal program or with the help of others are presented.

TERMS

stress The collective physiological and emotional responses to any stimulus that disturbs an individual's homeostasis, or equilibrium.

stressor Any physical or psychological event or condition that produces stress.

stress response The physiological changes associated with stress.

general adaptation syndrome (GAS) A pattern of stress responses consisting of three stages: alarm, resistance, and exhaustion.

sympathetic nervous system A division of the autonomous nervous system that reacts to danger or other challenges by almost instantly accelerating body processes.

autonomic nervous system The branch of the peripheral nervous system that, largely without conscious thought, controls basic body processes; subdivided into the sympathetic and parasympathetic nervous systems.

hormones Chemical messengers produced in the body and transported in the bloodstream to target cells or organs for specific regulation of their activities.

epinephrine A hormone secreted by the inner core of the adrenal gland; also called *adrenaline,* the "anger hormone."

norepinephrine A hormone secreted by the inner core of the adrenal gland; also called *noradrenaline,* the "fear hormone."

endorphins Brain secretions that have pain-inhibiting effects.

fight-or-flight reaction A defense reaction that prepares the individual for conflict or escape by triggering hormonal, cardiovascular, metabolic, and other changes.

homeostasis A state of stability and consistency in an individual's physiological functioning.

parasympathetic nervous system A division of the autonomic nervous system that moderates the excitatory effect of the sympathetic nervous system, slowing metabolism and restoring energy supplies.

adaptive energy Limited body reserves that are activated when the body is exhausted.

WHAT IS STRESS?

No one has explored the various aspects of stress more thoroughly than Hans Selye, an endocrinologist and biologist. Selye defines stress as "the nonspecific response of the body to any demand." A "nonspecific response" is the body's total physiological response, ranging from sweating palms to a pounding heart, to any stress-producing situation—be it a date, a final exam, or a flat tire. This response can vary in intensity, but it is the same response no matter what induces it.

One reason for the general confusion about stress is that the term is used in two different ways: to refer to the situations that trigger physical and emotional reactions as well as the reactions themselves. In this text, for the sake of clarity, we use the more precise term **stressor** to refer to triggers and the term **stress response** to refer to the physical and emotional reactions. We use the term *stress* to describe the general physical and emotional state that accompanies the stress response. Thus, a person taking a final exam (the stressor) responds with sweaty palms and a pounding heart (part of the stress response), which he or she experiences as stress.

The General Adaptation Syndrome (GAS)

Imagine a near-miss: A man steps off the curb, and a car suddenly careens around the corner just inches away from him. In that split second of danger, and in the moments following it, he experiences a predictable series of physiological reactions that Selye named the **general adaptation syndrome (GAS).** Selye divided GAS into three distinct stages: alarm, resistance, and exhaustion.

GAS: Alarm The instant the man senses the oncoming car, an internal alarm sounds, and the **sympathetic** division of his **autonomic nervous system** takes command. For the most part, this portion of the nervous system operates independently of conscious thought. It controls heart rate, breathing, blood pressure, digestion, and hundreds of other body functions. It also mobilizes the body to take physical action in response to a stressor.

As the car travels toward the man, he feels only fear, but outside his awareness, things happen to prepare him to meet the danger. Chemical messages cause the release of key **hormones,** including cortisol, **epinephrine,** and **norepinephrine.** These hormones trigger a series of profound physiological changes (Figure 10-1):

- Hearing and vision become more acute.
- The heart rate accelerates in order to pump more oxygen through the body.
- The liver releases extra sugar into the bloodstream to provide an energy boost to the muscles and the brain.
- Perspiration increases to cool the skin.
- **Endorphins** are released to relieve pain in case of injury.

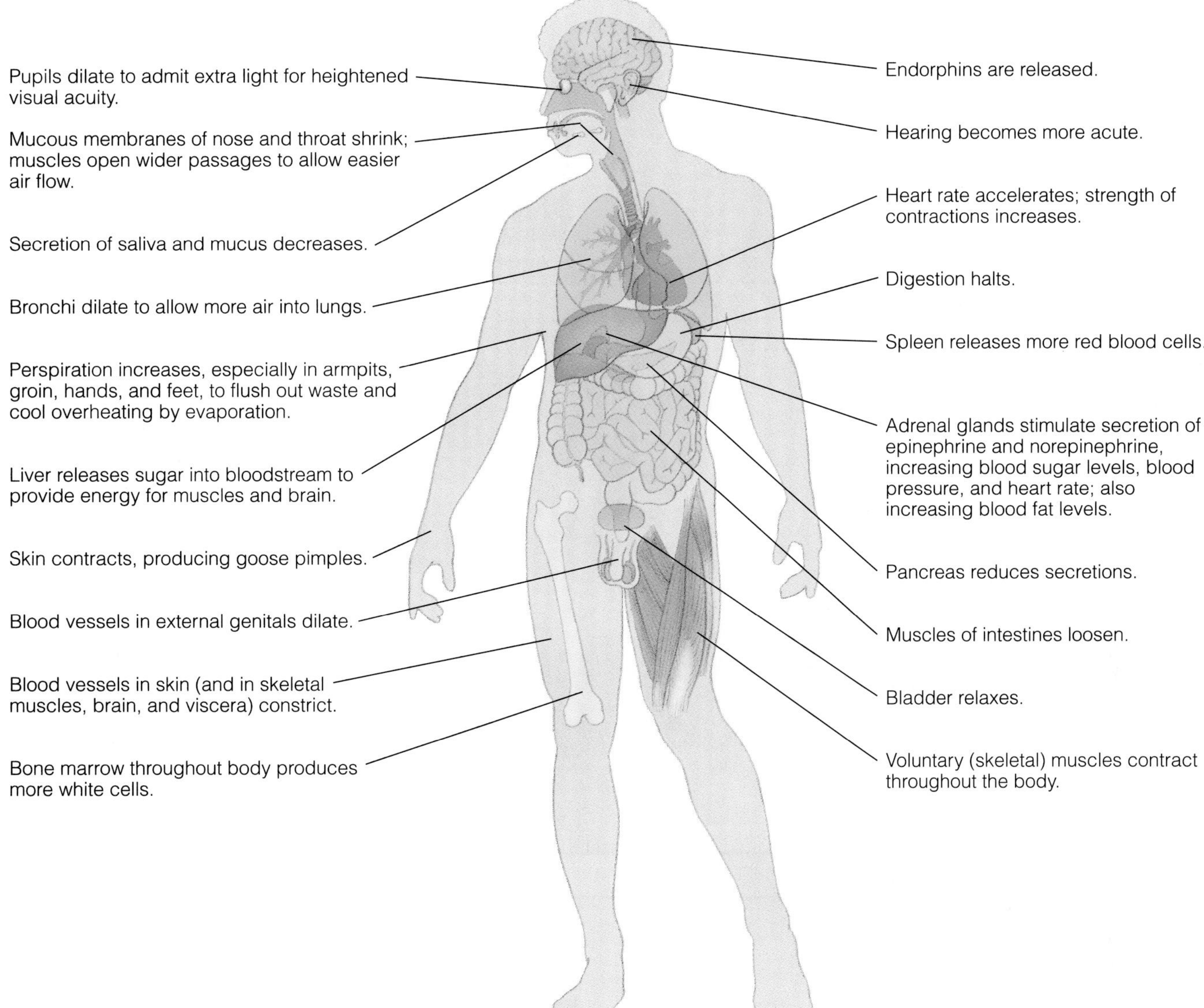

Pupils dilate to admit extra light for heightened visual acuity.
Mucous membranes of nose and throat shrink; muscles open wider passages to allow easier air flow.
Secretion of saliva and mucus decreases.
Bronchi dilate to allow more air into lungs.
Perspiration increases, especially in armpits, groin, hands, and feet, to flush out waste and cool overheating by evaporation.
Liver releases sugar into bloodstream to provide energy for muscles and brain.
Skin contracts, producing goose pimples.
Blood vessels in external genitals dilate.
Blood vessels in skin (and in skeletal muscles, brain, and viscera) constrict.
Bone marrow throughout body produces more white cells.
Endorphins are released.
Hearing becomes more acute.
Heart rate accelerates; strength of contractions increases.
Digestion halts.
Spleen releases more red blood cells.
Adrenal glands stimulate secretion of epinephrine and norepinephrine, increasing blood sugar levels, blood pressure, and heart rate; also increasing blood fat levels.
Pancreas reduces secretions.
Muscles of intestines loosen.
Bladder relaxes.
Voluntary (skeletal) muscles contract throughout the body.

Figure 10-1 ***The alarm reaction, the first stage of the general adaptation syndrome in response to a stressor.***

All these changes, together known as the **fight-or-flight reaction,** heighten reflexes and provide the added strength necessary to dodge the car. This response is a fundamental part of our biological inheritance, but in modern life it often occurs inappropriately. It can be triggered not just by a physical threat, but also by a party invitation, a sudden misstep on a flight of stairs, or even an insult. The alarm response prepares the body for physical action regardless of whether physical action is a necessary or appropriate response to a particular stressor.

GAS: Resistance The human body resists dramatic changes. Whenever normal function is disrupted, as during the alarm reaction, it strives to regain **homeostasis,** a state of balance and normality. Once the stressor recedes, the **parasympathetic** division of the autonomic nervous system halts the alarm reaction and initiates adjustments to restore homeostasis, calming the body down, slowing the heart rate, drying the sweaty palms, and returning the breathing to normal. The resistance stage of the GAS ends the alarm stage and permits the individual to get on with everyday life.

GAS: Exhaustion Both the alarm reaction and the return to equilibrium in the resistance stage use a considerable amount of energy. When severe stressors persist or occur in succession—as on a battlefield, for example—the alarm reaction is triggered repeatedly, and readily available stores of energy can be depleted. Worse, reserves of **adaptive energy** can be drained as well, resulting in exhaustion. This is not the sort of exhaustion people experience after a long, busy day. Rather, it is a life-threatening form of physiological depletion characterized by distorted and disorganized thinking.

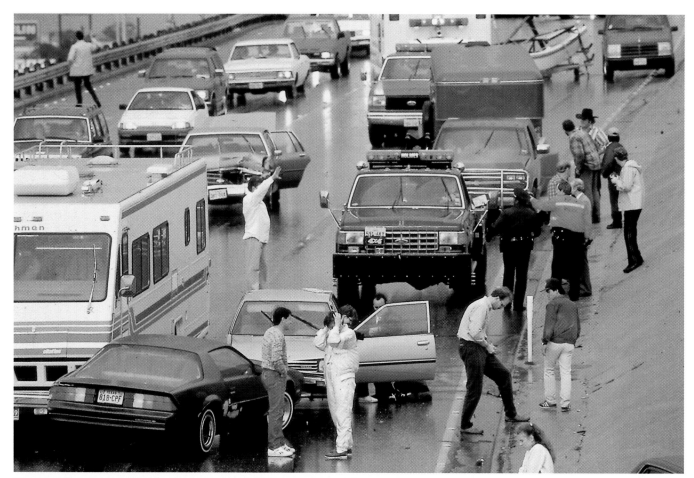

Heavy traffic on a rain-slick highway is a recipe for stress. Most of the people involved in this series of collisions have already experienced their peak alarm reaction and are in the process of returning to normal functioning.

Everyday stressors—such as noise, overcrowding, overwork, discrimination, and so on—don't usually lead to terminal exhaustion, but there is evidence that over the long term they can kill us just the same. When the body is subjected too often to the drastic demands of the stress response, health and wellness suffer. (The relationship between the stress response and disease risk is discussed in more detail later in this chapter.)

GAS is a survival mechanism intended to mobilize us in rare life-and-death emergencies, not on an ongoing basis. Ironically, the strains of modern life have transformed this life-saving mechanism into a potentially life-threatening one. Table 10-1 gives some of the signals of overstress, distinct warnings that the body is being taxed too greatly by the stress response.

somatic nervous system The branch of the peripheral nervous system that governs motor functions and sensory information; largely under our conscious control.

Individual Variations in Responses to Stress

Although everyone responds to stressors in the same way physically, individuals differ greatly in their emotional and behavioral responses. While one person feels relaxed and confident about taking a test, another may lie awake the night before, worrying about failure. Temperament, health, life experiences, beliefs and ideas, and coping skills all contribute to these individual variations.

Behavioral responses to stress—crying, talking, or hugging; exercising, meditating, or laughing; or, less appropriately, overeating or using drugs—are controlled by the **somatic nervous system,** which manages the body's conscious actions. This means that they fall under conscious control and, unlike the alarm reaction, can be voluntarily modified. Behavioral responses to stress are intimately related not only to the physical aspect of the GAS but to the emotional experience of it as well.

Consider the individual variations demonstrated by two students, David and Amelia, responding to the same stressor—the first exam of the semester. David enters the exam with a feeling of dread, and, as he reads the exam

TABLE 10-1 Signals of Stress

Emotional Signs	Behavioral Signs	Physical Signs
Tendency to be irritable or aggressive	Increased use of tobacco, alcohol, or other drugs	Pounding heart
Tendency to feel anxious, fearful, or edgy	Excessive TV watching	Trembling, with nervous tics
Hyperexcitability, impulsiveness, or emotional instability	Sleep disturbances (e.g., insomnia) or excessive sleep	Grinding of teeth
Depression	Overeating or undereating	Dry mouth
Frequent feelings of boredom	Sexual problems	Excessive perspiration
Inability to concentrate	Crying	Gastrointestinal problems (diarrhea, constipation, indigestion, queasy stomach)
Fatigue	Yelling	Stiff neck or aching lower back
	Job or school burnout	Migraine or tension headaches
	Spouse or child abuse	Frequent colds or low-grade infections
	Panic attacks	Cold hands and feet
		Allergy or asthma attacks
		Skin problems (e.g., hives, eczema, psoriasis)

questions, responds to his initial anxiety with more anxiety. The more emotionally upset he gets, the less he can remember and the more anxious he becomes. Soon he's staring into space, imagining what will happen if he fails the course.

Amelia, on the other hand, takes a deep breath to relax before she reads the questions, wills herself to focus on the answers she knows, and then goes back over the exam to deal with those questions she's not sure of. She leaves the room feeling calm, relaxed, and confident that she has done well.

It's not difficult to see that avoiding destructive responses to stress and adopting effective and appropriate ones can have a direct effect on emotional and physical well-being. But the adverse effects of stress that go unmanaged can be far greater and more consequential than just a few hours or days of psychological distress.

STRESS AND DISEASE

Although the role of stress in disease is complex, it is clear that people with too many stressors in their lives or who handle stressors poorly are at risk for a wide range of problems. In the short term, it might be a cold, a stiff neck, or a stomach ache. In the long term, however, the problems can be more severe: cardiovascular disease, high blood pressure, impairment of the immune system. As researchers continue to learn more about the connections between the mind and the body, the list grows.

Cardiovascular Disease

High blood pressure is probably the most serious long-term effect of stress on the body. In the alarm stage of the stress response, heart rate increases and blood vessels constrict, causing blood pressure to rise. Chronic high blood pressure is a major cause of atherosclerosis, a disease in which the blood vessels become blocked by fatty deposits. Atherosclerosis can lead to strokes, heart attacks, and death.

Recent research suggests that not only stress itself but also certain emotional responses it evokes can increase the risk of CVD. People who tend to react to stressful situations with hostility, anger, distrust, or cynicism are more likely to have heart attacks than people with less-explosive, more trusting personalities. This connection is discussed further in Chapter 11.

Impairment of the Immune System

A growing body of evidence suggests that stressors can have a direct bearing on the body's ability to fight off viruses and other disease agents. Studies have shown that anxiety, depression, anger, overexertion, and sleep deprivation are all associated with a temporary decline in immune function. Because of this decline, people with chronic ailments ranging from herpes to HIV infection

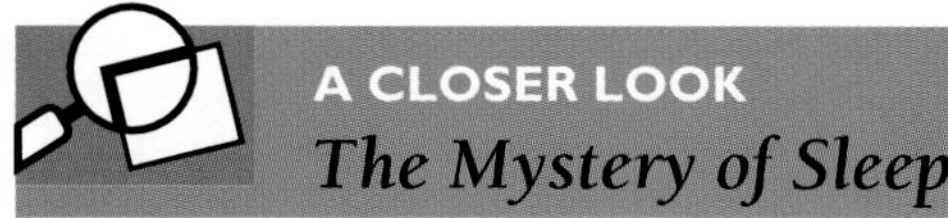

A CLOSER LOOK

The Mystery of Sleep

What is sleep, and why do we need it? Surprisingly enough, the answers to these questions are not completely known. What is known is that all animal species sleep, and must sleep. The need to sleep has an awesome power over us. Without sleep, our mental and physical processes steadily deteriorate. We get headaches, feel irritable, are unable to concentrate, forget things, and may even become more susceptible to illness. Extreme sleep deprivation can lead to hallucinations and other psychotic symptoms. In contrast, sufficient sleep improves mood, fosters feelings of competence and self-worth, and supports optimal mental and emotional functioning.

Many experts believe that most Americans don't get enough sleep. Studies have shown that many people fall asleep during the day in less than 5 minutes if stimulation is greatly reduced, indicating that they are sleep-deprived. When these people are encouraged or allowed to sleep extra hours, their daytime alertness and their intellectual abilities improve significantly. Although sleep requirements vary among individuals, some adults need as much as 9 hours of sleep to feel fully refreshed and alert.

Nearly everyone, at some time in life, has trouble falling asleep or staying asleep—a condition known as **insomnia.** Insomnia can last anywhere from a few nights to even years. The most common causes of insomnia are lifestyle factors, such as high caffeine or alcohol intake before sleep; medical problems, such as a breathing disorder; and psychological stress. Chronic sleep problems can themselves become a source of stress, as the person frets and worries about not getting enough sleep.

Most people can overcome insomnia by discovering the cause of poor sleep and taking steps to remedy the situation. Insomnia that lasts for more than 6 months and interferes with daytime functioning calls for consultation with a physician. Sleeping pills are not recommended for chronic insomnia because they can be habit-forming; they also lose their effectiveness over time.

If you're bothered by insomnia, here are some tips for getting a better night's sleep:

- Determine how much sleep you need to feel refreshed the next day, and don't sleep longer than that (but do make sure you get enough).
- Go to bed at the same time every night and, more importantly, get up at the same time every morning, 7 days a week, regardless of how much sleep you got. Don't nap during the day.
- Exercise every day, but not too close to bedtime. Your metabolism takes up to 6 hours to slow down after exercise.
- Avoid tobacco (nicotine is a stimulant), caffeine in the later part of the day, and alcohol before bedtime (it causes disturbed, fragmented sleep).
- Have a light snack before bedtime; you'll sleep better if you're not hungry.
- Deal with worries well before bedtime. Try writing them down, along with some possible solutions, and then allow yourself to forget about them until the next day.
- Use your bed only for sleep. Don't eat, read, study, or watch TV in bed.
- Relax before bedtime with a warm bath (not too close to bedtime; allow about 2 hours for your metabolism to slow down afterward), a book, music, or some relaxation exercises. Don't lie down in bed until you're sleepy.
- If you don't fall asleep within 15–20 minutes, or if you wake up and can't fall asleep again, get out of bed, leave the room if possible, and do something boring until you feel sleepy.
- Keep a perspective on your plight. Losing a night's sleep isn't the end of the world. Getting upset only makes it harder to fall asleep. Relax, and trust in your body's natural ability to drift off to sleep.

may experience flare-ups of symptoms during episodes of stress.

Other Health Problems

Other diseases and conditions that may be triggered or aggravated by stress include the following:

TERMS

insomnia The inability to obtain adequate sleep.

- *Colds and other infections.* Stress leaves people more vulnerable to contracting an infection and less capable of fighting one off.
- *Asthma and allergies.* Stress is a trigger or aggravator of asthma, eczema, and other allergies in people who normally suffer from allergic reactions.
- *Headaches, migraines, and stomach and muscle aches.* The complex biochemical reactions that accompany the stress response cause changes in muscle tension, digestion, and blood vessels, including vessels in the brain.
- *Insomnia and fatigue.* Stress puts the body into a state

of alarm, pumped with neurochemicals that maintain alertness—and ward off sleep. Sleep disruption in turn can produce fatigue (see the box "The Mystery of Sleep").

- *Anxiety and depression.* Chemicals released in the brain and other parts of the body during the stress response cause emotional as well as physical changes. Moreover, many stressors—an earthquake, for example, or the death of a loved one—are inherently anxiety-producing, depressing, or both. If stress is severe or prolonged, emotional symptoms can become chronic. Panic attacks or post-traumatic stress disorder develop in some individuals.
- *Injuries.* Faced with unaccustomed stress, people may forget to wear seat belts or to turn off the stove. On-the-job injuries, including repetitive-strain injuries such as carpal tunnel syndrome, are linked to job stress.
- *Cancer.* By compromising immune function, stress may increase a person's chance of developing cancer and decrease her or his chance of surviving it.

MANAGING STRESS

Stress is an inevitable part of life, and it's not going to go away. The issue is not how to avoid stress but rather how to manage it. While there are many approaches and specific techniques, in general the fundamental principles of physical and psychological fitness are themselves effective strategies for managing stress.

Exercise

One recent study found that taking a long walk can be effective at reducing anxiety and blood pressure. Another study showed that a brisk walk of as little as 10 minutes' duration can leave people feeling more relaxed and energetic for up to 2 hours. Regular exercise has even more benefits. Researchers have found that people who exercise regularly react with milder physical stress responses before, during, and after exposure to stressors, and that their overall sense of well-being increases as well. Although even light exercise—a brisk walk, an easy bike outing—can have a beneficial effect, stress reduction is a significant motivator for maintaining the integrated fitness program recommended in this book.

One warning: For some people, exercise can become just one more stressor in a highly stressed life. People who exercise compulsively risk overtraining, a condition characterized by fatigue, irritability, depression, and diminished athletic performance. An overly strenuous exercise program can even make a person sick by compromising immune function. For the details of a safe and effective exercise program, refer to Chapter 7.

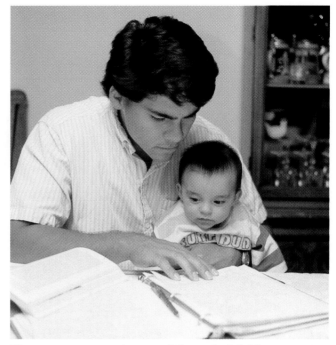

The commitments and responsibilities of adult life are ongoing sources of stress. Time-management skills, including careful planning and scheduling, can help people like this young father balance the challenges of work, school, and family.

Nutrition

As discussed in Chapters 8 and 9, a healthy, balanced diet designed in conjunction with a sensible exercise program and the principles of weight management will supply the energy needed to cope with stress. Two additional points are particularly important for stress management:

1. *Limit or avoid caffeine.* Although 1–2 cups of coffee a day probably won't hurt, caffeine is a mildly addictive stimulant that leaves some people jittery, irritable, and unable to sleep. Tea, cola, and some other soft drinks, chocolate, and more than a thousand over-the-counter drugs, including cold remedies, aspirin, and weight-loss preparations, also contain caffeine in varying amounts.
2. *Avoid the high-potency vitamin compounds and amino acid supplements designated as "stress formulas."* These capsules or tablets are worthless for reducing tension or anxiety and might actually increase stress through overdosing the body.

Time Management

Learning to manage your time successfully can be crucial to coping with everyday stressors. Overcommitment, procrastination, and even boredom are significant stressors for many people. Along with gaining control of nutrition and exercise to maintain a healthy energy balance, time management is an important element in a fitness and wellness program, leading indirectly, but nevertheless

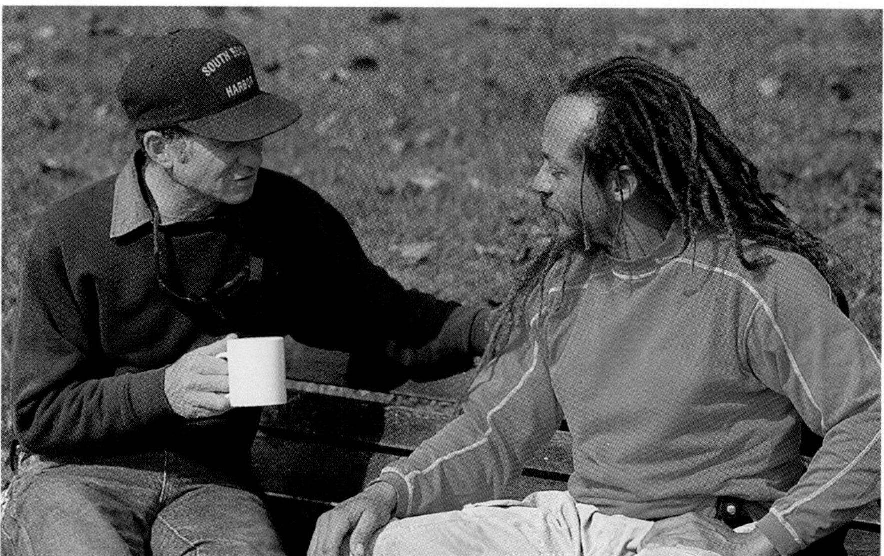

A strong social support network is an important part of stress management. By sharing their thoughts and feelings, these friends can help each other handle the stressors in their lives more successfully.

significantly, to physical fitness and mental health. The Behavior Change Activity at the end of this chapter provides strategies for improving your time-management skills.

Social Support

People need people. Sharing fears, frustrations, and joys not only makes life richer but also seems to contribute—like time management, indirectly but significantly—to the well-being of body and mind. Research supports this conclusion: One study of college students living in overcrowded apartments, for example, found that those with a strong social support system were less distressed by their cramped quarters than were the "loners" who navigated life's challenges on their own. Other studies have shown that married people live longer than single people and have lower death rates from a wide range of conditions. And people infected with HIV remain symptom-free longer if they have a strong social support network. The crucial common denominator in all these findings is the meaningful connection with others. For more on building up your social network, see the box "Social Support."

Relaxation Techniques

According to Herbert Benson of Harvard Medical School, relaxation techniques can trigger the **relaxation response,** a physiological state characterized by a feeling of warmth and quiet mental alertness. This response is the opposite of the fight-or-flight reaction. When the relaxation response is triggered, heart rate, breathing, and metabolism slow down; blood flow to the brain and skin increases; and brain waves shift from an alert beta rhythm to a relaxed alpha rhythm.

The techniques described below, and in the box "Stress-Management Techniques from Around the World" (p. 248), are among the most popular techniques and the easiest to learn. Other techniques, such as massage, self-hypnosis, and biofeedback, require a partner or professional training or assistance. Nevertheless, all these techniques take practice, sometimes several weeks before the benefits become noticeable in everyday life.

Progressive Relaxation In this simple relaxation technique, you simply tense, then relax, the muscles of the body, one by one. Also known as deep muscle relaxation, this technique focuses attention on the muscle tension that occurs when the body is experiencing stress. Consciously relaxing tensed muscles sends a message to other body systems to reduce the stress response.

To practice progressive relaxation, begin by inhaling as you contract your right fist. Then exhale as you release your fist. Repeat. Contract and relax your right bicep. Repeat. Do the same using your left arm. Then, working from forehead to feet, contract and relax other muscles. Repeat each contraction at least once, inhaling as you tense and exhaling as you relax. To speed up the process, tense and relax more muscles at one time—for example, both arms simultaneously. With practice you'll be able to relax quickly by simply clenching and releasing only your fists.

Visualization Visualization, also known as using imagery, is so effective in enhancing sports performance that it has become a part of the curriculum at training camps for U.S. Olympic athletes. This same technique can be

TERMS

relaxation response A physiological state characterized by a feeling of warmth and quiet mental alertness.

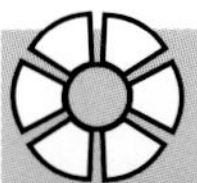

WELLNESS CONNECTION
Social Support

Social support can benefit both your emotional and your physical health. Meaningful connections with others can play a key role in stress management and overall wellness. A sense of isolation can lead to chronic stress, which in turn can increase one's susceptibility to temporary illnesses like colds and to chronic illnesses like heart disease and cancer. Social isolation can be as significant to mortality rates as such factors as smoking, high blood pressure, and obesity.

How strong is your social network? Read through the following statements relating to social support, and check those that are true for you:

____ I keep in daily contact with other people.

____ I have at least one friend or relative I can talk to about almost anything.

____ When I'm troubled or upset, I have a friend or relative I feel comfortable turning to for help and support.

____ I keep in regular contact with a group of friends and/or with members of my extended family.

____ I am active in a community, religious, or other service organization.

____ I am involved in a sports, hobby, or activity group.

If your responses indicate a lack of social contact and support, consider building up your social network. There are a variety of things you can do to strengthen your social ties:

- *Foster friendships.* Keep in regular contact with your friends. Offer respect, trust, and acceptance, and provide help and support in times of need. Express appreciation for your friends.
- *Keep your family ties strong.* Stay in touch with the family members you feel close to. Take time out to be involved in family activities and to attend family celebrations.
- *Get involved with a group.* Do volunteer work, take a class, attend a lecture series. These types of activities can give you a sense of security, a place to talk about your feelings or concerns, and a way to build new friendships. Choose activities that are meaningful to you and that include direct involvement with other people.
- *Build your communication skills.* The more you share your feelings with others, the closer the bonds between you will become. When others are speaking, be a considerate and attentive listener. (Chapter 15 includes more information on effective communication.)

Individual relationships will change over the course of your life, but it's never too late to build friendships or to become involved in your community. Your investment of time and energy in your social network will pay off—in a brighter outlook now and in better health for the future.

Sources: Social networks: The company you keep can keep you healthy. 1995. *Mayo Clinic Health Letter,* April. Ornish, D. 1991. The healing power of love. *Prevention,* February. House, J. S., K. R. Landis, and D. Umberson. 1988. Social relationships and health. *Science* 241: 540–544.

used to induce relaxation, to help change habits, or to improve performance on an exam, on stage, or on a playing field.

To practice visualization, imagine yourself floating on a cloud, sitting on a mountaintop, or lying in a meadow. Try to identify all the perceptible qualities of the environment—sight, sound, temperature, smell, and so on. Your body will respond as if your imagery were real.

An alternative is to close your eyes and imagine a deep purple light filling your body. Then change the color into a soothing gold. As the color lightens, so should your distress. Imagery can also enhance performance: Visualize yourself succeeding at a task that worries you.

Cognitive Techniques

Certain thought patterns and ways of thinking, including ideas, beliefs, and perceptions, can contribute to stress and have a negative impact on health. But other habits of mind, if practiced with patience and consistency, can help break unhealthy thought patterns. Below are some suggestions for changing destructive thinking:

- Reduce expectations; they often restrict experience and lead to disappointment. Try to accept life as it comes.
- Monitor your self-talk, and attempt to minimize hostile, critical, suspicious, cynical, and self-deprecating thoughts.
- Weed out trivia, keeping your memory free for essential details.
- Live in the present; clear your mind of old debris and fears for the future in order to enjoy life as it is now.
- "Go with the flow." Accept what you can't change, forgive faults, be flexible.
- Laugh. Seek out therapeutic humor (not dark, gruesome, or offensive humor, which is an unconscious means of dealing with fears). Laughter can temporarily elevate the heart rate, aid digestion, relax muscles, ease pain, and trigger the release of endorphins.

DIMENSIONS OF DIVERSITY
Stress-Management Techniques from Around the World

The origins of techniques for relaxation span many continents and many centuries. Three techniques that originated outside Western culture but are growing in popularity in the United States are meditation, hatha yoga, and t'ai chi ch'uan. Although you may not choose to adopt the philosophical bases of these techniques, all of them can help you manage stress by promoting the relaxation response.

Meditation

At its most basic level, meditation, or self-reflective thought, involves quieting or emptying the mind in order to achieve deep relaxation. Some practitioners of meditation view it on a deeper level as a means of focusing concentration, increasing self-awareness, and bringing enlightenment to their lives. The origins of meditation can be traced back to the sixth century B.C. in Asia. Meditation has been integrated into the practices of several religions—Buddhism, Hinduism, Confucianism, and Taoism—but it is not a religion itself, nor does its practice require any special knowledge, belief, or background.

There are two general styles of meditation, centered around different ways of quieting the mind. In exclusive meditation, one focuses on a single word or thought, eliminating all others. In inclusive meditation, the mind is allowed to wander uncontrolled from thought to thought, but one must observe these thoughts in a detached way, without judgment or emotion.

Exclusive meditation tends to be easier to learn. Several years ago, Herbert Benson developed a simple, practical technique for eliciting the relaxation response using exclusive meditation:

1. Pick a word, phrase, or object to focus on. You can choose a word or phrase that has a deep meaning for you, but any word or phrase will work. In Zen meditation, the word *mu* (literally, "absolutely nothing") is often used. Some meditators prefer to focus on their breathing.
2. Sit comfortably in a quiet place, and close your eyes if you're not focusing on an object.
3. Relax your muscles.
4. Breathe slowly and naturally. If you're using a focus word or phrase, silently repeat it each time you exhale. If you're using an object, focus on it as you breathe.
5. Keep your attitude passive. Disregard thoughts that drift in.
6. Continue for 10–20 minutes, once or twice a day.
7. After you've finished, sit quietly for a few minutes with your eyes closed, then open. Then stand up.

Allow relaxation to occur at its own pace; don't try to force it. Don't be surprised if you can't tune your mind out for more than a few seconds at a time. It's nothing to get angry about. The more you ignore the intrusions, the easier it will become.

If you want to time your session, peek at a watch or clock occasionally, but don't set a jarring alarm.

The technique works best on an empty stomach, before a meal or about 2 hours after eating. Avoid times of day when you're tired, unless you want to fall asleep.

Although you'll feel refreshed even after the first session, it may take a month or more to get noticeable results. Be pa-

Clear Communication

Clear, honest, open communication is a crucial component of healthy relationships. Poor communication can cause feelings of anger and frustration and significantly increase your levels of stress. The people who make up your social support system cannot respond to specific needs if they don't know what those needs are. To improve your communication skills, see the box "Clear Communication."

GETTING HELP

You can use the principles of behavioral self-management described in Chapter 1 to create a stress-management program tailored specifically to your needs. The starting point of a successful program is to listen to your body. When you learn to recognize the stress response and the emotions and thoughts that accompany it, you'll be in a position to take charge of how you handle stress. Labs 10-1 and 10-2 can guide you in identifying and finding ways to cope with stress-inducing situations.

If you have attempted to fashion a stress-management program to cope with the stressors in your life but still feel overwhelmed, you may want to seek outside help in the form of a peer counselor, a support group, or psychotherapy. Peer counseling, often available on college campuses, is usually staffed by volunteer students who have received special training that emphasizes confidentiality. Peer counselors can steer those seeking help to appropriate community resources, or just offer sympathetic listening.

Support groups are typically organized around a particular issue or problem; for example, all group members might be entering a new school, reentering school after a long interruption, struggling with single parenting, experiencing eating disorders, or coping with particular kinds of trauma. Simply voicing concerns that others share can relieve stress.

Psychotherapy, especially a short-term course of ses-

DIMENSIONS OF DIVERSITY
Stress-Management Techniques from Around the World (continued)

tient. Eventually the relaxation response will become so natural that it will occur spontaneously, or on demand, when you sit quietly for a few moments.

Hatha Yoga

Yoga is an ancient Sanskrit word meaning "union"; it refers specifically to the union of mind, body, and soul. The development and practice of yoga are rooted in the Hindu philosophy of spiritual enlightenment. The founders of yoga developed a system of physical postures, called *asanas,* designed to cleanse the body, unlock energy paths, and raise the level of consciousness.

There are many different yoga styles, each with its own interpretation of the path to enlightenment. Hatha yoga, the most common style practiced in the United States, emphasizes physical balance and breathing control. It integrates components of flexibility, muscular strength and endurance, and muscle relaxation; it also sometimes serves as a preliminary to meditation.

A session of hatha yoga typically involves a series of *asanas* that stretch and relax different parts of the body. The emphasis is on breathing, stretching, and balance. There are hundreds of different *asanas,* and they must be performed correctly in order to be beneficial. For this reason, qualified instruction is recommended, particularly for beginners. Yoga classes are offered through many community recreation centers, YMCAs and YWCAs, and private clubs. Regardless of whether an individual accepts the philosophy and symbolism of different *asanas,* the practice of yoga can induce the relaxation response as well as develop flexibility, muscular strength and endurance, and body awareness.

T'ai Chi Ch'uan

A martial art that developed in China, t'ai chi ch'uan is a system of self-defense that incorporates philosophical concepts from Taoism and Confucianism. An important part of this philosophy is *chi,* an energy force that surrounds and permeates all things. In addition to serving as a means of self-defense, the goal of t'ai chi ch'uan is to bring the body into balance and harmony with this universal energy, in order to promote health and spiritual growth. It teaches practitioners to remain calm and centered, to conserve and concentrate energy, and to harmonize with fear. T'ai chi ch'uan seeks to manipulate force by becoming part of it—"going with the flow," so to speak.

T'ai chi ch'uan is considered the gentlest of the martial arts. Instead of using quick and powerful movements, t'ai chi ch'uan consists of a series of slow, fluid, elegant movements, which reinforce the idea of moving *with* rather than *against* the stressors of everyday life. The practice of t'ai chi ch'uan promotes relaxation and concentration as well as the development of body awareness, balance, muscular strength, and flexibility. It usually takes some time and practice to reap the stress-management benefits of t'ai chi ch'uan, and, like yoga, it's best to begin with some qualified instruction.

Sources: Adapted from Seaward, B. L. 1994. *Managing Stress: Principles and Strategies for Health and Wellbeing.* Boston: Jones and Bartlett. Benson, H., with W. Proctor. 1984. *Beyond the Relaxation Response.* New York: Times Books.

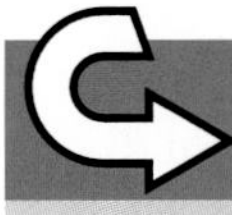

TACTICS AND TIPS
Clear Communication

- When you want to communicate with someone, state your case as clearly as you can. Use "I messages." Ask for what you want directly, instead of hoping that the other person will read your mind. Say what you feel and what you want to have happen.
- Be specific about the particular behaviors you like or don't like. Avoid generalizations such as, "You always . . ." and "You never . . . ."
- Avoid blaming, accusing, and belittling. Even if you are 100% right, you have little to gain by putting the other person down. Studies have shown that when people feel criticized or attacked, they are less able to think rationally or solve problems correctly.
- As a listener, don't make assumptions about what the other person is saying. Ask for clarifications. Don't play "fill in the blanks."
- Develop the skill of reflective listening. Don't judge, blame, or evaluate. Remember, the person may just need to have you there in order to sort out feelings. By jumping in right away to "fix" the problem, you may actually be cutting off communication.
- When you listen, be sure you are *really* listening, not off somewhere rehearsing your reply! Try to tune in to the other person's feelings and check them out as well. Do let the other person know that you value what he or she is saying and want to understand. Respect for the other person is the cornerstone of clear communication.

sions, can also be tremendously helpful in dealing with stress-related problems. Not all therapists are right for all people, so it's a good idea to shop around for a compatible psychotherapist with reasonable fees.

? COMMON QUESTIONS ANSWERED

Are there any relaxation techniques I can use in response to an immediate stressor? There are various strategies for dealing with stressors on the spot. Try some of the following to see which ones work best for you:

- Breathe slowly and deeply while concentrating on your breathing. Hold your breath for a few seconds after each inhalation, or exhale for a longer time than usual. Feel the muscles of your body relax more with each breath.
- Do a full-body stretch while standing or sitting. Stretch your arms out to the sides and then reach them as far as possible over your head. Rotate your body from the waist. Bend over as far as is comfortable for you.
- Do a partial session of progressive muscle relaxation. Tense and then relax some of the muscles in your body. Focus on the muscles that are stiff or tense. Shake out your arms and legs.
- Take a short, brisk walk (3–5 minutes). Breathe deeply.
- Engage in realistic self-talk about the stressor (see Chapter 9). Mentally rehearse dealing successfully with the stressor. As an alternative, focus your mind on some other activity.

Can stress cause a person to become depressed? Although not often the sole factor in the development of depression, poor stress-management skills can contribute to depression, and depression can be a sign of excess stress. Depression is more than just having a bad day; it is a serious disorder characterized by a negative self-concept, meaning that a person feels unloved and ineffective. Poor stress-management skills can reinforce a negative self-concept by sabotaging personal relationships and academic and professional performance. In addition to a negative self-concept, severe depression can include the following:

- Pervasive feelings of sadness and hopelessness
- Loss of pleasure in usual activities
- Poor appetite and weight loss
- Insomnia, especially early morning awakening
- Restlessness or lethargy
- Thoughts of worthlessness and guilt
- An inability to concentrate
- Thoughts of suicide

Not all of these symptoms are present in everyone who is depressed, but most do experience a loss of interest or pleasure in their usual activities. In some cases, depression, like severe stress, is a clear-cut reaction to specific events, such as the loss of a loved one or failing in school or work. In other cases, no trigger event is obvious.

Suicide is a primary danger of severe depression. Danger signals of suicide include expressing the wish to be dead; revealing contemplated suicide methods; increasing social withdrawal and isolation; and a sudden, inexplicable lightening of mood (which can indicate the person has finally decided to commit suicide). If you are severely depressed or know someone who is, expert help from a mental health professional is essential. Most communities have emergency help available, often in the form of a hotline telephone counseling service. Large colleges typically have health services and counseling centers that can provide help; professional therapists can also be located through the local telephone book.

SUMMARY

- Stress is the collective physiological and emotional responses to any stressor. Physiological responses to stressors are the same for everyone.
- The three stages of the general adaptation syndrome are controlled by the autonomic nervous system. In the alarm stage, the sympathetic nervous system mobilizes the body for action; in the resistance stage, the parasympathetic nervous system halts the alarm reaction and lets the body return to normal.
- The exhaustion stage occurs if the body's reserves of energy are depleted in successive stress responses; it is characterized by distorted perceptions and disorganized thinking.
- Behavioral responses to stress are controlled by the somatic nervous system and fall under a person's conscious control.
- People who have many stressors in their lives or who handle stress poorly are at risk for a wide range of health problems, including high blood pressure, atherosclerosis, and immune system impairment; in addition, many other conditions can be aggravated.
- Ways of managing stress include regular exercise; good nutrition; time management; support from other people; relaxation techniques such as progressive muscle relaxation, visualization, meditation, yoga, and t'ai chi ch'uan; modified thought patterns; and clear communication.
- If a personal program for stress management doesn't work, peer counseling, support groups, and psychotherapy are available.

BEHAVIOR CHANGE ACTIVITY

Managing Your Time Successfully

"Too little time" is a common excuse for not exercising or engaging in other healthy behaviors. Learning to manage your time successfully is crucial if you are to maintain a wellness lifestyle. The first step is to examine how you are currently spending your time. Use your health journal to track your current activities; use a grid broken into 15-, 20-, or 30-minute blocks. Next, list each category of activity and the total time you engaged in it on a given day on the chart below (for example, sleeping, 7 hours; eating, 1.5 hours; studying, 3 hours; working, 3 hours; and so on).

Take a close look at your list of activities. Successful time management is based on prioritization. Rank each of your activities according to how important it is to you: essential (A), somewhat important (B), or not important (C). Based on these priority rankings, make changes in your schedule by adding and subtracting hours from different categories of activities. Add your new activities to the list, and assign a priority and time period to each.

Activity	Current Total Duration	Priority	Goal Total Duration

Prioritizing in this manner will involve tradeoffs. For example, you may choose to reduce the amount of time you spend watching television, listening to music, and chatting on the telephone while you increase the amount of time you spend sleeping, studying, and exercising. Don't feel that you have to miss out on anything you enjoy. You can get more from less time by focusing on what you are doing. Strategies for managing time more productively and creatively include the following:

- *Schedule tasks for peak efficiency.* You've probably noticed that you're more productive at certain times of the day (or night). Schedule as many of your tasks for those hours as you can.
- *Avoid unnecessary distractions and interruptions.* Find a pleasant setting where you can focus on your current activity.
- *Listen actively and effectively.* Good communication can prevent misunderstandings and save time in the long run.
- *Set realistic goals.* Attainable goals will spur you on. Impossible goals, by definition, generate frustration and failure. Write down your goals, then fully commit yourself to achieving them.
- *Budget enough time.* For each project you undertake, calculate how long it will take to complete. Then add another 10–15% as a buffer against mistakes or unanticipated problems. If you wind up with extra free time, use it to do something you particularly enjoy.
- *Divide long-term goals into short-term ones.* Instead of waiting for or relying on large blocks of time, use short time periods to start a project or keep one going. For example, suppose you have a 50-page report due and are about to panic. Divide the assignment into three tasks: research, outlining, and writing. Then budget enough half-hour or hour-long time slots to complete each task. Steady progress will keep you encouraged and committed.
- *Visualize the achievement of your goals.* By mentally rehearsing your performance of a task, you can reach your goal more smoothly.

(continued)

- *Delegate responsibility.* Asking for help when you have too much to do is no cop-out; it's good time management. Just don't delegate to others the jobs you know you should do yourself. Believe that others can complete tasks as well as you can.
- *Say no when necessary.* If the demands made on you don't seem reasonable, say no—tactfully, but without guilt or apology.
- *Give yourself a break.* Allow time for fun—free, unstructured time when you ignore the clock. Don't consider this a waste of time. Fun activities renew you and enable you to work more efficiently.

FOR MORE INFORMATION

You'll probably find courses and seminars on your campus or in your community that teach ways of dealing with stress. Some may be specifically devoted to such issues as time management, test taking, or public speaking. The books listed below provide information on a variety of stress-related topics and tips for handling stress.

Antonovsky, A. 1990. *Learned Resourcefulness.* New York: Springer-Verlag. *Presents a variety of strategies for managing and coping with stress and increasing self-control and adaptive behavior.*

Dement, W. C. 1992. *The Sleepwatchers.* Stanford, Calif.: Stanford Alumni Association. *An entertaining discussion of sleep and dreams by one of the world's foremost authorities on sleep.*

Kabat-Zinn, J. 1990. *Full Catastrophe Living (Using the Wisdom of Your Body and Mind to Face Stress, Pain, and Illness).* New York: Dell. *Describes the program of the Stress Reduction Clinic at the University of Massachusetts Medical Center, which teaches the application of meditation to counteract the deleterious effects on health of stress from physical and emotional pain, work, other people, time pressure, and other sources.*

Matheny, K. B., and R. J. Riordan. 1992. *Stress and Strategies for Lifestyle Management.* Atlanta: Georgia State University Business Press. *Practical and realistic insights into managing stress and changing maladaptive lifestyles, with separate chapters on stress inoculation and creating stress-free relationships.*

Schafer, W. 1992. *Stress Management for Wellness.* 2d ed. Fort Worth: Harcourt Brace Jovanovich. *Basic information on stress and wellness and many different stress-management techniques, with a separate chapter on college stress.*

Seaward, B. L. 1994. *Managing Stress: Principles and Strategies for Health and Wellbeing.* Boston: Jones and Bartlett. *A comprehensive resource of stress-management techniques.*

Spiegel, D. 1993. *Living Beyond Limits.* New York: Random House. *A pioneering Stanford University School of Medicine researcher describes how he showed that support groups can help breast cancer patients live longer, higher-quality lives.*

If you're experiencing severe symptoms of stress or if your symptoms last for several weeks, you should consult a physician or counselor. Most campuses provide student psychological services that are free and informal. Your student health center may also provide peer counseling.

SELECTED BIBLIOGRAPHY

Adler, N., and K. Matthews. 1994. Health psychology: Why do some people get sick and some stay well? *Annual Review of Psychology* 45:229–259.

American College of Sports Medicine. 1990. *The Recommended Quantity and Quality of Exercise for Developing and Maintaining Cardiorespiratory and Muscular Fitness in Healthy Adults.* Indianapolis: American College of Sports Medicine.

Birmaher, B., et al. 1994. Cellular immunity in depresssed, conduct disorder, and normal adolescents: Role of adverse life events. *Journal of the American Academy of Child and Adolescent Psychiatry* 33(5): 671–678.

Burka, J. B. 1990. *Procrastination: Why You Do It, What to Do About It.* Reading, Mass.: Addison-Wesley.

Cohen, S., et al. 1991. Psychological stress and susceptibility to the common cold. *New England Journal of Medicine* 325(9): 606–612.

Flach, J., and L. Seachrist. 1994. Mind-body meld may boost immunity. *Journal of the National Cancer Institute* 86(4): 256–258.

Glaser, R., et al. 1993. Stress and the memory T-cell response to the Epstein-Barr virus in healthy medical students. *Health Psychology* 12(6): 435–442.

Hauri, P., and S. Linde. 1990. *No More Sleepless Nights.* New York: Wiley.

How to beat insomnia. 1994. *Consumer Reports on Health,* March.

Johansson, N. 1991. Effectiveness of a stress management program in reducing anxiety and depression in nursing students. *College Health* 40:125–129.

Lepore, S., et al. 1991. The dynamic role of social support in the link between chronic stress and psychological distress. *Journal of Personality and Social Psychology* 61(6): 899–909.

Lutgendorf, S. K., et al. 1994. Changes in cognitive coping strategies predict EBV-antibody titre change following a stressor disclosure induction. *Journal of Psychosomatic Research* 38(1): 63–78.

Mitler, E. A., and M. Merrill. 1990. *100 Questions About Sleep and Dreams.* Del Mar, Calif.: Wakefulness-Sleep Education and Research Foundation.

Ornstein, R., and D. Sobel. 1989. *Healthy Pleasures.* Reading, Mass.: Addison-Wesley.

Peterson, M. L., et al. 1991. Stress and the pathogenesis of infectious disease. *Reviews of Infectious Diseases* 13:710–720.

Selye, H. 1976. *The Stress of Life,* rev. ed. New York: McGraw-Hill.

Selye, H. 1979. Stress: The basis of illness. In *Inner Balance: The Power of Holistic Health,* ed. E. M. Goldwag. Englewood Cliffs, N.J.: Prentice-Hall.

Sleep: Are you getting enough? 1994. *Harvard Women's Health Watch,* March.

Name ______________________ Section ______________ Date ______________

LAB 10-1 *Identifying Your Stressors*

Signals of Stress

To identify the sources of stress in your life, you must first be able to identify the signals of stress. Put a check mark next to any of the following signs you have experienced in the last month.

Emotional Signs

_____ Tendency to be irritable or aggressive
_____ Tendency to feel anxious, fearful, or edgy
_____ Hyperexcitability, impulsiveness, or emotional instability
_____ Depression
_____ Frequent feelings of boredom
_____ Inability to concentrate
_____ Fatigue

Behavioral Signs

_____ Increased use of tobacco, alcohol, or other drugs
_____ Excessive TV watching
_____ Sleep disturbances or excessive sleep
_____ Overeating or undereating
_____ Sexual problems
_____ Crying or yelling
_____ Job or school burnout
_____ Spouse or child abuse
_____ Panic attack

Physical Signs

_____ Pounding heart
_____ Trembling with nervous tics
_____ Grinding of teeth
_____ Dry mouth
_____ Excessive perspiration
_____ Gastrointestinal problems (diarrhea, constipation, indigestion, queasy stomach)
_____ Stiff neck or aching lower back
_____ Migraine or tension headaches
_____ Frequent colds or low-grade infections
_____ Cold hands and feet
_____ Allergy or asthma attacks
_____ Skin problems (e.g., hives, eczema, psoriasis)

Possible Stressful Events

Listed below, in order of probable severity of effect, are 35 life events that cause stress. Put a check mark next to any item you have experienced recently or expect to experience soon. If you find you've checked several items, take time out from your daily routine to develop and cultivate your coping skills.

_____ Death of a close family member
_____ Divorce or separation from mate
_____ Detention in jail or other institution
_____ Major personal injury or illness
_____ Death of a close friend
_____ Divorce between parents
_____ Marriage
_____ Being fired from job or expelled from school
_____ Retirement
_____ Change in health of a family member
_____ Pregnancy
_____ Being a victim of crime
_____ Sexual difficulties
_____ Gaining new family members (through birth, adoption, older person moving in, etc.)
_____ New boyfriend or girlfriend
_____ Major business or academic readjustment (merger, change of job or major, failing course)
_____ Major change in financial state (a lot worse or a lot better off than before)
_____ Taking out a loan or mortgage for school or a major purchase
_____ Trouble with parents, spouse, or girlfriend or boyfriend
_____ Outstanding personal achievement
_____ Graduation
_____ First quarter/semester in college
_____ Denied admission to program or school
_____ Change in living conditions
_____ Serious argument with instructor, friend, or roommate
_____ Lower grades than expected
_____ Major change in working hours or conditions, or increased workload at school
_____ Major change in recreational, social, or church activities
_____ Major change in sleeping or eating habits
_____ Denied admission to required course
_____ Taking out a loan for a lesser purchase (e.g., a car, TV, or freezer)
_____ Chronic car trouble
_____ Change in number of family get-togethers
_____ Vacation
_____ Minor violation of the law (traffic tickets, etc.)

LABORATORY ACTIVITIES

Weekly Stress Log

Now that you are familiar with the signals of stress, complete the weekly stress log by assigning ratings for each hour of the day (use the key given below). Daily totals, as well as totals for specific times of the day, will indicate patterns in your stress levels and help you identify external and internal sources of stress. Your weekly total (the sum of the daily totals) will give you a sense of your overall level of stress.

	A.M.							P.M.												
	6	7	8	9	10	11	12	1	2	3	4	5	6	7	8	9	10	11	12	Total
Monday																				
Tuesday																				
Wednesday																				
Thursday																				
Friday																				
Saturday																				
Sunday																				
Total																				

Weekly Total____________

Key

1: No anxiety; general feeling of well-being
2: Mild anxiety; no interference with activity
3: Moderate anxiety; specific signal(s) of stress present
4: High anxiety; interference with activity
5: Very high anxiety and panic reactions; general inability to engage in activity

Identifying Sources of Stress

External stressors: List several people, places, or events that caused you a significant amount of discomfort this week.

____

____

____

Internal stressors: Make a list of any recurring thoughts or worries that produced feelings of discomfort this week.

____

____

____

To monitor your progress toward your goal, enter the results of this lab in the Preprogram Assessment column of Lab 15-2. After several weeks of a stress-management program, do this lab again and enter the results in the Post-program Assessment column of Lab 15-2. How do the results compare?

Name ______________________ Section ____________ Date ____________

LAB 10-2 *Stress-Management Techniques*

Equipment None
Preparation Wear comfortable clothing

Choose two relaxation techniques described in this chapter. If a taped recording is available for progressive relaxation or visualization, these techniques can be performed by your entire class as a group. Make sure you perform the techniques in a comfortable position in a quiet room.

List the techniques you tried:

1. ____

2. ____

How did you feel before you tried these techniques?

____

____

____

____

What did you think, or how did you feel, as you performed each of the techniques you tried?

1. ____

____

____

2. ____

____

____

How did you feel after you tried these techniques?

____

____

____

11

Cardiovascular Health

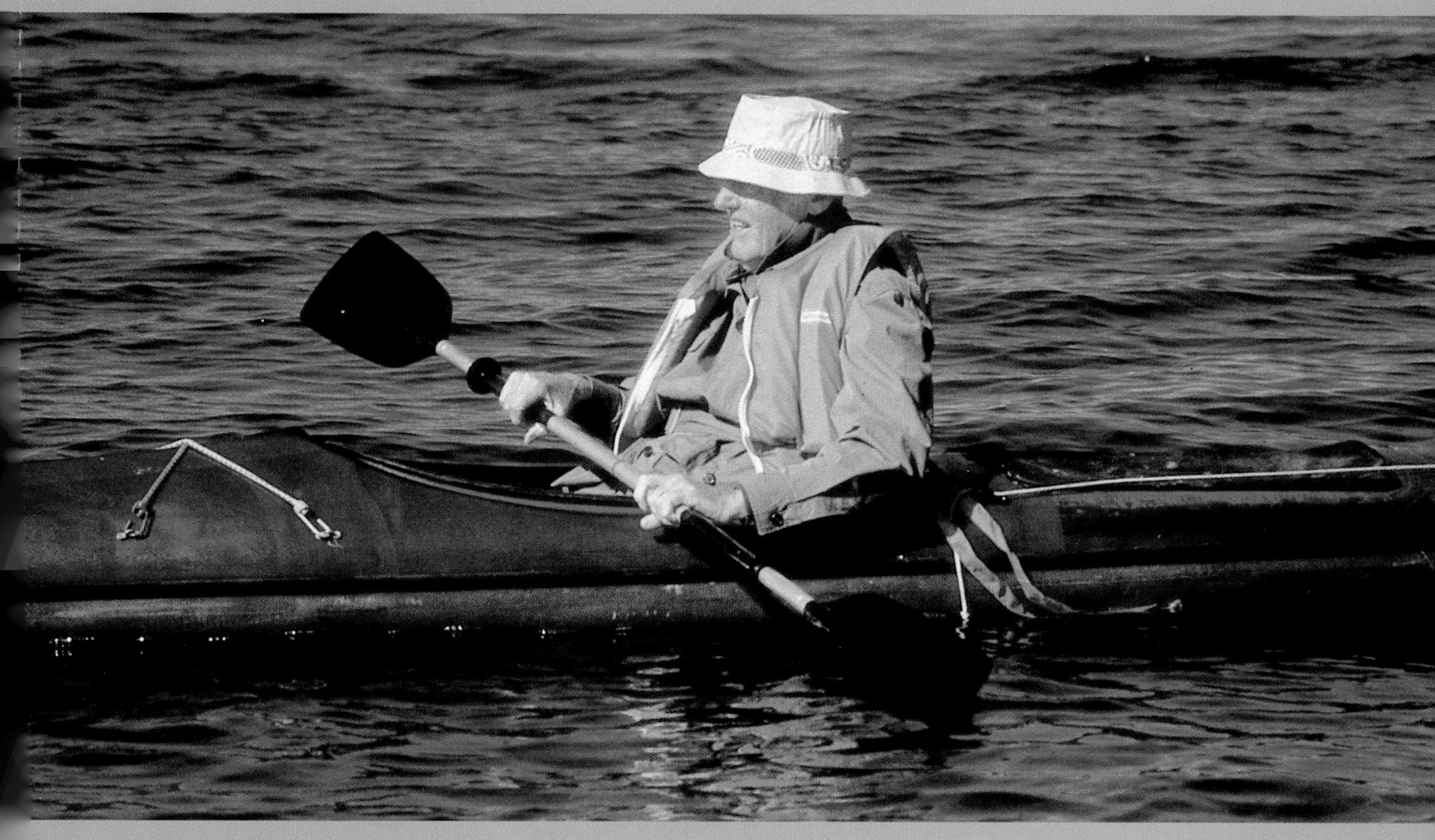

LOOKING AHEAD

After reading this chapter, you should be able to answer these questions about cardiovascular health and disease:

- How does the cardiovascular system pump and circulate blood throughout the body?
- What are the major forms of cardiovascular disease, and how do they develop?
- What controllable and uncontrollable risk factors are associated with cardiovascular disease?
- What steps can people take to keep their cardiovascular system healthy and avoid cardiovascular disease?

Cardiovascular disease (CVD) is the leading cause of death in the United States; nearly half of all Americans alive today will die from CVD. As discussed in Chapter 1, much of the incidence of CVD is attributable to the American way of life. Too many Americans eat a high-fat diet, are overweight and sedentary, smoke cigarettes, manage stress ineffectively, have uncontrolled high blood pressure or high cholesterol levels, and don't know the signs of CVD. Not all risk factors for CVD are controllable—some people have an inherited tendency toward high cholesterol levels, for example—but many are within the control of the individual.

This chapter explains the cardiovascular system and the major forms of CVD, including hypertension, atherosclerosis, and stroke. It also considers the factors that put people at risk for CVD. Most importantly, it explains the steps individuals can take to protect their hearts and promote cardiovascular health throughout their lives.

THE CARDIOVASCULAR SYSTEM

The cardiovascular system consists of the heart and blood vessels (veins, arteries, and capillaries); together, they pump and circulate blood throughout the body. A person weighing 150 pounds has about 5 quarts of blood, which is circulated about once every minute.

The heart is a four-chambered, fist-sized muscle located just beneath the ribs under the left breast (Figure 11-1). Its role is to pump oxygen-poor blood to the lungs and oxygenated (oxygen-rich) blood to the rest of the body. Blood actually travels through two separate circulatory systems: The right side of the heart pumps blood to and from the lungs in what is called **pulmonary circulation,** and the left side pumps blood through the rest of the body in **systemic circulation.**

Used, oxygen-poor blood enters the right upper chamber, or **atrium,** of the heart through the **vena cava,** the largest vein in the body (Figure 11-2). Valves prevent the blood from flowing the wrong way. As the right atrium fills, it contracts and pumps blood into the right lower chamber, or **ventricle,** which, when it contracts, pumps blood through the pulmonary artery into the lungs. There, blood picks up oxygen and discards carbon dioxide. Cleaned, oxygenated blood then flows through the pulmonary veins into the left atrium. As this chamber fills, it contracts and pumps blood into the powerful left ventricle, which pumps it through the **aorta,** the body's largest artery, to be fed into the rest of the body's blood vessels. The period of the heart's contraction is called **systole;** the period of relaxation is called **diastole.**

The heartbeat—the split-second sequence of contractions of the heart's four chambers—is controlled by electrical impulses. These signals originate in a bundle of specialized cells in the right atrium called the pacemaker. Unless it is speeded up or slowed down by the brain in response to such stimuli as danger or exhaustion, the heart produces electrical impulses at a steady rate.

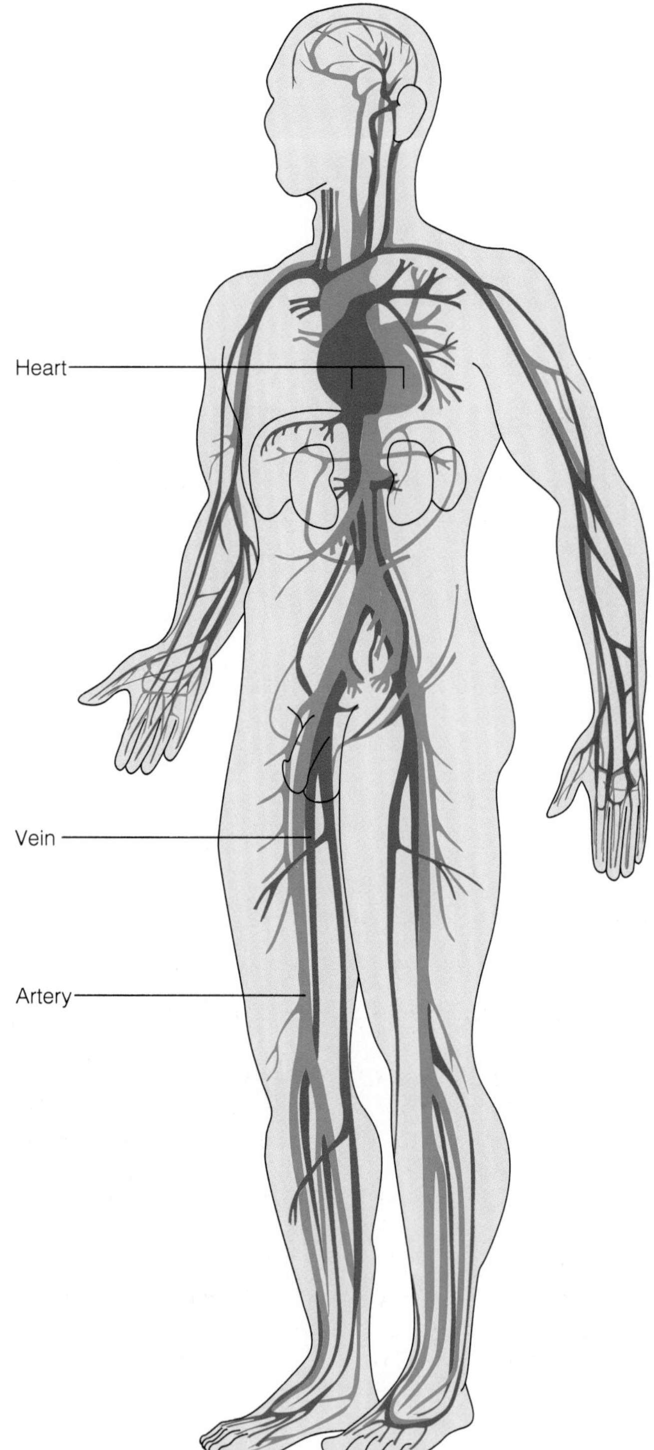

Figure 11-1 *Circulation in the body.*

Blood vessels are classified by size and function. **Veins** carry blood to the heart; **arteries** carry it away from the heart. Veins have thin walls, but arteries have thick elastic

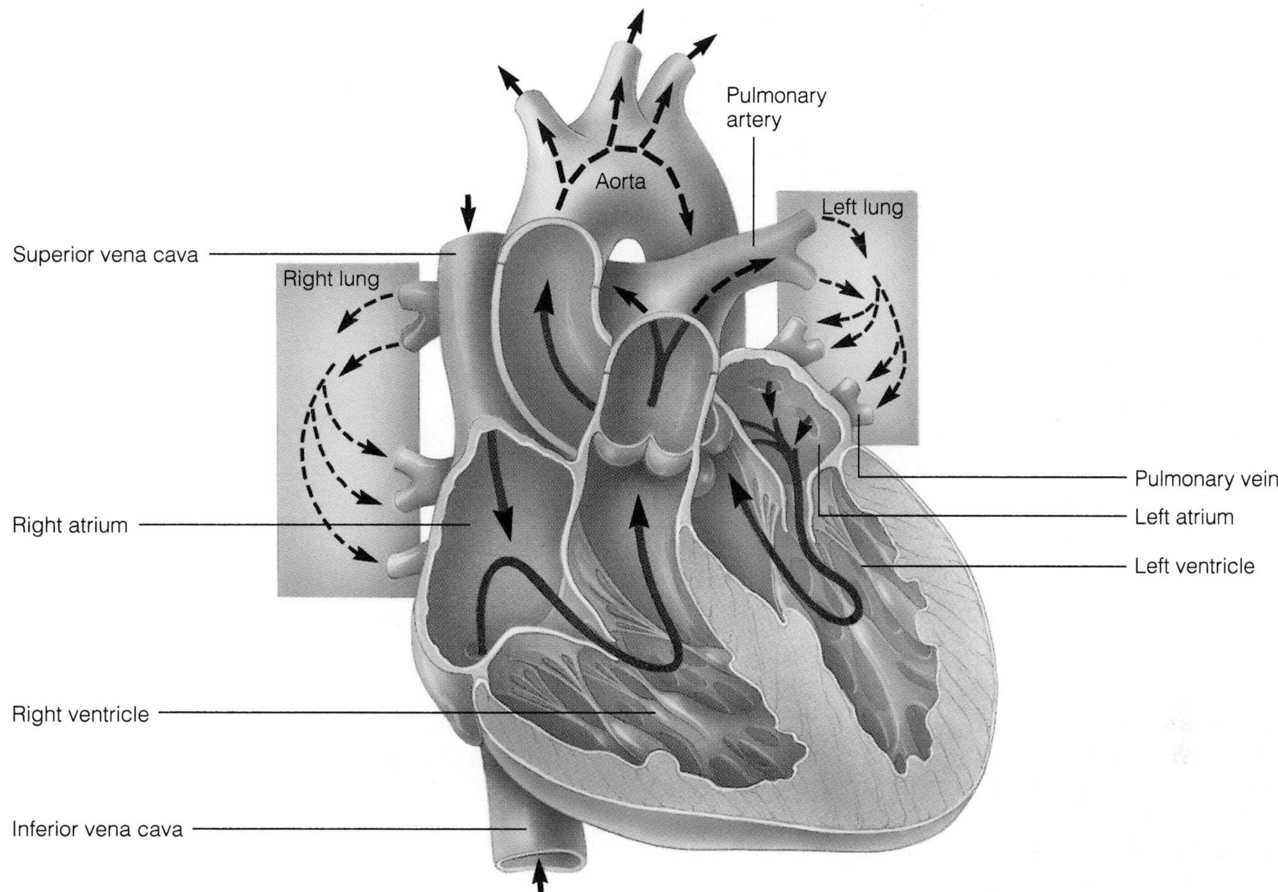

Figure 11-2 *Circulation in the heart.*

walls that enable them to expand and relax with the volume of blood being pumped through them. After leaving the heart, the aorta branches into smaller and smaller vessels. Two vital arteries, called the **coronary arteries,** branch off the aorta to carry blood back to the heart tissues themselves (Figure 11-3).

The smallest arteries branch still further into **capillaries,** tiny vessels only one cell thick. The capillaries deliver oxygen and nutrient-rich blood to the tissues and receive oxygen-poor, waste-carrying blood. From the capillaries, this blood empties into small veins and then into larger veins that return it to the heart to repeat the cycle.

RISK FACTORS FOR CARDIOVASCULAR DISEASE

Researchers have identified a variety of factors associated with an increased risk of developing cardiovascular disease. They are grouped into two categories: major risk factors and contributing risk factors. Some major risk factors are linked to controllable lifestyle factors, such as diet, exercise habits, and ways of managing stress. Other risk factors are beyond the individual's control.

TERMS

cardiovascular disease (CVD) Disease of the heart and blood vessels.

pulmonary circulation The part of the circulatory system that moves blood between the heart and the lungs; controlled by the right side of the heart.

systemic circulation The part of the circulatory system that moves blood between the heart and the rest of the body; controlled by the left side of the heart.

atria The two upper chambers of the heart in which blood collects before passing to the ventricles; also called auricles.

vena cava The large vein through which blood is returned to the right atrium of the heart.

ventricles The two lower chambers of the heart from which blood flows through arteries to the lungs and other parts of the body.

aorta The large artery that receives blood from the left ventricle and distributes it to the body.

systole Contraction of the heart.

diastole Relaxation of the heart.

veins Vessels that carry blood to the heart.

arteries Vessels that carry blood away from the heart.

coronary arteries Two arteries branching from the aorta that provide blood to the heart muscle.

capillaries Very small blood vessels that distribute blood to all parts of the body.

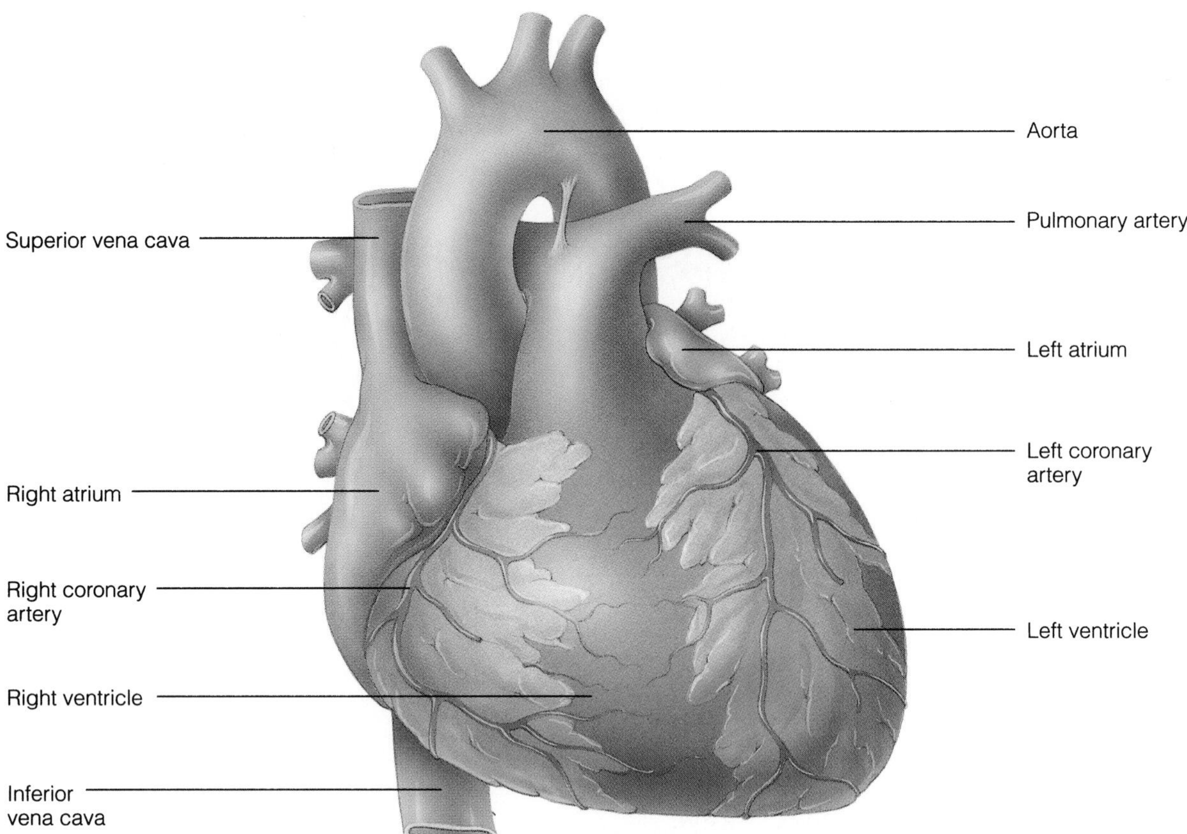

Figure 11-3 ***Blood supply to the heart.***

Major Risk Factors That Can Be Changed

The American Heart Association has identified four major risk factors for CVD that can be eliminated or controlled through lifestyle: tobacco use, high blood pressure, unhealthy blood cholesterol levels, and physical inactivity.

Tobacco Use Pack-a-day smokers have twice the heart attack risk of nonsmokers; smoking two or more packs daily triples the risk. And when smokers do have heart attacks, they are up to four times more likely than nonsmokers to die from them. Women who smoke and use oral contraceptives are up to 39 times more likely to have a heart attack and up to 22 times more likely to have a stroke than those who neither smoke nor take birth control pills.

Smoking has several harmful effects on the cardiovascular system. It can reduce levels of the "good" cholesterol in the bloodstream. Nicotine, the drug in tobacco, is a central nervous system stimulant that causes blood pressure and heart rate to rise. The carbon monoxide in cigarette smoke displaces oxygen in the blood, reducing the amount of oxygen available to the heart and other parts of the body. Cigarette smoking also causes the **platelets** in the blood to become sticky and cluster, thereby shortening platelet survival, decreasing clotting time, and thickening the blood. All these effects increase the risk of CVD.

It is not necessary to be a smoker to suffer the adverse effects of smoking. **Environmental tobacco smoke (ETS)**—"secondhand smoke"—in high concentrations has also been linked to the development of cardiovascular disease. Living or working with a smoker for a long period can be a significant CVD risk factor as well.

Regardless of how long they have smoked, smokers who quit lower their risk of developing CVD dramatically. Ten years after quitting, a person who smoked a pack a day or less has about the same CVD risk as a person who has never smoked.

High Blood Pressure High blood pressure, or **hypertension,** is a risk factor for many types of cardiovascular disease but is also considered a form of disease itself. High blood pressure occurs when there is resistance to normal flow of blood through the arteries or an increased output of blood from the heart. The higher the blood pressure, the harder the heart has to work to push the blood forward. Over time, a strained heart weakens and tends to enlarge, which weakens it further. Increased blood pressure also scars and hardens arteries, making them less elastic. Heart attacks, strokes, **atherosclerosis,** and kidney failure can result.

High blood pressure usually has no early warning signs, so yearly tests of blood pressure are important. Diet, weight control, exercise, and sometimes medication

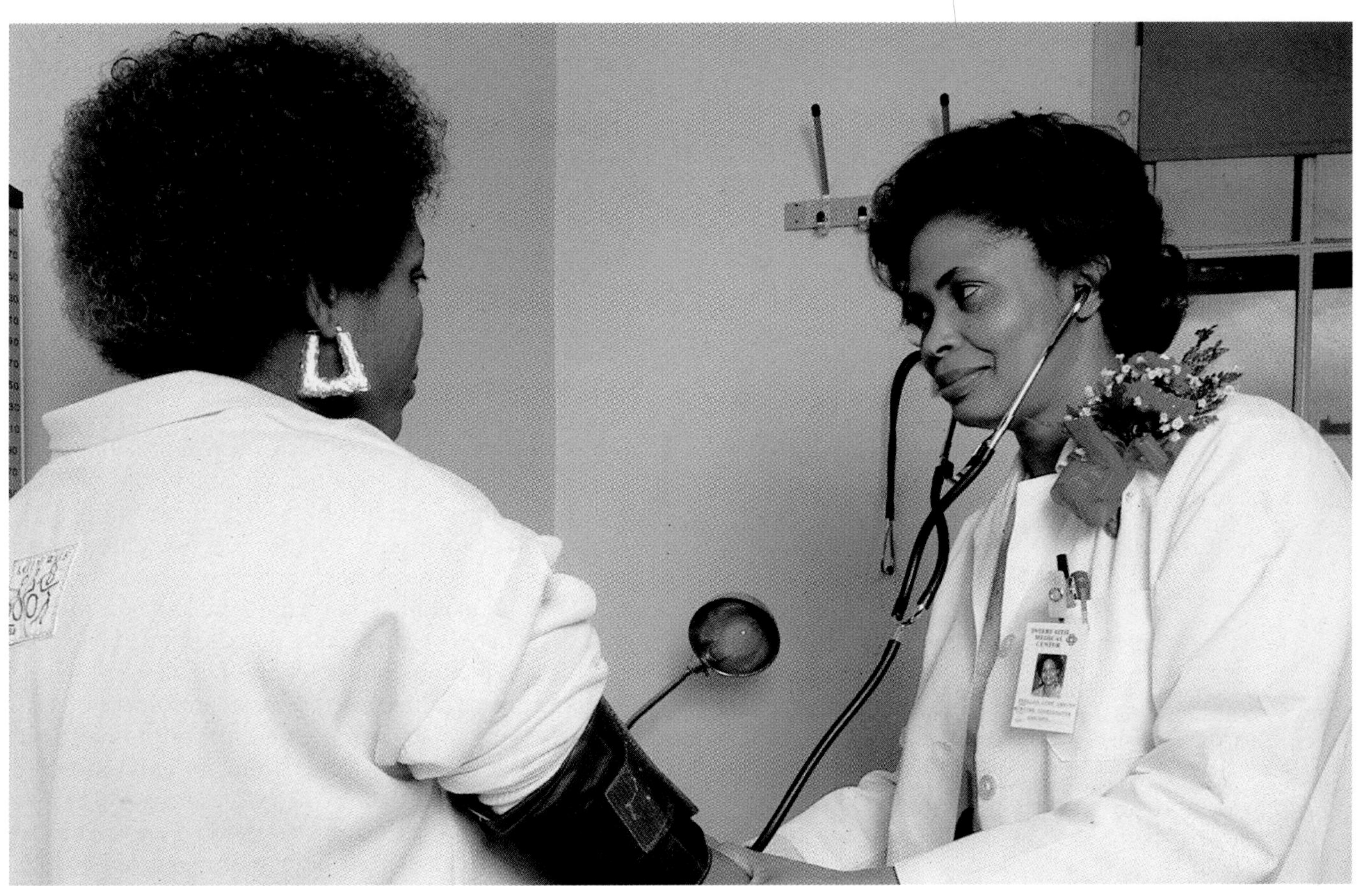

One of the most important steps individuals can take to guard against cardiovascular disease is having their blood pressure tested regularly. It is especially important for African Americans, because high blood pressure, both a disease in itself and a contributing factor to other forms of CVD, is much more common among African Americans than among Caucasian Americans.

are all means of controlling high blood pressure. (Hypertension and atherosclerosis are discussed in greater detail later in this chapter.)

Unhealthy Blood Cholesterol Levels Cholesterol, a fatty, waxlike substance that circulates through the bloodstream, is an important component of cell membranes, sex hormones, vitamin D, **lung surfactant,** and the protective sheaths around nerves. Adequate cholesterol is essential for proper body functioning, but, as mentioned in Chapter 8, too much cholesterol can clog arteries and increase the risk of cardiovascular disease.

The human body obtains cholesterol in two ways: from the liver, which manufactures it, and from foods. When blood contains more cholesterol than the body can use or dispose of, the excess is deposited on artery walls.

Cholesterol Testing The first step in gaining control of this risk factor is to have the blood tested to determine its cholesterol level. The National Cholesterol Education Program (NCEP) recommends testing for all adults at least once every 5 years, beginning at age 20, or, if there is a family history of heart disease, at least every 3 years. Table 11-1 shows how blood cholesterol levels (in milligrams per deciliter of blood) are rated.

The NCEP advises people with borderline high or high cholesterol levels to begin a cholesterol-lowering diet immediately. Experts calculate that people can cut heart at-

TERMS

platelets Microscopic disk-shaped cell fragments in the blood that disintegrate on contact with foreign objects and release chemicals necessary for the formation of blood clots.

environmental tobacco smoke (ETS) Smoke that enters the atmosphere from the burning end of a cigarette, cigar, or pipe, as well as smoke that is exhaled by smokers; also called secondhand smoke.

hypertension Sustained abnormally high blood pressure.

atherosclerosis Cardiovascular disease in which the inner layers of artery walls are made thick and irregular by deposits of a fatty substance; the internal channels of arteries become narrowed, and blood supply is reduced.

lung surfactant A chemical fluid coating the surface of the lung that lowers surface tension, aids in gas exchange, and helps keep the lungs from collapsing.

TABLE 11-1 *Cholesterol Guidelines**

Total Blood Cholesterol	Rating
Less than 200 mg/dl	Desirable**
200–239 mg/dl	Borderline high
240 mg/dl or more	High
LDL Cholesterol	
Less than 130 mg/dl	Desirable**
130–159 mg/dl	Borderline high
160 mg/dl or more	High
HDL Cholesterol	
More than 45 mg/dl	Desirable**
35–45 mg/dl	Borderline low
Less than 35 mg/dl	Low

*These guidelines are based on large-scale studies of middle-aged Americans; younger people should strive for somewhat lower levels. For example, for those age 19 and under, the desirable level for total blood cholesterol is below 170 mg/dl.
**For adults without known heart disease.

Sources: American Heart Association and National Cholesterol Education Program.

tack risk by 2% for every 1% of blood cholesterol reduction—for example, people whose level drops from 250 to 200 mg/dl lower their heart attack risk by 40%. Such a dietary reduction can also reverse deposits on artery walls.

Other tests, recommended for people with high total cholesterol, measure the proportions of different types of blood cholesterol.

LDLs and HDLs Cholesterol is carried to and from the liver in protein-lipid packages called **lipoproteins** (Figure 11-4). As noted in Chapter 3, **low-density lipoproteins (LDLs)** are known as "bad" cholesterol. They shuttle cholesterol from the liver to the organs and tissues that require it, and if they transport more cholesterol than the body can use, the excess is deposited in the blood vessels. There, accumulated cholesterol can block arteries, causing heart attacks and strokes.

High-density lipoproteins (HDLs), however, are referred to as "good" cholesterol because they shuttle unused cholesterol back to the liver for recycling. High LDL levels and low HDL levels are associated with a high CVD risk; low levels of LDL and high levels of HDL are associated with a lower risk.

Controlling Cholesterol As discussed in Chapter 8, most Americans can and should lower their total cholesterol level by cutting total fat intake and substituting unsaturated for saturated fats. To reiterate the recommended levels, the NCEP recommends that all Americans over the age of 2 consume a diet in which total fat consumption is 30% or less of total daily calories. Of this amount, no more than one-third should come from saturated fat, which is found in animal products, palm and coconut oil, and hydrogenated vegetable oils. Since saturated fat influences the production and excretion of cholesterol by the liver, limiting its intake is the most important dietary means of cholesterol control. One-third or more of total daily fat calories should come from monounsaturated fats, such as olive or canola oil, because these oils may raise HDL levels. And up to one-third of total daily fat calories should come from polyunsaturated fats, which may actually help lower total cholesterol without reducing HDLs. (See the box "Controlling Cholesterol Through Diet," p. 264, for specific suggestions.)

Vegetable products do not contain cholesterol, but animal products contain cholesterol as well as saturated fat. The NCEP recommends limiting dietary cholesterol to under 300 milligrams a day, which is slightly more than the amount in one egg.

Other dietary factors are linked to improving cholesterol levels. For example, as described in Chapter 8, dietary fiber can help reduce cholesterol by trapping the bile acids the liver needs to manufacture cholesterol and carrying them to the large intestine to be excreted. Good sources of fiber include wheat bran, oatmeal, psyllium, barley, legumes, apples, pears, figs, and the pulp of citrus fruits. Omega-3 fatty acids, found in fish and shellfish, may also be helpful in lowering cholesterol, and some experts recommend eating fish or seafood (but not taking fish-oil capsules) two or three times a week.

Besides controlling overall fat intake and balancing the proportions of the various types of fats, regular exercise and stopping smoking are two other steps in cholesterol control. Smoking lowers HDL level, while exercise raises it. But exercise has far more benefits in lowering CVD risk: It helps decrease blood pressure, maintain optimum body weight, and prevent or control diabetes. It might safely be said in this context, as well as many others, that physical exercise is the closest we can come to a "magic bullet" in our efforts to prevent disease.

TERMS

lipoproteins Blood fats formed in the liver that carry cholesterol throughout the body.

low-density lipoproteins (LDLs) Blood fats that transport cholesterol to organs and tissues; excess amounts result in the accumulation of deposits on artery walls.

high-density lipoproteins (HDLs) Blood fats that help transport cholesterol out of the arteries, thereby protecting against heart disease.

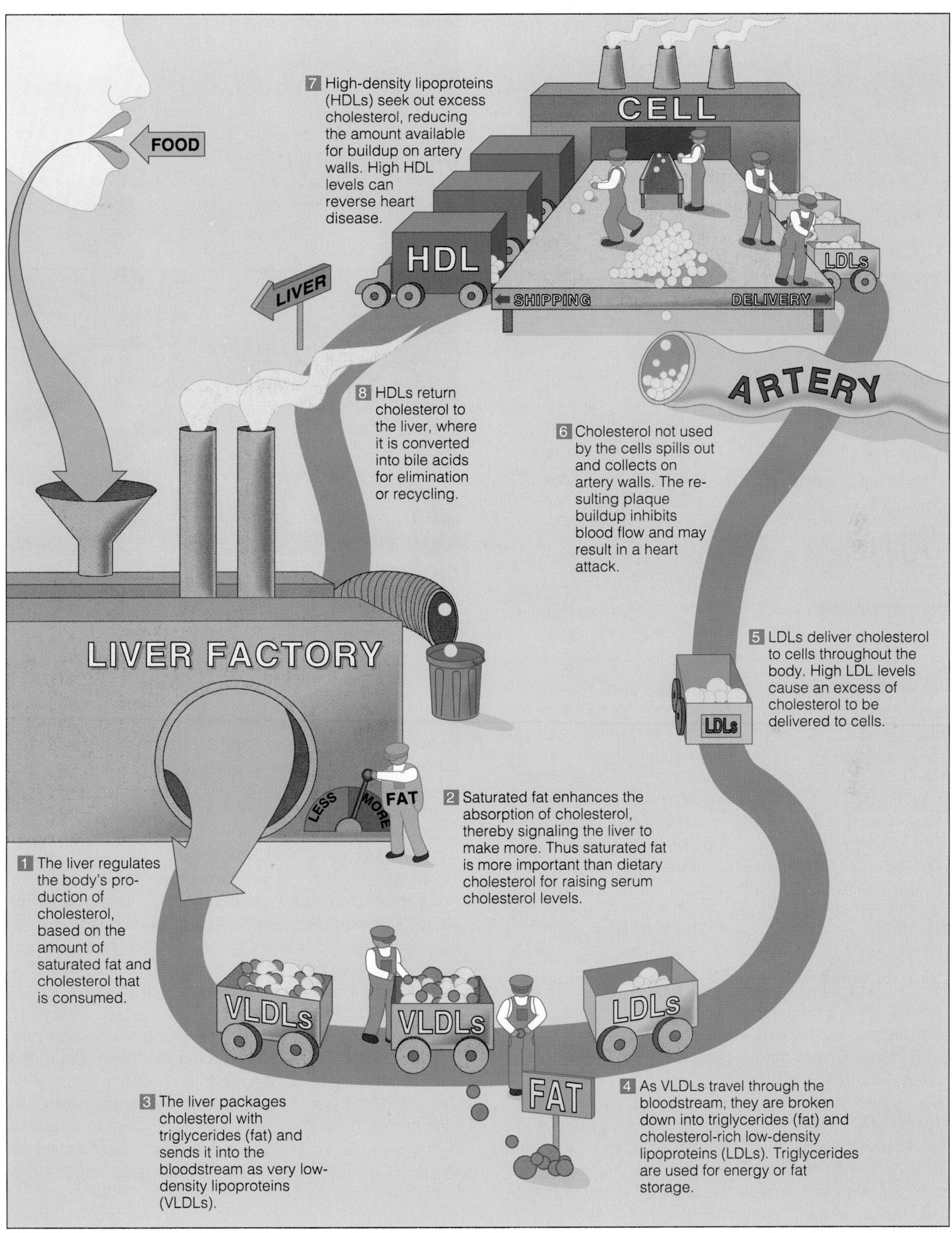

FOOD
7 High-density lipoproteins (HDLs) seek out excess cholesterol, reducing the amount available for buildup on artery walls. High HDL levels can reverse heart disease.
CELL
HDL
LIVER
SHIPPING
DELIVERY
LDLs
ARTERY
8 HDLs return cholesterol to the liver, where it is converted into bile acids for elimination or recycling.
6 Cholesterol not used by the cells spills out and collects on artery walls. The resulting plaque buildup inhibits blood flow and may result in a heart attack.
LIVER FACTORY
5 LDLs deliver cholesterol to cells throughout the body. High LDL levels cause an excess of cholesterol to be delivered to cells.
LDLs
LESS
MORE
FAT
2 Saturated fat enhances the absorption of cholesterol, thereby signaling the liver to make more. Thus saturated fat is more important than dietary cholesterol for raising serum cholesterol levels.
1 The liver regulates the body's production of cholesterol, based on the amount of saturated fat and cholesterol that is consumed.
VLDLs
VLDLs
LDLs
FAT
3 The liver packages cholesterol with triglycerides (fat) and sends it into the bloodstream as very low-density lipoproteins (VLDLs).
4 As VLDLs travel through the bloodstream, they are broken down into triglycerides (fat) and cholesterol-rich low-density lipoproteins (LDLs). Triglycerides are used for energy or fat storage.

Figure 11-4 *Travels with cholesterol.*

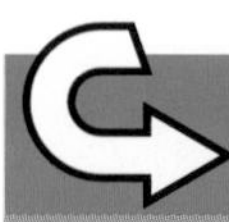

TACTICS AND TIPS
Controlling Cholesterol Through Diet

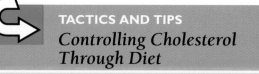

A diet that improves cholesterol levels is high in dietary fiber and low in fat, saturated fat, and cholesterol. To lower your CVD risk, try some of these dietary changes.

Decrease Intake	Increase Intake
Whole milk	Nonfat and low-fat milk
Hard cheeses, cream cheese	Low-fat cottage cheese, nonfat yogurt
Beef, pork, sausage, bacon	Fish, skinless chicken, turkey
Butter, high-fat mayonnaise	Mustard, vegetable oil
Ice cream	Sherbet, frozen yogurt
Palm and coconut oils	Olive and vegetable oils
Many luncheon meats	Turkey, chicken meats
Many prepared baked goods	Fruits, vegetables
Egg yolks (egg whites are OK)	Beans, cereals, pasta, bread

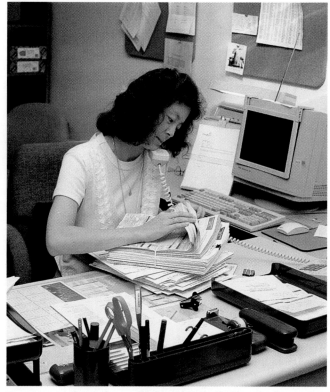

Too many tasks to do, too little time in which to do them, unexpected emergency situations—all create on-the-job stress. If appropriate stress-management techniques are not developed, stress can contribute to heart disease.

Physical Inactivity In 1992 the American Heart Association cited a sedentary lifestyle as on a par with smoking, unhealthy cholesterol levels, and high blood pressure as a major risk factor for cardiovascular disease. An estimated 35–50 million Americans live with this controllable risk factor. As little as 90 minutes a week of mild exercise—such as walking, gardening, or bowling—significantly reduces the risk of CVD. A moderate program, such as 30 minutes to 1 hour of brisk walking or cycling four times or more a week, would increase the benefit even more. See Chapter 7 for information on developing a complete, personalized exercise program.

Contributing Risk Factors That Can Be Changed

Various other modifiable factors have been identified as contributing to the risk of developing CVD. These include overweight, **diabetes mellitus,** responses to stress, and psychological and social factors.

Overweight When body weight is 30% or more above the recommended weight, the risk of heart disease and stroke is elevated even when no other risk factors are present. Excess weight strains the heart by contributing to high blood pressure, high cholesterol, and diabetes. As discussed in Chapter 6, the distribution of body weight is also significant: Fat that collects in the torso is more dangerous than fat that collects around the hips. A consistent, prudent diet and regular exercise are the recommended means of weight control. Some evidence suggests that yo-yo dieting (repeated loss and regaining) may be more harmful to the cardiovascular system than living with some excess weight.

Diabetes Diabetes, a metabolic disorder in which the body produces insufficient amounts of the hormone insulin to metabolize glucose, affects blood cholesterol levels and therefore raises CVD risk. Once again, weight control and regular exercise are preventive measures. (Refer to Chapter 6 for more information on diabetes.)

Responses to Stress Over time, excessive stress may contribute to CVD risk by straining the heart and blood vessels with repeated triggering of the alarm reaction of the stress response. In addition, many people adopt unhealthy habits such as smoking, overeating, or skipping meals as a means of dealing with severe stress. Chapter 10 discusses healthful strategies for managing stress effectively.

Psychological and Social Factors There is some evidence that certain psychological traits considered "toxic"

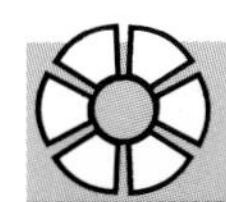

WELLNESS CONNECTION

Hostility and Cardiovascular Disease

Current research indicates that individuals who have a persistently hostile outlook, a quick temper, and a mistrusting, cynical attitude toward life are more likely to develop heart disease than people who have a calmer, more trusting attitude. Why is this true? What is the link between chronic hostility and the heart?

The connection is most likely to be found in the physiological mechanism of the stress response (see Chapter 10). Studies show that people who are prone to chronic hostility experience the stress response more intensely and frequently than individuals who are generally relaxed. When they encounter the irritations of daily life, their blood pressure increases much more than is the case for less hostile people. They also seem to have trouble shutting down the stress response. Less hostile people tend to calm down much more quickly, taking the stress off their body—especially their heart.

According to Redford Williams, noted researcher and author, hostile people can learn to change their attitude and, in doing so, reduce their risk of heart disease. Just as hostility increases the risk of developing CVD, having a trusting heart—being slow to anger, expecting the best of others, and spending minimal time feeling resentful, irritable, and angry—appears to prevent heart disease. Williams has created a 17-point behavior modification plan for developing a more trusting, and healthier, heart:

1. Reason with yourself. Try to talk yourself out of being upset. Then drop the matter.
2. Stop hostile thoughts, feelings, and urges. Silently shout "Stop!" at them.
3. Distract yourself. Look at a magazine when waiting in line. Sing along with a tape when stuck in traffic.
4. Meditate. Practice emptying your mind of thoughts 15 minutes a day. Use these skills when you become angry.
5. Avoid overstimulation. Cut back on nicotine, caffeine, and sweets. Exercise regularly.
6. Assert yourself. Learn to calmly and respectfully ask others to change a specific behavior.
7. Care for a pet.
8. Listen. Learning to listen to others will reduce misunderstandings and improve your relationships.
9. Practice trusting others. Begin with simple situations, such as letting a friend choose a restaurant.
10. Take on community service to reinforce your sense of connectedness with other people.
11. Increase your empathy. Learn to understand other people's needs and motivations.
12. Be tolerant. Intolerance is accompanied by anger.
13. Forgive. When you cannot change what was done, release your anger by forgiving the person who hurt you.
14. Have a confidant(e). Cultivate at least one relationship intimate enough that you can rely on each other for emotional support.
15. Learn to laugh at yourself when you feel yourself getting hostile.
16. Become more religious. Being an active participant in a religious community can help you achieve a more positive outlook.
17. Pretend this is the last day of your life. Does this argument matter in the long run?

Source: Adapted from Williams, R., and V. Williams. 1993. *Anger Kills: Seventeen Strategies for Controlling the Hostility That Can Harm Your Health.* New York: Times Books.

contribute to CVD risk. Hostility, anger, and cynicism may correlate with a greater danger of heart disease and stroke (see the box "Hostility and Cardiovascular Disease"). As with virtually all the strategies described here for managing identified risk factors, steps to control these negative emotional attitudes contribute to the quality of life in general. Along with smoking cessation, exercise, and dietary improvements, these include developing close ties with friends and family and learning to identify, share, and take action to deal with sources of anxiety and unhappiness.

Finally, socioeconomic status and educational attainment are also associated with CVD risk. People of low socioeconomic status and in lower educational brackets have higher blood pressure as well as higher death rates from heart disease. This association is probably related to a whole spectrum of factors, including education, lifestyle, the availability of healthy foods, stress levels, and access to health care.

Major Risk Factors That Cannot Be Changed

All the risk factors discussed above are controllable to one degree or another. Several other important variables are outside the realm of control:

TERMS

diabetes mellitus A disorder of glucose metabolism caused by an inadequate production or use of insulin, resulting in high blood glucose levels.

DIMENSIONS OF DIVERSITY

African Americans and CVD

African American men are 50% more likely to die from a heart attack than white men, and death from stroke is five times more common in African Americans than in other Americans. Hypertension, which is both a disease in and of itself and a risk factor for other forms of CVD, is twice as common in African Americans. What accounts for these higher levels of CVD among African Americans? Contributing factors can be grouped into three areas: biological/genetic factors, low income and discrimination, and lifestyle factors.

Biological/Genetic Risk Factors

Researchers are investigating a number of genetic factors that may contribute to CVD in blacks:

- *Sensitivity to lead and salt.* Both lead and salt can act in the body to raise blood pressure, and evidence suggests that African Americans may be more sensitive to these effects than other groups.
- *High cholesterol.* Studies have found that African Americans tend to have higher than average levels of LDL, the "bad" form of cholesterol, even when lifestyle factors are taken into account. This finding points to a genetic basis to unhealthy cholesterol levels among blacks.
- *Sickle-cell disease.* Sickle-cell disease is a genetic condition characterized by the malformation of oxygen-carrying red blood cells; it occurs almost exclusively in African Americans. Sickle-cell disease damages organs by impairing blood flow and can lead to heart failure.

Low Income and Discrimination

Another factor in the high incidence of CVD among African Americans is low income. One-third of blacks live below the official poverty line. Economic deprivation is usually accompanied by reduced access to adequate health care and poorer educational opportunities, which in turn often leads to less information about preventive health measures, such as diet and stress management.

Discrimination may also play a role in CVD among blacks. Research has shown that many physicians and hospitals treat the medical problems of African Americans differently than those of whites. Discrimination, along with low income and other forms of deprivation, may also increase stress, which is linked with hypertension and CVD.

Lifestyle Factors

Lifestyle choices also play a role in CVD rates. People with low income tend to smoke more, use more salt, and exercise less than those with higher incomes. In addition, almost half of African American women and one-third of African American men are severely overweight. Smoking cessation and weight loss could eliminate up to 45% of deaths from CVD among African Americans.

Some of these risk factors are far beyond the individual's control, but others are not. Medical experts advise all Americans to have their blood pressure checked regularly, exercise, eat a healthy diet, manage stress, and avoid smoking. These preventive strategies may be particularly important for African Americans.

Sources: Adapted from Gorman, C. 1991. Why do blacks die young? *Time,* 16 September, 50–52. Raloff, J. 1990. Lead heightens hypertension risk in blacks. *Science News,* 28 April, 261. Goldsmith, M. F. African lineage, hypertension linked. *Journal of the American Medical Association* 266(15): 2049. Alexander, W. 1991. Study links status, pressure. *Black Enterprise* 21(11): 40.

- *Heredity.* The tendency to develop CVD seems to be inherited. So do tendencies toward high cholesterol levels, abnormal blood-clotting problems, diabetes, and obesity. A tendency, however, is not the same as a certainty. People who have a genetic predisposition for CVD are not destined to develop it.
- *Aging.* The risk of heart attack increases dramatically after age 65, although many people in their thirties and forties, especially men, have heart attacks.
- *Being male.* Although CVD is the leading killer of both men and women in the United States, men face a greater risk of heart attack than women, especially earlier in life. Until age 55, men also have a greater risk of high blood pressure than women. The incidence of stroke is about 19% higher for males than females. However, when heart attacks occur, they are more deadly for women than for men: 39% of women who have heart attacks die within a year, compared to 31% of men.
- *Race/ethnicity.* African American men and women are more likely to have high blood pressure than whites, which puts blacks of both sexes at a greater risk of heart disease (see the box "African Americans and CVD"). Puerto Ricans, Cuban Americans, and Mexican Americans are also more likely to suffer from high blood pressure and angina (chest pains that are a warning sign of heart overload) than are non-Hispanic white Americans. Historically, Asian Americans have had far lower rates of CVD than Caucasian Americans. However, recent studies

TABLE 11-2 Blood Pressure Classification

Classification	Systolic*	Diastolic*	Examples	What to Do
Normal	Below 130	Below 85	120/80	Recheck in 2 years
High normal	130–139	85–89	135/85	Recheck in 1 year
Mild hypertension	140–159	90–99	145/95	Confirm within 2 months
Moderate hypertension	160–179	100–109	160/105	See physician within a month
Severe hypertension		110 or above	180/115	See physician immediately

*Based on an average of two or more readings on two or more occasions.

Sources: Adapted from National High Blood Pressure Education Program and the fifth report of the Joint National Committee on Detection, Evaluation, and Treatment of High Blood Pressure, *Archives of Internal Medicine,* 25 January 1993.

indicate that blood cholesterol levels among Asian Americans are on the rise, presumably owing to their adoption of the high-fat American diet.

Except for the dietary shifts, these variables fall largely outside the realm of personal control. Nevertheless, an awareness of them can reinforce one's commitment to gain control of those risk factors that can be managed.

MAJOR FORMS OF CARDIOVASCULAR DISEASE

The cluster of medical conditions that constitute the major cardiovascular diseases are hypertension, atherosclerosis, heart disease and heart attacks, and stroke. These forms of disease are interrelated but are discussed separately for the sake of clarity.

Hypertension

Blood pressure, the force exerted by the blood on blood vessel walls, is created by the pumping action of the heart. When the heart contracts (systole), blood pressure increases; when the heart relaxes (diastole), pressure decreases. Many factors affect blood pressure; for example, excitement or exercise causes the heart to pump more blood into the arteries, resulting in a rise in blood pressure. Short periods of high blood pressure are normal, but blood pressure that is continually at an abnormally high level is a condition of disease known as hypertension.

Blood pressure is measured with a stethoscope and an instrument called a **sphygmomanometer.** It is expressed as two numbers, such as 120 over 80, and measured in millimeters of mercury. The first and larger number is the systolic blood pressure; the second is the diastolic blood pressure. Average blood pressure readings for young adults in good physical condition are 110–120 systolic over 70–80 diastolic. High blood pressure in adults is defined as equal to or greater than 140 over 90 (Table 11-2).

High blood pressure results from either an increased output of blood by the heart, often as a result of overweight, or because of increased resistance to blood flow in the arteries because of narrowing and hardening. When a person has high blood pressure, the heart must work harder than normal to force blood through the arteries, and the arteries are under a greater strain than normal. Over time, high blood pressure causes the heart to enlarge and weaken, and the process of atherosclerosis speeds up.

High blood pressure is often called a "silent killer," because it usually has no symptoms or warning signs. In fact, it is possible to have high blood pressure for years without realizing it. Over that course of time, hypertension might be damaging vital organs (particularly the heart, brain, kidneys, and eyes) and increasing the risk of heart attack, congestive heart failure, stroke, and kidney failure. In about 90% of people with hypertension, the cause is unknown. Possible risk factors include low levels of the enzyme renin, problems with kidney function, atherosclerosis, chronic stress, diet, obesity, and heredity. The key to avoiding the complications of hypertension is having the blood pressure measured regularly.

Hypertension cannot be cured, but it can be treated and controlled through changes in diet, exercise, and medication. An estimated 50 million Americans have hypertension, though only a small percentage control it.

Atherosclerosis

Atherosclerosis is a slow, progressive hardening and narrowing of the arteries that can begin in childhood. Arteries become narrowed by deposits of fat, cholesterol, and

TERMS

sphygmomanometer An instrument for measuring blood pressure.

WELLNESS CONNECTION
Religion and Wellness

Of 212 clinical studies that evaluated the effect of religious commitment on Americans' health and well-being, 75% found a positive effect, according to research presented at the American Association for the Advancement of Science 1996 annual meeting. The report, sponsored by the National Institute for Health Care Research, found that religion was beneficial for both physical and psychological problems—including depression, hypertension, and heart disease—as well as overall quality of life.

The critical factor, says author Dale Matthews, M.D., of Georgetown University School of Medicine, seems to be the intensity of religious commitment: In general, those who had the greatest involvement with their church and the strongest devotion were the healthiest. For example, in one study of heart surgery patients, the death rate within six months of surgery was 5% for regular churchgoers—compared to a national average of 9%—and 0% for those who considered themselves "deeply religious." Overall, the report found these and other effects to be unrelated to a particular denomination.

The mechanism behind religion's apparent health benefits is still unclear, but Dr. Matthews speculates that the church provides a strong community that keeps people from becoming isolated and acts as a safety net when they are ill. Studies have consistently shown that social isolation contributes to poor health. In addition, people who are religious may follow a healthier lifestyle than the general population and be less inclined to smoke and drink excessive amounts of alcohol. Research has also found that the act of worship promotes relaxation, which itself confers other health benefits. And, of course, there is the possibility that all of this is outside the realm of medical science.

"I think religion *is* good for your health," Dr. Matthews says. "But we still need to do more research to understand how this works and whether there is a healing mechanism separate from the social one."

Source: Religion: Good for the body as well as the soul? 1996. *Healthnews* 2(5): 5.

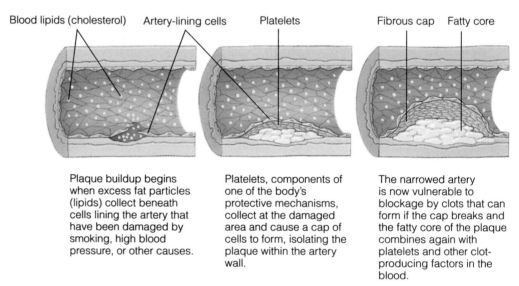

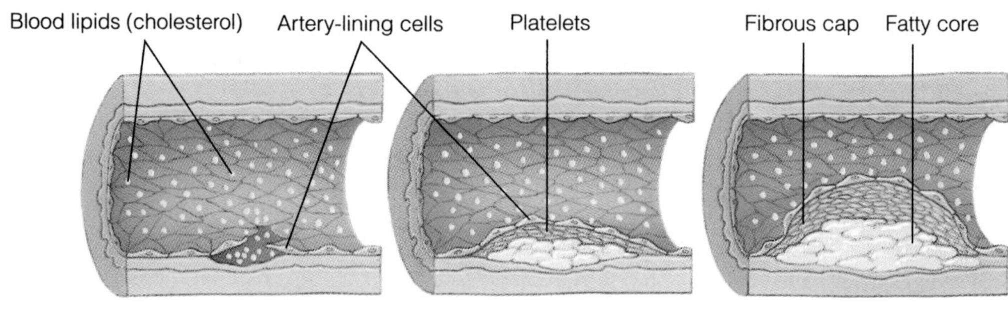

Blood lipids (cholesterol)
Artery-lining cells
Platelets
Fibrous cap
Fatty core
Plaque buildup begins when excess fat particles (lipids) collect beneath cells lining the artery that have been damaged by smoking, high blood pressure, or other causes.
Platelets, components of one of the body's protective mechanisms, collect at the damaged area and cause a cap of cells to form, isolating the plaque within the artery wall.
The narrowed artery is now vulnerable to blockage by clots that can form if the cap breaks and the fatty core of the plaque combines again with platelets and other clot-producing factors in the blood.

Figure 11-5 ***Stages of plaque development.***

other substances. As these deposits, called **plaques,** accumulate on artery walls, the arteries lose their elasticity and their ability to expand and contract, restricting blood flow. Once narrowed by a plaque, an artery is vulnerable to blockage by blood clots (Figure 11-5).

If the heart, brain, and/or other organs are deprived of blood, and thus the vital oxygen it carries, the effects of atherosclerosis can be deadly. Coronary arteries, which supply the heart with blood, are particularly susceptible to plaque buildup, a condition called coronary artery disease or coronary heart disease (CHD). Blockage of a coronary artery causes a heart attack. If a cerebral artery (leading to the brain) is blocked, the result is a stroke.

The three main risk factors for atherosclerosis are cigarette smoking, high levels of blood cholesterol, and high blood pressure.

Heart Disease and Heart Attacks

Every year, about 1.5 million Americans have a heart attack, usually as the end result of a long-term disease process. During a heart attack, part of the heart muscle may suffocate from lack of oxygen, leading to permanent

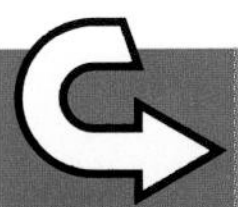

TACTICS AND TIPS

What to Do in the Event of a Heart Attack

When it comes to a heart attack, delay spells danger. Minutes make a difference, so it's vitally important to know what to do.

Know the Signals of a Heart Attack

- Uncomfortable pressure, fullness, squeezing, or pain in the center of the chest lasting 2 minutes or more.
- Pain may spread to the shoulders, neck, or arms.
- Severe pain, dizziness, fainting, sweating, nausea, or shortness of breath may also occur. Sharp, stabbing twinges of pain are usually not signals of a heart attack.

Know What Emergency Action to Take

- If you are having typical chest discomfort that lasts for 2 minutes or more, call the local emergency rescue service immediately.
- If you can get to a hospital faster by car, have someone drive you. Find out which hospitals have 24-hour emergency cardiac care, and discuss the choices with your physician. Plan in advance the route that's best from where you live and work.
- Keep a list of emergency rescue service numbers next to your telephone and in a prominent place in your pocket, wallet, or purse.

Know How to Help

- If you are with someone who is having the signals of a heart attack, take action even if the person denies there is something wrong.
- *Call* the emergency rescue service, or
- *Get* to the nearest hospital emergency room that offers 24-hour emergency cardiac care, and
- *Give* mouth-to-mouth breathing and chest compression (CPR) if it is necessary and if you are properly trained.

Source: American Heart Association.

damage. CHD, the most common form of heart disease leading to heart attack, is the leading killer of Americans.

Although heart attacks often occur without warning, some people experience pain or an abnormal heartbeat first. The chest pains known as **angina pectoris** are a signal that the heart isn't getting enough blood to meet its oxygen requirement. Although not actually a heart attack, angina pain is a warning that the heart is overloaded. **Arrhythmia,** or abnormal heartbeat, is another sign of impending heart attack. (The box "What to Do in the Event of a Heart Attack" provides information on how to respond to these signals.)

To determine a person's risk of heart attack, a physician may give a stress or exercise test in which the patient runs on a treadmill while being monitored with an electrocardiogram (EKG) for arrhythmias. Changes in the heart's electrical activity while under stress are associated with certain conditions, such as restricted blood flow to the heart. Other ways for physicians to assess an individual's risk of heart attack include the use of dye to obtain a visual image of the heart and major arteries, and the use of a radioactive tracer to determine whether blood flow is slowed by blocked arteries.

If tests indicate a problem or if a person has already had a heart attack, several treatments are possible, including coronary bypass surgery, percutaneous transluminal angioplasty (PCTA) (in which a balloon is inflated inside the blocked artery), and, for some patients, small, regular doses of aspirin to inhibit platelets from forming clots. Whatever the treatment, all patients with heart disease are advised to change their diet to lower their blood cholesterol levels, quit smoking, and begin a safe, personalized exercise program—all the measures, in fact, that are detailed in this book for achieving overall wellness.

Stroke

If the blood supply to part of the brain is cut off, the result is a **stroke.** Brain cells die if they are deprived of oxygen for more than a few minutes, and unlike the cells in other kinds of tissues, they do not regenerate. The blockages of blood flow that result in strokes can be blood clots or hemorrhages. High blood pressure and atherosclerosis (especially blockage of the cerebral arteries) greatly increase the risk of stroke.

When blood supply to the brain is interrupted, the nerve cells in the affected area stop functioning. Nerve

TERMS

plaque A deposit of fatty (and other) substances on the inner wall of the arteries.

angina pectoris A condition in which the heart muscle does not receive enough blood, causing severe pain in the chest and often in the left arm and shoulder.

arrhythmia An irregularity in the force or rhythm of the heartbeat that often precedes a heart attack.

stroke An impeded blood supply to some part of the brain resulting in the destruction of brain cells.

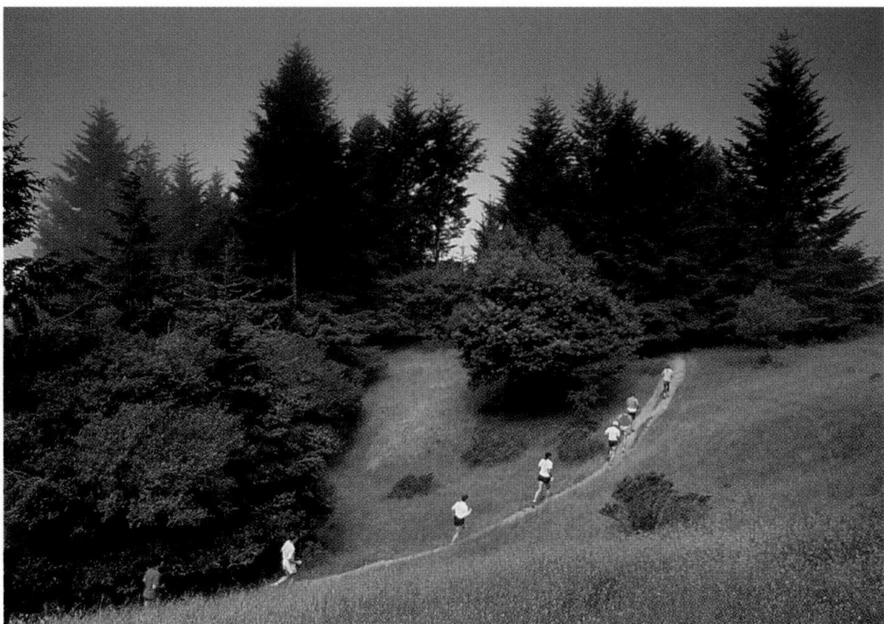

Exercising regularly is one of the most important things you can do to protect yourself from cardiovascular disease. For these runners in Marin County, California, a beautiful setting adds to the pleasure of exercising.

cells control sensation and most body movements; depending on the area of the brain that is affected, a stroke may cause paralysis, walking disability, speech impairment, or memory loss. Of the 500,000 Americans who have strokes each year, approximately one-third die within a year. Those who survive usually have some lasting disability.

For strokes to be treated effectively, the prompt recognition of symptoms is essential. Warning signs include sudden numbness or weakness of the limbs on one side of the body; loss of speech or difficulty speaking or understanding speech; dimming or loss of vision, especially in only one eye; and unexplained dizziness. Depending on the type of stroke, treatments include the use of clot-dissolving and antihypertensive drugs. If detection and medical intervention come too late, rehabilitation in the form of physical, speech and language, and occupational therapies is the only treatment.

Congestive Heart Failure

High blood pressure, heart attack, atherosclerosis, rheumatic fever, and birth defects can all reduce the efficiency of the heart. When the heart cannot maintain its regular pumping rate and force, fluids begin to back up and collect in the lungs and other parts of the body. This extra fluid seeps through capillary walls, causing swelling. Fluid accumulating in the lungs causes swelling there and shortness of breath. The entire process is called **congestive heart failure.** Treatments include reducing the heart's workload, modifying salt intake, and using drugs to help the body eliminate excess fluid.

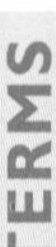

congestive heart failure A condition resulting from the heart's inability to pump out all the blood that returns to it. Blood backs up in the veins leading to the heart, causing an accumulation of fluid in various parts of the body.

PROTECTING YOURSELF FROM CARDIOVASCULAR DISEASE

Considering the scope and deadliness of CVD, it makes sense to begin now to take measures that will reduce your risk. Here are several important guidelines to follow:

- If you smoke, quit. If you live or work with smokers, encourage them to quit.
- Exercise regularly.
- Eat a healthy diet, one that is low in fat and high in complex carbohydrates.
- Maintain a healthy body weight.
- Develop effective ways to handle stress and anger.
- Have your blood pressure measured by a health care provider at least once a year, even if it has been normal in the past. If your blood pressure is high, follow your physician's advice on how to lower it.
- Have your blood cholesterol level measured. If your cholesterol is under 200 mg/dl, maintain a healthy lifestyle and get another test within 5 years. If your cholesterol is 200–239 mg/dl, have a second test performed and average the results. Begin a cholesterol-lowering diet, eliminate any other risk factors you may have, and get tested again in a year. Your physician may order a more detailed cholesterol

analysis. If your cholesterol is 240 mg/dl or higher, follow your physician's instructions.

- Manage medical conditions, such as diabetes, as recommended by your physician.
- If you have risk factors for CVD, ask your physician about taking small doses of aspirin.
- Know your risk factors for CVD. Lab 11-1 gives you the opportunity to evaluate your risks.

? COMMON QUESTIONS ANSWERED

Do women have a lower risk for cardiovascular disease than men, and, if so, why? Until about age 65, women have a significant advantage over men when it comes to CVD. Every year, about 700,000 people under the age of 65 have a heart attack; of these, 80% are men. Women who develop CVD tend to be about 10 years older than men when they first have symptoms and about 20 years older when they have a heart attack.

What explains this difference? Research thus far has focused on the beneficial effects of estrogen, which, prior to menopause, circulates in high concentrations in a woman's body. Estrogen improves blood cholesterol levels by raising the concentration of HDL and lowering levels of LDL. Women, on average, have much better blood cholesterol profiles than men. Estrogen also seems to prevent blood clots from forming in the body and to dissolve clots that do form. This is significant because clots can lead to heart attacks and strokes. And estrogen may also lower blood concentrations of the amino acid homocysteine, high levels of which may be linked with heart attacks and strokes.

But women should not be complacent about their risk of cardiovascular disease. CVD is the leading cause of death among women, killing five times as many women as breast cancer and significantly more women than all types of cancers combined. After menopause, estrogen levels fall and LDL cholestrol levels begin to rise. By age 65, heart attack risk for women is almost equal to that of men. And women are even less likely to survive an attack, perhaps because they tend to suffer heart attacks at an older age, or because CVD is less likely to be diagnosed in women.

As more studies of CVD among women are completed, scientists may learn more about how female biochemistry affects the development of CVD. In the meantime, it's important to note that the major risk factors for CVD are the same for both women and men. The general advice for preventing CVD presented in this chapter—exercising regularly, managing stress, eating a lowfat diet, and so on—is appropriate for everyone.

I know what foods to avoid to prevent CVD, but are there any foods I should eat to protect myself from CVD? The most important dietary change for CVD prevention is a negative one: cutting back on foods high in fat, particularly saturated fat. However, research indicates that certain foods can be helpful. Eating foods high in soluble fiber, for example, can lower cholesterol levels because soluble fiber binds cholesterol and helps eliminate it from the body. (Foods rich in soluble fiber include beans, oat bran, barley, and cereals made with psyllium.) Foods rich in monounsaturated fatty acids, such as olive oil, may also have a protective effect by raising HDL levels.

The evidence for other foods is more preliminary. Studies are ongoing about the effects of certain B vitamins on homocysteine levels. The amino acid homocysteine may raise CVD risk by scarring artery walls and increasing the development of plaques. High homocysteine levels are associated with a low intake of folic acid, vitamin B-6, and vitamin B-12. All of these B vitamins convert homocysteine to other, less harmful compounds. (Refer to Table 8-2 for listings of foods rich in these vitamins.) Other substances under study that may help protect against CVD include the polyphenols found in tea, vitamin C, vitamin E, and soy protein (found in tofu, textured vegetable protein, and soy flour and milk).

More research is needed to clarify the effects of these compounds on CVD risk. Meanwhile, you can't go wrong by increasing your intake of fruits, grains, and vegetables.

The advice I hear from the news about protecting myself from CVD seems to be changing all the time. What am I supposed to believe? Health-related research is now described in popular newspapers and magazines rather than just medical journals, meaning that more and more people have access to the information. Researchers do not deliberately set out to mislead or confuse people. However, news reports may oversimplify the results of research studies, leaving out some of the qualifications and questions the researchers present with their findings. In addition, news reports may not differentiate between a preliminary finding and a result that has been verified by a large number of long-term studies. And researchers themselves must strike a balance between reporting promising preliminary findings to the public, thereby allowing people to act on them, and waiting 10–20 years until long-term studies confirm (or disprove) a particular theory.

This can leave you in a difficult position. You cannot become an expert on all subjects, able to effectively evaluate all the available health news. However, there are some general strategies you can use to better assess the health advice that appears in the media; see the box "Evaluating Health News" (p. 272).

SUMMARY

- The cardiovascular system, which includes the pulmonary and systemic circulations, pumps and

CRITICAL CONSUMER
Evaluating Health News

Americans face an avalanche of health information from newspapers, magazines, books, and television programs. It's not always easy to decide which news to believe and which news to ignore. The following questions can help you evaluate health news:

1. *Is the report based on research or on an anecdote?* Information or advice based on one or more carefully designed research studies has more validity than one person's experiences.
2. *What is the source of the information?* A study in a respected publication has been reviewed by editors and other researchers in the field—people who are in a position to evaluate the merits of a study and its results. Information put forth by government agencies and national research organizations is also usually considered fairly reliable.
3. *How big was the study?* A study that involves many subjects is more likely to yield reliable results than a study involving only a few people. Another indication that a finding is meaningful is if several different studies yield the same results.
4. *Who were the people involved in the study?* Research findings are more likely to apply to you if you share important characteristics with the subjects of the study. For example, the results of a study on men over age 50 who smoke may not be particularly meaningful for a 30-year-old nonsmoking woman.
5. *What kind of study was it?* Epidemiological studies involve observation or interviews in order to trace the relationship among lifestyle, physical characteristics, and diseases. While epidemiological studies can suggest links, they cannot establish cause-and-effect relationships. Experiments or interventional studies involve testing the effects of different treatments on groups of people who have similar lifestyles and characteristics. They are more likely to provide conclusive evidence of a cause-and-effect relationship. The best interventional studies share the following characteristics:
   - *Controlled.* A group of people who receive the treatment is compared with a matched group who do not receive the treatment.
   - *Randomized.* The treatment and control groups are selected randomly.
   - *Double-blind.* Researchers and participants are unaware of who is receiving the treatment.
   - *Multicenter.* The experiment is performed at more than one institution.
6. *What do the statistics really say?* First, are the results described as "statistically significant"? If a study is large and well designed, its results can be deemed statistically significant, meaning there is less than a 5% chance that the findings resulted from chance. Second, are the results stated in terms of relative or absolute risk? Many findings are reported in terms of relative risk—how a particular treatment or condition affects a person's disease risk. Consider the following examples of relative risk:
   - According to some estimates, taking estrogen without progesterone can increase a postmenopausal woman's risk of dying from endometrial cancer by 233%.
   - Giving AZT to HIV-infected pregnant women reduces prenatal transmission of HIV by 66%.

   The first of these two findings seems far more dramatic than the second—until one also considers absolute risk, the actual risk of the illness in the population being considered. The absolute risk of endometrial cancer is 0.3%; a 233% increase based on the effects of estrogen raises it to 1%, a change of 0.7%. Without treatment, about 25% of infants born to HIV-infected women will be infected with HIV; with treatment, the absolute risk drops to about 8%, a change of 17%. Because the absolute risk of an HIV-infected mother passing the virus to her infant is so much greater than a woman's risk of developing endometrial cancer (25% compared with 0.3%), a smaller change in relative risk translates into a much greater change in absolute risk.
7. *Is new health advice being offered?* If the media report new guidelines for health behavior or medical treatment, examine the source. Government agencies and national research foundations usually consider a great deal of evidence before offering health advice. Above all, use common sense, and check with your physician before making a major change in your health habits based on news reports.

Sources: Adapted from Ten tips for judging the medical news. 1993. *Harvard Women's Health Watch,* October. Health headlines. 1994. *Mayo Clinic Health Letter,* December. Balancing risks and benefits. 1993. *Consumer Reports on Health,* September.

circulates blood throughout the body. The ventricles contract (systole) to pump blood to the lungs and body; the ventricles relax (diastole) to receive blood from the atria.

- The major controllable risk factors for CVD are smoking, hypertension, unhealthy cholesterol levels, and a sedentary lifestyle.
- Contributing factors for CVD that can be changed include overweight, diabetes, inadequate stress management, a hostile personality, lack of social support, and poverty.
- Hypertension weakens the heart and scars and hardens arteries, causing resistance to blood flow. It is defined as blood pressure equal to or higher than 140 over 90.
- Atherosclerosis is a progressive hardening and narrowing of arteries that can lead to restricted blood flow and even complete blockage; high blood pressure and high levels of blood cholesterol are contributing factors.
- Heart attacks, strokes, and congestive heart failure are the results of a long-term disease process; hypertension and atherosclerosis are usually involved.
- To prevent CVD, it's important to begin early to avoid or change lifestyle risk factors and to be aware of inherited risks.

BEHAVIOR CHANGE ACTIVITY

Involving the People Around You

Your behavior change program will be more successful if the people around you are supportive and involved—or at least are not sabotaging your efforts. Use your health journal to track how other people influence your target behavior and your efforts to change it. For example, do you always goof off and skip exercising when you're with certain people? Do you always drink or eat too much when you socialize with certain friends? Are friends and family members offering you enthusiastic support for your efforts to change your behavior, or do they make jokes about it? Have they even noticed? Summarize the reactions of those around you in the chart below.

Target behavior: ______________________________

Person	Typical Effect on Target Behavior	Involvement in/Reaction to Program

It may be difficult to change the actions and reactions of the people who are close to you. For them to be involved in your program, you may need to develop new ways of interacting with them (for example, taking a walk rather than going out to dinner as a means of socializing). Most of your friends and family members will want to help you—if they know how. Ask for exactly the type of help or involvement you want. Do you want feedback, praise, or just cooperation? Would you like someone to witness your contract, or be involved more directly in your program? Do you want someone to stop sabotaging your efforts by inviting you to watch TV, eat rich desserts, and so on? Look for ways that the people who are close to you can share in your behavior change program. They can help to motivate you and to maintain your commitment to your program. Develop a way that each individual you listed above can become involved in your program in a positive way.

Person	Target Involvement in Behavior Change Program

FOR MORE INFORMATION

American Heart Association. *Heart and Stroke Facts.* Dallas, Tex.: American Heart Association. *An annually updated text that describes the different types of cardiovascular diseases, including incidence, symptoms, risks, and treatments.*

American Heart Association Cookbook, 5th ed. 1993. New York: Random House. *Recipes and easy-to-follow advice for heart-healthy eating.*

Fortmann, S., and P. Breitrose. 1996. *The Blood Pressure Book: How to Get It Down and Keep It Down.* Palo Alto, Calif.: Bull Publishing. *A step-by-step guide for making lifestyle changes to control blood pressure.*

Ornish, D. 1990. *Dr. Dean Ornish's Program for Reversing Heart Disease.* New York: Random House. *A practical program for reducing cholesterol and reversing atherosclerosis that includes dietary changes, exercise, and stress management.*

Ornish, D. 1993. *Eat More, Weigh Less.* New York: Harper-Collins. *Recipes and advice for losing weight and controlling dietary risk factors for cardiovascular disease.*

Smith, J. S., and S. D. Smith. 1993. *The Low-Fat Supermarket.* Lancaster, Pa.: Starburst Publications. *A practical guide to cutting down on fat by a registered dietitian and a physician.*

Ulene, A., and V. Ulene. 1994. *Count Out Cholesterol.* Berkeley, Calif.: Ulysses Press. *A step-by-step plan for changing your eating habits to lower cholesterol.*

Williams, R., and V. Williams. 1993. *Anger Kills: Seventeen Strategies for Controlling the Hostility That Can Harm Your Health.* New York: Times Books. *A discussion of the biological correlates of anger and hostility that can lead to heart disease, and strategies for recognizing and controlling hostility, by experts in behavioral medicine.*

For additional information, contact the following agencies and organizations:

American Dietetic Association
216 W. Jackson Blvd.
Chicago, IL 60606-6995
312-899-0040

American Heart Association
7320 Greenville Ave.
Dallas, TX 75231
214-373-6300

Check your phone book for the local American Heart Association Office.

National Heart, Lung, and Blood Institute
Cardiovascular Disease Education Program
7200 Wisconsin Ave., Box 329
Bethesda, MD 20814-4820
301-951-3260

For more resources, refer to the For More Information listings in Chapters 3, 8, and 10.

SELECTED BIBLIOGRAPHY

American Heart Association. 1992. *Physicians' Cholesterol Education Handbook.* Dallas, Tex.: American Heart Association.

American Heart Association. 1996. *Heart and Stroke Facts.* Dallas, Tex.: American Heart Association.

American Heart Association. 1995. *Heart and Stroke Facts: 1995 Statistical Supplement.* Dallas, Tex.: American Heart Association.

American Medical Association. 1992. *Position Paper on Exercise.* Chicago: American Medical Association.

Blair, S. N., H. W. Kohl, R. S. Paffenbarger, D. G. Clark, K. H. Cooper, and L. W. Gibbons. 1989. Physical fitness and all-cause mortality: A prospective study of healthy men and women. *Journal of the American Medical Association* 262: 2395–2401.

Caralis, P. V. 1991. Coronary artery disease in Hispanic Americans: How does ethnic background affect risk factors and mortality rates? *Postgraduate Medicine* 91(4): 179–182, 185–188, 193.

Centers for Disease Control and Prevention. 1994. *Advance Report of Final Mortality Statistics, 1992. Monthly Vital Statistics Report,* 8 December, 43(6): 51.

Centers for Disease Control and Prevention. Office on Smoking and Health. 1994. *Facts About Second-Hand Smoke.*

Coronary artery disease: Diagnosis and treatment. 1994. *Harvard Heart Letter, A Special Report.* November.

Douglas, P. S., et al. 1992. Exercise and atherosclerotic heart disease in women. *Medicine and Science in Sports and Exercise* 6 Suppl.: S266–276.

Goldsmith, M. F. 1991. African lineage, hypertension linked. *Journal of the American Medical Association* 26(15): 2049.

Haskell, W. L., et al. 1992. Cardiovascular benefits and assessment of physical activity and physical fitness in adults. *Medicine and Science in Sports and Exercise* 6 Suppl.: S201–220.

Haskell, W. L., et al. 1992. Role of water-soluble dietary fiber in the management of elevated plasma cholesterol in healthy subjects. *American Journal of Cardiology* 69(5): 433–439.

Keil, J. E., et al. 1992. Does equal socioeconomic status in black and white men mean equal risk of mortality? *American Journal of Public Health* 82(8): 1133–1136.

Laragh, J. H., and B. M. Brenner, eds. 1996. *Hypertension: Pathophysiology, Diagnosis and Management.* New York: Raven.

Leaf, A. 1992. Health claims: Omega-3 fatty acids and cardiovascular disease. *Nutrition Reviews* 50(5): 150–154.

Mayo Clinic Heart Book. 1993. New York: Morrow.

More on aspirin. 1995. *Harvard Health Letter,* January, 2.

Musante, L., et al. 1992. Hostility: Relationship to lifestyle behaviors and physical risk factors. *Behavioral Medicine* 18(1): 21–26.

Pashkow, F. J., and C. Libov. 1994. *The Women's Heart Book: The Complete Guide to Keeping Your Heart Healthy and What to Do If Things Go Wrong.* New York: Penguin.

Shakespeare, C. F. 1992. Recent advances in cardiology. *Postgraduate Medical Journal* 68(799): 327–337.

The truth about secondhand smoke. 1995. *Consumer Reports,* January, 27–33.

Treasure, C. B., et al. 1995. Beneficial effects of cholesterol-lowering therapy on the coronary endothelium in patients with coronary artery disease. *New England Journal of Medicine* 332: 481–487.

Name ______________________ Section ____________ Date ______________

LAB 11-1 *Risk Factors for Cardiovascular Disease*

Your chances of suffering an early heart attack or stroke depend on a variety of factors, many of which are under your control. To help identify your risk factors, circle the response for each risk category that best describes you.

1. Sex
   - 0 Female
   - 2 Male
2. Heredity
   - 0 Neither parent suffered a heart attack or stroke before age 60.
   - 3 One parent suffered a heart attack or stroke before age 60.
   - 7 Both parents suffered a heart attack or stroke before age 60.
3. Smoking
   - 0 Never smoked
   - 1 Quit more than 2 years ago
   - 2 Quit less than 2 years ago
   - 8 Smoke less than ½ pack per day
   - 13 Smoke more than ½ pack per day
   - 15 Smoke more than 1 pack per day
4. Environmental Tobacco Smoke
   - 0 Do not live or work with smokers
   - 2 Exposed to ETS at work
   - 3 Live with smoker
   - 4 Both live and work with smokers
5. Blood Pressure

   The average of the last three readings:
   - 0 130/80 or below
   - 1 131/81–140/85
   - 5 141/86–150/90
   - 9 151/91–170/100
   - 13 Above 170/100
6. Total Cholesterol

   The average of the last three readings:
   - 0 Lower than 190
   - 1 190–210
   - 2 Don't know
   - 3 211–240
   - 4 241–270
   - 5 271–300
   - 6 Over 300
7. HDL Cholesterol

   The average of the last three readings:
   - 0 Over 65 mg/dl
   - 1 55–65
   - 2 Don't know HDL
   - 3 45–54
   - 5 35–44
   - 7 25–34
   - 12 Lower than 25
8. Exercise
   - 0 Aerobic exercise three times a week
   - 1 Aerobic exercise once or twice a week
   - 2 Occasional exercise less than once a week
   - 7 Rarely exercise
9. Diabetes
   - 0 No personal or family history
   - 2 One parent with diabetes
   - 6 Two parents with diabetes
   - 9 Non–insulin-dependent diabetes (Type 2)
   - 13 Insulin-dependent diabetes (Type 1)
10. Weight
    - 0 Near ideal weight
    - 1 6 pounds or less above ideal weight
    - 3 7–19 pounds above ideal weight
    - 5 20–40 pounds above ideal weight
    - 7 More than 40 pounds above ideal weight
11. Stress
    - 0 Relaxed most of the time
    - 1 Occasional stress and anger
    - 2 Frequently stressed and angry
    - 3 Usually stressed and angry

Scoring

Total your risk factor points. Refer to the list below to get an approximate rating of your risk of suffering an early heart attack or stroke.

Score	*Estimated Risk*
Less than 20	Low risk
20–29	Moderate risk
30–45	High risk
Over 45	Extremely high risk

To monitor your progress toward your goal, enter the results of this lab in the Preprogram Assessment column of Lab 15-2. After several weeks of a program to reduce CVD risk, do this lab again and enter the results in the Postprogram Assessment column of Lab 15-2. How do the results compare?

12

Cancer

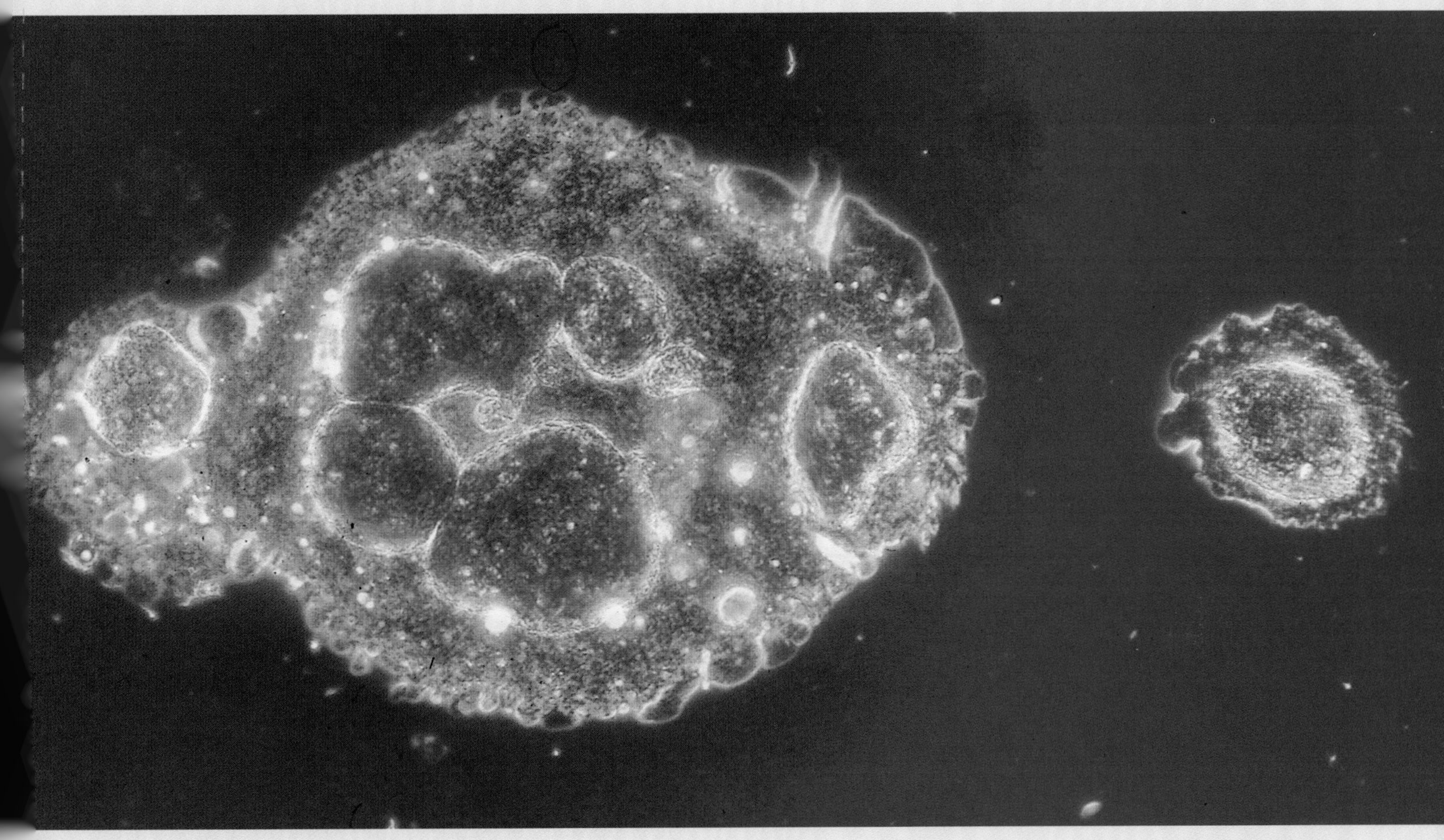

LOOKING AHEAD

After reading this chapter, you should be able to answer these questions about cancer:

- What is cancer? How does it spread?
- What are the most common forms of cancer, and what are the risk factors associated with each form?
- What are the signs and symptoms of cancer in its early stages?
- What causes cancer?
- What can an individual do to lower his or her risk of cancer?

Cancer is probably the most feared illness in the United States, although cardiovascular death is the leading cause of death. About 85 million Americans, or approximately one in three, will develop cancer. New cancer-causing agents and risks are constantly being identified, and yet to many people the disease continues to seem mysterious and untreatable. In fact, there are many steps most individuals can take to protect themselves from cancer and, if those fail, to detect it in its earliest, most treatable stages.

This chapter provides basic information about common cancers, specific guidelines for prevention, and treatment strategies. It describes how to integrate a preventive point of view into your daily life and your general health awareness.

WHAT IS CANCER?

Cancer is an abnormal and uncontrollable growth of cells or tissue that leads to death if untreated. Most cancers take the form of tumors, although not all tumors are cancers. A tumor is simply a mass of new tissue that serves no physiological purpose. **Benign tumors** are made up of cells similar to surrounding cells and are enclosed in a membrane that prevents them from penetrating other tissues. They are dangerous only if their presence interferes with the functioning of the body. **Malignant tumors,** or cancer, are capable of invading surrounding tissues and spreading to distant sites via blood and lymphatic circulation. A few cancers—such as **leukemia,** cancer of the blood—do not produce masses but still have the fundamental property of rapid and inappropriate growth.

Every case of cancer begins as a change in a cell that allows it to grow and divide when it should not. A malignant cell divides without regard for normal control mechanisms and gradually produces a mass of abnormal cells—a tumor. Eventually the tumor becomes detectable. Detection can be earlier in an accessible site such as a breast than in a relatively inaccessible one such as a lung, where the tumor may not be noticed until it has produced indirect symptoms like a persistent cough or pain.

Metastasis, the spread of cancer cells from one part of the body to another, occurs because cancer cells break away from each other more easily than normal cells. They can invade nearby tissue or drift to distant parts of the body and establish new colonies of cancer cells. This breakaway ability is what makes early detection critical. Death is preventable only by removing every cancerous cell. Once cancer cells have entered the lymph system or bloodstream, stopping their spread is particularly difficult.

TERMS

benign tumor A tumor that is not malignant or cancerous.

malignant tumor A tumor that is cancerous and capable of spreading.

leukemia A malignant disease of the blood-forming system.

metastasis The spread of cancer cells from one part of the body to another.

remission A condition in which there are no symptoms or any other evidence of disease.

carcinogen Any substance that causes cancer.

INCIDENCE OF CANCER

Overall cancer rates, as well as deaths from cancer, have increased over the last 35 years. Lung cancer and melanoma, a serious form of skin cancer, account for the greatest increases. Figure 12-1 shows a breakdown of cancer incidence and deaths by site and sex.

In 1996, about 1,400,000 people in the United States were diagnosed with cancer. More than half will be cured, but about 44% will eventually die as a result of their cancer. These grim statistics exclude more than 800,000 cases of the easily curable types of skin cancer.

Although the incidence of cancer is increasing numerically, when cancer death rates are adjusted to reflect the presence of more older people in the population, they appear to be leveling off or even decreasing. The only major exception to this trend involves lung cancer, which is increasing rapidly in women. The death rate in women from lung cancer today parallels the increase in the rate of smoking among women beginning about 25 years ago. Since 1987, lung cancer has surpassed breast cancer as the leading cause of cancer death in women.

In all types of cancer, the earlier the abnormal growth is detected, the greater the chances of survival. For this reason, alert, informed self-monitoring of the major cancer sites is a part of any overall fitness and wellness program.

COMMON CANCERS

It is beyond the scope of this book to discuss all the known types of cancers. We will describe some of the most common cancers and look at their causes and modes of prevention.

Lung Cancer

Lung cancer is the most common cause of cancer death in the United States (Table 12-1, p. 280). A signal such as a persistent cough, chest pain, or recurring bronchitis may be the first indication of the presence of a tumor. However, these symptoms usually do not appear until the disease has advanced to the invasive stage, making early detection very difficult. This difficulty, plus the fact that most cancer cells in the lungs are resistant to treatment, explains the fact that only 13% of lung cancer patients are

Male

INCIDENCE	DEATH	
3%	2%	Skin (melanoma)
3%	2%	Oral
13%	32%	Lung
2%	5%	Pancreas
9%	9%	Colon and rectum
41%	14%	Prostate
7%	5%	Urinary
6%	9%	Leukemia and lymphomas
16%	22%	All other

Female

	INCIDENCE	DEATH
Skin (melanoma)	3%	1%
Oral	2%	1%
Breast	31%	17%
Lung	13%	25%
Pancreas	2%	5%
Colon and rectum	11%	10%
Ovary	5%	6%
Uterus	6%	2%
Urinary	4%	3%
Leukemia and lymphomas	6%	8%
All other	17%	22%

VITAL STATISTICS

Figure 12-1 ***Cancer incidence by site and sex, and cancer deaths by site and sex.*** The Incidence column indicates what percentage of all cancers occurred in each site; the Death column indicates what percentage of all cancer deaths were attributed to each type. *Source:* American Cancer Society. 1996. *Cancer Facts and Figures, 1996.* New York: American Cancer Society.

alive 5 years after diagnosis. However, about 25% of lung cancers do respond to chemotherapy. These cancers, called small-cell lung cancers, often respond to chemotherapy and radiation with **remission,** a cessation of growth that can last for years.

The chief risk factor for lung cancer is smoking, which is implicated in 87% of cases. When smoking is combined with exposure to other environmental **carcinogens,** such as radioactive radon gas or asbestos particles, the risk of cancer can increase by a factor of 10 or more. Long-term exposure to environmental tobacco smoke (ETS, or secondhand smoke) increases lung cancer risk.

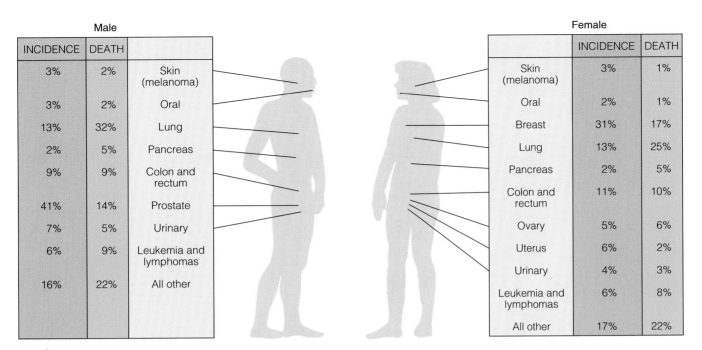

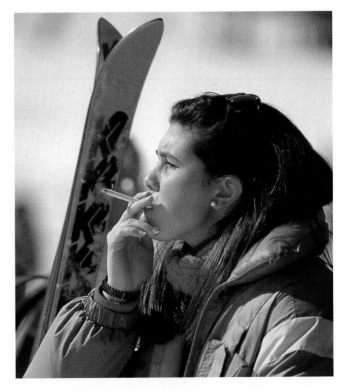

Cigarette smoking is the primary cause of lung cancer and is implicated in numerous other kinds of cancer. Many people begin smoking as teenagers, believing that the habit makes them look sophisticated or will help them lose weight. Tobacco advertising is designed to encourage such beliefs.

Colon and Rectal Cancer

The second most common cause of cancer death in the United States is colon and rectal cancer (also known as colorectal cancer). Most of these cancers arise from preexisting polyps, small growths on the wall of the colon that may gradually become malignant. The tendency to form polyps appears to be hereditary, although after age 50 there is a higher risk of this type of cancer, regardless of health profile or family background.

Colon and rectal cancer is clearly linked to both diet and genetic predisposition. In countries where people eat a low-fat, high-fiber diet, its incidence is notably low: only 10–20% of the incidence in the United States. Polyps may bleed as they progress, and if such bleeding is detected in time, a polyp can be tested and even removed

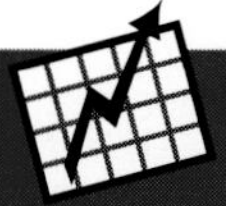

VITAL STATISTICS

*TABLE 12-1 Leading Cancer Sites, 1996**

Site	Estimated New Cases in 1996	Estimated Deaths in 1996	Warning Signals	Comment
Lung	177,000	158,700	Persistent cough or lingering respiratory ailment	The leading cause of cancer death among both men and women.
Colon and rectum	133,500	54,900	Change in bowel habits; bleeding	Considered a highly curable disease when digital and proctoscopic examinations are included in routine checkups.
Breast	185,700	44,560	Lump or thickening in the breast	Until recently, the leading cause of cancer death in women; now surpassed by lung cancer.
Prostate	317,100	41,400	Urinary difficulty	Occurs mainly in men over 60; the disease can be detected by digital rectal exams at annual checkups.
Kidney and bladder	83,500	23,700	Urinary difficulty; bleeding (in which case consult physician at once)	Protective measures for workers in high-risk industries are helping eliminate one of the important causes of these cancers.
Stomach	22,800	14,000	Unexplained indigestion continuing for more than a week	A 40% decline in mortality in 25 years, for unknown reasons.
Uterus (including cervix)	49,700**	10,900	Unusual bleeding or discharge	Cervical cancer mortality has declined 70% during the last 40 years because of early detection by Pap tests. Postmenopausal women with abnormal bleeding should be checked.
Oral (including pharynx)	29,500	8,300	Sore that does not heal; difficulty swallowing	Many more lives should be saved because the mouth is easily accessible to visual examination by physicians and dentists.
Skin	38,300[†]	7,300	Sore that does not heal; change in wart or mole	Melanoma is readily detected by observation and diagnosed by simple biopsy.
Leukemia	27,600	21,000	Leukemias are cancers of blood-forming tissues and are characterized by the abnormal production of immature white blood cells. Acute leukemia occurs mostly in children and is treated by drugs that have extended lives from a few months to as much as 10 years. Chronic leukemia strikes usually after age 25 and progresses less rapidly.	
Other blood and lymph tissues	74,600	35,210	Cancers arising in the lymph system include Hodgkin's disease and lymphosarcoma. Some patients with lymphatic cancers can lead normal lives for many years. Five-year survival rate for Hodgkin's disease increased from 40% to 79% over the last 30 years.	

*All figures are rounded to the nearest 100 and include both sexes.
**Totals do not include cases in which the carcinoma is confined to the epithelium.
[†]Totals do not include nonmelanoma skin cancers (800,000 new cases annually).

Source: Incidence estimates are based on rates of cancer in the United States from American Cancer Society. 1996. *Cancer Facts and Figures, 1996.* New York: American Cancer Society.

without major surgery. The standard warning signs of colon cancer are bleeding from the rectum or a change in bowel habits. However, a rectal exam can detect some rectal tumors, and testing for blood in the stool, performed during a routine physical exam, can detect small amounts of blood long before bleeding becomes obvious. The American Cancer Society recommends that this examination be performed annually after age 40.

Even for those who have a genetic predisposition to colon and rectal cancer, lifestyle can make a significant difference. Just as stopping smoking can reverse precancerous changes in the lungs, a high-fiber diet can slow or even reverse precancerous changes in colon cells. Regular exercise is also associated with a lower risk of colon and rectal cancer. In addition, recent research has shown that regular aspirin use reduces the risk. In a study of 90,000 nurses, those who regularly took aspirin (at least three tablets a week) for at least 10 years had nearly a 40% lower risk of colon and rectal cancer than those who did not.

Colon and rectal cancer is more curable than lung cancer, particularly if it is caught before it spreads beyond the bowel. The 5-year survival rate is 61% overall; about 91% if the tumor is localized, but only 40% if it has spread.

Breast Cancer

Breast cancer is the most common cancer in women (although lung cancer is the most common cause of cancer death). Breast cancer occurs in men only rarely but will afflict about one American woman in nine. In 1996, breast cancer was diagnosed in about 184,000 American women; 45,000 died from the disease. About 79% of patients survive at least 5 years after diagnosis, and most of them are completely cured.

Only a small percentage of breast cancer cases occur before the age of 30, but a woman's risk doubles every 5 years between ages 30 and 45. After that, the risk grows more slowly, by 10–15% every 5 years after age 45.

Although there is a strong genetic factor in breast cancer, only about 20% of cases occur in women with a family history of the disease. Because the incidence of breast cancer is high in developed Western countries but low in developing non-Western countries, it has been called a "disease of civilization." The distribution of cancer throughout the world has led some researchers to postulate a link between breast cancer and the sedentary Western lifestyle and its high-fat, low-fiber diet.

Other risk factors include alcohol use, certain kinds of benign breast disease, obesity, the use of oral contraceptives, early first menstruation (thought to be due to the robustness of well-nourished children), late menopause, and late first childbirth. These risk factors may be linked by the female sex hormone estrogen. Estrogen circulates in a woman's body in high concentrations during the years between puberty and menopause and promotes the growth of responsive cells in a variety of sites. Fat cells also produce estrogen, and estrogen levels are higher in obese women. Alcohol can interfere with the metabolism of estrogen in the liver and can increase the hormone's levels in the blood. And evidence suggests that estrogen is a promoter of cancer in sites that are estrogen-responsive, including breast and uterine tissue.

The links between breast cancer and diet and exercise are still being explored. Recent studies suggest that a high-fat diet alone may not increase the risk of breast cancer, but women may be more likely to get breast cancer if their diet is low in fiber, if they have a sedentary lifestyle, or if they are obese.

The American Cancer Society recommends a three-part program for the early detection of breast cancer:

1. Monthly breast self-examination for all women over age 20 (see the box "Breast Self-Examination," p. 282).
2. A clinical breast exam by a physician every 3 years.
3. **Mammograms** (low-dose breast x-rays) every 1–2 years for most women over 40 and annually for most women over 50 (individual risk factors must be considered in determining the frequency of mammograms).

If a lump is detected, it may be scanned by **ultrasonography** (imaging through sound waves) and **biopsied** (excised and microscopically examined) to determine whether it is cancerous. In 90% of cases, breast lumps turn out to be harmless. But if the lump does contain cancer cells, it may be treated by lumpectomy, removal of the lump and surrounding tissue, or by mastectomy, removal of the breast. Chemotherapy or radiation may also be used. In addition, recent studies have shown that social support can have a significant impact on the course of the disease (see the box "Support Groups and Cancer Survival," p. 284).

At the time of surgery, lymph nodes from the armpit may be removed and examined to determine whether the cancer has spread. The chances of surviving breast cancer vary depending on both the nature of the tumor and whether it has metastasized. If the tumor is discovered early, before it has spread to the adjacent lymph nodes, the patient has about a 96% chance of surviving for more than 5 years.

TERMS

mammogram An x-ray of the breasts used for the early detection of breast cancer.

ultrasonography An imaging method in which inaudible high-pitched sound (ultrasound) is bounced off body structures to create an image on a monitor.

biopsy The removal and examination of a small piece of body tissue for the purpose of diagnosis.

TACTICS AND TIPS
Breast Self-Examination

All women over 20 should practice monthly breast self-examination (BSE) to help in the early detection of breast cancer. Examine your breasts when they are least tender, usually 7 days after the start of your menstrual period. If you discover a lump or detect any changes, seek medical attention. Most breast changes are not cancerous.

For a complete BSE, remember these seven Ps: positions, perimeter, **palpation,** pressure, pattern, practice with feedback, and plan of action.

1. *Positions.* The first part of BSE is a visual inspection while standing in front of a mirror. Examine your breasts with your arms raised. Look for changes in contour and shape of the breasts, color and texture of the skin and nipple, and evidence of discharge from the nipple. Repeat the visual examination with your arms at your side, with your hands on your hips, and while bending slightly forward.

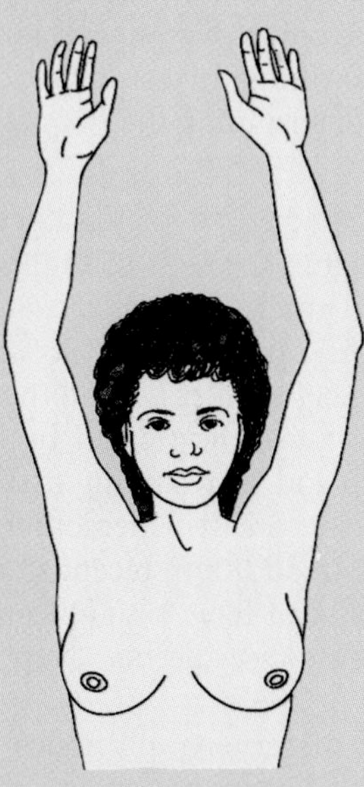

The remainder of the examination involves palpation of your breasts. Two positions are possible: *side-lying* or *flat.* The side-lying position is particularly recommended for women with large breasts: Lie on your side and rotate one shoulder back to the flat surface. You will be examining the breast on the side that is rotated back. If you use the flat position, place a pillow or folded towel under the shoulder of the breast to be examined.

2. *Perimeter.* The area you should examine is bounded by a line that extends down from the middle of the armpit to just beneath the breast, continues across along the underside of the breast to the middle of the breastbone, then moves up to and along the collarbone and back to the middle of the armpit (shaded area). Most cancers occur in the upper outer area of the breast.

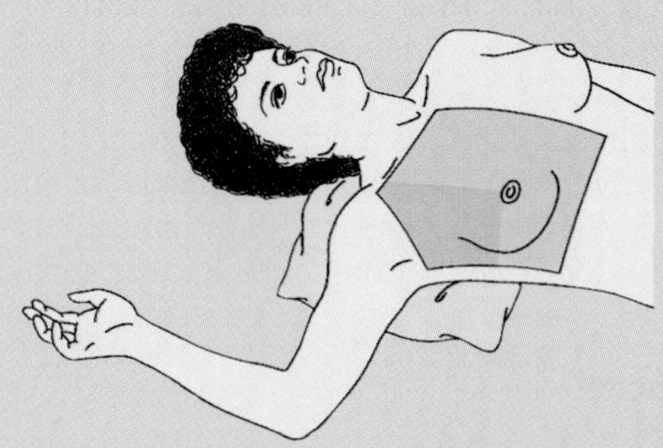

3. *Palpation.* Use your left hand to palpate the right breast, while holding your right arm at a right angle to the rib cage, with your elbow bent. Repeat the procedure on the other side. Use the pads of three or four fingers to examine every inch of your breast tissue. Move your fingers in circles about the size of a dime. Do not lift your fingers from your breast between palpations. You can use powder or lotion to help your fingers glide from one spot to the next.
4. *Pressure.* Use varying levels of pressure for each palpation, from light to deep, to examine the full thickness of your breast tissue. Using pressure will not injure the breast.

Prostate Cancer

Cancer of the prostate gland is the most common cancer in men. More than 240,000 new cases are diagnosed each year, 80% of which are men over age 65. The prostate gland, which produces seminal fluid, is situated at the base of the bladder. When it is enlarged, it can block the flow of urine. Diet and lifestyle probably influence the occurrence of this type of cancer, but compared to other cancers, the risk factors are somewhat obscure. For reasons not completely understood, African American men have the highest incidence of prostate cancer in the world.

Early detection is the best method of control. Most cases are first detected by rectal examination during a routine physical exam. A promising new blood test measures the amount of prostate-specific antigen (PSA) in the blood, which can help signal early prostate cancer, as well as other benign prostate conditions. And ultrasonography

TACTICS AND TIPS
Breast Self-Examination (continued)

5. *Pattern of search.* Use one of the following search patterns to examine all of your breast tissue:
   - *Vertical strip.* Start in the armpit and proceed downward to the lower boundary. Move a finger's width toward the middle, and continue palpating upward until you reach the collarbone. Repeat this until you have covered all breast tissue. Make at least six strips before the nipple and four strips after the nipple.

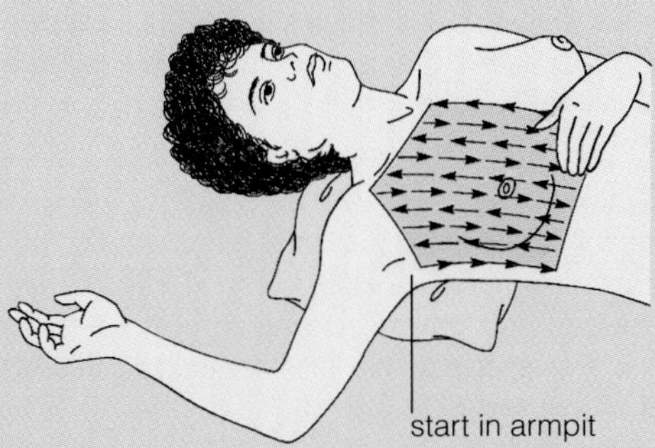

   - *Wedge.* Imagine your breast divided like the spokes of a wheel. Examine each separate segment, moving from the outside boundary toward the nipple. Slide your fingers back to the boundary, move over a finger's width, and repeat this procedure until you have covered all breast tissue. You will need 10–16 segments.

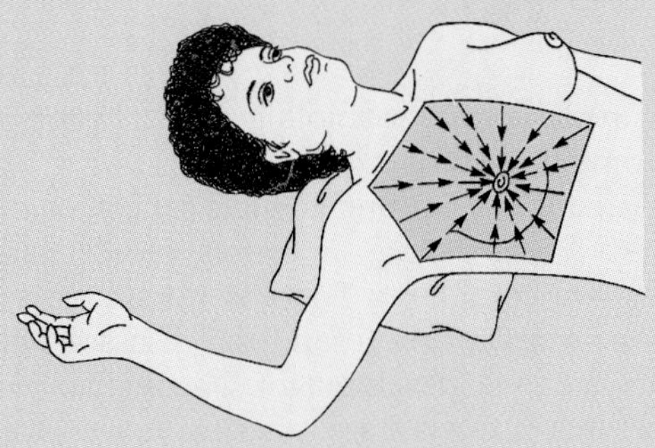

   - *Circle.* Imagine your breast as the face of a clock. Starting at 12:00, palpate along the boundary of each circle until you return to your starting point. Then move down a finger's width, and continue palpating in increasingly smaller circles until you reach the nipple. Depending on the size of your breast, you will need 8–10 circles.

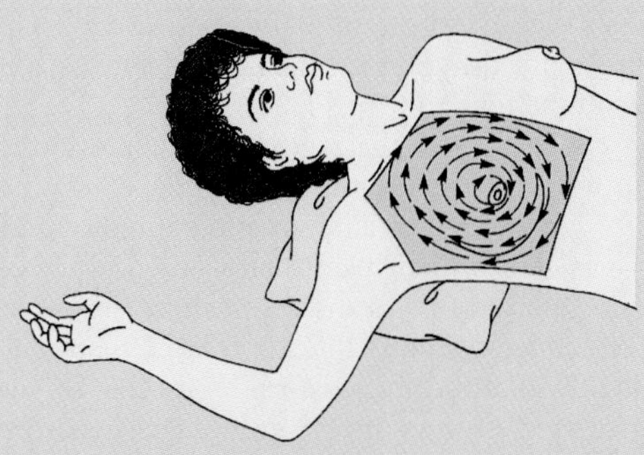

Once you have completed the pattern, perform two additional exams: (1) squeeze your nipples to check for discharge (some women have a normal discharge), and (2) examine the breast tissue that extends into your armpit while your arm is relaxed at your side.

6. *Practice with feedback.* Have your BSE technique checked by your physician or another health care professional. Practice under supervision until you feel comfortable and confident.
7. *Plan of action.* Your personal breast health plan of action should include the following: (1) discuss the American Cancer Society breast cancer detection guidelines with your physician, (2) schedule clinical breast examinations and mammograms as appropriate, (3) do monthly BSEs, and (4) report any changes to your health care professional.

Source: American Cancer Society. 1992. *Breast Self-Examination: A New Approach,* May.

is used increasingly to detect lumps that are too small to be felt.

If a lump is found, a pathologist studies the cells gathered in a needle biopsy to determine whether they are malignant or benign. If the cells are malignant, the prostate is usually removed surgically. Alternative treatments include radiation, hormone therapy, and anticancer drugs. Survival rates for all stages of this cancer have improved steadily since 1940; over the last 30 years, the 5-year survival rate has increased from 50% to 85%.

Uterine, Cervical, and Ovarian Cancer

Because the uterus, cervix, and ovaries are subject to similar hormonal influences, the cancers of these organs can be discussed as a group. The cervix is the narrow end of

TERMS

palpation Examination by touch.

WELLNESS CONNECTION

Support Groups and Cancer Survival

Stanford University psychiatrist Dr. David Spiegel and his colleagues carried out a 3-year study on women with advanced breast cancer to determine how participation in a support group would affect their psychological health. Women in the experimental group not only received standard medical care but also participated in weekly group therapy sessions. In the support group, women shared their fears, planned means of coping with the threat of death, grieved over the loss of group members, learned to control their pain with self-hypnosis, and looked for ways to live more fully in the time they had left.

At the conclusion of the study, researchers found that women in the study had, indeed, been helped by the support group. They were less anxious and depressed and were better able to control their pain than women in the control group, who received only standard medical treatment. The real surprise came several years later when Dr. Spiegel reexamined the data from this study. He found that the women who participated in the support group also lived on average more than twice as long from the start of the study than women in the control group.

How might support groups improve the survival as well as the psychological health of participants? Researchers have hypothesized several ways in which psychosocial support could be translated into changes in physical health:

- Social support may affect behavior, making patients in a support group more likely to engage in healthy behaviors such as eating well, exercising regularly, and getting plenty of sleep.
- Cancer patients who benefit from group support might interact more effectively with their physicians, eliciting more vigorous medical treatment.
- Support groups may buffer people against stress, cushioning the body from the effects of the stress response.
- In light of the close relationship between the brain and the immune system, feeling understood and supported may affect the functioning of the immune system in some way that enables the body to fight cancer more effectively.

Additional research should help clarify how support groups benefit cancer patients. In the meantime, this study can serve as a reminder of the powerful effects that social support has on our physical and emotional well-being, whether we are coping with a life-threatening illness or the challenges of everyday life.

Sources: Adapted from Spiegel, D. 1993. *Living Beyond Limits: New Hope and Help for Facing Life-Threatening Illness.* New York: Random House. Spiegel, D., J. R. Bloom, H. C. Kraemer, and E. Gottheil. 1989. Effect of psychosocial treatment on survival of patients with metastatic breast cancer. *Lancet* ii:888–891.

the uterus that opens into the vagina, and the uterus itself is in contact with the ovaries, which are deep in the abdomen. Uterine cancer is the most common cancer of the reproductive system, but ovarian cancer and cervical cancer are more deadly.

Cancer of the uterus, also called endometrial cancer, is usually diagnosed in women between ages 55 and 69. The risk factors are a history of infertility, obesity, and prolonged estrogen therapy. Fortunately, uterine cancer is often detectable during a standard pelvic exam and is curable by surgery. About 83% of patients are apparently healthy 5 years after diagnosis.

Cervical cancer, in contrast, attacks younger women, eventually killing one-third of those who are diagnosed with it. Nevertheless, cervical cancer is one of the great success stories in cancer control during the last few decades. The diagnostic tool known as the **Pap test** has become nearly universal in the United States over the last 40 years, and during that same period the cervical cancer death rate has dropped by more than 70%. The risk factors for cervical cancer are different from those for uterine cancer. They include early age at first intercourse, multiple sex partners, cigarette smoking, and a history of sexually transmissible diseases.

Compared to uterine and cervical cancer, ovarian cancer is rare. Nevertheless, it causes more deaths than the other two combined. There is no simple screening method for ovarian cancer, and the disease is often noticed only late in its development. The incidence of ovarian cancer increases with age, peaking at ages over 60.

Skin Cancer

When the highly curable forms are counted, skin cancer is the most common cancer of all. More than 800,000 cases were diagnosed in 1996, but only 38,000 of these were the most serious type. Treatments are usually simple and successful when the cancers are caught early.

Almost all types of skin cancer can be traced to excessive direct exposure to **ultraviolet (UV) radiation** from the sun, especially during childhood. Skin cancer may also be caused by exposure to coal tar, pitch, creosote, arsenic, and radioactive materials, but sunlight accounts for the largest proportion of cases by far. In particular, melanoma in later life is linked to severe sunburns in

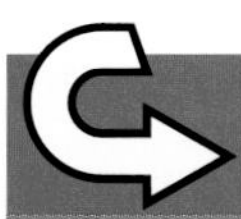

TACTICS AND TIPS

Protecting Your Skin from the Sun

With proper clothing and use of sunscreens, you can lead an active outdoor life *and* protect your skin against most sun-induced damage.

Clothing

- Wear long-sleeved shirts made of tightly woven cotton fabric to protect your forearms, chest, and back. Thin, white shirts and wet clothing that clings to the body will not protect you sufficiently.
- Wear a wide-brimmed hat to protect your ears, forehead, and upper cheeks.

Sunscreen

- Use a sunscreen with an SPF (sun protection factor) of 15 or higher. (An SPF rating refers to the amount of time you can stay out in the sun before you burn, compared to using no sunscreen; for example, a product with an SPF of 15 would allow you to remain in the sun without burning 15 times longer, on average, than if you didn't apply sunscreen.) If you're fair-skinned or will be outdoors for long hours, use a sunscreen with a high SPF. Look for the seal of approval from the Skin Cancer Foundation, which tests sunscreens with SPF 15 or higher for safety and effectiveness.
- Choose a "broad-spectrum" sunscreen for maximum protection against the full range of UV radiation from the sun. Many combinations of ingredients work together to block a broader range of light rays, and they also wash off less easily.
- Apply sunscreen 30–45 minutes before exposure, to allow time for the sunscreen to penetrate the skin.
- Reapply sunscreen frequently and generously. Most people use less than half as much as they should in order to benefit from the full SPF rating. Use a water-resistant sunscreen if you swim or sweat quite a bit.
- If you're taking medication, ask your physician or pharmacist about possible reactions to sunlight and interactions with sunscreens.

Time of Day and Location

- Try to avoid sun exposure between 10:00 A.M. and 3:00 P.M., when the sun's rays are most intense.
- Ultraviolet rays can penetrate at least 3 feet into water, so swimmers should wear water-resistant sunscreen.
- Locations near the equator have more intense sunlight, so stronger sunscreens should be used and applied often. High elevations also have intense sunlight, because there is less atmosphere to filter the UV rays.
- Snow reflects the sun's rays, so don't forget to apply sunscreen before skiing and other snow activities. Sand and water also reflect the sun's rays, so you still need to apply a sunscreen if you are under a beach umbrella. Concrete and white-painted surfaces are also highly reflective.

Sources: Adapted from Sunscreens: Everything new under the sun. 1994. *Consumer Reports on Health,* July. Protecting yourself against the sun. 1992. *Healthline,* June.

childhood, but chronic low-level reactions to the sun from regular suntanning can lead to forms of skin cancer as well (see the box "Protecting Your Skin from the Sun").

Men and women are equally at risk for skin cancer, but people with naturally heavy skin pigmentation are relatively protected. Conversely, people with fair skin have less natural protection against sun damage and a higher risk of certain skin cancers.

There are three main types of skin cancer, named for the types of skin cell from which they develop:

- **Basal cell carcinomas** and **squamous cell carcinomas** account for about 95% of the skin cancers diagnosed each year. Found in chronically sun-exposed areas, such as the face, neck, hands, and arms, they usually appear as pale, waxlike, pearly nodules or red, scaly, sharply outlined patches. They are often painless but may form open sores.
- **Melanoma** is by far the most dangerous skin cancer, because it spreads rapidly. Since 1973, the incidence of melanoma has increased about 4% annually. It can

TERMS

Pap test A scraping of cells from the cervix for examination under a microscope to detect cancer; also called Pap smear.

ultraviolet (UV) radiation Light rays of a specific wavelength emitted by the sun; most UV rays are blocked by the ozone layer in the upper atmosphere. Exposure to ultraviolet A (UVA) and/or ultraviolet B (UVB) rays is linked to the development of skin cancer.

basal cell carcinoma Cancer of the deepest layers of the skin.

squamous cell carcinoma Cancer of the surface layers of the skin.

melanoma A malignant tumor of the skin that arises from pigmented cells, usually a mole.

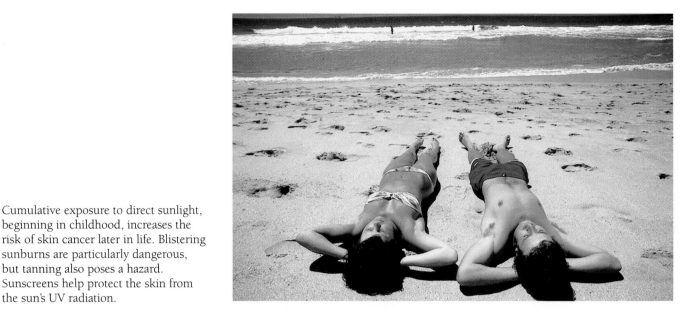

Cumulative exposure to direct sunlight, beginning in childhood, increases the risk of skin cancer later in life. Blistering sunburns are particularly dangerous, but tanning also poses a hazard. Sunscreens help protect the skin from the sun's UV radiation.

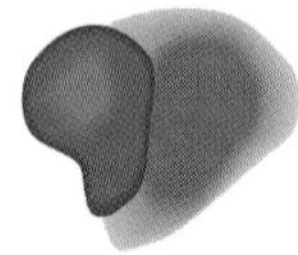

A—Asymmetry: Is one half unlike the other?

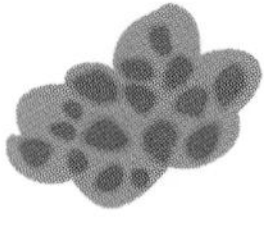

B—Border irregularity: Does it have an uneven, scalloped edge rather than a clearly defined border?

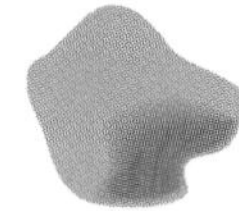

C—Color variation: Is the color uniform, or does it vary from one area to another, from tan to brown to black, or from white to red to blue?

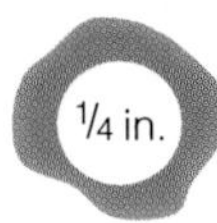

D—Diameter larger than 1/4 inch: At its widest point, is the growth as large as, or larger than, a pencil eraser?

Figure 12-2 ***ABCD test for melanoma.*** *Source:* American Academy of Dermatology.

occur anywhere on the body but is most common on the back, chest, abdomen, and lower legs. A melanoma usually appears at the site of a preexisting mole, which begins to enlarge and become mottled or varied in color; it may develop an irregular surface or irregular borders.

People of every age, including babies and children, need to be protected from sun exposure by **sunscreens** and protective clothing. As with other cancers, when skin cancers are diagnosed, early detection offers the most promise for a good prognosis.

If a skin lesion is cancerous, it is usually removed surgically. Occasionally, other forms of treatment are used. Even for melanoma, the outlook after removal in the early stages is good, with a 5-year survival rate of 94% and a 10-year survival rate of 90%. If the tumor is removed after it has begun to invade the surrounding tissues, the survival rate drops sharply, so it is important to monitor the body for unusual growths, discolorations, or sores that do not heal. For a list of characteristics that may signal melanoma, see Figure 12-2.

Kaposi's sarcoma, a rare form of skin cancer, is seen almost exclusively in men with HIV infection (see Chapter 14).

Oral Cancer

Cancers of the lip, tongue, mouth, and throat can be traced principally to cigarette, cigar, or pipe smoking; the use of snuff and chewing tobacco; and excessive alcohol use. These risk factors work together to multiply an individual's risk of oral cancer.

Oral cancers are fairly easy to detect, but they are often hard to cure. The principal methods of treatment are surgery and radiation. The overall 5-year survival rate from oral cancer is about 52%.

TERMS

sunscreen A substance used to protect the skin from UV radiation; usually applied as an ointment or cream.

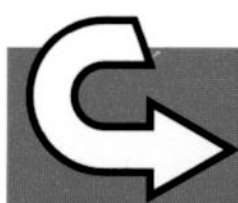

TACTICS AND TIPS

Testicle Self-Examination

To detect testicular cancer, the American Cancer Society recommends the following self-examination:

1. The best time to perform the examination is after a warm bath or shower, when the scrotal skin is most relaxed. (*Scrotal* refers to the scrotum, the pouch in which the testicles normally lie.)
2. Roll each testicle gently between the thumb and fingers of both hands. A normal testicle is smooth, egg-shaped, and somewhat firm to the touch. At the rear of each testicle is a tube called the epididymis, which carries sperm away from the testicle; this is a normal part of your body.
3. If you find any hard lumps or nodules, or if there is any change in the shape, size, or texture of the testicles, consult a physician promptly. These signs may not indicate a malignancy, but only your physician can make a diagnosis.

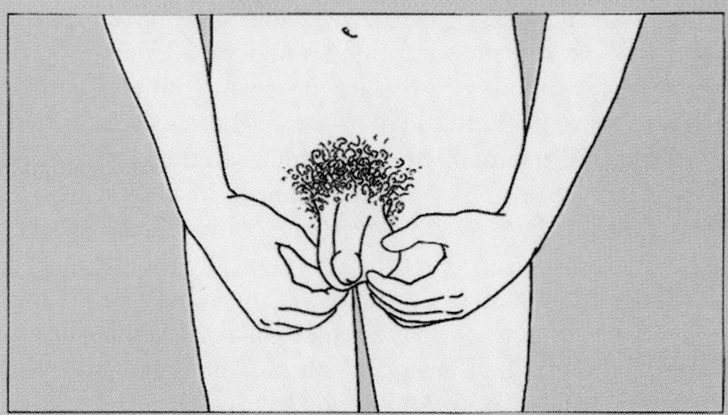

Repeat this examination every month. It is important that you know what your own testicles feel like normally so that you will recognize any changes.

Source: American Cancer Society. 1990. *For Men Only: Testicular Cancer and How to Do TSE (a Self-Exam)*. New York: American Cancer Society.

Testicular Cancer

Although relatively rare overall, testicular cancer is the most common form of cancer in men age 29–35. Regular self-examination to feel the testicles for lumps is a means of early detection (see the box "Testicle Self-Examination"). Men with undescended testicles are at an increased risk for testicular cancer, which is one reason this condition should be treated in early childhood. Treatment of testicular cancer has improved dramatically over the past 25 years, during which time 5-year survival rates have risen from 63% to 93%.

Other Cancers

Bladder cancer occurred in about 53,000 people in 1996. This disease is four times as common in men as in women, and smoking is responsible for about half of all cases in men. People in cities and those exposed to large amounts of dye, rubber, or leather are at increased risk. The first symptoms are likely to be blood in the urine and/or increased frequency of urination. The survival rate for early stage bladder cancer is 93%.

Pancreatic cancer is the fifth leading cause of death from cancer, with about 28,000 deaths in the United States in 1996. This cancer is both hard to detect and almost always deadly. The major environmental risk factor is, again, smoking; there is also a link to a high-fat diet. The disease often takes a "silent" course, and by the time symptoms occur, it is usually far advanced.

WHAT CAUSES CANCER?

Although scientists don't know everything about what causes cancer, they have identified genetic, environmental, and lifestyle factors. In many cases, these work together (see the box "Can Poverty Cause Cancer?" on p. 288).

Genetic Factors

Certain types of cancer have a genetic basis; in other words, an individual may inherit an increased risk for a particular type of cancer from one or both parents. This genetic predisposition seems to involve a special class of genes called suppressor genes, which normally act as a brake on cell growth. If a person is born with a damaged suppressor gene, or if a suppressor gene is damaged by an environmental agent, there is a higher likelihood that the person will experience more rapid cell growth, a precondition for the development of cancer.

Dietary Factors

The foods we eat contain not only carcinogens but also compounds that protect us from cancer.

Fat and Fiber A diet high in saturated fats, such as those found in red meat, appears to contribute to colon, prostate, and other cancers. People in Scotland, for example, consume a great deal of fatty red meat (over 40% of total daily calories from fat), and Scotland has the highest

DIMENSIONS OF DIVERSITY

Can Poverty Cause Cancer?

Along with the well-publicized warning signs of cancer another less-often-mentioned one should be added: poverty. Americans with low incomes are more susceptible to cancer and also more likely to die of it—even if the extent of their condition and treatment are both similar to those of wealthier cancer victims. As National Cancer Institute director Samuel Broder has stated, "Poverty is a carcinogen."

Why does cancer afflict the economically disadvantaged so disproportionately? A principal factor is lifestyle: People of low socioeconomic status are more likely to smoke, abuse alcohol, and eat high-fat food—all of which are associated with developing cancer. Another reason is lack of knowledge and information. Studies have found that low-income people are less exposed to information about cancer, less aware of its early warning symptoms, and less likely to seek medical care when they have such symptoms. A third reason may be an inability to respond to health information and health needs. Many low-income people know they should eat nutritious foods and get regular checkups, but they still may not be able to afford proper nutrition and may not have transportation or access to health care clinics.

In fact, many of the cancer-related threats that people with low incomes face are difficult or impossible to avoid. They may be forced to live and work in unsafe or unhealthy environments. They may have jobs, for example, in which they come into daily contact with carcinogenic chemicals, and they may not have been trained in handling them properly. They face similar risks in their homes and schools, where they may be exposed to asbestos or other cancer-causing hazards daily.

But even poor health habits and dangerous living and working conditions don't completely explain the high cancer mortality rates among the economically disadvantaged. Although scientists don't have a full explanation for it, there's something about economic deprivation that makes cancer deadlier. In a study of cancer patients at two New York City hospitals, it was found that chemotherapy was less effective on the tumors of the poorer patients. They had a lower rate of cancer remission than wealthier patients, even when the latter had more extensive disease.

One possible explanation for these results can be found in the high levels of stress associated with poverty. Stress can impair the immune system, the body's first line of defense against cancer, and experiments with animals have shown that a stressful environment can enhance the growth of a variety of tumors. The link between poverty, stress, and cancer mortality in humans has not been proven, but studies have shown a link between stress and other illnesses.

What can be done about reducing the rate of cancer and cancer mortality among low-income populations? Educating people about prevention is clearly important, and elementary schools and high schools are places where people can be reached in time to encourage healthy habits and prevent bad habits before they begin. However, people from lower socioeconomic groups tend to have high dropout rates. Furthermore, most people have a difficult time worrying about a disease they might get in 10 or 20 years when their immediate concern is basic survival.

For these reasons, some medical researchers look to policy-makers for solutions. They maintain that living and working conditions in the inner cities must be improved. Then, even without new miracle drugs or medical breakthroughs, the United States will see a real decrease in cancer rates among low-income populations.

Source: Adapted from Grabmeier, J. 1992. Poverty can cause cancer. *USA Today*, July.

incidence of colon and rectal cancer in the world. The Japanese, by contrast, eat much less fat (less than 20% of total daily calories) because fish, rather than fatty meat, is the staple dietary protein; and colon and rectal cancer is uncommon in Japan. These patterns cannot be explained by genetic factors. Japanese who have emigrated to the United States, where meat is a major part of the diet, are as susceptible to colon and rectal cancer as other Americans.

Some groups of people, particularly vegetarians, have a low incidence of colon and rectal cancer. The vegetarian diet is typically low in fat and high in insoluble fiber. This link, backed up by laboratory evidence, suggests that colon and rectal cancer may also be related to a lack of fiber in the diet. While fiber does not supply nutrition, it has many other useful properties. It provides bulk, which dilutes any carcinogens that may be present. It reduces the transit time of waste through the intestine, so that carcinogens have less time to act on cells. Fiber also binds bile acids and other lipids that promote the development of colon and rectal cancer.

Alcohol Alcohol is associated with an increased incidence of several types of cancer. The link between alcohol intake and breast cancer is not well understood, but it is dramatic. An average alcohol intake of three drinks per day is associated with a doubling of breast cancer risk. As mentioned earlier, alcohol and tobacco (cigarettes or smokeless tobacco) interact as risk factors for oral cancer. The combination of the two multiplies the carcinogenic effect of each substance. Heavy users of both alcohol and tobacco have a risk for oral cancer up to 15 times greater than that of people who don't drink or smoke.

Anticancer Agents in the Diet Some dietary compounds—**anticarcinogens**—have the ability to act against carcinogens; others prevent the development and spread of cancer through different means. Certain dietary compounds prevent carcinogens from forming in the first place or block them from reaching or acting on target cells. Others boost enzymes in the body that detoxify carcinogens, thereby rendering them harmless. Yet other anticancer agents act on cells that have already been exposed to carcinogens, slowing the development of cancer or starving cancer cells of oxygen and nutrients by cutting off their blood supply. Although much more research needs to be done, preliminary evidence is strong that there are many substances in common foods that can help protect against cancer.

Some essential nutrients also act as anticarcinogens. For example, vitamin C, vitamin E, and selenium may help prevent cancer by acting as **antioxidants.** As described in Chapter 8, antioxidants react with **free radicals** and prevent them from damaging DNA in body cells. Vitamin C may also block the conversion of nitrites and nitrates (food preservatives) into cancer-causing agents. The B vitamin folic acid may inhibit the transformation of normal cells into malignant cells and strengthen immune function. And additional protection against some cancers may be provided by calcium, which inhibits the growth of cells in the large intestine, thereby slowing the spread of potentially cancerous cells.

Many other anticancer agents in the diet fall under the heading of **phytochemicals**—substances in plants that are not essential nutrients but that do affect health. One of the first to be identified was **sulforaphane**, a potent anticarcinogen that has been purified from broccoli. Sulforaphane can turn on the body's natural detoxifying enzymes, which in turn render some carcinogens harmless. In animal studies, sulforaphane has been shown to reduce the risk of breast tumors. Although broccoli and other **cruciferous vegetables** have received the most publicity, most fruits and vegetables contain beneficial phytochemicals. Cancer researchers are just beginning to identify all of the substances found in plant foods and to investigate their potential anticancer properties. Some of the most promising compounds are listed in Table 12-2.

If you want to increase your intake of these potential cancer fighters, it is best to obtain them by eating a variety of foods rather than by relying on supplements. Many of these compounds are not available in supplement form, and optimal intakes have not been determined for those that are. Like many vitamins and minerals, isolated phytochemicals may be harmful if taken in high doses. In addition, it is likely that the anticancer effects of many foods are the result of chemical substances working in combination. Consuming whole foods known to be rich in vitamins, minerals, and beneficial phytochemicals is the best strategy. Suggestions for maximizing your intake of anticancer agents are included in the box "A Dietary Defense Against Cancer" (p. 291).

Inactivity

Several common types of cancer appear to be associated with an inactive lifestyle, and research has shown a relationship between increased physical activity and a reduction in cancer risk. Exercise is helpful in preventing obesity, a risk factor for several different types of cancer. Exercise also seems to have a direct effect on cancer risk. There is good evidence that exercise reduces the risk of colon cancer, perhaps by speeding the movement of food through the digestive tract, enhancing immune function, and reducing blood fats. Exercise is also associated with a lower risk of cancer of the breast and reproductive organs in women.

Environmental Factors

Many carcinogens occur naturally in the environment, such as UV rays from the sun. Others are manufactured or synthetic substances that show up occasionally in the general environment but more often occur in the work environment of specific industries.

Ingested Chemicals The food industry adds many substances to foods to preserve and stabilize them. Some of these additives may actually decrease any carcinogenic properties the food may have, but others are potentially dangerous. For example, sodium nitrate and sodium nitrite are often added to foods such as beer and ale, ham,

TERMS

anticarcinogen An agent that destroys or otherwise blocks the action of carcinogens.

antioxidant A substance that inhibits reactions promoted by oxygen, usually by reacting with it itself, thereby providing protection against the damaging effects of oxidation.

free radical An electron-seeking compound that can react with fats, proteins, and DNA, damaging cell membranes and mutating genes in their search for electrons; free radicals can be produced through chemical reactions in the body and through exposure to environmental factors such as sunlight.

phytochemical A naturally occurring substance found in plant foods that is not an essential nutrient but does have health benefits (such as preventing cancer and heart disease).

sulforaphane A compound found in cruciferous vegetables that activates detoxifying enzymes in the body.

cruciferous vegetables Vegetables of the cabbage family, including cabbage, broccoli, brussels sprouts, kale, and cauliflower; the flower petals of these plants form the shape of a cross, hence the name.

TABLE 12-2 *Selected Phytochemicals and Their Potential Anticancer Effects*

Compound	Potential Anticancer Effects	Dietary Sources
Allyl sulfides	Increase levels of enzymes that break down potential carcinogens; boost activity of cancer-fighting immune cells	Garlic, onions, leeks, shallots, chives
Capsaicin	Neutralizes the effect of nitrosamines; may block carcinogens in cigarette smoke from acting on cells	Chili peppers (the hotter the pepper, the more capsaicin it contains)
Carotenoids	Act as antioxidants; enhance communication between cells, thereby inhibiting the spread of cancer cells	Orange, yellow, and green vegetables and some fruits
Catechins	Prevent cancer cells from multiplying; help speed the excretion of carcinogens from the body	Green, oolong, and black teas (Note: drinking tea that is burning hot may *increase* cancer risk)
Chlorogenic and *p*-coumaric acid	Bind with nitric oxides in foods and remove them from the body before they turn into cancer-causing nitrosamines	Tomatoes, green peppers, strawberries, carrots
Ellagic acid	Blocks the production of enzymes used by cancer cells; prevents carcinogens from altering DNA in cells	Grapes, strawberries, raspberries, apples
Flavonoids	Act as antioxidants; block the access of carcinogens to cells; suppress malignant changes in cells	Citrus fruits (orange, lemons, limes), onions, apples, grapes, wine
Genistein and other isoflavones	Bind to estrogen receptors, blocking estrogen from acting on target cells; prevent small blood vessels from forming around cancer cells, thereby cutting off oxygen and nutrients	Soybeans, tofu, soy milk and flour, miso, mung beans, peanuts, alfalfa sprouts
Glucarase	Inactivates carcinogens and speeds their removal from the body	Citrus fruits, celery, cardamom, caraway seeds, fennel seeds
Isothiocyanates and indoles	Block carcinogens from reaching target cells; suppress tumor growth; stimulate the production of forms of estrogen that don't promote breast cancer	Cruciferous vegetables: broccoli, cabbage, bok choy, cauliflower, kale, brussels sprouts, turnips
Limonene	Increases the production of enzymes that help rid the body of carcinogens	Citrus fruits
Lycopene	Lowers the levels of cancer-promoting enzymes and other substances in the body	Tomatoes, watermelons, red peppers, carrots
Phytic acid	Binds iron, which may prevent iron from creating cell-damaging free radicals	Grains, legumes
Phytosterols	Slow the reproduction of cells in the large intestine, which may prevent colon cancer	Soybeans, legumes

bacon, and processed lunch meats to inhibit the growth of bacteria. Nitrates and nitrites are not themselves carcinogenic, but they may combine with substances in the body to produce **nitrosamines**, which are potent carcinogens. Foods cured with nitrites as well as those cured by salt or smoke have been linked to esophageal and stomach cancer and should be eaten only in modest amounts.

TERMS

nitrosamines Chemical substances formed in the body from nitrate and nitrite food preservatives that can cause cancer.

Environmental and Industrial Pollution Pollutants in urban air have long been suspected of causing lung cancer. The products of oil and gasoline combustion have

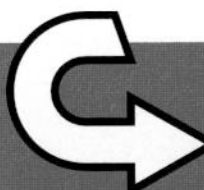

TACTICS AND TIPS

A Dietary Defense Against Cancer

The National Cancer Institute estimates that about one-third of all cancers are in some way linked to what we eat. This means that you can affect your risk of developing cancer by changing your diet in certain ways. The following dietary changes are recommended as a way of reducing your chances of getting cancer:

- Eat a varied diet.
- Eat 5–9 servings of fruits and vegetables every day. (Less than one-third of Americans currently meet this recommendation.) Chose a wide variety, including foods from each of the following categories:

  Cruciferous vegetables

  Citrus fruits

  Dark-green leafy vegetables

  Dark-yellow, orange, or red fruits or vegetables
- Eat other high-fiber foods such as legumes, whole-grain cereals, breads, and pasta.
- Cut down on your intake of fat and saturated fat.
- Be moderate in your consumption of salt-cured, smoked, and nitrite-cured foods.
- Be moderate in your consumption of alcoholic beverages.

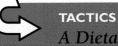

been of special concern. Although smoking has a much greater role, evidence suggests that atmospheric pollution plays a limited but measurable role in lung cancer.

Exposure to carcinogens in particular occupations is a more serious problem. Workers in the rubber, plastics, paint and dye, and petrochemical industries have historically been at greater risk for cancer than the rest of the population.

Radiation All sources of radiation are potentially carcinogenic. These include medical x-rays, radioactive substances, and the ultraviolet rays of the sun. Another source of environmental radiation is radon gas, a radioactive decomposition product of radium, which is found in small quantities in some rocks and soils. In enclosed spaces, such as mines, some basements, and airtight houses built of brick or stone, radon can rise to dangerous levels. Radon and smoking together create a more-than-additive risk of lung cancer.

Sunlight is a "surface" carcinogen, since its rays penetrate only a millimeter or so into the skin. As noted earlier, excessive sun exposure and severe sunburn in early childhood apparently boost the risk of melanoma later in life.

A great many substances produce cancer-causing changes in cells, and in our highly complex society it is impossible to escape them all. Reducing and controlling carcinogens is a major global environmental concern. However, by learning to recognize known carcinogens, learning how they affect our bodies, and doing what we can to avoid them, each of us can to a significant degree make cancer prevention a matter of individual, personal control. Lab 12-1 will help you assess your risk of developing cancer.

DETECTING CANCER

Early detection is the key to effective cancer treatment, and self-monitoring is the first line of defense. It is advisable, therefore, that in your total wellness program you regularly check your body for the following seven warning signs, identified by the American Cancer Society and made easy to remember by the acronym CAUTION:

1. Change in bowel or bladder habits
2. A sore that does not heal
3. Unusual bleeding or discharge
4. Thickening or lump in the breasts or elsewhere
5. Indigestion or difficulty swallowing
6. Obvious change in a wart or mole
7. Nagging cough or hoarseness

Although none of these signs is a sure indication of cancer, any one of them should trigger a visit to a physician, who will administer diagnostic tests, the second factor in a program of early detection. For an overview of the recommended cancer screening tests for healthy people, see Table 12-3 (p. 292).

PREVENTING CANCER

Because behavior significantly influences cancer risk, every person can take specific measures not only to detect possible cancers but also to avoid cancer-causing agents. The American Cancer Society recommends the following guidelines, most of which are components of the approach to general wellness discussed in other chapters of this book:

TABLE 12-3 Cancer Screening Tests for Asymptomatic People

Site of Cancer	Test or Procedure	Population		
		Sex	*Age*	*Frequency*
Colon or rectum	Sigmoidoscopy	M & F	Over 50	Every 3–5 years
	Stool occult blood test	M & F	Over 50	Every year
	Digital rectal examination	M & F	Over 40	Every year
Prostate	Digital rectal examination	M	50 and over	Every year
	PSA blood test	M	50 and over	Every year
Uterus or cervix	Pap test	F	18–65; under 18, if sexually active	At least every 3 years after three negative exams 1 year apart
	Pelvic examination	F	18–39; under 18, if sexually active	Every 3 years
			40 and over	Every year
	Endometrial tissue sample	F	At menopause; women at high risk*	At menopause
Breast	Breast self-examination	F	20 and over	Every month
	Breast physical examination	F	20–40	Every 3 years
			Over 40	Every year
	Mammography	F	Under 40	Baseline
			40–49	Every 1–2 years
			50 and over	Every year
Lung	Chest x-ray		Not recommended	
	Sputum cytology		Recommended for people at risk	
Other**	Health counseling and cancer checkup	M & F	20–39	Every 3 years
		M & F	40 and over	Every year

*History of infertility, obesity, failure of ovulation, abnormal uterine bleeding, or estrogen therapy.
**To include examination for cancers of the thyroid, testicles, prostate, ovaries, lymph nodes, oral region, and skin.

Source: American Cancer Society.

- Stop smoking, avoid secondhand smoke, and avoid smokeless tobacco such as chewing tobacco and snuff.
- To protect your skin against excessive sun exposure, wear protective clothing and use a sunscreen with an SPF rating of 15 or higher.
- Control your weight. Obesity is a risk factor for certain cancers.
- Exercise regularly.
- Maintain the high-fiber, low-fat diet and nutritional standards discussed in Chapter 8, and avoid salt-cured, nitrite-cured, and smoked foods.
- If you drink alcohol, do so only in moderation.
- Avoid excessive radiation exposure—limit medical x-rays to those absolutely necessary and explore the possibility that you might be exposed to radon in your home. If the latter is the case, remedial steps are possible.

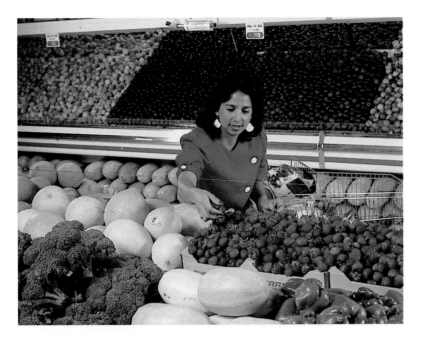

The American Cancer Society recommends a high-fiber diet that contains cruciferous vegetables and is rich in vitamins A and C. Broccoli, strawberries, and red and green peppers are all excellent choices.

- Avoid occupational exposure to carcinogens.
- Follow the cancer screening test recommendations of the American Cancer Society.

? COMMON QUESTIONS ANSWERED

Is it true that a sexually transmissible disease can cause cervical cancer? Yes. Research strongly suggests that the critical event in the development of cervical cancer is infection of the cervical cells by one of the human papillomaviruses (HPV). This is a large group of viruses that cause common warts as well as genital warts. HPV can cause normally well-behaved cells to divide and grow rapidly. The initial infection begins when the virus is introduced into the cervix by an infected sex partner.

Only a very small fraction of HPV-infected women ever get cervical cancer; other factors work with the HPV infection to produce a cancer. It seems that the two most important other factors are smoking and infection with another common sexually transmitted virus, the genital type of herpesvirus. Both smoking and herpesvirus can speed and intensify the cancerous changes begun by HPV. Nicotine and other mutagenic chemicals in tobacco smoke, carried from the lungs by the blood, can be identified in the cervical secretions of women who smoke.

To protect yourself from cervical cancer, avoid infection with HPV and herpesvirus. This can be done through sexual abstinence, mutually monogamous sex with an uninfected partner, or the regular use of condoms. Women who are infected with one or both viruses may need to have more frequent Pap tests in order to track potentially cancerous changes in cervical cells.

What is a biopsy? A biopsy is the removal and examination of a small piece of body tissue. Biopsies enable cancer specialists to carefully examine cells that are suspected of having turned cancerous. Some biopsies are fairly simple to perform, such as those on tissue from moles or skin sores. Other biopsies may require the use of a needle or probe to remove tissue from inside the body, such as in the breast or stomach. Some biopsies require more extensive surgery.

If a biopsy determines that a sample of tissue is malignant, other tests may be performed to determine the exact location, type, and degree of malignancy. New high-technology diagnostic imaging techniques have replaced exploratory surgery for many patients. In magnetic resonance imaging (MRI), a huge electromagnet is used to detect tumors by mapping, on a computer screen, the vibrations of different atoms in the body. Computerized tomography (CT) uses x-rays to create cross-sectional images of the brain and other parts of the body. Ultrasonography, or ultrasound, in which sound waves are bounced off body structures to create an image on a monitor, can also be used to visualize tumors.

How is cancer treated? Treatment methods for cancer are based primarily on surgery (removing the tumor), chemotherapy, and radiation therapy. In the last two techniques, cancer cells that can't be surgically removed are killed either by interfering chemically with their growth or by killing them directly with concentrated ionizing radiation. Newer and still experimental methods also show promise. Immunotherapy, for instance, uses the body's own immune system to control cancer; interferon, interleukin-2, and other substances that stimulate immune function are under study. Other techniques being studied include bone marrow transplants, vaccines, and genetic engineering.

SUMMARY

- Cancer is an abnormal and uncontrollable growth of cells or tissue; cancer cells can metastasize.
- Cancer rates may be leveling off or decreasing when adjusted for an aging population; survival rates increase with early detection.
- Many cancers have specific risk factors that can be avoided. Lung cancer and oral cancer are strongly associated with tobacco use, which is also a risk factor in cervical, bladder, and pancreatic cancer. Ultraviolet radiation is the major risk factor in skin cancer. A high-fat, low-fiber diet plays a major role in colon and rectal cancer, as well as breast cancer and pancreatic cancer.
- Other carcinogens include environmental and industrial pollution, ingested chemicals, alcohol, and radiation. Sexually transmissible diseases and estrogen play a role in female reproductive system cancers.
- Genetic factors in cancer probably involve damage to suppressor genes.
- Anticarcinogens in food, including antioxidants and phytochemicals, can inhibit cancer cell development.
- Early detection, which involves both self-examination and screening tests, leads to effective treatment; the acronym CAUTION can be used to remember the signs of possible cancer.
- Prevention involves avoiding tobacco; excessive radiation from the sun, medical equipment, and radon; excessive alcohol intake; and industrial carcinogens. It also requires weight control, regular exercise, a diet that meets nutritional standards, and adherence to a schedule for screening tests.

BEHAVIOR CHANGE ACTIVITY

Maintaining Your Program Away from Home

It's particularly challenging to stick to your behavior change program when you are away from home and your usual routine. These three key strategies can help:

- *Plan ahead, and stick with your plans.* Run through the schedule of events you'll be involved in while you are away from home, and plan where your new or changed behavior will fit. Resolve to stick with your plan.
- *Maintain your motivation and commitment.* Carry a list of your goals, a copy of your contract, or some other reminder to help keep your program in your mind.
- *Be flexible and creative.* You will probably need to make some adjustments in your program to accommodate the new setting.

Take the example of maintaining an exercise program while on a trip for business or pleasure. There are numerous tactics for keeping up with your program:

- Find out ahead of time about the exercise possibilities where you will be staying. Does your motel or hotel have fitness facilities? Is your friend's house near a park, a trail, or a gym?
- Pack your exercise shoes and clothing.
- Schedule free time during the time of day you typically exercise, or plan to exercise during the free time you'll have.
- Do push-ups, sit-ups, and other calisthenic exercises in place of weight training to maintain your muscular strength and endurance. You can also create makeshift free weights from items in your luggage or in a typical motel room. Flexibility exercises can be done anywhere with no equipment.
- Walk. If you don't have access to the exercise equipment or facilities you usually use, you can always walk. If the area in which you are staying isn't particularly safe or if you only have free time in the evening, walk indoors. Walking down hotel corridors and up stairs can provide an excellent cardiorespiratory workout.

Remember that it's OK to take a few days off—as long as you maintain your commitment to continue with your program when you return to your usual schedule.

Take a few minutes now to devise some strategies to help you maintain your behavior change program while you are away from home.

Target Behavior ________________________________

Strategies for Maintaining My Program

1. ________________________________

____

2. ________________________________

____

3. ________________________________

____

4. ________________________________

____

FOR MORE INFORMATION

The American Cancer Society (1-800-ACS-2345) publishes a wide range of materials on the prevention and treatment of cancer, all available free of charge. Titles include *Nutrition and Cancer, How to Examine Your Breasts, Cancer Facts for Women, Facts on Ovarian Cancer,* and *Sexuality and Cancer.*

The National Cancer Institute (NCI) maintains a database of the latest published information about cancer. Operators will perform a search for callers on specific subjects and send along relevant materials (1-800-4-CANCER). NCI also publishes a wide range of cancer materials, available free of charge. Sample titles are *Cancer Prevention, Cancer Rates and Risks, Breast Biopsy: What You Should Know, What You Need to Know About Colon and Rectal Cancer, When Someone In Your Family Has Cancer,* and *The Future of Cancer Therapy.* Publications may be ordered by writing to Public Inquiries Section, Office of Cancer Communications, NCI, Bldg. 31, Room 10A16, 9000 Rockville Pike, Bethesda, MD 20892.

Your library will have many books on cancer-related topics. A few of interest include the following:

American Cancer Society. 1996. *Cancer Facts and Figures, 1996.* New York: American Cancer Society. *Available in every library, this is a condensed and authoritative summary of the current cancer statistics, renewed each year.*

Dollinger, M., E. H. Rosenbaum, and G. Cable. 1991. *Everyone's Guide to Cancer Therapy: How Cancer Is Diagnosed, Treated, and Managed Day to Day.* Toronto: Somerville House. *An authoritative lay guide to cancer diagnosis and treatment written by top cancer specialists.*

National Cancer Institute. 1994. *National Cancer Institute Fact Book.* Bethesda, Md.: Office of Cancer Communications. *A sourcebook of detailed and up-to-date information on the cancer problem.*

Sohn, W., and S. Corngold. 1992. *Colorectal Cancer: Reducing Your Risk.* New York: Bantam Books. *A guide to understanding the hereditary factors in bowel cancer and to controlling environmental risk factors.*

Whelan, E. 1994. *The Complete Guide to Preventing Cancer.* New York: Prometheus Books. *Up-to-date information in nontechnical language.*

SELECTED BIBLIOGRAPHY

Ames, B. N., and L. S. Gold. 1992. Animal cancer tests and cancer prevention. *Monographs/National Cancer Institute* 12: 125–132.

Baghurst, P. A., and T. E. Rohan. 1994. High-fiber diets and reduced risk of breast cancer. *International Journal of Cancer* 56:173–176.

Banks, B. A., et al. 1992. Attitudes of teenagers toward sun exposure and sunscreen use. *Pediatrics* 89(1): 40–42.

Blair, S. N., H. W. Kohl, R. S. Paffenbarger, D. G. Clark, K. H. Cooper, and L. W. Gibbons. 1989. Physical fitness and all-cause mortality: A prospective study of healthy men and women. *Journal of the American Medical Association* 262: 2395–2401.

Blamey, A., N. Mutrie, and T. Aitchison. 1995. Health promotion by encouraged use of stairs. *British Medical Journal* 311: 289–290.

Bosch, F. X., et al. 1995. Prevalence of humanpapillomavirus in cervical cancer: A worldwide perspective. International Biological Study on Cervical Cancer (IBSCC) Study Group. *Journal of the National Cancer Institute* 87(11): 796–802.

Connolly, G. N., et al. 1992. Snuffing tobacco out of sport. *American Journal of Public Health* 82(3): 351–353.

Giovannucci, E., et al. 1995. Aspirin and the risk of colorectal cancer in women. *New England Journal of Medicine* 333(10): 609–614.

Glantz, S. A., and W. W. Parmley. 1992. Passive smoking causes heart disease and lung cancer. *Journal of Clinical Epidemiology* 45(8): 815–919.

Harris, J. R., et al. 1992. Breast cancer: Medical progress. *New England Journal of Medicine* 327(5): 319–327.

Hirayama, T. 1992. Life-style and cancer: From epidemiological evidence to public behavior change to mortality reduction of target cancers. *Monographs/National Cancer Institute* 12: 65–74.

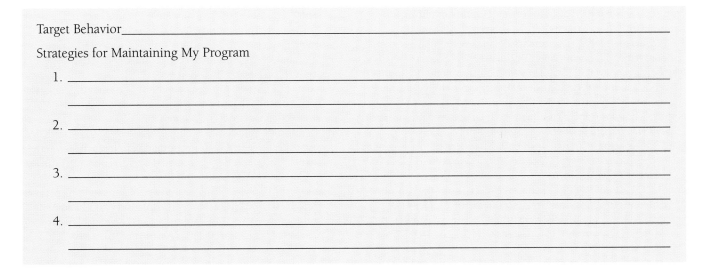

Jaret, P. 1995. Foods that fight cancer. *Health,* March/April.

Lamb, D. R. 1994. Exercise for the traveler. *Healthline,* July.

La Vecchia, C. 1992. Cancers associated with high-fat diets. *Monographs/National Cancer Institute* 12:79–85.

Nagasawa, H., et al. 1995. The effects of lycopene on spontaneous mammary tumour development in SHN virgin mice. *Anticancer Research* 15(4): 1173–1178.

Napier, K. 1995. Cancer-fighting foods: Green revolution. *Harvard Health Letter Special Supplement,* April.

National Research Council. 1989. *Diet and Health: Implications for Reducing Chronic Disease Risk.* Washington, D.C.: National Academy Press.

Peters, C., et al. 1995. Exercise, cancer, and the immune response of monocytes. *Anticancer Research* 15:175–179.

Schapira, D. V., et al. 1991. Estimate of breast cancer risk reduction with weight loss. *Cancer* 67(10): 2622–2625.

Schardt, D. 1994. Phytochemicals: Plants against cancer. *Nutrition Action Health Letter* 21(3): 10–11.

Schreinemachers, D. M., and R. B. Enerson. 1994. Aspirin use and lung, colon, and breast cancer incidence in a prospective study. *Epidemiology* 5: 138–146.

Wynder, E. L. 1992. Cancer prevention: Optimizing life-styles with special reference to nutritional carcinogenesis. *Monographs/National Cancer Institute* 12:87–91.

Vail-Smith, K., and D. M. White. 1992. Risk level, knowledge, and preventive behavior for human papillomaviruses among sexually active college women. *Journal of American College Health* 40(5): 227–230.

Zhang, Y., et al. 1992. A major inducer of anticarcinogenic protective enzymes from broccoli: Isolation and elucidation of sulforaphane structure. *Proceedings of the National Academy of Sciences of the United States of America* 89(6): 2399–2403.

Name ______________________ Section ______________ Date ______________

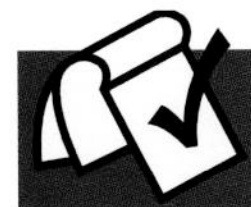

LAB 12-1 *Risk Factors for Cancer*

Are you doing all you can to avoid cancer? You can directly influence some risk factors, such as diet and exposure to cigarette smoke; others are beyond your control. The following statements relate to factors that can put you at increased risk for cancer. To identify your risk factors, check any statements that are true for you.

_____ I have a family history of cancer. Check any of the following family members who have had cancer; list the type(s):

- _____ Mother ______________________
- _____ Father ______________________
- _____ Sister ______________________
- _____ Brother ______________________
- _____ Paternal grandfather ______________________
- _____ Paternal grandmother ______________________
- _____ Maternal grandfather ______________________
- _____ Maternal grandmother ______________________

_____ I smoke cigarettes.

_____ I am constantly exposed to cigarette smoke at work or at home.

_____ I use smokeless tobacco.

_____ I live in a heavily polluted urban area.

_____ I work in one of the following industries:

- _____ Rubber
- _____ Paint and dye
- _____ Petrochemical
- _____ Plastics
- _____ Cable

_____ I am regularly exposed to one of the following substances:

- _____ Arsenic
- _____ Benzene
- _____ Coal combustion products
- _____ Radiation
- _____ Asbestos
- _____ Benzidine
- _____ Nickel compounds
- _____ Vinyl chloride

_____ My home, office, or school has high levels of radon gas.

_____ I have frequently gotten blistering, peeling sunburns.

_____ I am frequently exposed to sunlight and get a tan whenever possible.

_____ I have fair skin.

_____ I rarely use sunscreens.

_____ I am overweight or obese (I weigh more than 20% over my upper weight limit on a standard height-weight chart or have a measured percent body fat above 25% [males] or 32% [females]).

_____ I am sedentary (I do not exercise at least three times a week).

_____ I eat a diet that is high in fat overall.

_____ I eat a diet that is low in fiber overall.

_____ My diet often includes the following:

- _____ Whole milk and milk products
- _____ Beer, wine, liquor
- _____ Grilled or barbecued meats
- _____ Beef, pork, poultry skin, egg yolks
- _____ Bacon, hot dogs, sausages, ham
- _____ Old peanuts, old peanut butter, or corn that may be moldy (aflatoxin, the mold on peanuts and other crops, is linked to liver cancer)

_____ My diet seldom includes the following:

- _____ Cruciferous vegetables (cabbage, broccoli, cauliflower, brussels sprouts)
- _____ Yellow and orange fruits (apricots, cantaloupe, cherries, peaches, nectarines, mangoes, watermelon, persimmons, papayas)
- _____ Yellow and orange vegetables (carrots, yams, sweet potatoes, winter squash, pumpkin)
- _____ Dark-green leafy vegetables (broccoli, spinach, Swiss chard, kale, collard greens)
- _____ Citrus fruits, tomatoes, strawberries, red peppers
- _____ Nuts and vegetable oils
- _____ Whole grains and dried beans (brown rice, kasha, bulgur, whole-grain breads, garbanzo beans, lentils, pinto beans)

_____ I seldom/never perform breast self-examination (females) or testicle self-examination (males).

_____ I do not know the seven warning signs of cancer designated by the acronym CAUTION.

For Women Only (Check statements that are true for you; ignore those that are not applicable.)

_____ I had early first menstruation.

_____ My first pregnancy occurred late in life, or I have never had a child.

_____ I had a child and did not breastfeed.

_____ I had prolonged high-dose estrogen treatment.

_____ I had late onset of menopause.

_____ I have had genital warts (exposure to human papillomavirus).

_____ I have genital herpes.

_____ I do not have regular Pap tests.

Your answers here can help you identify behaviors that you should change. Consider planning a behavior change program to alter one or more of your risky behaviors.

13

Substance Use and Abuse

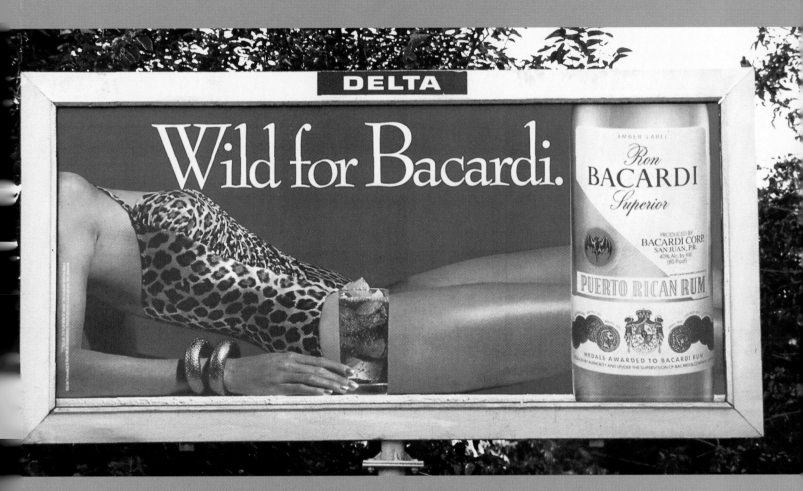

LOOKING AHEAD

After reading this chapter, you should be able to answer these questions about substance use and abuse:

- What are psychoactive drugs, and why do people use them?
- What are the health hazards associated with tobacco use and environmental tobacco smoke, and how can people quit smoking?
- What are the short-term and long-term effects of alcohol use, and how can alcoholism be treated?
- What techniques can help a person drink in moderation?
- What are the principal psychoactive drugs in use in the United States today?
- How can drug abuse and dependence be treated and prevented?
- How can a person help a friend or family member who is dependent on alcohol or other drugs?

The use of drugs for both medical and social purposes is common and widespread in the United States. The prevailing attitude among many people is that all problems, no matter how big or small, have chemical solutions. Our expectations about drugs are fed by medical research findings, advertisements, social pressures, and personal hopes for quick answers to difficult questions.

Drugs are defined as chemicals other than food intended to affect the structure or function of the body. They include prescription medicines; over-the-counter remedies; legal substances such as tobacco, alcohol, and caffeine; and illegal substances such as marijuana, cocaine, and heroin.

This chapter focuses on **psychoactive drugs,** chemicals that can alter a person's thoughts, sensations, feelings, or nervous system functioning. The chapter explains the action and effects of these substances and explores their relation to overall wellness. This information is designed to help individuals make healthy, informed decisions about personal drug use.

TOBACCO

Smoking is hazardous to everyone's health—smoker and nonsmoker alike. Smoking causes more ill health than any other behavior. According to the U.S. Surgeon General, smoking is the leading preventable cause of illness and death in the United States. Tobacco in any form—cigarettes, cigars, pipes, chewing tobacco, clove cigarettes, or snuff—is unsafe. Despite its well-known hazards, however, tobacco use is still widespread in our society, particularly among certain groups (Table 13-1). A major objective of *Healthy People 2000,* a U.S. government report of health goals to achieve by the year 2000, is to reduce the proportion of Americans who smoke to 15% by the end of the decade.

Tobacco Addiction

If smoking is so dangerous, why is it so widespread? Regular tobacco use, and especially cigarette smoking, is not just a habit but a full-blown addiction, involving physical **dependence** on the psychoactive drug **nicotine.** Addicted tobacco users must keep a steady amount of nicotine circulating in the blood and going to the brain. If that amount falls below a certain level, they experience **withdrawal symptoms:** muscular pains, headaches, nausea, insomnia, irritability, and other discomforts. Many heavy smokers continue to smoke not for pleasure but in order to avoid the unpleasantness of withdrawal.

Health Hazards

Tobacco has negative effects on nearly every part of the body and increases the risk of many dangerous diseases.

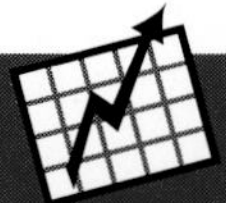

VITAL STATISTICS

TABLE 13-1 Who Smokes? Percentage of American Adults Who Smoke Cigarettes by Sex, Race, and Education

	Men	Women	Total
Race/ethnic group (all ages)			
White	29%	26%	27%
Black	36	25	30
Asian/Pacific Islander	24	8	16
American Indian/ Alaskan Native	38	36	37
Hispanic	29	17	23
Education (young adults age 18–24)			
≤12 years	35%	31%	NA
≥13 years	12	15	NA
Total population	28	24	26

Source: Adapted from U.S. Centers for Disease Control and Prevention. 1994. Surveillance for selected tobacco-use behaviors: United States, 1900–1994. *Morbidity and Mortality Weekly Report,* 18 November.

Some of the many damaging chemicals in tobacco are carcinogens and cocarcinogens (agents that can combine with other chemicals to promote cancer). Others irritate the tissues of the respiratory system. Carbon monoxide, the deadly gas in automobile exhaust, is present in cigarette smoke in concentrations 400 times greater than the safety threshold set in workplaces. Table 13-2 lists some of the other hazardous substances in tobacco smoke.

The effects of nicotine on smokers vary, depending on the size of the dose and the smoker's past smoking behavior. Nicotine can either excite or tranquilize the nervous system, generally resulting in stimulation that gives way to tranquility and then depression. Figure 13-1 (p. 302) summarizes the immediate effects of smoking.

In the short term, smoking interferes with the functions of the respiratory system and often leads rapidly to shortness of breath and the conditions known as smoker's throat, smoker's cough, and smoker's bronchitis. Other common short-term complaints are loss of appetite, diarrhea, fatigue, hoarseness, weight loss, stomach pains, insomnia, and impaired visual acuity, especially at night. These effects generally disappear when a person quits smoking.

Long-term effects fall into two general categories. The first is reduced life expectancy: A male who takes up smoking before age 15 and continues to smoke is only

TABLE 13-2 Selected Substances in Cigarette Smoke

Carcinogens		
Nitrosamines	Benzo(a)pyrene	Toluidine
Crysenes	Polonium	Urethane
Cadmium	Nickel	
Metals		
Aluminum	Mercury	Titanium
Zinc	Gold	Lead
Magnesium	Silver	

Other Substances

Chemical	*Typical Use or Source*
Acetone	Nail polish remover
Ammonia	Floor or toilet cleaner
Arsenic	Poison
Butane	Cigarette lighter fluid
Carbon monoxide	Car exhaust fumes
DDT/dieldrin	Insecticides
Formaldehyde	Body tissue and fabric preserver
Hydrogen cyanide	Gas chamber poison
Methane	Swamp gas
Methanol	Rocket fuel
Naphthalene	Mothballs
Nicotine	Insecticide, addictive drug
Toluene	Industrial solvent
Vinyl chloride	Makes PVC

Source: California Medical Association, 1995.

half as likely to live to age 75 as one who never smokes. Female smokers, too, experience dramatic losses in life expectancy.

The second category of long-term effects involves quality of life. Both male and female smokers have higher rates of acute and chronic diseases than those who have never smoked. The more people smoke, and the deeper and more often they inhale, the greater the risk of disease. Cardiovascular disease, respiratory diseases such as emphysema and lung cancer, and other types of cancer are the most costly smoking-related diseases (Table 13-3, p. 303).

People who don't smoke but use other forms of tobacco also face health hazards. Chewing tobacco and snuff both lead to nicotine addiction. Users of these smokeless tobacco products are at increased risk for cancers of the lip, mouth, larynx, and esophagus; tooth decay; inflammation and recession of the gums; and high blood cholesterol levels.

When smokers quit, many health improvements begin almost immediately, including the following:

- Food is absorbed more efficiently.
- Appetite increases.
- The senses of smell and taste improve.
- Cardiorespiratory function improves.
- Circulation improves.
- Breathing capacity increases.

The younger people are when they stop smoking, the more pronounced are their health improvements (see the box "The Benefits of Quitting Smoking," p. 304).

Environmental Tobacco Smoke

Every year, more laws are passed to protect nonsmokers from secondhand smoke, or **environmental tobacco smoke (ETS)**—both **mainstream smoke,** the smoke exhaled by smokers, and **sidestream smoke,** the smoke that enters the atmosphere from the burning end of the cigarette, cigar, or pipe. Undiluted sidestream smoke is unfiltered by a cigarette filter or a smoker's lungs, so it contains significantly higher concentrations of toxic and carcinogenic compounds than mainstream smoke. Nearly 85% of the smoke in a room where someone is smoking is sidestream smoke. Even though such smoke is diffuse, the concentrations can be considerable. In rooms where people are smoking, levels of carbon monoxide, for instance, can exceed those permitted by Federal Air Quality Standards for outside air.

Effects of ETS Studies show that up to 25% of nonsmokers subjected to ETS develop coughs, 30% develop headaches and nasal discomfort, and 70% suffer eye

TERMS

drug A chemical other than food intended to affect the structure or function of the body.

psychoactive drug Any chemical other than food that, when taken into the body, can alter the user's cognitive and emotional functioning.

dependence The pathological use of a drug or impairment in functioning due to both drug use and tolerance or withdrawal; addiction.

nicotine A poisonous substance found in tobacco and responsible for many of the effects of tobacco.

withdrawal symptoms Unpleasant physical and mental sensations experienced when abstaining from a drug upon which one is dependent.

environmental tobacco smoke (ETS) Smoke that enters the atmosphere from the burning end of a cigarette, cigar, or pipe, as well as smoke that is exhaled by smokers; the combination of mainstream and sidestream smoke; also called secondhand smoke.

mainstream smoke Smoke that is inhaled by a smoker and then exhaled into the atmosphere.

sidestream smoke Smoke that comes from the burning end of a cigarette, cigar, or pipe.

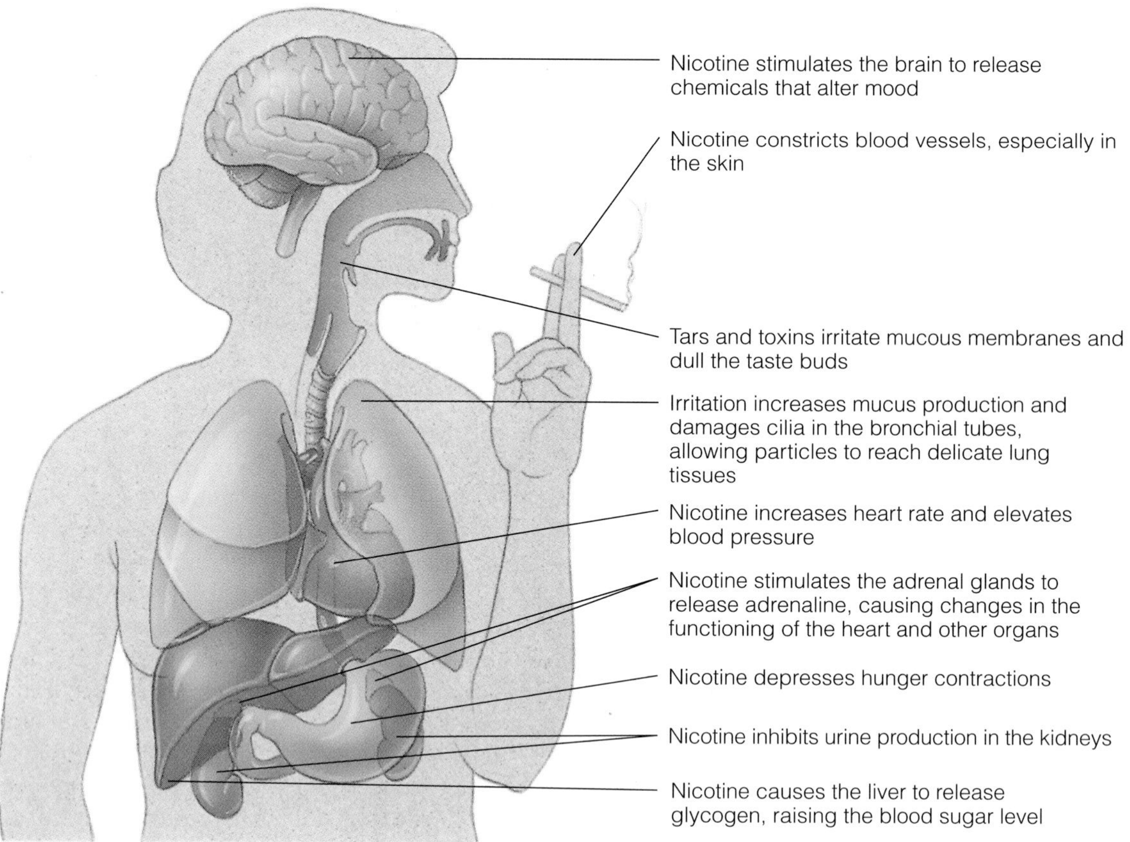
Nicotine stimulates the brain to release chemicals that alter mood
Nicotine constricts blood vessels, especially in the skin
Tars and toxins irritate mucous membranes and dull the taste buds
Irritation increases mucus production and damages cilia in the bronchial tubes, allowing particles to reach delicate lung tissues
Nicotine increases heart rate and elevates blood pressure
Nicotine stimulates the adrenal glands to release adrenaline, causing changes in the functioning of the heart and other organs
Nicotine depresses hunger contractions
Nicotine inhibits urine production in the kidneys
Nicotine causes the liver to release glycogen, raising the blood sugar level

Figure 13-1 *How smoking a cigarette affects your body.*

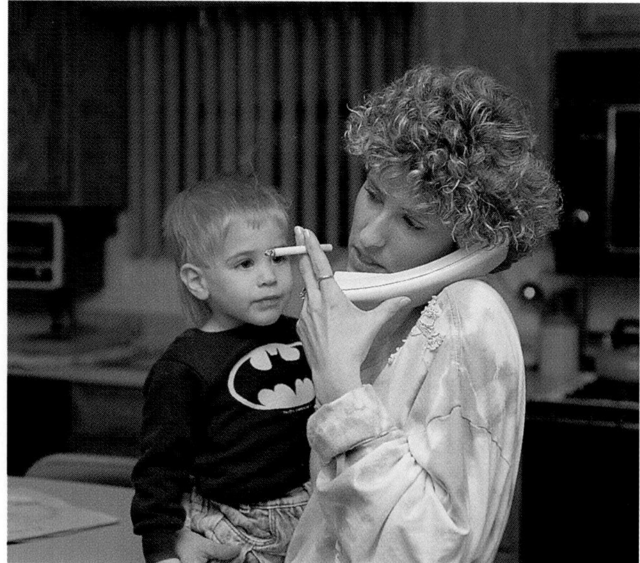

It is estimated that 9 million American children are regularly exposed to environmental tobacco smoke. ETS can trigger respiratory infections, cause or aggravate asthma, contribute to middle-ear infections, and impair development.

irritation. Other symptoms range from breathlessness to sinus problems. People with allergies tend to have the worst symptoms. Tobacco odor, which clings to the skin and clothes, is another unpleasant effect of ETS.

But ETS has far more serious effects as well. The EPA estimates that people who live or work among smokers face a 20–30% increase in lung cancer risk, and that 3000 Americans die from lung cancer caused by ETS each year. ETS also contributes to heart disease—about 35,000 heart disease deaths are attributed to this cause annually—and aggravates respiratory conditions such as asthma. Scientists have been able to measure changes capable of contributing to lung tissue damage and potential tumor promotion in the bloodstreams of healthy young test subjects who spent just 3 hours in a smoke-filled room.

Children and ETS Infants and children are particularly vulnerable to the harmful effects of ETS. Because they breathe faster than adults, they inhale more air—and more of the pollutants in the air. And because they weigh less than adults, children inhale proportionately more pollutants per unit of body weight.

The U.S. Environmental Protection Agency (EPA) estimates that secondhand smoke triggers 150,000–300,000 cases of bronchitis, pneumonia, and other respiratory infections in infants and toddlers up to 18 months of age each year, resulting in 7500–15,000 hospitalizations. Older children suffer, too. The EPA has labeled ETS a risk factor for asthma in children who have not previously exhibited symptoms of the disease, and has blamed ETS for aggravating the symptoms of the 200,000 to 1 million

TABLE 13-3 Adverse Effects of Cigarette Smoking

Disease and Death Risks

Cardiovascular disease
- Coronary heart disease
- Atherosclerosis
- Heart attack
- Stroke
- High blood pressure
- High cholesterol

Lung disease
- Emphysema
- Chronic bronchitis
- Hoarseness

Cancer
- Lung
- Trachea
- Larynx
- Esophagus
- Liver
- Colon and rectal
- Pancreas
- Kidney
- Bladder
- Cervix

Dental disease
- Tooth decay
- Gum disease
- Periodontal disease
- Halitosis (bad breath)

Other diseases
- Peptic and duodenal ulcers
- Osteoporosis
- Diabetes

Maternal/Child Risks

Delayed conception or infertility
Increased fetal death
- Miscarriage
- Ectopic pregnancy

Preterm birth
Stillbirth
Low birth weight
Sudden infant death syndrome (SIDS)
Slow growth rate
Learning delays

Effects of ETS on Healthy Nonsmokers

In adults
- Increased risk of lung cancer, cardiovascular disease, and other diseases

In children
- Increased frequency of asthma and respiratory infection
- Increased risk of hospitalization for bronchitis and pneumonia
- Increased ear infections
- Exacerbation of allergies

Other Health and Cosmetic Concerns

Circulatory problems
Complications from diabetes
Acceleration of multiple sclerosis
Menstrual disorders
Increased risk of impotence
Infertility in men and women
Early menopause
Shortness of breath
Decreased sense of taste and smell
Decreased energy level
Increased susceptibility to colds
Increased hair loss
Increased facial wrinkling
Stained teeth
Discolored fingers
Increased risk of fire
Increased risk of auto accidents

Economic Costs

Average of $2.00 per pack of cigarettes, or $730 per year for a pack-a-day habit
Increased health and home insurance premiums
More frequent dry cleaning of clothes
More frequent cleaning of teeth
More frequent cleaning of house, office, and car
Burnt clothing, upholstery, and carpeting

Sources: American Lung Association; U.S. Centers for Disease Control and Prevention; Environmental Protection Agency; U.S. Surgeon General.

children who already have asthma. The EPA also links ETS to reduced lung function and identifies it as a cause of fluid buildup in the middle ear, a contributing factor in middle-ear infections, a leading reason for childhood surgery. Approximately 9 million American children are regularly exposed to ETS, usually in the home.

As research reveals more about ETS and its effects, nonsmokers are asserting their right to breathe clean air. Many people feel that this right supersedes the right of smokers to smoke when the two conflict.

Smoking and Pregnancy

Smoking almost doubles a pregnant woman's chance of suffering a miscarriage, and women who smoke also face an increased risk of **ectopic pregnancy** (see the box "Special Risks for Women Who Smoke"). Maternal smoking causes an estimated 4600 infant deaths in the United States each year, primarily due to premature delivery and smoking-related problems with the placenta, the organ that delivers blood, oxygen, and nutrients to the fetus. Infants whose mothers smoked during pregnancy are also more likely to die from sudden infant death syndrome (SIDS). Maternal smoking causes fetal growth retardation, too. It is a major factor in low birth weight, which puts newborns at high risk for infections and other potentially fatal problems. Babies born to mothers who smoke more than two packs per day perform poorly on developmental

TERMS

ectopic pregnancy A pregnancy in which the fertilized egg implants itself in an oviduct rather than in the uterus; the embryo must be surgically removed.

A CLOSER LOOK

The Benefits of Quitting Smoking

Within 20 minutes of your last cigarette:

- You stop polluting the air.
- Blood pressure drops to normal.
- Pulse rate drops to normal rate.
- Temperature of hands and feet increases to normal.

8 hours:

- Carbon monoxide level in blood drops to normal.
- Oxygen level in blood increases to normal.

24 hours:

- Chance of heart attack decreases.

48 hours:

- Nerve endings adjust to the absence of nicotine.
- Ability to smell and taste things is enhanced.

72 hours:

- Bronchial tubes relax, making breathing easier.
- Lung capacity increases.

2–3 months:

- Circulation improves.
- Walking becomes easier.
- Lung function increases up to 30%.

1–9 months:

- Coughing, sinus congestion, fatigue, and shortness of breath all decrease.
- Cilia regrow in lungs, reducing the potential for infection.
- Body's overall energy level increases.

1 year:

- Heart disease death rate is halfway back to that of a nonsmoker.

5 years:

- Heart disease rate drops to the rate for nonsmokers.
- Lung cancer death rate decreases halfway back to that of nonsmokers.

10 years:

- Lung cancer death rate drops almost to the rate for nonsmokers.
- Precancerous cells are replaced.
- Incidence of other cancers (mouth, larynx, esophagus, bladder, kidney, and pancreas) decreases.

Source: California Medical Association. 1995.

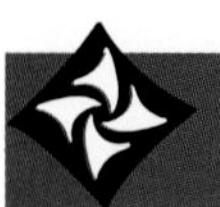

DIMENSIONS OF DIVERSITY

Special Risks for Women Who Smoke

Everyone knows that smoking is dangerous to your health. It shortens life expectancy and increases the risk of cancer, lung disease, and heart disease. But smoking also carries special risks for women. Many of these risks are associated with reproduction and the reproductive organs. The risk of cervical cancer, for example, is higher in women who smoke than in women who don't. For women trying to become pregnant, smoking may impair fertility. For pregnant women, smoking increases the risk of ectopic pregnancy, miscarriage, and stillbirth.

Smoking interacts with oral contraceptives in dangerous ways; women who smoke and take birth control pills have a higher risk of developing potentially fatal blood clots. They are also at greater risk for heart attacks and strokes.

Smoking increases a woman's chance of developing osteoporosis. Estrogen is often prescribed to prevent bone loss after menopause, but estrogen works less well in preventing osteoporosis when a woman smokes. Older women who smoke are thus more likely to suffer hip fractures from falls.

Right now, for the first time in U.S. history, teenage girls are taking up smoking in greater numbers than teenage boys. If the trend continues, female smokers will outnumber male smokers in the adult population by the year 2000. We can expect to see a corresponding increase in tobacco-related diseases among women. Already, lung cancer has surpassed breast cancer as the most common cause of cancer death in American women. Unfortunately, we can also expect to see more of these debilitating and life-threatening tobacco-related diseases that are unique to women.

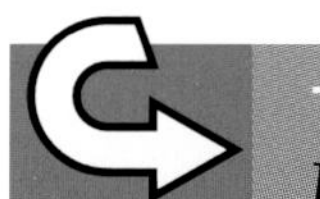

TACTICS AND TIPS

How You Can Help a Tobacco User Quit

The National Cancer Institute recommends a "Four A's" approach for physicians who want to help patients quit using tobacco. The approach can be adapted for anyone who wants to help a friend quit.

1. *Ask* about tobacco use. "How long have you been smoking? How many cigarettes a day do you smoke?"
2. *Advise* tobacco users to stop. "As your friend, I hate to see you jeopardize your health. I've noticed you cough a lot already, and your voice is raspy. You should stop." Studies show the cumulative messages tobacco users get about quitting do help motivate them to stop.
3. *Assist* the tobacco user who is willing to stop. To coincide with your friend's quit date, invite him or her on a camping trip, hike, or other outing far from any stores selling tobacco. Be tolerant if the quitter is irritable and unpleasant. Introduce the quitter to nonsmoking restaurants. Offer to be an exercise partner; exercise can increase a quitter's chance of success. Call the quitter once a day to offer encouragement and help. Bring gifts of low-calorie snacks or crafts that occupy the hands. Offer to take a relaxation course with him or her. If the quitter lapses, be encouraging. A lapse doesn't have to become a relapse.
4. *Arrange* follow-up. Maintaining abstinence is an ongoing process. Every month or so, congratulate quitters again on their success. Note how much better their cars and rooms smell, how they get winded less easily and cough less often, and how much you appreciate not having to breathe their smoke. Continue to engage quitters in exercise and to help them find new ways to enjoy life that don't revolve around tobacco.

tests in the first hours after birth when compared with babies of nonsmoking mothers. Later in life, hyperactivity, short attention span, and lower scores on spelling and reading tests all occur more frequently in children whose mothers smoked throughout pregnancy than in those born to nonsmoking mothers. In addition, animal research suggests certain cancers are more common in animals that were exposed to cigarette smoke as fetuses. Nevertheless, 20–25% of pregnant American women continue to smoke throughout pregnancy.

Giving Up Tobacco

Giving up tobacco is a long-term process that involves breaking both the physical and the psychological addiction to nicotine. Although most ex-smokers have stopped using tobacco on their own, some smokers benefit from stop-smoking programs and support groups. Programs that combine several approaches—pharmacological, psychological, behavioral, and so on—tend to work best.

Certain prescription options help in the quitting process. Physicians can now prescribe nicotine in gum or skin-patch form to help ease a user's withdrawal symptoms. Clonidine, a drug used to help heroin addicts during drug withdrawal, is also prescribed to help some smokers quit. Meanwhile, researchers are investigating the usefulness of antidepressant and antianxiety medications in smoking cessation and are experimenting with nicotine nose drops and sprays.

If you use tobacco and decide to quit, use the behavioral self-management plan described in Chapter 1. The quiz in Lab 13-1 can provide clues about your smoking behavior that will be helpful as you plan a strategy for quitting. Begin by completing a personal contract for quitting that specifies the day and time when you will stop using tobacco, as well as some rewards for quitting. You may be unsure whether to quit "cold turkey" or gradually. Research favors the cold turkey approach, but with enough time set aside to learn and practice effective quitting skills.

Your first few days without tobacco will probably be the most difficult. Nicotine is a powerfully addictive drug, and its use quickly becomes a deeply ingrained habit. But remember that 44 million Americans have quit—and you can too. Plan and rehearse the steps you'll take when you experience a strong craving for tobacco. For example, try drinking a glass of water, chewing gum, taking a walk or a shower, going swimming, or practicing a relaxation technique. Avoid or control situations that you strongly associate with tobacco use.

Social support can be a big help. Arrange with a friend to encourage you in difficult moments, and call him or her when you feel overwhelmed by a craving for tobacco. (If you are in the position of helping a friend quit, follow the advice given in the box "How You Can Help a Tobacco User Quit.") Tell people you've just quit. You may discover many former tobacco users who can reassure you that it's possible to quit and lead a healthier life.

Maintaining abstinence from tobacco over time is the ultimate goal of any cessation program. Tracking and controlling any lingering urges make relapses less likely. Keeping track of them in a health journal helps you deal

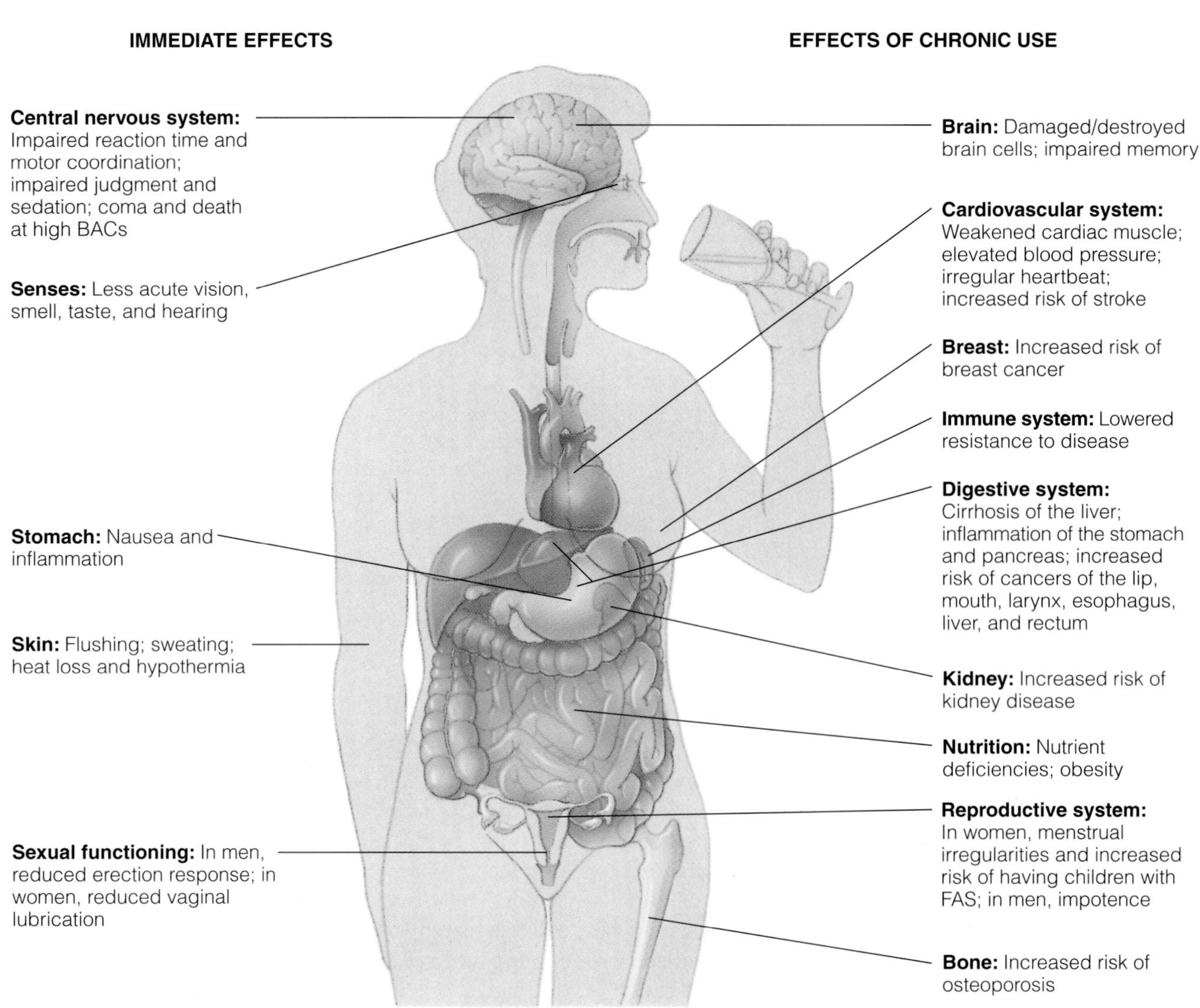
IMMEDIATE EFFECTS
EFFECTS OF CHRONIC USE
Central nervous system: Impaired reaction time and motor coordination; impaired judgment and sedation; coma and death at high BACs
Senses: Less acute vision, smell, taste, and hearing
Stomach: Nausea and inflammation
Skin: Flushing; sweating; heat loss and hypothermia
Sexual functioning: In men, reduced erection response; in women, reduced vaginal lubrication
Brain: Damaged/destroyed brain cells; impaired memory
Cardiovascular system: Weakened cardiac muscle; elevated blood pressure; irregular heartbeat; increased risk of stroke
Breast: Increased risk of breast cancer
Immune system: Lowered resistance to disease
Digestive system: Cirrhosis of the liver; inflammation of the stomach and pancreas; increased risk of cancers of the lip, mouth, larynx, esophagus, liver, and rectum
Kidney: Increased risk of kidney disease
Nutrition: Nutrient deficiencies; obesity
Reproductive system: In women, menstrual irregularities and increased risk of having children with FAS; in men, impotence
Bone: Increased risk of osteoporosis

Figure 13-2 *Immediate and long-term effects of alcohol use.*

with them. When you have an urge to use tobacco, use a relaxation technique, take a brisk walk, chew gum, or substitute some other activity. Practice time management so you don't get overwhelmed at school or work. Exercise regularly, eat sensibly, and get enough sleep. These habits will not only ensure your success at remaining free from tobacco use but will also serve you well in stressful times throughout your life.

ALCOHOL

Used moderately, alcohol can enhance social occasions by loosening inhibitions and inducing relaxation; it may also lower the risk of heart attack in some people. However, the excessive use of alcohol can damage health and dangerously impair functioning. Deciding whether or how to use alcohol requires serious consideration, with a full understanding of the complex ways in which alcohol affects the body and mind.

Chemistry and Metabolism

Ethyl alcohol is the common psychoactive ingredient in wine, beer, and hard liquor. The concentration of alcohol in a beverage is indicated by the proof value, which equals twice the concentration percentage. So if a beverage is 100 proof, it contains 50% alcohol. A 12-ounce bottle of beer, a 5-ounce glass of wine, and a cocktail containing 1.5 ounces of liquor contain about 0.6 ounces of alcohol each.

When consumed, alcohol is absorbed into the bloodstream from the stomach and small intestine. Once in the bloodstream, alcohol is distributed through the body's tissues. When it reaches the liver, a certain amount of it

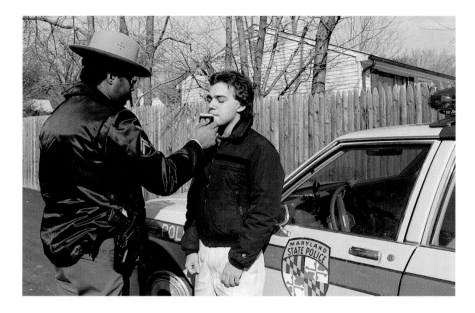

Alcohol interferes with judgment, perception, coordination, and other areas of mental and physical functioning. Not surprisingly, it is a factor in a majority of all fatal motor vehicle crashes. This driver is being given a breathalyzer test to determine his blood alcohol concentration.

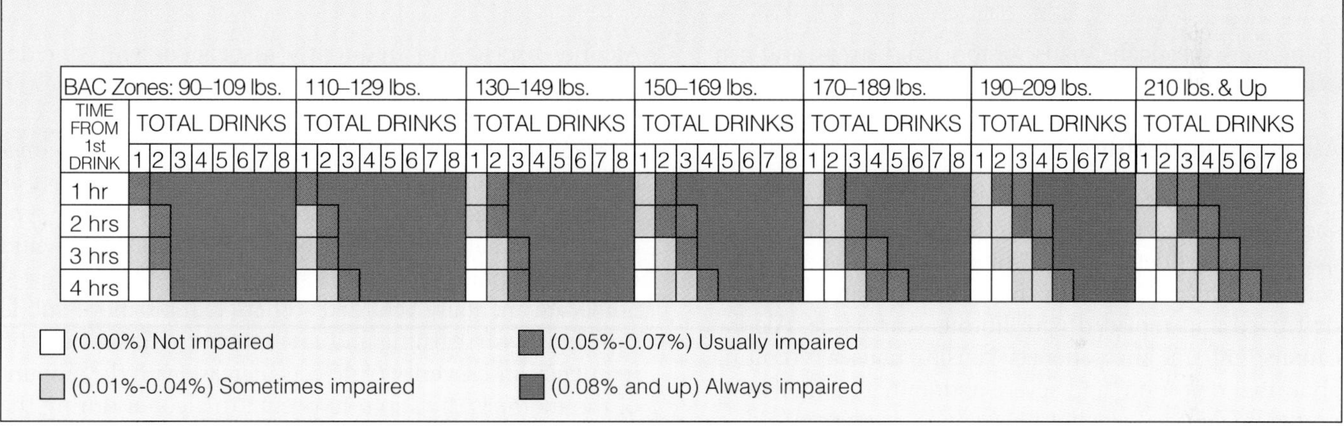

Figure 13-3 ***Approximate blood alcohol concentration and body weight.*** This chart illustrates the BAC an average person of a given weight would reach after drinking the specified number of drinks in the time given. *Source:* California Department of Motor Vehicles.

passes into the liver cells, where it is transformed into energy and other products. Alcohol affects virtually every body system, both in the short term and in the long term (Figure 13-2).

The body can metabolize approximately half a bottle of beer or half an ordinary drink in about an hour. If a person drinks slightly less than that each hour, the **blood alcohol concentration (BAC)** remains low. By drinking slowly, people can drink large amounts over time without becoming intoxicated. But if more is consumed than is metabolized, the BAC will steadily increase, as will the level of **intoxication.** A BAC of 0.08 is considered legally drunk in some states, and a BAC of 0.10 is considered legally drunk in most other states (Figure 13-3). However, alcohol impairs the user even at much lower BACs.

As mentioned, low doses of alcohol induce relaxation and release inhibitions. Higher doses lead to less pleasant effects, including interference with motor coordination, intellectual functioning, and judgment (Table 13-4). Other effects of alcohol include flushing and sweating; compromised sexual performance; disturbed sleep patterns; and

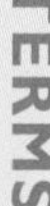

ethyl alcohol The ingredient in fermented liquors that causes intoxication; a colorless, pungent liquid.

blood alcohol concentration (BAC) The amount of alcohol in the blood in terms of weight per unit volume.

intoxication The state of being mentally affected by a chemical.

TABLE 13-4 Effects of Alcohol Use

Blood Alcohol Concentration (%)	Common Behavioral Effects	Hours Required for Alcohol to Be Metabolized
0.00–0.05	Slight change in feelings, usually relaxation and euphoria; decreased alertness.	2–3
0.05–0.10	Emotional lability with exaggerated feelings and behavior; reduced social inhibitions; impairment of reaction time and fine motor coordination, increasing while driving. Legally drunk at BAC 0.08 in many states and BAC 0.10 in others.	4–6
0.10–0.15	Unsteadiness in standing and walking; loss of peripheral vision. Driving is extremely dangerous. Legally drunk at BAC 0.15 in all states.	6–10
0.15–0.30	Staggering gait; slurred speech; impairment of pain perception and other sensory perceptions.	10–24
More than 0.30	Stupor or unconsciousness; anesthesia. Can result from rapid or binge drinking with few earlier effects. Death possible at BAC 0.35 and above.	More than 24

"hangover" (headache, nausea, stomach distress, and general discomfort).

Alcohol and Health

The average life span of alcohol abusers is 10–12 years shorter than that of nonabusers. **Cirrhosis** of the liver, a major cause of death in the United States, is one result of continued alcohol use. In this condition, liver cells are destroyed and replaced with fibrous scar tissue. Alcohol can also inflame the pancreas, causing nausea, vomiting, abnormal digestion, and severe abdominal pain. Though moderate doses of alcohol (one to two drinks a day) may slightly reduce the chances of heart attack in some people, high doses are associated with cardiovascular problems, including high blood pressure and a weakening of the heart muscles. Chronic alcohol abuse has also been linked to certain cancers, asthma, gout, diabetes, recurrent infections, nutritional deficiencies, and nervous system diseases. Psychiatric problems associated with excessive alcohol use include paranoia and memory gaps. Alcohol use is also frequently associated with suicide, homicide, and fatal injuries on and off the road (see the box "Protecting Yourself on the Road").

Maternal drinking during pregnancy can result in miscarriage, stillbirth, or a cluster of symptoms known as **fetal alcohol syndrome (FAS).** Children with this syndrome are small at birth, likely to have heart defects, and often have abnormal features such as small, wide-set eyes. Some are mentally retarded; others exhibit more subtle problems with learning and fine motor coordination. The frequency and severity of defects increase with the amount of the mother's drinking. Exposure to alcohol during the first 12–13 weeks of pregnancy is particularly hazardous, because this is a critical time for the formation of the central nervous system (CNS, the brain and spinal cord), the heart, and other organs.

Alcohol Abuse

According to the current edition of the *Diagnostic and Statistical Manual of Mental Disorders* (1994) of the American Psychiatric Association, **alcohol abuse** involves one or more of the following occurring within a 12-month period:

- Recurrent alcohol use resulting in a failure to fulfill major role obligations at work, school, or home
- Recurrent alcohol use in situations in which it is physically hazardous
- Recurrent alcohol-related legal problems
- Continued alcohol use despite having persistent or recurrent social or interpersonal problems caused by or exacerbated by the effects of alcohol

The term alcohol dependence, or **alcoholism,** refers to

TERMS

cirrhosis A disease caused by excessive and chronic drinking, in which liver cells are first damaged and then destroyed and replaced by fibrous scar tissue.

fetal alcohol syndrome (FAS) A characteristic group of birth defects caused by excessive alcohol consumption by the mother.

alcohol abuse The use of alcohol to a degree that causes physical damage, impairs functioning, or results in behavior harmful to others.

alcoholism A chronic psychological and nutritional disorder from excessive and compulsive drinking; alcohol dependence.

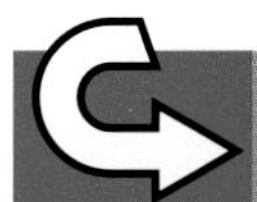

TACTICS AND TIPS

Protecting Yourself on the Road

People who drink and drive are unable to drive responsibly because their judgment is impaired, their reaction time is slower, and their coordination is compromised. No one can drive skillfully and safely when under the influence of alcohol.

What can you do to protect yourself from alcohol-related auto crashes? If you are out of your home and drinking, follow the practice of having a designated driver, an individual who refrains from drinking in order to provide safe transportation home for others in the group. To reduce your chances of being involved in a collision caused by someone else, learn to be alert to the erratic driving that signals an impaired driver. Warning signs include the following:

- Unusually wide turns
- Straddling the center line or lane marker
- Driving with one's head out the window or with the window down in cold weather
- Nearly striking an object or another vehicle
- Weaving or swerving
- Driving on other than the designated roadway
- Stopping with no apparent cause
- Following too closely
- Responding slowly to traffic signals
- Abrupt or illegal turns
- Rapid acceleration or deceleration
- Driving with headlights off at night

If you see any of these warning signs, what should you do?

- If the driver is ahead of you, maintain a safe following distance. Do not try to pass, because the driver may swerve into your car.
- If the driver is behind you, turn right at the nearest intersection. Let the driver pass, then return to your route.
- If the driver is approaching your car, move to the shoulder and stop. Avoid a head-on collision by sounding your horn or flashing your lights.
- When approaching an intersection, slow down and expect the unexpected.
- Fasten your seat belt, place children in approved safety seats, and keep your doors locked.
- Report suspected impaired drivers to the nearest police station by phone. Give a description of the vehicle, license number, location, and direction the vehicle is headed.

Source: Adapted from "The Designated Driver: Being a Friend." 1986. *Healthline,* December.

more extensive problems with alcohol use, usually involving tolerance and withdrawal.

Other authorities use different definitions to describe problems associated with drinking. The important point is that one does not have to be an alcoholic to have problems with alcohol. Any person who drinks only once a month, perhaps after an exam, but then drives while intoxicated *is* an alcohol abuser.

Below is a list of warning signs for alcohol abuse:

- Drinking alone or secretively
- Using alcohol deliberately and repeatedly to perform or get through difficult situations
- Discomfort at social occasions where no alcohol is available
- Escalating alcohol consumption beyond an already-established drinking pattern
- Heavy consumption in risky situations, such as before driving
- Getting drunk regularly or more frequently than in the past
- Drinking in the morning or at other unusual times

Binge Drinking

Binge drinking is a common form of alcohol abuse on college campuses. In a survey of over 17,000 students on 140 U.S. college campuses, 44% reported binge drinking, defined as having five drinks in a row for men or four in a row for women on at least one occasion in the 2 weeks prior to the survey. Nineteen percent of all students were found to be frequent binge drinkers, defined as having at least three binges during the 2-week period. The prevalence of binge drinking was highest among students who lived in fraternity and sorority houses and at residential colleges in northeastern and northcentral states. Black colleges and women's colleges have historically had lower rates of binge drinking.

Binge drinking has a profound effect on students' lives. Frequent binge drinkers were found to be 7–10 times more likely than non–binge drinkers to engage in unplanned sex, to have unprotected sex, to drive after drinking, to get into trouble with campus police, to damage property, and to get hurt or injured. Binge drinkers were also more likely to miss classes, get behind in schoolwork, and argue with their friends. The more frequent the

TACTICS AND TIPS

Responsible Drinking Behavior

- *Drink slowly.* Sip drinks rather than gulping them. Don't drink alcoholic beverages to quench your thirst.
- *Space your drinks.* Drink nonalcoholic beverages at parties (juices or tonic waters), or intersperse them with alcoholic drinks. It's OK to refuse a round.
- *Eat before and while drinking.* Don't drink on an empty stomach. Food in your stomach will not prevent alcohol absorption, but it will slow the rate somewhat, lowering your peak blood alcohol level.
- *Know your limits and your drinks.* Individuals respond differently to alcohol and to different kinds of alcoholic drinks. Drink cautiously if you aren't sure how alcohol affects you. Learn from experience.
- *Provide nonalcoholic alternatives.* When you're the host, have nonalcoholic beverages on hand, and make them accessible and attractive. Serve food along with alcohol, and stop serving alcohol an hour or more before people leave. If a guest has had too much to drink, insist that he or she take a taxi, ride with someone else, or stay at your house rather than drive.
- *Cultivate and model responsible attitudes toward drinking.* Don't be afraid to express disapproval to someone who has had too much to drink.
- *Hold the drinker responsible for the consequences of his or her drinking.* Pardoning unacceptable behavior fosters the attitude that the behavior is due to alcohol and not the responsibility of the drinker.
- *Learn about school or community alcohol abuse prevention programs.* Are programs available for students who are at increased risk for alcohol abuse, such as those whose parents abuse alcohol? Are counseling or self-help programs such as Alcoholics Anonymous available for students who are having problems with alcohol? Don't hesitate to use these services yourself or recommend them to a friend.

binges, the more problems the students encountered. Despite their experiences, less than 1% of the binge drinkers identified themselves as problem drinkers.

Binge drinking also affects students who don't binge drink. At schools with high rates of binge drinking, nonparticipating students were up to three times as likely to report being bothered by the drinking-related behaviors of others than students at schools with lower rates of binge drinking. These problems included being pushed, hit, or assaulted; having property damaged; having sleep or studying disrupted; and experiencing unwanted sexual advances.

The *Healthy People 2000* report set the goal of reducing binge drinking to 32% of college students by the year 2000. Unfortunately, little progress has been made toward this goal. Binge drinking is a difficult problem to address. Many students arrive at college with drinking patterns already established. And many colleges have drinking "cultures" that may perpetuate binge-drinking patterns. On many campuses, drinking behavior that would be classified as alcohol abuse in another setting may be viewed as socially acceptable or even socially attractive, despite the documented evidence that such behavior leads to automobile crashes, injuries, violence, suicide, and high-risk sexual behavior.

TERMS

tolerance Lower sensitivity to a drug such that a given dose no longer exerts the usual effect and larger doses are needed.

DTs (delirium tremens) A state of confusion brought on by the reduction of alcohol intake in a person addicted to alcohol. Other symptoms are sweating, trembling, anxiety, disorientation, and hallucinations.

Alcoholism

Alcoholism is similar to nicotine dependence in usually being characterized by tolerance and withdrawal. Everyone who drinks—even nonalcoholics—develops tolerance to alcohol after repeated use. Developing a **tolerance** means needing increasingly more alcohol to achieve intoxication or the desired effect, that the effects of continued use of the same amount of alcohol are diminished, or that the drinker can function adequately at doses or blood alcohol levels that would produce significant impairment in a casual drinker. When alcoholics stop drinking or cut their intake significantly, they have withdrawal symptoms, which can range from unpleasant to serious and even life-threatening distress. The jitters, or "shakes," are the most common withdrawal symptoms and may last as long as 2 weeks. Seizures are less common but more serious, and still less common is the severe reaction known as the **DTs (delirium tremens),** characterized by confusion and vivid, usually unpleasant, hallucinations.

It is estimated that 13 million Americans are alcoholics, and that 4 million 14- to 17-year-olds show signs of potential alcohol dependence. The cost to society and to the personal well-being of its citizens is inestimable. Despite media attention on cocaine and other chemicals, alcohol remains our society's number-one drug problem.

Some alcoholics recover without professional help, but

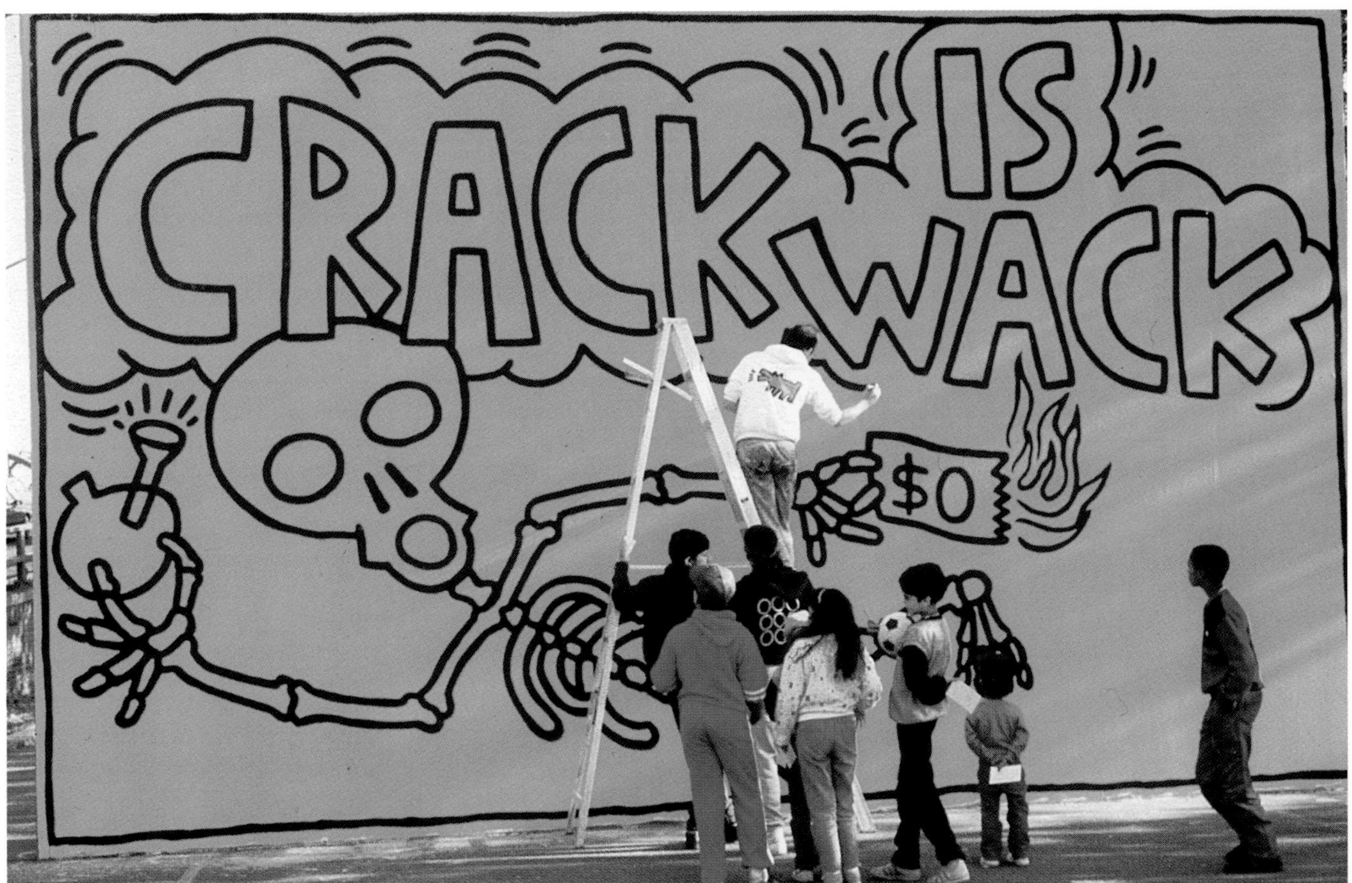

With the introduction of crack cocaine in the 1980s, the use of drugs rose dramatically in the United States. This playground mural, painted by the late Keith Haring, attempts to raise awareness among young people about the dangers of crack use.

the majority do not. Treatment is difficult. However, many different kinds of programs exist, including those that emphasize group and "buddy" support, those that stress lifestyle management, and those that use drugs and chemical substitutes as therapy. Although not all alcoholics can be treated successfully, considerable optimism has replaced the older view that nothing can be done. One encouraging note is that many alcoholics have drinking patterns that fluctuate widely over time, indicating that their alcohol abuse is influenced by environmental factors and therefore may respond to treatment.

Drinking and Responsibility

The responsible use of alcohol means drinking in a way that keeps your BAC low and your behavior under control. If you do drink, know your reasons for doing so. Are you being sociable? Giving in to peer pressure? Or are you attempting to satisfy underlying needs that could best be met by other means? Lab 13-2 gives you an opportunity to examine your drinking behavior in greater detail so you can make informed decisions about it. Additional suggestions are given in the box "Responsible Drinking Behavior."

OTHER PSYCHOACTIVE DRUGS

Illegal drugs are big business in America, with sales ranging upwards from $100 billion annually—all supported by the dependencies and recreational habits of large segments of the population. This volume of drug traffic is associated with major health problems, including overdoses, drug-related injuries and violence, HIV infection (from the sharing of needles), cocaine- and HIV-affected babies, and skyrocketing health care costs. As with tobacco and alcohol, occasional drug use can develop into physical and psychological dependence. Table 13-5 (p. 312) lists the common psychoactive drugs and describes their effects and uses. Figure 13-4 (p. 314) ranks the addictive quality of some common psychoactive drugs.

Use, Abuse, and Dependence

People begin using drugs for a variety of reasons—experimenting, giving in to peer pressure, excitement. Distinguishing drug *use* from drug *abuse* is not always easy, but many experts describe the latter as a maladaptive pattern of use of any substance that persists despite adverse social, psychological, or medical consequences. As with

TABLE 13-5 Effects and Uses of Psychoactive Drugs

Drug Group and Examples	Typical Short-Term Effects	Medical Uses	Comments
Opiates Opium, morphine, heroin, methadone, codeine, meperidine	Pain relief; euphoria; lethargy, apathy, and inability to concentrate; lowered responsiveness to frustration, hunger, and sexual stimulation; nausea and vomiting	Some opiates are used to control pain.	• Use of opiates often leads to physical and psychological dependence.
Central nervous system depressants Alcohol, barbiturates (Seconal, Nembutal, Amytal, Tuinal), methaqualone (Quaalude), diazepam (Valium)	Reduced anxiety; mood changes (obstinacy, irritability, and abusiveness are common); muscular incoordination; slurring of speech; drowsiness or sleep	Some CNS depressants are prescribed for insomnia and anxiety, to control seizures, and to calm patients before operations and other medical or dental procedures.	• Long-term use of CNS depressants can lead to dependence even at prescribed dosages. Withdrawal symptoms are severe and resemble the DTs of alcoholism. • Many CNS depressant drugs show cross-tolerance, in which an individual who has developed tolerance to the effects of one drug can tolerate higher-than-normal doses of another. • Barbiturate overdose is a frequent method of suicide. Many unintended deaths result from the use of barbiturates and alcohol together.
Central nervous system stimulants Cocaine, amphetamine, nicotine, caffeine	Accelerated heart rate; increased blood pressure; constriction of blood vessels; dilation of pupils of the eyes and bronchial tubes; increased gastric and adrenal secretions; greater muscular tension; increased motor activity; euphoria; increased alertness; reduced fatigue; disturbed sleep patterns	Amphetamines are sometimes used to curb appetite. Amphetaminelike drugs have been used to treat children and young adults who have attention-deficit disorder with hyperactivity. Caffeine is available without a prescription and is commonly taken to reduce fatigue.	• Tolerance to cocaine develops rapidly. • In large doses, cocaine can cause excessive CNS stimulation and death. • Babies of women who use cocaine in any form during pregnancy are more likely to have birth defects and other problems than the babies of women without a cocaine habit. • The repeated use of moderate doses of amphetamines often leads to tolerance; the result can be severe disturbances in behavior, including hostility, delusions of persecution, and unprovoked violence. • Taking amphetamines to cope with a passing situation, such as cramming for exams or driving long distances, can be dangerous because judgment is impaired and the user may suddenly fall asleep when the effects wear off. • High doses of caffeine can cause nervousness, irritability, headache, disturbed sleep, gastric irritation, and aggravation of the symptoms of premenstrual syndrome. Caffeine *is* a dependence-producing drug; withdrawal symptoms include headache and irritability.

TABLE 13-5 *Effects and Uses of Psychoactive Drugs (continued)*

Drug Group and Examples	Typical Short-Term Effects	Medical Uses	Comments
Marijuana and other cannabis products	Increased heart rate; dilation of certain blood vessels in the eyes; euphoria, heightened subjective sensory experiences, and sensory distortion; slowing down of time sense; relaxation; impaired memory function; disturbed thought patterns; attention lapses; subjective feelings of depersonalization	Marijuana is sometimes used to reduce nausea and improve appetite during cancer chemotherapy; it is being studied for possible use in certain forms of glaucoma, an eye disease that causes blindness.	• Marijuana is the most widely used illegal drug in the United States (cocaine is second). • The unpleasant side effects, throat and lung irritation, make the development of tolerance unlikely; but a chronic user of marijuana is more likely to be a heavy user of tobacco, alcohol, and other dangerous drugs. The effects of long-term use of marijuana are largely unknown. • Marijuana use during pregnancy can result in impaired growth and development.
Psychedelics LSD, mescaline, psilocybin, STP, DMT	Altered states of consciousness (changes in mood, thinking, and perception); dilation of the pupils; dizziness, weakness, nausea, panic; intellectual impairment; psychological disturbances	The therapeutic potential of hallucinogens has not been clearly determined.	• Many psychedelics induce tolerance within a few days of use. • Even after the chemical effects of a psychedelic have worn off, spontaneous flashbacks and other psychological disturbances can occur.
Deliriants Phencyclidine (PCP), inhalants (chemicals found in some glues, gases in aerosols, kerosene, gasoline, butyl nitrate, nitrous oxide)	Impairment of brain function characterized by mental confusion, emotional excitement, and distortion of sensory input; convulsions; memory impairment; coma	PCP is used as an animal anesthetic.	• High concentrations of inhalants in the blood can cause brain, liver, and kidney damage or even asphyxiation.
Designer drugs Fentanyl derivatives, including "China white"; meperidine derivatives; mescaline-methamphetamine derivatives, including MDA and MDMA, or "Ecstasy"; and PCP derivatives	Similar to the drugs they are designed to mimic	These substances are made illegally and are intended solely as "street" drugs. They have no known therapeutic effects.	• Each of the designer drugs has its own set of risks; parkinsonism, including drooling, shuffling, tremor, and other neurological symptoms, is associated with analogs of the drug meperidine; an overdose of MDMA can cause life-threatening disturbances in heart rhythm, high blood pressure, and seizures.

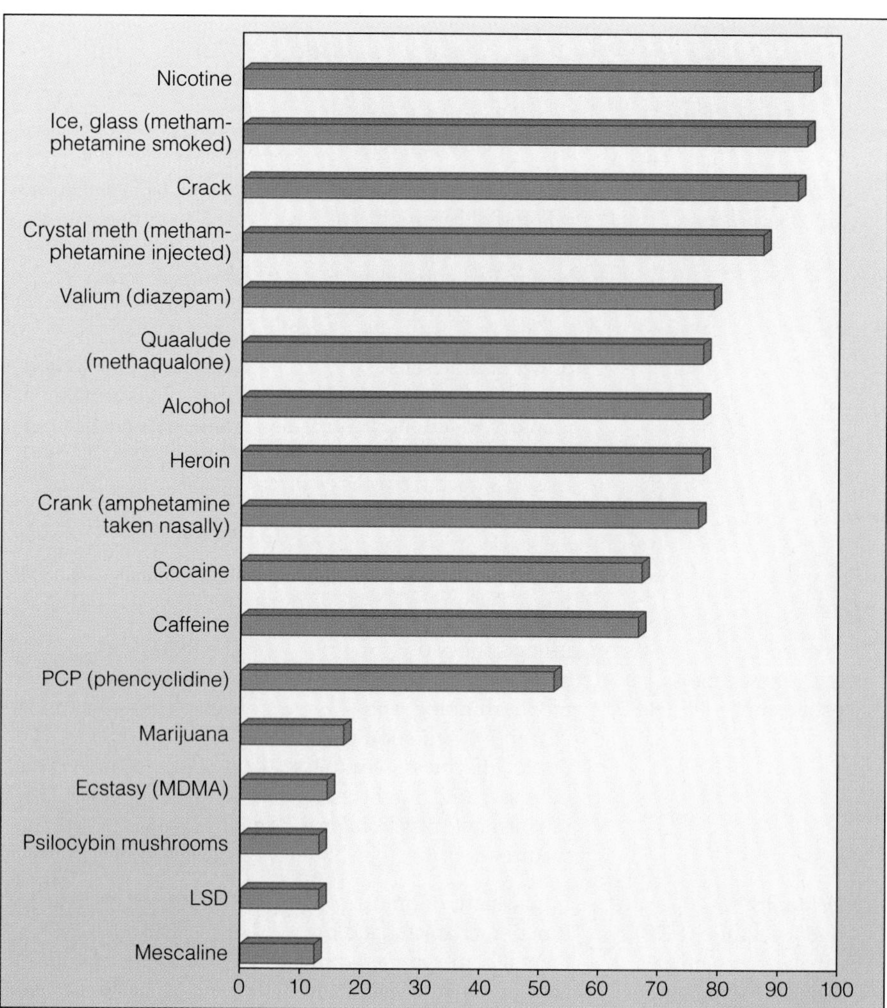

Figure 13-4 ***How easy is it to get hooked on drugs?*** The numbers at the bottom of the chart are relative rankings. *Source:* Davis, L. 1990. Why do people take drugs? *In Health,* November/December.

alcohol, the pattern of abuse may be constant or intermittent, and physical dependence may or may not occur. Where physical drug dependence exists, its hallmarks are the same as for alcoholism: tolerance and withdrawal. Substance dependence also typically involves compulsive drug taking and strong cravings.

Why do some people, but not others, become drug dependent? The answer seems to be a combination of physical, psychological, and social factors. For example, some people have more difficulty than others controlling their impulses and have a strong need for excitement, stimulation, and immediate gratification. Feelings of rejection, hostility, aggression, anxiety, or depression are also associated with drug dependence. People who grow up in a family in which drugs are abused are at higher risk for drug dependence, as are those who belong to a peer group that encourages drug abuse.

Drug Treatment

A variety of programs is available to help people break their drug habits. Professional treatment programs usually take the form of drug substitution programs or programs operated by rehabilitation centers. Nonprofessional self-help groups and peer counseling are also available. As with treatment for alcoholism, there is no single best method of treatment for drug abuse, and the relapse rate is high for all types of treatment. To be successful, a treatment program must deal with the reasons behind people's drug abuse and help them develop behaviors, attitudes, and a social support system that will help them remain drug-free.

Young people with drug problems are often unable to seek help on their own. In such a case, friends and family members may need to act on their behalf. The following is a list of signals suggesting drug dependence:

- Sudden withdrawal or emotional distance
- Rebellious or unusually irritable behavior
- Loss of interest in usual activities or hobbies
- A decline in school performance
- A sudden change in group of friends
- Changes in sleeping or eating habits
- Frequent borrowing of money

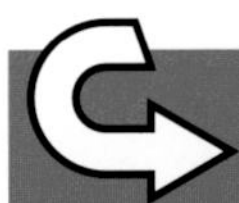

TACTICS AND TIPS
What to Do Instead of Drugs

- *Bored?* Go for a walk or a run; stimulate your senses at a museum or a movie; challenge your mind with a new game or book; introduce yourself to someone new.
- *Stressed out?* Practice relaxation or visualization; try to slow down and open your senses to the natural world; get some exercise.
- *Shy, lonely?* Talk to a counselor; enroll in a shyness clinic; learn and practice communication techniques.
- *Feeling low self-esteem?* Focus on the areas in which you are competent; give yourself credit for the things you do well.
- *Depressed, anxious?* Talk to a friend, parent, or counselor.
- *Apathetic, lethargic?* Force yourself to get up and get some exercise to energize yourself; assume responsibility for someone or something outside yourself; volunteer.
- *Searching for meaning?* Try yoga or meditation; explore spiritual experiences through religious groups, church, prayer, or reading.
- *Afraid to say no?* Take a course in assertiveness training; get support from others who don't want to use drugs; remind yourself that you have the right and the responsibility to make your own decisions.
- *Still feeling peer pressure?* Begin to look for new friends or roommates. Take a class or join an organization that attracts other health-conscious people.

Preventing Drug Abuse

As with every health issue covered in this book, the best solution to the drug-abuse problem is prevention. While the government tends to focus on stopping the production, importation, and distribution of illicit drugs, it is equally important to develop creative and persuasive antidrug educational programs and to disseminate accurate information about the adverse health effects of drugs. Viewed in terms of a lifestyle devoted to achieving and maintaining wellness, drug abuse becomes another challenge to be met with behavior modification, time and stress-management techniques, a healthy diet, and regular exercise.

The Role of Drugs in Your Life

What role do drugs play in your life? Lab 13-3 gives you an opportunity to examine your drug-related behaviors and determine whether you show any signs of developing drug dependence. If you are concerned about your recreational use of drugs, first pinpoint your reasons for using drugs, then substitute healthier coping behaviors. The box "What to Do Instead of Drugs" suggests some alternative behaviors for dealing with certain feelings or situations.

? COMMON QUESTIONS ANSWERED

Is smokeless ("spit") tobacco as dangerous as cigarettes? No, but it carries many health risks. There are two main categories of smokeless tobacco products: chewing tobacco and snuff. In chewing tobacco, the tobacco leaf may be shredded, pressed into bricks or cakes, or twisted into ropelike strands; it is usually treated with molasses and other flavorings. The user places a wad of tobacco in his or her mouth, then chews or sucks it to release the nicotine. In snuff, the leaf is processed into a coarse, moist powder. The user places a pinch of tobacco between the cheek and gum. All types of smokeless tobacco cause an increase in saliva production, and the resulting juice is spit out or swallowed. The nicotine in smokeless tobacco—along with flavorings, additives, and carcinogenic chemicals—is absorbed through the gums and lining of the mouth. The dose of nicotine that the user of smokeless tobacco products receives is similar to that provided by cigarettes, and smokeless tobacco is highly addictive.

After only a few weeks of use, the gums and lips of a smokeless tobacco user can become dried and irritated and may bleed. Precancerous white or red patches may appear inside the mouth. Long-term snuff use may increase the risk of cancer of the cheek and gums by as much as 50 times. Smokeless tobacco use causes bad breath, tooth decay, and gum problems; the senses of taste and smell are usually dulled. It may also have dangerous effects on the cardiovascular system, increasing the risk of heart disease.

The use of smokeless tobacco products has increased in recent years, especially among young adults. The Centers for Disease Control and Prevention estimate that nearly one out of every five male high-school seniors uses smokeless tobacco.

Can a person predict how he or she will respond to a particular psychoactive drug? No, not with any certainty.

WELLNESS CONNECTION

The Power of Belief: The Placebo Effect

A placebo is a chemically inactive substance or ineffective procedure that a patient believes is an effective medical therapy for his or her condition. Researchers frequently give placebos to the control group in an experiment testing the efficacy of a particular treatment. By comparing the effects of the actual treatment with the effects of the placebo, researchers can judge whether or not the treatment is effective. The so-called placebo effect occurs when a patient improves after receiving a placebo. In such cases, the effect of the placebo on the patient cannot be attributed to the specific actions or properties of the drug or procedure.

Researchers have consistently found that 30–40% of all patients given a placebo show improvement. This result has been observed for a wide variety of conditions or symptoms, including coughing, seasickness, migraines, and angina. For some conditions, placebos have been effective in up to 70% of patients. In some cases, people given a placebo even report having the side effects associated with an actual drug. Placebos are particularly effective when they are administered by a physician whom the patient trusts.

A clear demonstration of the placebo effect occurred in a recent study that examined the effectiveness of a type of beta blocker, a drug used in the treatment of heart attacks. The men who participated in the study were randomly assigned to one of two groups: One group received the beta blocker, the other received a placebo (a sugar pill with no chemical effects). Patients did not know to which group they had been assigned. Researchers found that the likelihood of the patient surviving a year was 2.6 times higher among the men who took their pills as prescribed. This may not seem surprising, until you learn that it did not matter which pill they took, the beta blocker or the sugar pill. The act of taking the pill, regardless of whether it contained the drug, had a greater impact on the health of the patient than the chemical effect of the drug itself.

Placebo-like effects have also been observed in people using psychoactive drugs. People given a punchlike drink that they had been told contained alcohol reported feeling symptoms of intoxication. A study of people dependent on heroin found that many experienced the expected level of euphoria after injecting a placebo; one participant in the study even exhibited the contraction of the pupils that typically accompanies heroin injection. In another study, regular users of marijuana reported a moderate level of intoxication after using a cigarette that smelled and tasted like marijuana but contained no THC, the active ingredient in marijuana.

The placebo effect does not work for everyone or in all circumstances, and it does not mean you can improve your medical condition if you believe or do just anything, regardless of how irrelevant. Getting well, like getting sick, is a complex process. Anatomy, physiology, mind, emotions, and the environment are all inextricably entwined. But the placebo effect does show that belief can have both psychological and physical effects.

Sources: Turner, J. 1995. Placebo effects on pain. *Healthline,* April. The power of hope. 1994. *University of California at Berkeley Wellness Letter,* September. Spiegel, D. 1993. *Living Beyond Limits: New Hope and Help for Facing Life-Threatening Illness.* New York: Random House.

Psychoactive drugs have complex and variable effects. The same drug may affect different users differently, or the same user in different ways under different circumstances. A wide variety of factors relating both to the drug and the user influence a person's reaction. For example, increasing the dose of a drug may not simply lead to an increase in the intensity of its effect; rather, the effect can change. An example of this is a person who becomes friendly after one drink but belligerent and hostile after four. The method by which a drug is administered can also have a significant impact: Injecting a drug often produces stronger effects than swallowing the same drug because it reaches the brain more quickly.

Other influences stem from an individual's physical characteristics, past history of drug use, and biochemistry. For example, the effects of certain drugs on a 100-pound person will be twice as great as the effect of the same amount of the drug on a 200-pound person. A habitual user of heroin can tolerate doses that would kill a novice user. And some people have severe, unpredictable reactions to cocaine in which their heart rhythm is disrupted, leading to cardiac failure and death.

An individual's response to a drug can be strongly influenced by his or her mood, expectations, and surroundings. For example, the dose of alcohol that produces mild euphoria and stimulation at a noisy, active party might induce sleepiness and slight depression when taken at home while alone. In the case of LSD and other psychedelics, a fearful person who takes the drug in a loud, darkened room may be more likely to have a bad experience than someone in a nonthreatening environment. This is not to say that the actual dose and chemical effects of a drug are not important—they are. But the expectations and mood of the user can also influence his or her response to a drug. See the box "The Power of Belief: The Placebo Effect" for more information.

Does drinking benefit health? Studies have shown that moderate drinking—one drink per day for women and two drinks per day for men—is associated with a lower risk of coronary heart disease. The precise mechanism isn't entirely clear, but it appears that moderate drinking raises levels of beneficial HDL cholesterol. Researchers have found that blood levels of HDL are 10–15% higher in moderate drinkers than in abstainers. Alcohol also appears to make platelets less likely to stick together—an important protection against heart attacks and some types of strokes because platelets that stick together can form dangerous clots.

The bottom line is that limited, regular consumption of alcohol appears to safely reduce the risk of heart disease for some adults. However, it's not for everyone. A major risk of moderate drinking is that it won't stay moderate. People who avoid alcohol because they've had problems with dependence in the past or come from families with a history of alcoholism should not start drinking for their health. In addition, people with medical conditions such as peptic ulcer, diabetes, or depression that are worsened by alcohol use should also probably avoid even moderate drinking. And because some studies have found an association between moderate drinking and an increased risk of breast cancer, women with other breast cancer risk factors should discuss the potential risks and benefits of alcohol with their physician before taking up moderate drinking. Nor should excessive drinkers use this information as an excuse to overindulge. There is a narrow window of benefit, and excessive drinking causes serious health problems.

Does drinking coffee help an intoxicated person sober up more quickly? No. Once alcohol is absorbed into the body, there are no ways of appreciably accelerating its breakdown. The rate of alcohol metabolism varies among individuals, largely as a result of heredity, but it is not affected by caffeine, exercise, fresh air, or other stimulants. It is the same whether a person is asleep or awake. To sober up, you simply have to wait until your body has had sufficient time to metabolize all the alcohol you have consumed.

SUMMARY

- The use of psychoactive drugs, which can alter a person's thoughts, sensations, feelings, or nervous system functioning, becomes abuse when the use continues despite adverse psychological, social, or medical consequences; even sporadic use can be abuse if it is physically hazardous. Dependence on drugs occurs when symptoms of withdrawal and/or tolerance exist.
- Addiction to tobacco results from dependence on nicotine. Tobacco contains carcinogens; smoking both excites and depresses the nervous system, interferes with respiration, and is a major factor in cardiovascular disease. Improvements in health begin immediately when smoking stops.
- Environmental tobacco smoke contains toxic and carcinogenic compounds in high concentrations; it not only causes allergy problems and discomfort but is also implicated in cancer and cardiovascular disease in nonsmokers exposed to it—especially infants, children, and fetuses.
- Alcohol affects nearly every body system, and excessive use damages the liver, pancreas, and heart; cancer, nutritional deficiencies, and psychological problems can result from continued use. Pregnant women who drink risk having children with fetal alcohol syndrome.
- Intoxication can be avoided by consuming less than the body can metabolize within a given period.
- Success rates for treatment vary; substitute drugs are sometimes used, and social support and behavioral self-management techniques are especially helpful.
- Drug dependence is associated with a strong need for stimulation and immediate gratification; feelings of hostility, rejection, aggression, anxiety, or depression; and a family or peer group that abuses drugs. Symptoms include changes in a variety of usual behaviors.

BEHAVIOR CHANGE ACTIVITY

Dealing with Feelings

Long-standing habits are difficult to change in part because many represent ways people have developed to cope with certain feelings. For example, people may overeat when they're bored, skip their exercise session when they feel frustrated, or drink alcoholic beverages when anxious. Developing new ways to deal with feelings can help improve the chance that a behavioral self-management program will succeed.

Review the records on your target behavior that you kept in your health journal. Identify the feelings that are interfering with the success of your program, and develop new strategies for coping with them. Some common prob-

(continued)

lematic feelings are listed below, along with one possible coping strategy for each. Put a check mark next to those that are influencing your target behavior, and fill in additional strategies. Add the other feelings that are significant roadblocks in your program to the bottom of the chart, along with coping strategies for each.

✔	Feeling	Coping Strategies
	Stressed out	Go for a 10-minute walk.
	Anxious	Do one of the relaxation exercises described in Chapter 10.
	Bored	Call a friend for a chat.
	Tired	Take a 20-minute nap.
	Frustrated	Identify the source of the feeling, and deal with it constructively.

FOR MORE INFORMATION

On campus, the student health center or student counseling center may have information or special programs about tobacco, alcohol, and other drugs.

Check your phone book for local chapters of the American Cancer Society, American Heart Association, American Lung Association, Alcoholics Anonymous, and Al-Anon. These agencies can provide information and materials on tobacco, alcohol, and other drugs. Some have special programs to help you break dependencies.

The following books, available in most libraries, may also be helpful:

Alcoholics Anonymous. 5th ed. 1991. New York: Alcoholics Anonymous World Services. *This is the "Big Book," the basic text for AA. It includes the founding principles of AA and vivid histories of recovering alcoholics.*

Beattie, M. 1990. *Codependents' Guide to the Twelve Steps*. New

York: HarperCollins. *A useful book for friends and loved ones of substance abusers by the writer who first popularized the now-trendy term "codependent."*

Cahalan, D. 1991. *An Ounce of Prevention: Strategies for Solving Tobacco, Alcohol, and Drug Problems.* San Francisco: Jossey-Bass. *A cogent analysis of proposed solutions to the problem of tobacco and other drug addictions.*

Consumer Reports Books. 1993. *The Facts About Drug Use: Coping with Drugs and Alcohol in Your Family, at Work, in Your Community.* Binghampton, NY: Haworth Press. *An authoritative, unbiased book that addresses the social, psychological, and physical effects of various drugs, including comprehensive information on available resources and strategies for coping with problems related to drugs and alcohol.*

Dorris, M. 1992. *The Broken Cord.* New York: HarperCollins. *A personal story and a current source of information on fetal alcohol syndrome.*

Hilts, P. J. 1994. Embattled tobacco: Cigarette makers debated the risks they denied. *New York Times,* 15 June. *A fascinating look behind the congressional hearings on tobacco regulation.*

Keller-Phelps, J., and A. E. Nourse. 1992. *The Hidden Addiction.* Boston: Little, Brown. *Straightforward information from two physicians about a range of addicting substances, from caffeine to cocaine, along with advice for avoiding or overcoming dependence problems.*

Krogh, D. 1992. *Smoking: The Artificial Passion.* New York: W. H. Freeman. *Probes the roots of smoking.*

A Lifetime of Freedom from Smoking. 1989. New York: American Lung Association. *Useful for anyone who wants to quit, or wants anyone else to quit.*

Mooney, A. J. 1992. *The Recovery Book.* New York: Workman. *Written by a physician, a helpful guide that covers family relationships, support groups, work, money, and other issues involved in chemical dependence.*

U.S. Journal, Inc. 1992. *The Treatment Directory: National Directory of Alcohol, Drug Addiction and Other Addiction Treatment Programs.* Deerfield Beach, Fla.: U.S. Journal, Inc. *A helpful reference for people seeking information about treatment options for themselves or loved ones.*

The following organizations and agencies provide pamphlets, books, films, videos and/or other types of educational materials about smoking, drinking, and drug use:

Alcoholics Anonymous (212-870-3400)

American Heart Association (214-373-6300)

National Cancer Institute (800-4-CANCER)

National Council on Alcoholism and Drug Dependency (800-NCA-CALL)

National Clearinghouse for Alcohol and Drug Information (800-729-6686)

National Heart, Lung, and Blood Institute (301-496-1051)

National Institute on Drug Abuse (301-443-6245)

Office on Smoking and Health (404-488-5705)

Helpful information is also available at the following toll-free numbers:

800-COCAINE A round-the-clock information and referral service.

800-NCA-CALL National Council on Alcoholism and Drug Dependency Information Line, providing information and referrals to families and individuals seeking help with an alcohol or other drug problem.

800-662-HELP National Institute on Drug Abuse information and referral line, providing written materials on drug use and treatment referrals.

SELECTED BIBLIOGRAPHY

American Psychiatric Association. 1994. *Diagnostic and Statistical Manual of Mental Disorders (DSM-IV),* 4th ed. Washington, D.C.: American Psychiatric Association.

Blot, W. J. 1992. Alcohol and cancer. *Cancer Research* 52(7 suppl): 2119s–2123s.

Brook, J. S., et al. 1992. Childhood precursors of adolescent drug use: A longitudinal analysis. *Genetic, Social and General Psychology Monographs* 118(2): 195–213.

Centers for Disease Control and Prevention. 1994. Medical-care expenditures attributable to cigarette smoking: United States, 1993. *Morbidity and Mortality Weekly Report* 40(20).

Centers for Disease Control and Prevention. 1994. Reasons for tobacco use and symptoms of nicotine withdrawal among adolescent and young adult tobacco users: United States, 1993. *Morbidity and Mortality Weekly Report* 43(41).

Centers for Disease Control and Prevention, Office on Smoking and Health. 1994. *Facts About Second-Hand Smoke.*

Day, N. L., and G. A. Richardson. 1991. Prenatal marijuana use: epidemiology, methodologic issues and infant outcome. *Clinics in Perinatology* 18(1): 77–91.

Environmental Protection Agency. 1993. *Respiratory Health Effects of Passive Smoking: Fact Sheet.* EPA-43-F-93-003.

Forty-four percent of college students are binge drinkers, poll says. 1994. *New York Times.* 7 December.

Hecht, M. L., et al. 1992. Resistance to drug offers among college students. *International Journal of the Addictions* 27(8): 995–1017.

Imperato, P. J. 1992. Syphilis, AIDS and crack cocaine. *Journal of Community Health* 17(2): 69–71.

Johnston, L. D., et al. 1994. National survey results on drug use. *The Monitoring the Future Study, 1975–1993.* National Institute on Drug Abuse. NIH Volume 1(61).

Lando, H. A., et al. 1991. A comparison of self-help approaches to smoking cessation. *Addictive Behaviors* 16:183–193.

National Center for Health Statistics. 1994. *Healthy People 2000 Review, 1993.* Hyattsville, Md.: Public Health Service.

National Institute on Drug Abuse. 1993. *NIDA Capsules: Designer Drugs.*

Rave drug could damage brain. 1995. *New York Times,* 15 August.

Roeleveld, N., et al. 1992. Mental retardation associated with parental smoking and alcohol consumption before, during, and after pregnancy. *Preventive Medicine* 21(1): 110–119.

Schatzkin, A., and M. P. Longnecker. 1994. Alcohol and breast cancer. *Cancer Supplement* 74(3): 1101–1110.

Teenage marijuana use nearly doubled since 1992. 1995. *San Francisco Chronicle,* 13 September.

The Truth About Secondhand Smoke. 1995. *Consumer Reports,* January.

Transdermal Nicotine Study Group. 1991. Transdermal nicotine for smoking cessation. *Journal of the American Medical Association* 266(22): 3133–3138.

U.S. Department of Health and Human Services. 1993. *Alcohol, Tobacco, and Other Drugs May Harm the Unborn.* Public Health Service. Alcohol, Drug Abuse, and Mental Health Administration: PH291.

U.S. Department of Health and Human Services. 1994. *National Survey Results on Drug Use from the Monitoring the Future Study, 1975–1993.* Volume 1. National Institutes of Health.

Wechsler, H., et al. 1994. Health and behavioral consequences of binge drinking in college. *Journal of the American Medical Association* 272(21): 1672–1677.

Werch, C. E. 1990. Behavioral self-control strategies for deliberately limiting drinking among college students. *Addictive Behaviors* 15:119–128.

Westermeyer, J. 1992. Substance abuse disorders: Predictions for the 1990s. *American Journal of Drug and Alcohol Abuse* 18(1): 1–11.

Name ______________________ Section ____________ Date ______________

LAB 13-1 *For Smokers Only: Why Do You Smoke?*

Although smoking cigarettes is physiologically addictive, people smoke for reasons other than nicotine craving. What kind of smoker are you? Knowing what your motivations and satisfactions are can ultimately help you quit. This test is designed to provide you with a score on each of six factors that describe many people's smoking. Read the statements, then circle the number that represents how *often* you feel this way when you smoke cigarettes. Be sure to answer each question.

		Always	Frequently	Occasionally	Seldom	Never
A.	I smoke cigarettes in order to keep myself from slowing down.	5	4	3	2	1
B.	Handling a cigarette is part of the enjoyment of smoking it.	5	4	3	2	1
C.	Smoking cigarettes is pleasant and relaxing.	5	4	3	2	1
D.	I light up a cigarette when I feel angry about something.	5	4	3	2	1
E.	When I have run out of cigarettes, I find it almost unbearable until I can get them.	5	4	3	2	1
F.	I smoke cigarettes automatically without even being aware of it.	5	4	3	2	1
G.	I smoke cigarettes to stimulate me, to perk myself up.	5	4	3	2	1
H.	Part of the enjoyment of smoking a cigarette comes from the steps I take to light up.	5	4	3	2	1
I.	I find cigarettes pleasurable.	5	4	3	2	1
J.	When I feel uncomfortable or upset about something, I light up a cigarette.	5	4	3	2	1
K.	I am very much aware of the fact when I am not smoking a cigarette.	5	4	3	2	1
L.	I light up a cigarette without realizing I still have one burning in the ashtray.	5	4	3	2	1
M.	I smoke cigarettes to give me a "lift."	5	4	3	2	1
N.	When I smoke a cigarette, part of the enjoyment is watching the smoke as I exhale it.	5	4	3	2	1
O.	I want a cigarette most when I am comfortable and relaxed.	5	4	3	2	1
P.	When I feel "blue" or want to take my mind off cares and worries, I smoke cigarettes.	5	4	3	2	1
Q.	I get a real gnawing hunger for a cigarette when I haven't smoked for a while.	5	4	3	2	1
R.	I've found a cigarette in my mouth and didn't remember putting it there.	5	4	3	2	1

How to Score

Enter the numbers you have circled in the spaces provided. Total the scores on each line. Total scores can range from 3 to 15. Any score of 11 or above is high; any score of 7 or below is low.

			TOTALS
________ +	________ +	________ =	________________
A	G	M	Stimulation
________ +	________ +	________ =	________________
B	H	N	Handling
________ +	________ +	________ =	________________
C	I	O	Pleasurable relaxation
________ +	________ +	________ =	________________
D	J	P	Crutch: tension reduction
________ +	________ +	________ =	________________
E	K	Q	Craving: strong physiological or psychological addiction
________ +	________ +	________ =	________________
F	L	R	Habit

What Your Scores Mean: A Summary

The six factors measured by this test describe ways of experiencing or managing certain kinds of feelings. A high score on any factor indicates that this factor is an important source of satisfaction for you. The higher your score, the more important a particular factor is in your smoking, and the more useful the discussion of that factor can be in your attempt to quit.

Stimulation: If you score high on this factor, it means you are stimulated by a cigarette—you feel that it helps wake you up, organize your energies, and keep you going. If you try to give up smoking, you may want a safe substitute—a brisk walk or moderate exercise, for example—whenever you feel the urge to smoke.

Handling: Handling things can be satisfying, but there are many ways to keep your hands busy without lighting up or playing with a cigarette. Try doodling or toying with a pen, pencil, or other small object.

Pleasurable relaxation: Those who do get real pleasure out of smoking often find that an honest consideration of the harmful effects of their habit is enough to help them quit. They substitute social or physical activities and find they do not seriously miss their cigarettes.

Crutch: Many smokers use cigarettes as a kind of crutch in moments of stress or discomfort, and occasionally it may work; but heavy smokers are apt to discover that cigarettes do not help them deal with their problems effectively. When it comes to quitting, this kind of smoker may find it easy to stop when everything is going well but may be tempted to start again in a time of crisis. Physical exertion or social activity may serve as useful substitutes for cigarettes.

Craving: Quitting smoking is difficult for people who score high on this factor. It may be helpful for them to smoke more than usual for a day or two, so that the taste for cigarettes is spoiled, and then isolate themselves completely from cigarettes until the craving is gone.

Habit: These smokers light up frequently without even realizing it; they no longer get much satisfaction. They may find it easy to quit and stay off if they can break the habit patterns they have built up. The key to success is becoming aware of each cigarette when it's smoked. Ask, "Do I really want this cigarette?"

Source: National Institutes of Health.

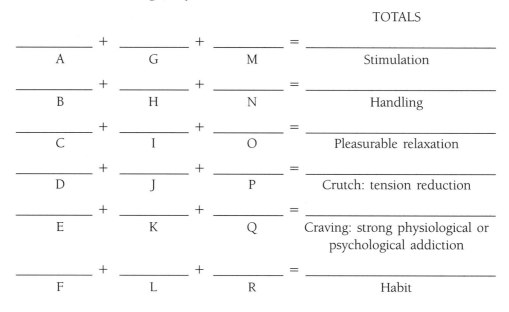

Name ______________________ Section ____________ Date ____________

LAB 13-2 *A Personal Drinking Guide*

Evaluate Your Reasons for Drinking

Be honest with yourself. It is necessary for you to know why you drink in order to control your alcohol-related behavior. Put a check mark next to the statements that are true for you.

I drink to tune myself in, so that I can

____ enhance my enjoyment of people, activities, and special occasions

____ promote social ease by relaxing my inhibitions, aiding my ability to talk to others

____ complement and add to my enjoyment of food

____ relax after a period of hard work and/or tension

I drink to tune myself out, so that I can

____ escape my problems

____ mask fears when courage and self-confidence are lacking

____ block out my painful loneliness, self-doubt, and/or feelings of inadequacy

____ substitute for close relationships or a challenging activity

____ mask a sense of guilt about drinking

Alcohol Content

Drinks differ in the amount of pure alcohol they contain. A proof value indicates the alcohol concentration in a particular drink; the proof value is equal to twice the percentage of alcohol in a drink. A higher-proof drink has more alcohol per ounce of liquid than a lower-proof drink. To calculate the number of ounces of pure alcohol in a drink, multiply the size of the drink by the percentage of alcohol it contains (one-half proof value). For example, a 12-oz beer (10 proof) has 0.6 oz of pure alcohol (10 proof = 5% alcohol concentration; 0.05 × 12 oz = 0.6 oz).

Calculate the number of ounces of pure alcohol in each of the drinks below.

Drink	Size (oz)	Proof Value	Ounces of Pure Alcohol
beer	12	10	________
wine	6	24	________
sherry	4	40	________
liquor	1.5	80	________

Try the calculations on drinks of different sizes and drinks of different alcohol content.

________	________	________	________
________	________	________	________
________	________	________	________
________	________	________	________

Maintenance Rate (How Long to Sip a Drink)

Remember that the effects of alcohol will be greater when your BAC is rising than when you keep it stable or allow it to fall. BAC is directly proportional to the rate of ethyl alcohol intake. Assuming a general maintenance rate (rate at which the body rids itself of alcohol) of 0.1 oz of pure alcohol per hour per 50 pounds of body weight, you can calculate the approximate length of time it takes you to metabolize a given drink by applying this formula:

$$\frac{2.5 \times \text{proof of drink} \times \text{volume (size in oz) of drink}}{\text{body weight}} = \text{time in hours per drink}$$

For example, to calculate how long it should take to drink one can (12 oz) of 10-proof beer for a person weighing 150 pounds:

$$\frac{2.5 \times 10 \times 12}{150} = 2 \text{ hours}$$

It takes this 150-pound person 2 hours to completely metabolize one 12-oz can of 10-proof beer.

Choose your favorite three drinks (or choose three of the examples from the previous page), and use this formula to calculate your maintenance rate for each drink:

1. $\frac{(\quad) \times (\quad) \times (\quad)}{(\quad)}$ = ______ hours/drink

2. $\frac{(\quad) \times (\quad) \times (\quad)}{(\quad)}$ = ______ hours/drink

3. $\frac{(\quad) \times (\quad) \times (\quad)}{(\quad)}$ = ______ hours/drink

In Case of Excess

To sober up, the only remedy that works is to stop drinking and allow time to pass. For any type of drink, the amount of time would be the number of drinks you have consumed multiplied by your maintenance rate for that drink. For the example given above, if the 150-pound individual had consumed three 12-oz cans of 10-proof beer, he or she would have to wait 6 hours before the alcohol would be metabolized. Calculate the amount of time that would have to elapse for you to metabolize all the alcohol if you had consumed three of one of the types of drinks you calculated a maintenance rate for above:

3 × (   ) = ______ hours

Given this consumption level, your answer here indicates the number of hours you should wait before driving.

Name ______________________ Section ______________ Date ______________

LAB 13-3 *Abusing Psychoactive Drugs*

Signs of Drug Dependence

If you are wondering whether you're becoming dependent on a drug, answer the questions below. The more times you answer yes, the more likely it is that you are developing a physical or psychological dependence on the drug. If you answer yes to more than two or three of these questions, you should seek professional help.

Yes	No	
____	____	1. Do you take the drug regularly?
____	____	2. Have you been taking the drug for a long time?
____	____	3. Do you always take the drug in certain situations or when you're with certain people?
____	____	4. Do you find it difficult to stop using the drug? Do you feel powerless to quit?
____	____	5. Have you tried repeatedly to cut down or control your use of the drug?
____	____	6. Do you need to take a larger dose of the drug in order to get the same high you're used to?
____	____	7. Do you feel specific symptoms if you cut back or stop using the drug?
____	____	8. Do you frequently take another psychoactive substance to relieve withdrawal symptoms?
____	____	9. Do you take the drug to feel "normal"?
____	____	10. Do you go to extreme lengths or put yourself in dangerous situations to get the drug?
____	____	11. Do you hide your drug use from others?
____	____	12. Do you think about the drug when you're not high, figuring out ways to get it?
____	____	13. If you stop taking the drug, do you feel bad until you can take it again?
____	____	14. Does the drug interfere with your ability to study, work, or socialize?
____	____	15. Do you skip important occupational, social, or recreational activities in order to obtain or use the drug?
____	____	16. Do you continue to use the drug despite a physical or mental disorder, or despite a significant problem that you know is worsened by drug use?
____	____	17. Have you developed a mental or physical condition or disorder because of prolonged drug use?

Reasons for Drug Use

If you have tried a psychoactive drug in the past, describe the circumstances of your first use of the drug. What were your reasons for trying the drug? Did other people have an impact on your decision to try the drug? Did you seek out the experience, or did you find yourself in a situation where the drug was available?

____

____

____

If you have continued to use a psychoactive drug, what are your reasons? Which of the following apply to you?

_____ 1. Taking drugs allows me to escape boredom or depression.

_____ 2. Drug use enables me to socialize with a group of people with whom I want to socialize.

_____ 3. Using drugs makes me feel daring.

_____ 4. Using drugs is exciting because they're illegal.

_____ 5. Drug use allows me to feel better about myself.

_____ 6. Taking drugs enables me to alter my mood or see the world in a way I can't without the drugs.

_____ 7. Drug use is a natural part of my society.

_____ 8. I take drugs to rebel against my parents or society.

_____ 9. Drug use is enjoyable.

_____ 10. Drugs enable me to socialize more easily.

_____ 11. Drug use allows me to be a more spiritual person.

_____ 12. I take drugs when I am angry or upset.

List other reasons that apply to you.

____

____

____

If you have never tried a psychoactive drug, give your reasons for this choice.

____

____

____

If you have been in a situation where you were offered a psychoactive drug and turned it down, what reasons did you give? What would you say to someone who asked you why you were refusing the drug? Can you offer suggestions to someone who does not want to use psychoactive drugs but feels self-conscious about refusing them when they are offered?

____

____

____

14

Sexually Transmissible Diseases

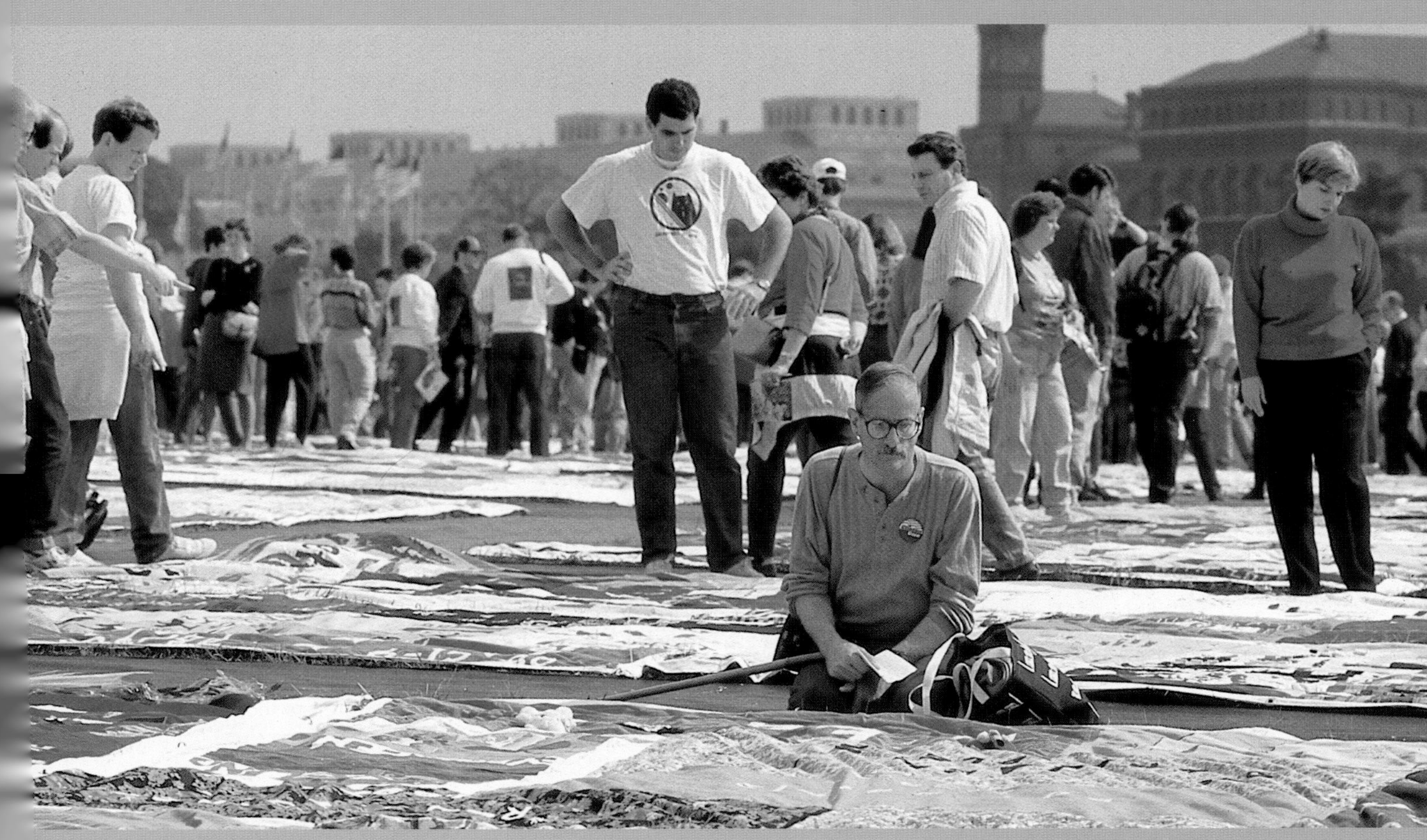

LOOKING AHEAD

After reading this chapter, you should be able to answer these questions about sexually transmissible diseases (STDs):

- In what ways do STDs pose a threat to wellness?
- What is AIDS, and how is it transmitted, diagnosed, and treated?
- What are the symptoms, risks, and treatments of the other major STDs?
- How can individuals protect themselves from STDs?

No health issue has commanded as much public attention in recent years as **acquired immunodeficiency syndrome,** or **AIDS.** This fatal, incurable disease is the leading cause of death in the United States among men 25–44 years of age and the fifth leading cause for women in the same age group. People between the ages of 18 and 25 are at the highest risk of acquiring **HIV infection.** The epidemic of HIV infection is considered the number-one health priority in the United States. Although recent public education campaigns have focused primarily on HIV infection, they deserve to be repeated for all the **sexually transmissible diseases (STDs)**—gonorrhea, chlamydia, herpes, syphilis, and others—because they continue to have a high incidence among Americans. Worldwide, more than 18 million people are believed to have HIV infection, and 250 million people are affected by the other STDs each year.

STDs are a particularly insidious group of diseases because they are often silent in the early stages of infection. A person can be infected—and therefore be capable of transmitting the disease to others—and still not look or feel sick. Not until years later does the cost of unprotected sexual activity become apparent. By then, an infected person may find that an undiagnosed STD has caused infertility, contributed to the development of cancer, or caused a birth defect in a child. In the case of HIV infection, the immune system becomes fatally weakened and can no longer provide protection from disease.

It is important that everyone have a clear understanding of what STDs are, how they are transmitted, and, most importantly, how they can be prevented. The crucial message is that they *can* be prevented. And many can also be cured if they are treated early and properly.

This chapter is designed to provide information about healthy, safe sexual behavior and to help you understand what you can do to reduce the risk of contributing to the further spread of and damage caused by these diseases. Lab 14-1 will help you evaluate your risk of contracting an STD by helping you examine your attitudes and behaviors.

TERMS

acquired immunodeficiency syndrome (AIDS) A fatal, incurable, sexually transmissible viral disease.

HIV infection A chronic, progressive disease that damages the immune system; caused by the human immunodeficiency virus (HIV).

sexually transmissible disease (STD) A disease that can be transmitted by sexual contact; some STDs can also be transmitted by other means.

hemophilia A hereditary blood disease in which blood fails to clot and abnormal bleeding occurs, requiring transfusions of blood with a specific factor to aid coagulation.

THE MAJOR STDs

In general, seven different STDs pose major health threats: HIV infection/AIDS, hepatitis, syphilis, chlamydia, gonorrhea, genital warts, and herpes. These diseases are considered "major" because they are serious in themselves, cause serious complications if left untreated, and/or pose risks to a fetus or newborn. In addition, pelvic inflammatory disease (PID) is a common complication of gonorrhea and chlamydia and merits discussion as a separate disease.

HIV Infection/AIDS

HIV infection is one of the most serious and challenging problems facing the United States and the world today. Despite the intense efforts of health professionals worldwide, HIV infection continues to spread. By 1996, more than 500,000 Americans had been diagnosed with AIDS, and more than 1 million were believed to be infected with HIV. Worldwide, more than 6 million people are believed to have AIDS, and it is estimated that by the year 2000, 40–120 million people will be infected with the virus.

HIV infection is a chronic disease that progressively damages the body's immune system, making an otherwise healthy person susceptible to a variety of infections and disorders. Under normal conditions, when a virus or other disease-causing agent enters the body, it is destroyed by the body's immune system. But HIV attacks and disarms the immune system itself so that it can no longer respond adequately to infection. See Figure 14-1 for a graphic representation of the general pattern of HIV infection.

Transmission HIV is transmitted by blood and blood products, semen, and vaginal and cervical secretions. It cannot live in air, water, or on objects such as toilet seats, eating utensils, or telephones. There are three main routes for HIV transmission:

1. Particular kinds of sexual contact; primarily unprotected anal or vaginal intercourse and, to a lesser degree, oral-genital contact
2. Direct exposure to infected blood
3. From an HIV-infected woman to her fetus during pregnancy or childbirth or, possibly, to her infant during breastfeeding

The unprotected sexual activities in the first category above carry the greatest risks. HIV can be transmitted through minute tears in the fragile lining of the vagina, cervix, penis, anus, and mouth and through direct infection of cells in some of these areas. (Refer to Figures 14-2 and 14-3 on pp. 330–331 for basic information about human sexual anatomy.) The presence of lesions or blisters from other STDs in the genital, anal, or oral areas facilitates transmission. During vaginal intercourse, male-to-

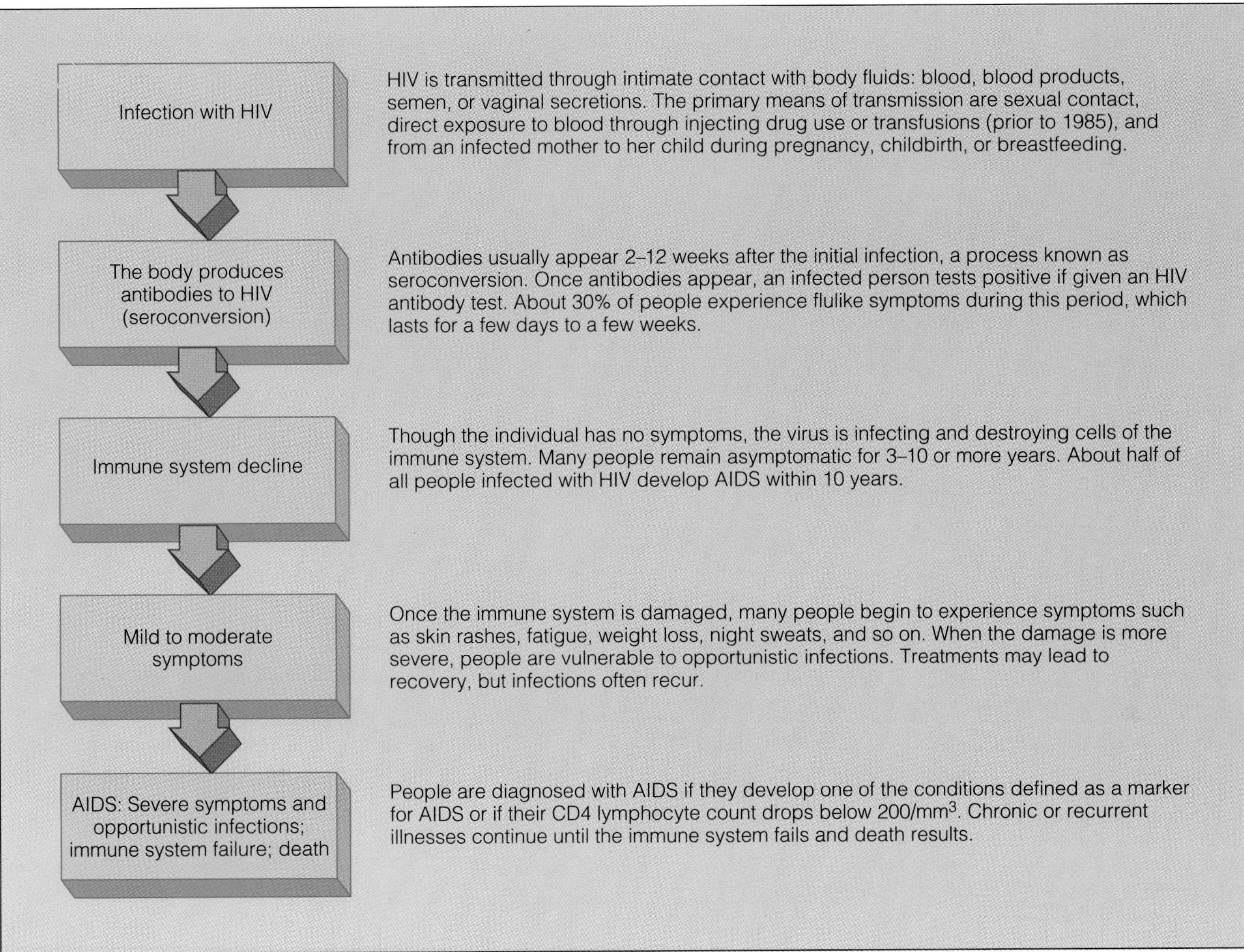

Infection with HIV
HIV is transmitted through intimate contact with body fluids: blood, blood products, semen, or vaginal secretions. The primary means of transmission are sexual contact, direct exposure to blood through injecting drug use or transfusions (prior to 1985), and from an infected mother to her child during pregnancy, childbirth, or breastfeeding.
The body produces antibodies to HIV (seroconversion)
Antibodies usually appear 2–12 weeks after the initial infection, a process known as seroconversion. Once antibodies appear, an infected person tests positive if given an HIV antibody test. About 30% of people experience flulike symptoms during this period, which lasts for a few days to a few weeks.
Immune system decline
Though the individual has no symptoms, the virus is infecting and destroying cells of the immune system. Many people remain asymptomatic for 3–10 or more years. About half of all people infected with HIV develop AIDS within 10 years.
Mild to moderate symptoms
Once the immune system is damaged, many people begin to experience symptoms such as skin rashes, fatigue, weight loss, night sweats, and so on. When the damage is more severe, people are vulnerable to opportunistic infections. Treatments may lead to recovery, but infections often recur.
AIDS: Severe symptoms and opportunistic infections; immune system failure; death
People are diagnosed with AIDS if they develop one of the conditions defined as a marker for AIDS or if their CD4 lymphocyte count drops below 200/mm^3. Chronic or recurrent illnesses continue until the immune system fails and death results.

Figure 14-1 ***The general pattern of HIV infection.*** The pattern of HIV infection is different for every person, and not everyone infected with HIV will go through all the stages shown here. *Sources:* Adapted from Schwarz, R. 1992. *AIDS Medical Guide.* San Francisco: San Francisco AIDS Foundation. DeVita, V. T., Jr., et al., eds. 1996. *AIDS: Etiology, Diagnosis, Treatment and Prevention.* Philadelphia: Lippincott-Raven.

female transmission is more likely to occur than female-to-male transmission. HIV has been found in preejaculatory fluid, so transmission can occur before ejaculation.

Direct bloodstream contact with the blood of an infected person is the second major route of HIV transmission. Needles used to inject drugs are routinely contaminated by the blood of the user, so if needles are shared, small amounts of one person's blood can be directly injected into another person's bloodstream. HIV may also be transmitted from needles or blades used in acupuncture, tattooing, ritual scarring, and piercing of the earlobes, nose, lip, or nipple.

HIV has been transmitted in blood and blood products used in the medical treatment of **hemophilia,** injuries, and serious illnesses. All licensed blood banks and plasma centers in the United States now screen for HIV. The Centers for Disease Control and Prevention (CDC) estimate that the current risk of transfusion-related HIV transmission is about one in 450,000–660,000 transfusions, or about 30 blood recipients per year.

The mother-to-child transmission route, called vertical transmission, results in the infection of about 25–30% of the babies born to HIV-infected mothers. Most of these infections seem to occur during pregnancy, but a few may happen during childbirth or breastfeeding. By 1996, more than 7000 babies had been infected in the United States. Recent research has revealed that giving the drug AZT to HIV-infected pregnant women greatly reduces the risk of vertical transmission; therefore, this route of infection may be somewhat controllable.

Trace amounts of HIV have been found in the saliva and tears of some infected people, but researchers believe that these fluids do not carry enough virus to infect another person. Contact with the urine or feces of infected people may carry some risk; contact with an infected person's sweat is believed to hold no risk. For a summary of

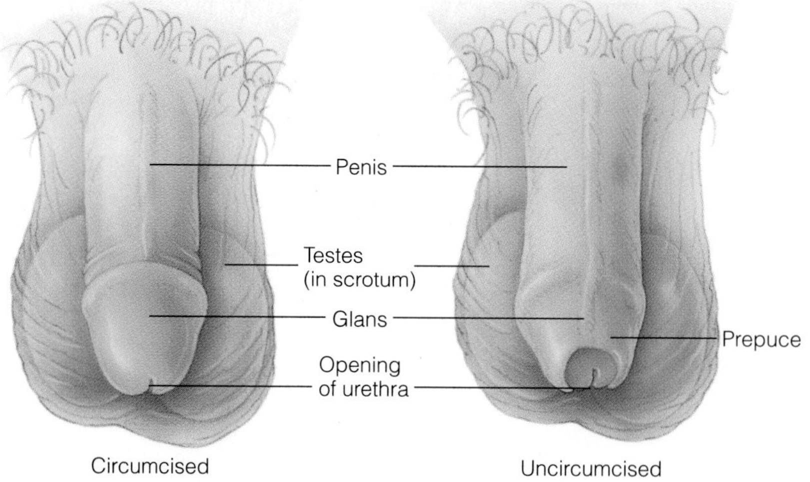

External structures

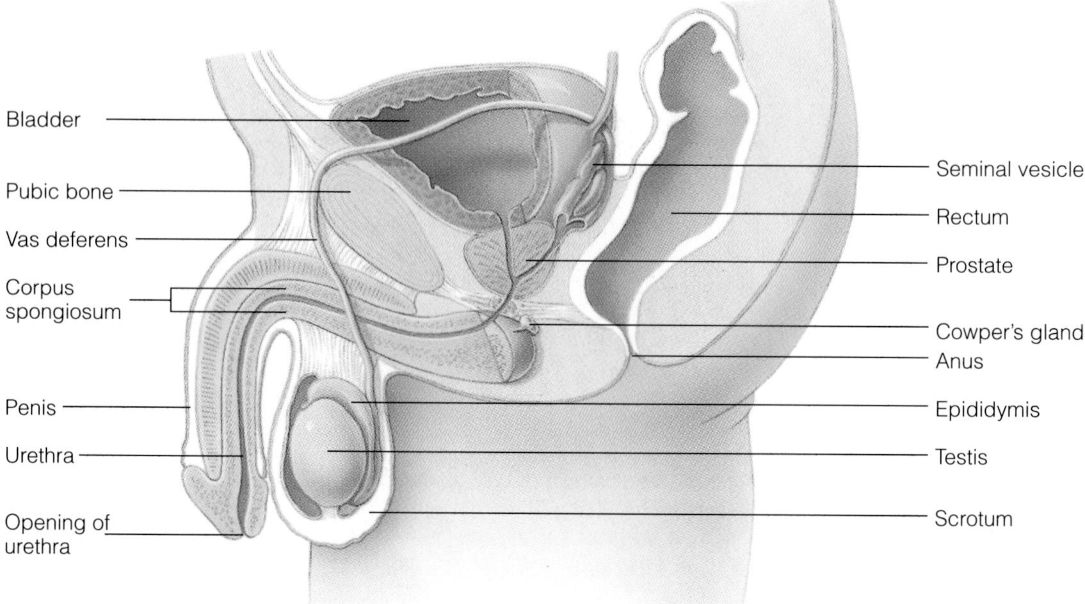

Internal structures (cross section)

Figure 14-2 ***Male sexual anatomy.***

the routes of HIV transmission among adults, see Figure 14-4 (p. 332).

Symptoms The signs and symptoms that suggest HIV infection include the following:

- Persistent swollen glands
- Lumps, rashes, sores, or other growths on or under the skin or on the mucous membranes of the eyes, mouth, anus, or nasal passages
- Persistent yeast infections
- Unexplained weight loss (unrelated to illness, dieting, or increased physical activity) of more than 10 pounds or 10% of body weight in less than 2 months
- Fever and drenching night sweats
- Dry cough and shortness of breath
- Persistent diarrhea
- Easy bruising and/or unexplained bleeding
- Profound fatigue, sometimes accompanied by light-headedness or dizziness
- Memory loss
- Tremors, seizures, unstable balance
- Change in vision, hearing, taste, or smell
- Difficulty swallowing
- Mood changes and other psychiatric symptoms
- Persistent or recurrent pain

Obviously, some of these symptoms can also occur with minor colds, flu, or other illnesses.

Because of a weakened immune system, people with HIV infection are highly susceptible to infections and

Mons pubis
Labia majora
Prepuce of clitoris
Clitoris (glans)
Labia minora
Urethral opening
Vaginal opening
Anus

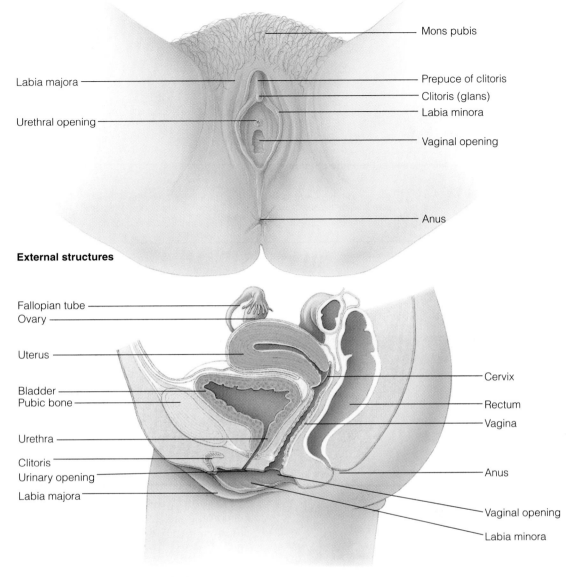

External structures

Fallopian tube
Ovary
Uterus
Cervix
Bladder
Pubic bone
Rectum
Vagina
Urethra
Clitoris
Urinary opening
Anus
Labia majora
Vaginal opening
Labia minora

Internal structures (cross section)

Figure 14-3 *Female sexual anatomy.*

other disorders, both common and uncommon. The most common ones seen in people with HIV include *Pneumocystis carinii* pneumonia, Kaposi's sarcoma, tuberculosis, AIDS dementia, cryptosporidiosis, and invasive cervical cancer. Most of these conditions are rare among people with healthy immune systems and are not contagious. However, tuberculosis is spread through the air and may pose a risk for both non–HIV-infected people and other HIV-infected people who associate with an HIV-infected person who has an active case of TB.

Diagnosis and Treatment Minimizing the impact of HIV/AIDS depends on early diagnosis. The surest diagnosis of HIV infection is the detection of the virus itself by means of laboratory tissue cultures. The most commonly used screening test is the **HIV antibody test,** which determines whether a person has **antibodies** to HIV in his or her blood or tissue. An individual who repeatedly tests positive on this test is considered both infected and infectious. Another test, the HIV-1 or P-24 antigen test, measures the actual HIV particles in the blood.

AIDS is the most severe form of HIV infection. People are diagnosed with AIDS if they are **HIV-positive** and either have developed an infection defined as an AIDS indi-

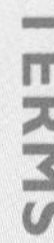

HIV antibody test A blood test currently being used to determine whether an individual has been infected by HIV.

antibody A globular protein produced in the blood in response to a foreign substance.

HIV-positive The condition of being infected with HIV.

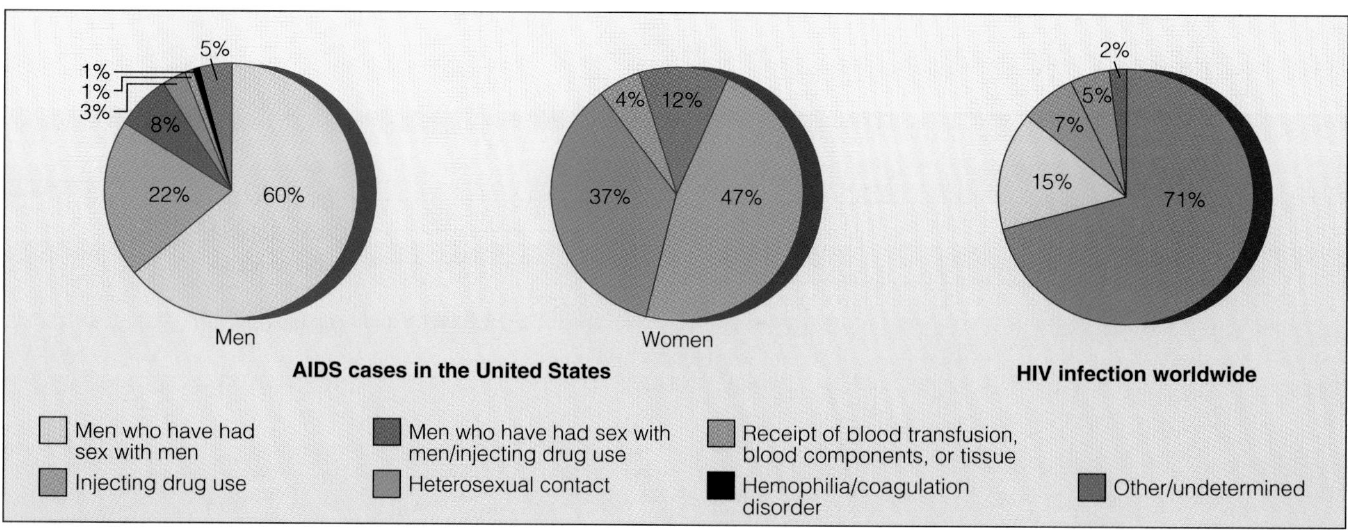

Figure 14-4 ***Routes of HIV transmission among adults.*** *Sources:* Centers for Disease Control and Prevention. 1995. *HIV/AIDS Surveillance Report,* 7(2). Mann, J., J. M. Tarantola, and T. W. Netter, eds. 1992. *AIDS in the World.* Cambridge, Mass.: Harvard University Press.

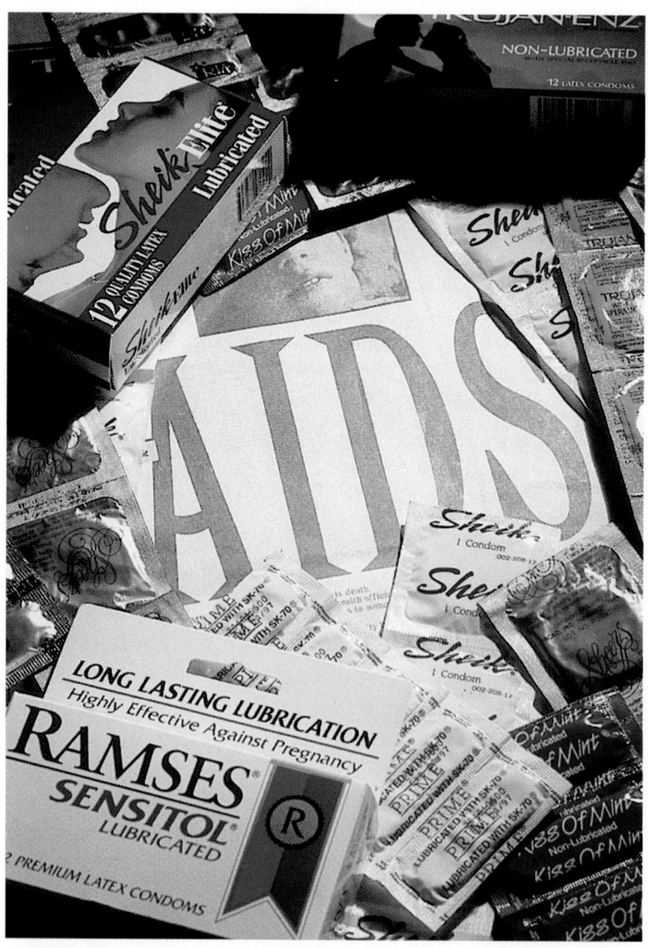

Condoms are gaining in popularity because they provide protection not only against pregnancy but also against STDs, which birth control pills and most other forms of contraception do not.

cator or have a severely damaged immune system, as measured by counts of CD4 lymphocytes (cells that kill disease-causing agents).

There is no known cure for HIV infection, but new drugs have been developed to slow the advance of the virus and treat some of the individual infections that arise when the immune system is compromised. Lifestyle measures such as a proper diet, regular exercise, and stress management can also help maintain healthy immune function (see the box "Stress and the Immune System"). People infected with HIV can live 10 years or more before becoming sick with AIDS. Researchers hope that before too long, AIDS will be a manageable chronic disease that people will control with medication.

Prevention Although currently incurable and fatal, AIDS is preventable. You can avoid it by making careful choices about sexual activity and drug use:

- If you are uninfected and in a mutually monogamous relationship with another uninfected person, you are not at risk for HIV.
- If you are not involved in a long-term, mutually monogamous relationship, abstain from any sexual activity that involves the exchange of body fluids, or always use a latex condom (see the box "Male Condoms," p. 334). Condoms are not 100% reliable and therefore do not guarantee risk-free sex, but used properly a latex condom provides a high level of protection against the transmission of HIV. Condoms should also be used during oral sex. Some experts also suggest the use of latex squares and dental dams, rubber devices that can be used as barriers during oral-genital sex or oral-anal sexual contact. Limiting

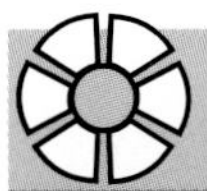

WELLNESS CONNECTION

Stress and the Immune System

Many people believe, on an intuitive level, that excessive amounts of stress make them more susceptible to illness. Studies have shown that rates of illness are higher for weeks or even months among people who have experienced the severe emotional trauma of divorce or the death of a loved one. Can more commonplace anxieties and stresses also cause significant, measurable changes in the immune system? And can common stress-management techniques actually boost the immune system?

Results of studies conducted at Ohio State University suggest that poor emotional well-being suppresses the body's ability to fight disease. Medical students taking final exams were tested for their ability to mount an immune response to a hepatitis vaccination. Compared to students who received the vaccine under unstressed conditions, the stressed students showed much weaker immune responses.

Additional research suggests that anxiety and depression may affect a person's susceptibility to disease long after the distress is alleviated. The Ohio State team studied the immune systems of people who cared for loved ones with Alzheimer's disease. The stress of caring for an Alzheimer's patient depressed the caregiver's immune system, even 2 years after the patient had died.

Other researchers have studied the opposite side of the relationship between stress and immunity—whether therapies that induce positive emotions can boost immune function. Relaxation and imagery of a powerfully functioning immune system increased T-cell levels for some people. (T-cells are white blood cells vital to the functioning of the immune system.) Other stress-management techniques may boost the immune system in different ways.

In seeking to explain these effects, researchers are looking at the connections among emotions, stress, hormones, and immunity—an area of study known as **psychoneuroimmunology,** or PNI. Some hormones, such as cortisol, have been found to impair the ability of immune cells to multiply and function. Others, such as prolactin, seem to give immune cells a boost. By matching stress levels and hormonal changes to the ups and downs of immune function, researchers hope to gain a better grasp of the shifting chemistry of mind and immunity.

What can you do to give your immune system a boost? In addition to developing techniques for successfully managing the stress in your life, adopt other parts of a wellness lifestyle that have a positive effect on immunity: Eat a balanced diet and maintain moderate weight; get enough sleep, 6–8 hours per night; engage in moderate endurance exercise; don't smoke; drink alcohol only in moderation; and, of course, protect yourself from HIV infection.

Sources: Adapted from Flach, J., and L. Seachrist. 1994. Mind-body meld may boost immunity. *Journal of the National Cancer Institute* 86(4): 256–258. Jaret, P. 1992. Mind over malady. *Health,* November/December.

the number of sex partners and openly discussing sexual issues and sexual histories can contribute to reducing the risk of HIV exposure, but the proper use of latex barriers is most effective.

- Do not mix sexual activity with alcohol or drug use. The use of these substances can lower inhibitions and affect judgment, making unsafe sex more likely. Surveys show that the majority of college students do not use safer sex practices. Many students report a willingness to lie about past sexual activity in order to obtain sex; they also tell researchers that they believe their risk of contracting HIV depends on "who they are" rather than on their sexual behavior. Such misconceptions and behaviors put college students at high risk for contracting HIV.
- Do not share drug needles. Needles can be decontaminated with a solution of bleach and water, but even this is not foolproof (boiling needles and syringes does not necessarily destroy HIV either). For injecting drug users, however, the most effective prevention is to obtain drug treatment and to quit using drugs.
- Participate in an HIV education program. Education is all we have to combat the prevalent myth that "bad things happen only to other people." Until we have a vaccine and a cure, education and individual responsibility will be the cornerstones of any program to control this devastating epidemic.

Hepatitis

Hepatitis is an inflammation of the liver usually caused by one of three different viruses:

- Hepatitis A virus causes the mildest form and is usually transmitted by food or water contaminated by sewage or by anal-oral contact with an infected person.
- Hepatitis B lives in all body fluids and is easily transmitted through sexual activity involving the exchange of body fluids. It can also be transmitted via

TERMS

psychoneuroimmunology The study of the interactions among the brain, the endocrine system, and the immune system.

hepatitis Inflammation of the liver, caused by one of a group of viruses that can be transmitted through certain types of sexual and nonsexual contact.

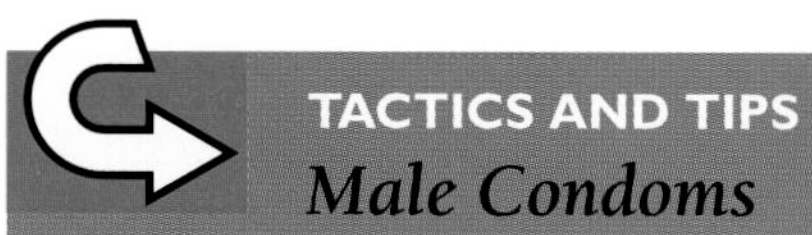

TACTICS AND TIPS
Male Condoms

Although they're not 100% effective as a contraceptive or as protection from STDs—only abstinence is—condoms improve your chances on both counts. Use them properly by following these guidelines:

- *Buy only latex.* If you're allergic to rubber, try wearing a lambskin condom under a latex one.
- *Buy them fresh.* Don't use condoms that are more than a year old. Don't remove the condom from its individual sealed wrapper until you're ready to use it. Don't use it if it's gummy, dried out, or discolored.
- *Buy an effective design.* Condoms with a reservoir tip are preferable.
- *Use a water-based lubricant.* Oil-based lubricants such as petroleum jelly, baby oil, and hand lotion make condoms break.
- *Use them correctly.* Roll the condom down over the penis as soon as it's erect. Squeeze the air out of the reservoir tip or the top quarter-inch of the condom as you unroll it to leave room for semen. Make sure there are no air bubbles (which are the biggest reason condoms break). Remove it after ejaculation before the penis becomes flaccid. Use a new condom every time you have intercourse.
- *Store them correctly.* Too much heat or cold can damage condoms. Don't leave them in your wallet longer than overnight.
- *Practice.* Condoms aren't hard to use, but practice helps. Take one out of the wrapper; examine it and stretch it to see how strong it is. Practice by yourself and with your partner.

If you feel awkward discussing condoms with your partner, try bringing up the subject when AIDS is in the news. You can talk about its effect on sexual practices and how more and more people are using condoms. Or you can talk about caring for each other. Open the discussion *before* you have sex. If he or she still resists the idea of using condoms, try some of the approaches listed below.

If your partner says . . .	Try saying . . .
"They're not romantic."	"Worrying about AIDS isn't romantic. With condoms, we won't need to worry." OR "If we put one on together, it can be romantic."
"You don't trust me."	"It's not a matter of trust. It's a matter of health." OR "It's important to me that we're both protected."
"I don't use condoms."	"I use condoms every time." OR "I don't have sex without condoms."
"But I love you."	"Being in love can't protect us against AIDS." OR "I love you, too. We still need to use condoms."
"But we've been having sex without condoms."	"I want to start using condoms now so we won't be at any more risk." OR "We can still prevent infection or reinfection."

Sources: The Condom Buyer's Guide and *Condoms for Couples,* San Francisco AIDS Foundation.

contaminated razor blades, toothbrushes, and eating utensils. The primary risk factors are heterosexual exposure and intravenous drug use; having multiple sex partners greatly increases risk, and pregnant women can transmit hepatitis B to their unborn children.

- Hepatitis C used to be the leading form of hepatitis following blood transfusions, but the blood supply is now screened for both hepatitis B and C. Hepatitis C is transmitted in the same way as hepatitis B, but sexual transmission has not been confirmed.

Symptoms Many people with hepatitis never develop symptoms. Others get flulike symptoms such as fever, body aches, chills, and loss of appetite. As the illness progresses, there may be nausea, vomiting, dark-colored urine, abdominal pain, and **jaundice.** Some people also develop a skin rash and joint pain or arthritis. Most cases of hepatitis A are of short duration, but people with hepatitis B or C, even when they recover completely, can become chronic carriers, capable of infecting others for the rest of their lives. Chronic hepatitis can cause cirrhosis of the liver, liver failure, and a deadly form of liver cancer. Hepatitis kills about 6000 Americans every year.

Diagnosis and Treatment Hepatitis is diagnosed through blood tests. There is no cure, and treatment is designed to minimize damage to the liver. Preventive measures for hepatitis A involve avoiding contaminated water and infected food, careful hand washing, and avoiding oral-anal sexual contact. Preventive measures for the B and C forms of hepatitis are similar to those for HIV infection: avoiding sexual contact that involves the sharing of body fluids—in this case, including saliva; using latex barriers to make sex safer; and avoiding the sharing of hypodermic needles.

There is a safe and highly effective vaccine for hepatitis B. All pregnant women should be tested for this form of hepatitis, and all infants of infected mothers must be vaccinated immediately after birth. Many physicians recommend immunization of all infants and adolescents as well as adults in high-risk groups; these include health care workers, homosexually active men, injecting drug users, and heterosexually active people with multiple sex partners.

Syphilis

Although death and disability from **syphilis** have declined dramatically worldwide since the introduction of penicillin treatment in 1943, there are about 100,000 new cases every year in the United States. Syphilis is caused by a bacterium called ***Treponema pallidum,*** which requires warmth and moisture to survive. This disease is usually acquired through sexual contact, although unborn children can contract it through the placenta from an infected mother. The organism can pass through any break or opening in the skin or mucous membranes and can be transmitted by kissing, vaginal or anal intercourse, or oral-genital contact.

Symptoms Syphilis is characterized by sores or lesions known as **chancres** that contain large numbers of bacteria; they make the disease highly contagious when they are present. If untreated, an individual can remain contagious for as long as 18 months. In later stages, although the lesions have disappeared and the person is no longer contagious, the disease can cause devastating damage to almost any body system.

Syphilis progresses through three stages as the organism becomes established in the body:

1. *Primary syphilis.* About 3 weeks after contact with an infected partner, a single chancre less than the size of a dime appears at the site of entry, most commonly the genital area. Chancres can also appear in the mouth or armpit or on the tongue, lips, breasts, or fingers. The sores are painless unless they become infected.
2. *Secondary syphilis.* Approximately 6 weeks after the chancre first appears, an untreated person begins to experience fever, malaise, sore throat, headache, hoarseness, a depressed appetite, swollen lymph glands, and hair loss. A rash may appear anywhere on the body, including the mucous membranes of the lips, cheeks, tongue, tonsils, throat, and vocal chords, but most typically on the palms of the hands and soles of the feet. These sores break down and ooze a clear fluid that contains a large number of bacteria, making this stage highly contagious. With or without antibiotic treatment, skin lesions of secondary syphilis usually heal in 2–10 weeks, although relapses are possible.
3. *Latent syphilis.* By definition, people without symptoms but with evidence of having had syphilis in the past have latent syphilis. In this stage, the organism invades the internal organs and the central nervous system. The principal manifestation of CNS damage is **paresis,** which involves partial or complete paralysis and chronic, progressive mental degeneration, leading to death. Symptoms may include facial tremors, slurred speech, impaired vision, headaches, epileptic convulsions, exaggerated reflexes, defective memory, delusions, depression, and insanity.

An infected pregnant woman who is not treated before the eighteenth week of pregnancy usually experiences stillbirth or gives birth to a child with a congenital deformity.

Diagnosis and Treatment To diagnose primary syphilis, clinicians microscopically examine a specimen from the surface of a chancre. Diagnosis of secondary syphilis is made from blood tests and clinical observation. Penicillin is the preferred treatment for syphilis in all stages, but for infected people who are allergic to penicillin, tetracycline and erythromycin can be effective substitutes. All sex partners of individuals diagnosed with syphilis should be treated as well, and follow-up tests after treatment are necessary.

A person who has had syphilis should abstain from all sexual contact with others until at least 1 month after treatment is completed. As with any serious illness, it is absolutely vital that the entire course of prescribed medication be completed and all evidence of disease has disappeared.

Regular self-examinations can help detect syphilis, in addition to other STDs (see the box "A Genital Self-Examination Guide"). As with all STDs, responsible, safer sex practices are the most effective means of prevention.

TERMS

jaundice Increased bile pigment levels in the blood, characterized by yellowing of the skin and the whites of the eyes.

syphilis An STD caused by a spiral-shaped bacterium called a spirochete.

Treponema pallidum The spiral-shaped bacterium that causes syphilis.

chancre A sore produced by syphilis in its earliest stage (pronounced "shang-ker").

paresis Central nervous system damage, sometimes a result of syphilis, involving paralysis and mental degeneration.

TACTICS AND TIPS
A Genital Self-Examination Guide

Although only a physician can make a proper diagnosis of an STD, you can examine yourself to determine whether you have any of the signs or symptoms that might indicate an infection.

General Instructions

If you're sexually active, see your physician regularly for examinations. Between checkups, use GSE periodically to check yourself for early warning signs. Throughout the exam, look for bumps, sores, blisters, or warts on the skin. Bumps or blisters may be red or light-colored; they may look like pimples, or they may develop into open sores. Genital warts may appear as very small bumpy spots, or they may have a fleshy, cauliflowerlike appearance. You should see your physician if you see anything that resembles a sore, blister, bump, or wart; if you feel any bumpy growth; or if you have any of the other symptoms described below. In addition, if you've had contact with someone whom you think might have an STD, see your physician even if you don't have any symptoms.

GSE for Women

Undress and assume a comfortable position. You may want to use a mirror; position it so you can see your entire genital area. You may find it difficult to see the area from your urinary opening down; do the best you can without making yourself uncomfortable.

Start by spreading your pubic hair apart and examining the area covered by pubic hair (the mons and the outer lips). Look for any bumps, sores, blisters, or warts. Next, spread your outer vaginal lips apart and take a close look at the hood of your clitoris. Then gently pull the hood up to examine your clitoris.

Next, look at both sides of your inner lips for the same signs. Then move on to examine the area around your urinary and vaginal openings. This is as far up as we recommend that you look. Signs of STDs may appear out of view (up in your vagina or on your cervix), so it's important to see your physician if you think you've been exposed to an STD, even if you don't discover any signs or symptoms during your GSE.

In addition to examining your entire genital area, be alert to other symptoms that can be associated with STDs: abnormal vaginal discharge (possibly thicker than usual, yellow, or with an unpleasant odor); a painful or burning sensation when urinating; pain in your pelvic area; bleeding between menstrual periods; or an itchy rash around the vagina.

GSE for Men

Once undressed, hold your penis in your hand. Start by examining the head of the penis from the urinary opening down to where it extends out a little just above the shaft. If you are not circumcised, pull down the foreskin to examine the head. Look over the entire head of the penis in a clockwise direction, checking carefully for any bumps, sores, blisters, or warts on the skin.

Next, move down the shaft and look for the same signs. Then go on to the base. At the base, try to separate your pubic hair with your fingers so you can get a good look at the skin underneath. After careful examination here, move on to the underside of the penis. You may want to use a mirror to be sure that you've seen the entire underside. A mirror can also be helpful as you examine the scrotum. Handling each testicle gently, examine the scrotum for bumps, blisters, sores, and warts. Also be aware of any lump, swelling, or soreness in the testicle.

In addition to examining your entire genital area, be alert to other symptoms that can be associated with STDs. STDs may cause burning or pain when you urinate. Some STDs cause a drip or discharge from the penis. The discharge may be thick and yellow, or it could be watery or very slight.

Source: Adapted from *Genital Self-Examination Guide*. Research Triangle Park, N.C.: Burroughs Wellcome Co. To receive a copy of the guide in English or Spanish, call 1-800-234-1124.

Chlamydia

Gonorrhea and chlamydia have similar symptoms and are often mistaken for each other, but chlamydia is now the more common disease. In fact, ***Chlamydia trachomatis*** currently causes the most prevalent bacterial infection in the United States: 3–4 million new cases occur every year.

Although everyone is susceptible to chlamydia, women bear the greatest burden because of the possible complications and consequences of the disease. In men, chlamydia is the leading cause of urinary tract infection and is also responsible for approximately 50% of the 500,000 cases of **epididymitis** (inflammation of the testicles) seen annually in the United States. But in most women, chlamydia produces no early symptoms, a factor that contributes to its devastating effects. If left undetected for 2 months or more, chlamydia may result in pelvic inflammatory disease (PID), discussed later in this chapter.

Infants of infected mothers can acquire the infection during birth. In newborns, chlamydia can cause eye in-

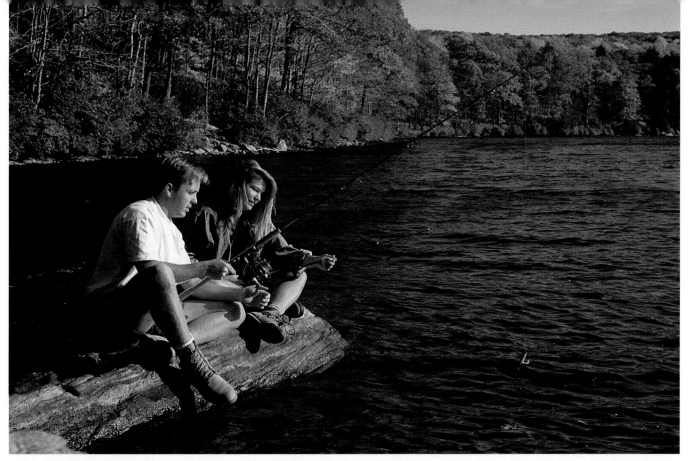

Although both men and women can contract STDs, women face a higher risk of serious long-term consequences, including pelvic inflammatory disease and infertility. If this couple's relationship includes sexual intimacy, using condoms can help protect both partners from disease.

fections, pneumonia, and (less often) ear infections. Screening for chlamydia and treating infected mothers are highly effective ways of preventing the infection of babies during birth.

Symptoms In men, chlamydia symptoms include painful urination and a slight watery discharge from the penis. In women, symptoms include a discharge from the cervix, painful urination, and a painful inflammation of the oviducts, which is symptomatic of PID. However, most people experience few or no symptoms, increasing the likelihood that they will inadvertently spread the infection to their partners.

Diagnosis and Treatment Chlamydia is diagnosed by means of a microscopic antibody test. Because of the seriousness of an undetected infection, some physicians may include a laboratory test for chlamydia with a routine Pap test.

Once diagnosed, chlamydia is treated in the affected person and his or her sex partners with antibiotics. To prevent reinfection and complications, as with all STDs, it is imperative that the full course of medication be completed. It is also important to refrain from sexual intercourse until treatment is finished.

Gonorrhea

In the United States, 400,000–600,000 cases of **gonorrhea,** also known as "drip" or "the clap," are reported each year, with the highest incidence among 20- to 24-year-olds. Like chlamydia, untreated gonorrhea can cause PID in women and epididymitis in men, leading to sterility. It can also cause **dermatitis** (inflammation of the skin) and a type of arthritis. An infant passing through the birth canal of an infected mother may contract **gonococcal conjunctivitis,** an eye infection that can lead to blindness. In some states, all newborn babies are routinely treated with antimicrobial eyedrops to prevent infection.

TERMS

Chlamydia trachomatis A sexually transmissible organism that produces a wide variety of infections.

epididymitis An inflammation of the small body of ducts that rests on the testes.

gonorrhea An STD caused by a bacterium that usually affects mucous membranes.

dermatitis An inflammation of the skin.

gonococcal conjunctivitis An inflammation of the mucous membrane lining of the eyelids, caused by the gonococcus bacterium.

Gonorrhea is caused by a bacterium, ***Neisseria gonorrhoeae,*** which thrives in the mucous membranes. It cannot live long outside the warm, moist environment of the human body and dies within moments of exposure to air and light. Consequently, gonorrhea cannot be contracted by contact with toilet seats, towels, or other objects.

Symptoms In men, the **incubation period** is about 5 days. The first symptoms are a form of urethritis (inflammation of the urethra) that causes discomfort on urination and a thick, yellowish-white or yellowish-green discharge from the penis. The lips of the urethral opening may become inflamed and swollen. In some men, the lymph glands in the groin become enlarged and swollen. Some 10–30% of men will have very minor symptoms or none at all.

Approximately 80% of women with gonorrhea have no symptoms whatsoever and therefore do not know they are infected. When symptoms do appear in women, they are similar to those in men, including an irritating discharge and discomfort on urination. After 2 months or more, symptoms may include lower abdominal cramping or pain, fever, and vaginal bleeding, a possible indication of PID.

Gonorrhea bacteria can also infect the throat or rectum of infected people who engage in oral or anal sex. The symptoms of gonorrhea in the throat may be a sore throat or pus on the tonsils, and those of gonorrhea in the rectum may be pus in the feces or rectal irritation, pain, and itching. As with other infections, gonorrhea is often accompanied by a fever and swollen glands.

Diagnosis and Treatment Gonorrhea is diagnosed by examining a laboratory culture of the discharge. Accurate diagnosis of gonorrhea is especially important because new strains of the gonococcal organism have arisen that are antibiotic-resistant. When gonorrhea is diagnosed early, treatment with broad-spectrum antibiotics is relatively easy and effective. Following treatment, sexual activity should not be resumed until follow-up testing shows no evidence of the disease.

Pelvic Inflammatory Disease

If gonorrhea is left untreated in women, it can spread internally and, like chlamydia, cause **pelvic inflammatory disease (PID),** an infection of the oviducts that may extend to the ovaries. This condition is often serious enough to require hospitalization and can result in a continuing susceptibility to recurrent infection, ectopic pregnancy (pregnancy in an oviduct rather than the uterus), sterility, and chronic menstrual problems. PID is the leading cause of infertility in young women.

The infectious agents for both gonorrhea and chlamydia can be sexually transmitted by an infected partner. During or just after menstruation, these organisms appear to increase in the uterine cavity, where they may cause inflammation or pass directly into the oviducts. The inflammation spreads easily into the pelvic cavity, where it can cause further infection and pelvic abscess.

Symptoms Most women remain asymptomatic for some time, usually until the next menstrual cycle after infection. Once the organisms reach the oviducts, symptoms can develop within 7 days. These include chills, fever, loss of appetite, nausea and/or vomiting, and abdominal pain on both sides (though sometimes more intense on one side). Some women have prolonged menstruation, abnormal vaginal bleeding, or abnormal discharge.

Diagnosis and Treatment PID is usually diagnosed on the basis of symptoms. **Laparoscopy** may be used to isolate the suspected organism and grow it in a culture medium. Cultures from the rectum or cervix may also be taken to help identify the specific organism. All sex partners of a woman who has been diagnosed with PID should be treated for infection. The complications of PID are serious and irreversible: scarring of the oviducts, often as a result of abscesses; adhesions; chronic pelvic pain; and ectopic pregnancies.

Genital Warts

Genital warts, or condyloma, is the most common STD for which students seek treatment at campus health clinics. The disease has increased rapidly in recent years and appears to be most prevalent in people age 16–25. This increase has serious implications because the precancerous condition known as cervical dysplasia often occurs

TERMS

Neisseria gonorrhoeae The bacterium that causes gonorrhea.

incubation period A period during which bacteria or viruses are actively multiplying inside the body's cells, usually without symptoms of illness.

pelvic inflammatory disease (PID) An infection that progresses from the vagina and cervix to infect the oviducts and pelvic cavity.

laparoscopy A method of examining the internal organs by inserting a tube containing a small light through an abdominal incision.

genital warts An STD caused by a virus and characterized by the appearance of growths on the genital area of both men and women.

human papillomavirus (HPV) The organism that causes genital warts; certain strains of HPV are associated with the development of cervical dysplasia and cervical cancer.

podophyllin An acid used in the treatment of warts.

herpes A type of virus, or the disease produced by the virus, such as cold sores; considered sexually transmissible.

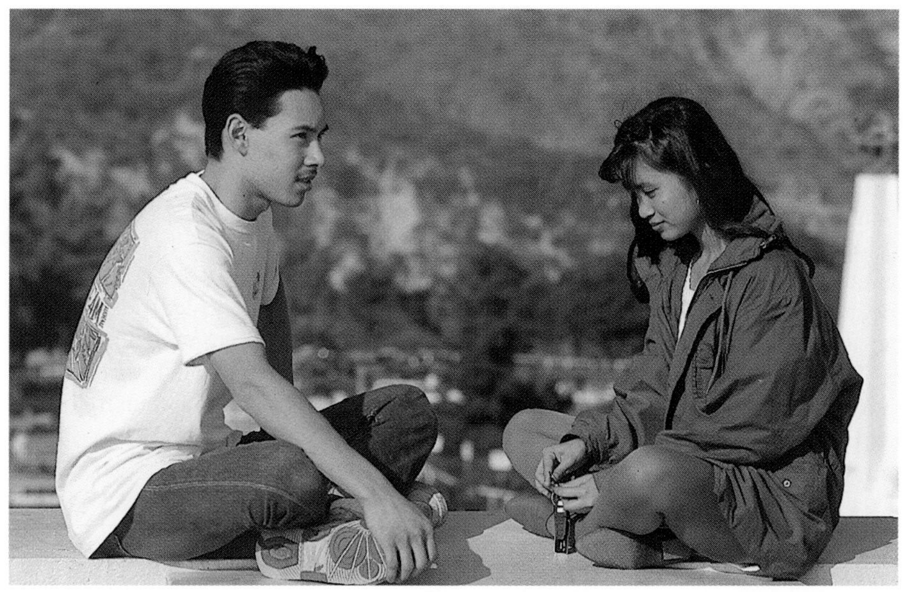

Sexual activity has many consequences, including pregnancy, disease, and emotional changes in the relationship. Honest communication is a crucial part of responsible sexual behavior.

among women with untreated genital warts. Condyloma is caused by a large family of viruses known as **human papillomavirus (HPV).**

Symptoms Symptoms are dry, painless growths, rough in texture and gray or pink in color, flat or raised and varied in size. Untreated warts can grow together to form cauliflowerlike clumps. In males they appear on the penis, more commonly in circumcised men. They often involve the urethra, appearing first at the opening and then spreading. The growths may cause irritation and bleeding, leading to painful urination and urethral discharge. Warts may also appear around the anus or within the rectum. In women, warts may appear on the labia or vulva and spread to the perineum. They may also appear on the cervix. If the warts are small and flat, they can be difficult for a physician to see.

Diagnosis and Treatment A genital wart infection is very contagious through contact with the lesions, but infected people can transmit the disease to their sex partners without having any symptoms themselves. Early diagnosis and effective treatment are often impeded by a long incubation period (averaging 4–6 weeks but sometimes extending up to 8–12 weeks following infection), a lack of awareness of symptoms in women, and a complex, not-always-effective treatment approach. Although the risk is not clear, newborns can be infected during delivery.

The traditional treatment is **podophyllin,** a toxic agent, applied directly to the lesions. Other treatments include removal of the lesions by electrocautery, cryosurgery (freezing), surgery, and laser therapy. Drug therapy with alpha interferon is administered in a series of injections, but long-term effects of this treatment are still under study. Even after treatment, however, genital warts can recur, so follow-up care is especially important, along with the avoidance of sexual contact until healing is complete and open discussion to inform sex partners of exposure. Because of the relationship between HPV and cervical cancer, women who have had genital warts should have Pap tests every 6 months.

Herpes

Herpes is an extremely common viral infection for which there is no cure and no preventive vaccine. It is a difficult condition to deal with because a variety of factors can trigger recurrent outbreaks. Adding to the infection's complexity and the lack of clarity how it is transmitted is the fact that there are six different viruses in the herpes family that infect humans, all with different manifestations:

- Herpes simplex, type I, which causes cold sores and fever blisters around the lips, mouth, face, and, as a result of oral-genital contact, the genital area.
- Herpes simplex, type II, also known as genital herpes, which is usually seen in the genital area; as a result of oral-genital contact, it is sometimes also responsible for infections of the lips, mouth, and face.
- Varicella zoster, which causes chicken pox in children and shingles in adults.
- Epstein-Barr virus (EBV), which is implicated as the cause of infectious mononucleosis and has recently been linked with certain cancers.
- Cytomegalovirus (CMV), which can cause severe infections of the lungs, brain, colon, and eyes in people with suppressed immune systems (including those with HIV infection) and can also cause birth defects.

- Human herpesvirus 6 (HHV6), which has only recently been identified.

Herpes simplex I and II, CMV, and HHV6 are all sexually transmissible.

Symptoms Herpes infections of types I and II are extremely contagious and appear 2–20 days after the initial exposure. Symptoms can include one or more blisterlike sores on or around the mouth, face, or genitals. The sores are painful, fluid-filled lesions and may be accompanied by swollen glands, general muscle pains, fever, a mild burning sensation during urination in men, and a vaginal discharge in women. Some women may have internal lesions on the vagina or the cervix, but because the cervix has no nerve endings, an infected woman may be completely unaware that lesions are present.

Complications Women with genital herpes are five times more likely to develop cancer of the cervix. Any woman who has had genital herpes should have a Pap test every 6 months.

Because their immune system is immature, newborns are particularly susceptible to herpes, which can cause severe brain damage and sometimes death. Newborns should never have contact with cold sores. Pregnant women with herpes must be monitored near the time of delivery to ensure that the newborn is protected from exposure to the virus. If the woman's infection becomes active, the baby will usually be delivered by cesarean section to protect it from contact with lesions in the birth canal or genital area.

One of the most frustrating aspects of a herpes infection is its ability to recur. After the first infection, the virus lies dormant in the nerve pathways in the area of initial infection, but exposure to sun, temperature extremes, high levels of stress, acute illness, certain foods, lowered resistance, or other factors can trigger a recurrence. Because herpes is chronic, it has a long-lasting effect on sexuality. A person with an active infection is contagious and has an obligation to prevent the spread in others. Maintaining good general health and fitness can help prevent repeated bouts of infection.

Diagnosis and Treatment Most cases of herpes are diagnosed from the presence of the lesions, but cultures can be grown from a tissue sample. There is no cure for herpes, and at present treatment is directed at relieving pain, itching, and burning and, where possible, preventing recurrences and spread of the disease.

OTHER STDs

Although far less serious than those described above, a few other diseases can be sexually transmitted.

- **Trichomoniasis,** commonly called "trich," is caused by a protozoan. It is possible to contract trich by nonsexual means, but sexual contact with an infected partner is the most likely means of transmission. Women infected with trich develop a greenish, foul-smelling vaginal discharge within 4 days after contact. The discharge causes severe itching and irritates the vagina and vulva, causing redness and pain. Although most males do not have any symptoms, some may experience slight itching, clear discharge, and painful urination.
- ***Candida albicans*** is a very common fungus normally found in the vaginal tract. If the fungus increases, however, the result is candidiasis, commonly called a yeast infection, characterized by discomfort and itching. Symptoms can then be passed to a sex partner. Candidiasis is a common opportunistic infection in people with HIV infection. Sometimes a runaway yeast infection is symptomatic of a more extensive condition—for example, diabetes or metabolic changes due to pregnancy. Increased fungus production can also result from oral contraceptive use, antibiotic therapy, and the general lowering of body resistance to infection.

  Intense vaginal and vulval itching and a thick, cottage-cheese–like discharge are common symptoms of candidiasis. This infection can also manifest itself in the mouth (where it is called thrush) and show as whitish patches on the mucous membrane of the insides of the cheeks and back of the throat, making eating very difficult.
- **Pubic lice** are parasitic organisms that attach to the pubic hairs. Commonly known as "crabs," they are often difficult to see but are the color of small freckles until they have fed, when they become dark brown. They feed on human blood. These organisms are easily passed sexually from person to person, but they are also transmitted via infested bedding, towels, clothing, sleeping bags, and even toilet seats. Intense itching is the usual symptom, and with careful examination both the parasite and its eggs can be seen.
- **Scabies** is another common parasite that burrows and deposits eggs beneath the skin. When the eggs hatch, the new mites congregate around the hair follicles. The symptom of scabies is intense itching, especially at night. The itching usually occurs between the

TERMS

trichomoniasis A protozoan vaginal infection that may be transmitted to sex partners.

Candida albicans The organism that causes candidiasis, or yeast infection.

pubic lice Parasites that infest the hair of the pubic region.

scabies A contagious skin disease caused by a type of mite.

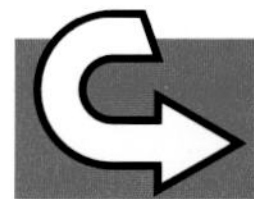

TACTICS AND TIPS

Prevention and Treatment of STDs

The surest way to avoid STDs is to abstain from sex.

If you are sexually active:

- Have sex with only one uninfected partner who has sex only with you (mutual monogamy).

If you have more than one sex partner:

- Limit the number of partners you have.
- Always use a condom.
- Use condoms with a water-based lubricant.
- Discuss STDs and prevention with new partners before having sex.
- Perform genital self-examination regularly.

If you or any partners have a sign or symptom of an STD:

- See your physician immediately for diagnosis and treatment.
- Take all medications as prescribed.
- Return for follow-up examinations as directed by your physician.
- Do not engage in sexual activity until treatment is complete and tests confirm you are cured.
- Inform all sex partners of your condition, and tell them to be tested and treated.

fingers, on the wrists, in the armpits, under the breasts, along the inner surfaces of the thigh, penis, scrotum, and occasionally the female genitals. Scabies is easily spread from person to person through any direct or close contact.

WHAT YOU CAN DO

As emphasized throughout this chapter, undetected and untreated STDs can lead to serious medical complications and even death. In asymptomatic cases, the only way infected people can find out they have a disease is by being tested. For this reason, open, honest communication between sex partners is essential. The responsibility of informing partners is an ethical task too important to disregard.

With the exception of some AIDS treatments, available STD treatments are safe, effective, and generally inexpensive. If you are being treated, follow the instructions carefully, and complete all medications as prescribed. Don't stop taking the medication just because you feel better or your symptoms have disappeared. Above all, don't give any of your medication to your partner or anyone else. Doing so will only make your treatment incomplete and reinfection more likely (see the box "Prevention and Treatment of STDs"). Being cured of an STD doesn't mean that you will not get it again, so stay informed, alert, and open with your partners. And always practice safer sex.

? COMMON QUESTIONS ANSWERED

Who should have an HIV test? Anyone at risk for HIV infection should consider being tested. Early treatment for HIV infection can help keep an infected person free of symptoms for a longer period of time. In addition, if you know you are HIV-positive, you can inform your sex partners and encourage them to consider testing. You can also avoid transmitting HIV to others by abstaining from sex or limiting your sexual activity to safer practices. Testing is particularly important for pregnant women because there is now a treatment that can significantly lower the risk of HIV transmission from mother to child.

Researchers believe that HIV has been in the United States since the middle to late 1970s. You are potentially at risk for HIV infection if any of the following apply to you since that time: you have had unprotected sexual contact with more than one partner or with a partner who was not in a mutually monogamous relationship with you; you have used or shared syringes, bulbs, works, or needles to inject drugs (including steroids); or you received a blood transfusion prior to 1985.

If you decide to be tested for HIV, look for a testing program that offers counseling as well as testing. If you have doubts about whether to be tested, get counseling; then you can decide whether to go ahead with testing. Some states offer anonymous testing, where no one asks your name and you are the only one who can reveal the test results to others. Other states provide confidential testing, where your record is kept secret from everyone except medical personnel and, in some states, the state health department. To find out where you can receive counseling, check with your physician, your local or state health department, or the national AIDS hotline (800-342-AIDS, 800-344-SIDA for Spanish speakers, or 800-243-7889 for TTY, deaf access). A home-use HIV test kit, which provides anonymous results and counseling by phone, received FDA approval in 1996.

The test itself involves a blood sample that is analyzed in the laboratory for the presence of antibodies to HIV. If the first stage of testing proves positive, it is followed by a confirmatory test. The accuracy of the combined tests is high. However, it usually takes about 22–25 days (possibly as long as 6 months in some individuals) after exposure to HIV for antibodies to appear; therefore, a person may need to be retested at a later date to be absolutely certain of his or her HIV status.

Which contraceptive methods protect best against STDs? The only sure way to avoid STDs is to abstain from sexual activity or to be in a mutually monogamous relationship with an uninfected partner. If you choose to be sexually active, male condoms are the best known protection against HIV and other STDs. (The recently developed female condom should theoretically reduce the risk of STDs, but research results are not yet available.) Condoms are not foolproof, however, and they do not protect against the transmission of diseases from sores or lesions that aren't covered by condoms.

You can increase their effectiveness by using them properly. Latex condoms are about 88% effective as a contraceptive; researchers estimate that when condoms are used properly, failure rates can be as low as 1–2%. Failure rates vary from brand to brand and batch to batch, as well as according to the user's age, education, and the amount of experience he's had with condoms. Breakage is most often caused by inadequate lubrication, use of an improper (oil-based) lubricant, and failure to smooth out air bubbles, which may pop and break the condom during sexual activity. Condoms slipping off during withdrawal is another common cause of failure. Refer to the box on p. 334 for more information on proper condom use.

Some other contraceptive methods may provide some protection against certain STDs. The diaphragm and cervical cap cover the cervix and may provide some protection against diseases that involve the infection of cervical cells. Spermicides reduce the risk of cervical gonorrhea, chlamydia, and PID; but if vaginal irritation occurs from the use of spermicides, the risk of infection with HIV and other STDs may increase. Hormonal methods such as oral contraceptives do not protect against STDs in the lower reproductive tract but do provide some protection against PID. For sexually active people, the consistent and correct use of latex male condoms provides the best protection against STDs currently available; combining condom use with another method can provide even greater protection.

SUMMARY

- Sexually transmissible diseases, which are increasing in incidence, are insidious because infection is not always obvious and can be passed on without either partner knowing about it.
- HIV infection progressively damages the immune system; it is transmitted through unprotected sexual contact, through direct exposure to infected blood, and from mother to fetus or newborn. Diagnosis is usually by means of an antibody test. Drugs can slow the progression of the disease and treat particular infections. Prevention involves the use of latex condoms and other safer sex practices and avoiding injecting drug use, as well as awareness of all risks.
- Hepatitis, usually caused by one of three different viruses, can be transmitted sexually; it is an infection of the liver that can lead to cirrhosis and cancer. Prevention of sexual transmission is similar to that for HIV; a vaccine for hepatitis B is available.
- Syphilis, contracted through sexual contact or the placenta of an infected mother, is diagnosed through a chancre specimen and treated with penicillin.
- Both chlamydia and gonorrhea can lead to pelvic inflammatory disease if not treated with antibiotics. PID can lead to sterility.
- Genital warts are a risk factor for cervical cancer; toxic agents are used in treatment once diagnosis is made by examination of the lesions.
- Herpes is especially difficult to treat because the virus lies dormant and recurrences are common; it is especially dangerous to newborns.
- Less serious STDs include trichomoniasis, candidiasis, pubic lice, and scabies.
- Responsible sexual behavior includes examining oneself for symptoms of STDs, getting and completing treatment when infected, informing partners, and avoiding sexual activity until treatment is complete.

BEHAVIOR CHANGE ACTIVITY

Overcoming Peer Pressure: Communicating Assertively

- Julia is trying to give up smoking; her friend Marie continues to offer her cigarettes whenever they are together.
- Emilio is planning to exercise in the morning; his roommates tell him he's being antisocial by not having brunch with them.
- Tracy's boyfriend told her that in high school he once experimented with drugs and shared needles; she wants him to have an HIV test, but he says he's sure the people he shared needles with did not have AIDS.

Peer pressure is the common ingredient in these situations. To successfully maintain your behavior change program, you must develop effective strategies for standing up to peer pressure. Assertive communication is one such strategy. By communicating assertively—firmly, but not aggressively—you can stick with your program even in the face of pressure from others.

To determine whether peer pressure is a problem to be addressed in your behavior change program, use your health journal to track how other people affect your target behavior. If you find that you often do give in to peer pressure, try the following strategies for communicating more assertively:

- Collect your thoughts, and plan in advance what you will say. You might try out your response on a friend to get some feedback.
- State your case—how you feel, and what you want—as clearly as you can.
- Use I messages—statements about how you feel—rather than statements beginning with "You."
- Focus on the behavior rather than the person. Suggest a solution, such as asking the other person to change his or her behavior toward you. Avoid generalizations. Be very specific about what you want.
- Make clear, constructive requests. Focus on your needs ("I would like . . .") rather than on the mistakes of others ("You always . . .").
- Avoid blaming, accusing, and belittling. Treat others with the same respect you'd like to receive yourself.
- Ask for action ahead of time. Tell others what you would like to happen; don't wait for them to do the wrong thing and then get angry at them.
- Ask for a response to what you have proposed. Wait for an answer, and listen carefully to it. Try to understand other people's points of view, just as you would hope that others would understand yours.

With these strategies in mind, review your health journal and identify three instances in which peer pressure interfered with your behavior change program. For each of these instances, write out what you might have said to deal with the situation more assertively. (If you can't find three situations from your own experiences, choose one or more of the three scenarios described at the beginning of this section.)

1. ______________________________

____

____

2. ______________________________

____

____

3. ______________________________

____

____

Assertive communication can help you achieve your behavior change goals in a direct way by helping you keep your program on track. It can also provide a boost for your self-image and increase your confidence in your ability to successfully manage your own behavior.

FOR MORE INFORMATION

There are many sources of information about STDs:

- Your school probably offers courses that contribute to a broader understanding of sexual behavior.
- Free pamphlets and other literature are available from public health departments, health clinics, physicians' offices, student health centers, and Planned Parenthood. Literature about AIDS is available from the National AIDS Clearinghouse (1-800-458-5231) or Impact AIDS, the distributor for the San Francisco AIDS Foundation (415-861-3397).
- The National STD hotline provides free, confidential information and referral services to callers anywhere in the country. Call 1-800-227-8922 between 8:00 A.M. and 11:00 P.M. (Eastern time), Monday through Friday.

- The National AIDS hotline provides free, confidential information and can direct you to local counseling and testing centers. Call 1-800-342-AIDS, 24 hours a day, 7 days a week. The service is available in Spanish (1-800-344-SIDA) and for the hearing impaired (1-800-AIDS-TTY).
- Easy-to-understand books are available in libraries and bookstores. Helpful resources include the following:

Burroughs Wellcome Co. 1990. *What You Need to Know About Sexually Transmitted Diseases, HIV Disease and AIDS.* Distributed at the American Medical Association Conference on STDs: Risk Assessment, Diagnosis and Treatment. Research Triangle Park, N.C.: Burroughs Wellcome, November. *An easy-to-read survey of the STDs.*

Channing L. Bete Co., Inc. 1995. *What Do You Know About HIV?* South Deerfield, Mass.: Channing L. Bete Co., Inc. *Basic information, written for the general public.*

Hatcher, R. A., et al. 1994. *Contraceptive Technology, 1994–1996,* 16th ed. New York: Irvington. *Updated every 2 years, an informational handbook that provides a scientific overview of reproductive health, including STDs.*

Mass, L. 1989. *Medical Answers About AIDS.* New York: Gay Men's Health Crisis. *A comprehensive, understandable book about AIDS.*

Sacks, S. L. 1989. *The Truth About Herpes.* West Vancouver: Gordon Soules. *A complete overview of the disease that makes a good reference for self-care information.*

Shilts, R. 1987. *And the Band Played On: Politics, People and the AIDS Epidemic.* New York: St. Martin's Press. *A highly readable account of the AIDS epidemic and the political response it has evoked, written by a concerned and committed reporter; as powerful now as it was when it was first published.*

U.S. Department of Health and Human Services. 1993. *Surgeon General's Report to the American Public on HIV Infection and AIDS.* Washington, D.C.: U.S. Public Health Service.

SELECTED BIBLIOGRAPHY

Altman, L. 1995. AIDS is now the leading killer of Americans from 24 to 44. *New York Times Science,* 31 January.

American College Health Association. 1990. *HIV Infection and AIDS: What Everyone Should Know.* Baltimore, Md.: American College Health Association.

Basen-Enquist, K. 1992. Psychosocial predictors of safer sex behaviors in young adults. *AIDS Education and Prevention* 4(2): 120–134.

Bosch, F. X., et al. 1995. Prevalence of humanpapillomavirus in cervical cancer: A worldwide perspective. International Biological Study on Cervical Cancer (IBSCC) Study Group. *Journal of the National Cancer Institute* 87(11): 796–802.

Centers for Disease Control. 1988. Condoms for the prevention of STDs. *Mortality and Morbidity Weekly Report* 37:133.

Centers for Disease Control. 1991. Revised classification system for HIV infection and expanded AIDS surveillance case definition for adolescents and adults. Atlanta: Centers for Disease Control, Draft Report, 15 November.

Centers for Disease Control and Prevention. 1993. Update: Barrier protection against HIV infection and other sexually transmitted diseases. *Morbidity and Mortality Weekly Report* 42:589–591, 597.

Centers for Disease Control and Prevention. 1995. Update: AIDS among women—United States, 1994. *Morbidity and Mortality Weekly Report* 44:5.

DeBuono, B. A., S. H. Zinner, M. Daamen, and W. M. McCormack. 1990. Sexual behavior of college women in 1975, 1986, and 1989. *New England Journal of Medicine* 322:821–825.

Doucett, M., M. Perry, and B. Winterbottom. 1992. AIDS education of college students: The effect of an HIV positive lecturer. *AIDS Education and Prevention* 4(2): 160–171.

Evans, D. L., et al. 1995. Stress-associated reductions of cytotoxic T lymphocytes and natural killer cells in asymptomatic HIV infection. *American Journal of Psychiatry* 152(4): 543–550.

Felts, W. M., and S. M. Knight. 1992. The nature and prevention of viral hepatitis: What health educators should know. *Journal of Health Education* 23(5): 267–274.

Goldsmith, M. F. 1992. Critical moment at hand in HIV/AIDS pandemic, new global strategy to arrest its spread proposed. *Journal of the American Medical Association* 268(4): 445.

Holmes, K. K., P. March, P. F. Sparling, and P. J. Weisner, eds. 1990. *Sexually Transmitted Diseases,* 2d ed. New York: McGraw-Hill.

Kitchen, V. S., et al. 1995. Safety and activity of saquinavir in HIV infection. *Lancet* 345(8955): 952–955.

MacDonald, N. E., et al. 1990. High-risk STD/HIV behavior among college students. *Journal of the American Medical Association* 263:3155–3159.

O'Leary, A., F. Goodhart, L. S. Jermmott, and D. Boccher-Lattimore. 1992. Predictors of safer sex on the college campus: A social-cognitive theory analysis. *Journal of American College Health* 40, May.

San Francisco AIDS Foundation. 1992. *AIDS Medical Guide,* 3d ed. San Francisco: Impact AIDS.

Sarracco, A., et al. 1993. Man-to-woman sexual transmission of HIV: Longitudinal study of 343 steady partners of infected men. *Journal of Acquired Immune Deficiency Syndrome* 6: 497–502.

Schochetman, G., and J. R. George. 1994. *AIDS Testing: A Comprehensive Guide to Technical, Medical, Social, Legal, and Management Issues,* 2d ed. New York: Springer-Verlag.

Smith, K. V., and D. M. White. 1992. Risk level knowledge and prevention behavior for human papillomaviruses among sexually active college women. *Journal of American College Health* 40, March.

Swanson, J. M., S. L. Dibble, and K. Trocki. 1995. A description of gender differences in risk behaviors in young adults with genital herpes. *Public Health Nursing* 12:99–108.

Taylor, D. N. 1995. Effects of a behavior stress-management program on anxiety, mood, self-esteem, and T-cell count in HIV-positive men. *Psychological Reports* 76(2): 451–457.

U.S. Department of Health and Human Services. 1995. News Release: FDA approves first protease inhibitor drug for treatment of HIV, 7 December.

Weber, J. T., and R. E. Johnson. 1995. New treatments for chlamydia trachomatis genital infection. *Clinical Infectious Diseases* 20(S1): S66–S71.

Name ______________________ Section ____________ Date ______________

LAB 14-1 *Behaviors and Attitudes Related to STDs*

All sexually transmissible diseases are preventable. You have control over the behaviors that put you at risk for contracting STDs and for increasing their negative effects on your health. To identify your risk factors for STDs, read the following list of statements, and indicate whether they're true or false for you.

True or False

______ 1. I have never been sexually active. (If false, continue. If true, you are not at risk; respond to the remaining statements based on how you realistically believe you would act.)

______ 2. I am in a mutually faithful relationship with an uninfected partner or am not currently sexually active. (If false, continue. If true, you are at minimal risk now; respond to the remaining statements according to your attitudes and past behaviors.)

______ 3. I have only one sex partner.

______ 4. I always use a latex condom for each act of intercourse.

______ 5. I use a water-based lubricant with condoms.

______ 6. I discuss STDs and prevention with new partners before having sex.

______ 7. I do not use alcohol or another mood-altering drug in sexual situations.

______ 8. I would tell my partner if I thought I had been exposed to an STD.

______ 9. I am familiar with the signs and symptoms of STDs.

______ 10. I regularly perform genital self-examination.

______ 11. When I notice any sign or symptom of any STD, I consult my physician immediately.

______ 12. When diagnosed with an STD, I inform all recent partners.

______ 13. When I have a sign or symptom of an STD that goes away on its own, I still consult my physician.

______ 14. I do not use drugs prescribed for friends or sex partners or left over from other illnesses to treat STDs.

______ 15. I do not share syringes or needles to inject drugs.

False answers indicate attitudes and behaviors that put you at risk for contracting STDs or for suffering serious medical consequences from them.

The time to think about prevention is before you have sex.

1. List three ways to bring up the subject of STDs with a new partner. How would you ask whether or not he or she has been exposed to any STDs or engaged in any risky behaviors? (Remember that because many STDs can be asymptomatic, it is important to know about past behaviors even if no STD was diagnosed.)

a. ____

____

LABORATORY ACTIVITIES

b. ______________________________

____

c. ______________________________

____

2. List three ways to bring up the subject of condom use with your partner. How might you convince someone who does not want to use a condom?

a. ______________________________

____

b. ______________________________

____

c. ______________________________

____

3. If you had had an STD in the past that you might possibly still pass on (e.g., herpes), how would you tell your partner(s)?

____

____

____

4. If you were diagnosed with an STD that you believe was given to you by your current partner, how would you begin a discussion about STDs with him or her?

____

____

____

15

Wellness for Life

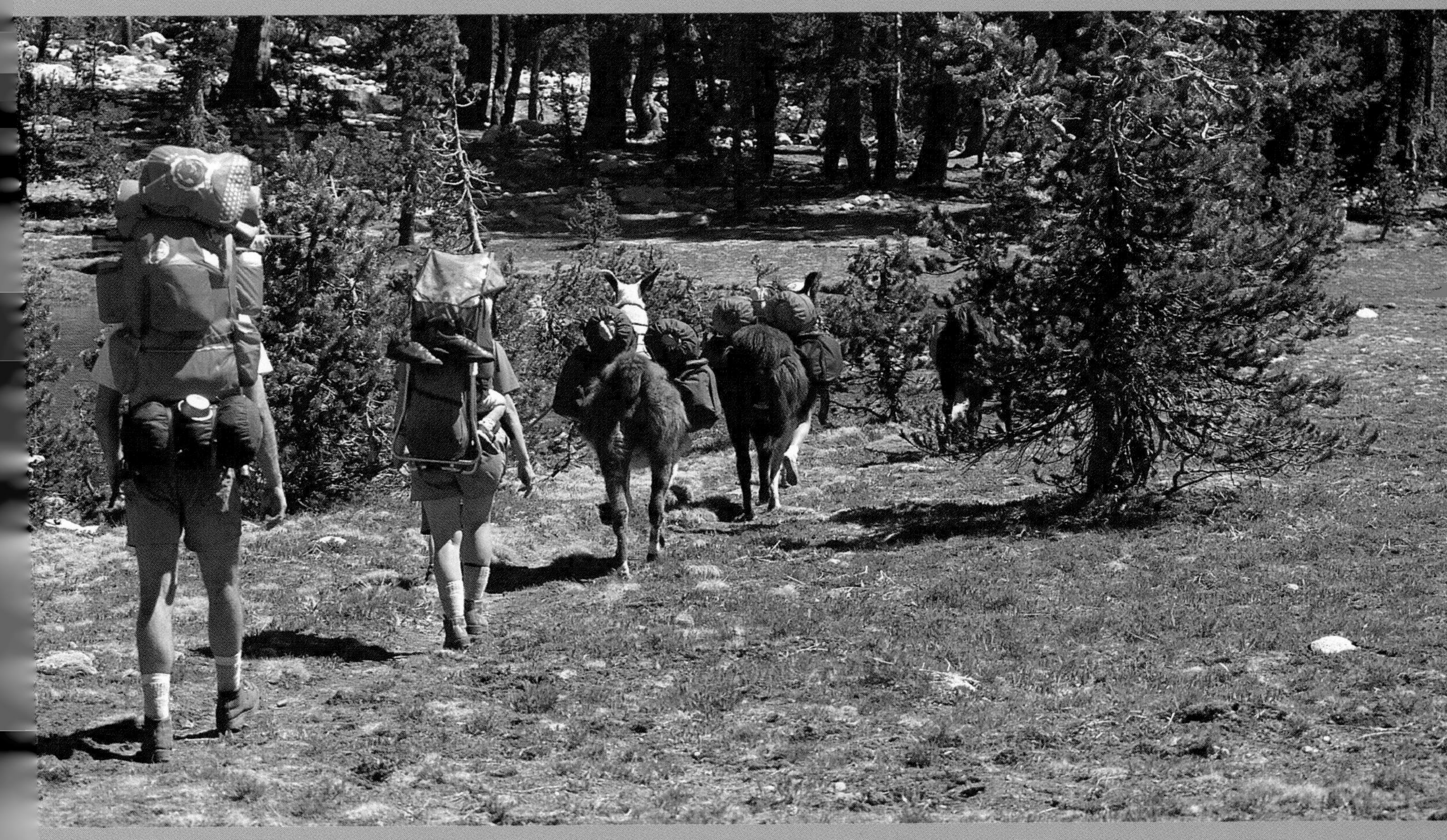

LOOKING AHEAD

After reading this chapter, you should be able to answer these questions about wellness:

- Why are healthy interpersonal relationships important for wellness?
- What are the characteristics of healthy relationships, satisfying partnerships, and strong families? What characteristics, skills, and behaviors support successful relationships?
- What physical changes are associated with aging? What can people do to promote healthy aging?
- What are the components of effective self-care? What skills contribute to effective use of the health care system?
- What role does the environment play in personal health and wellness? What can individuals do to improve the environment?
- What steps are involved in creating and maintaining an effective behavior change program?

The goal of this book has been to introduce the concept of wellness and to provide the knowledge and skills you need to live a fit and well lifestyle. Knowing the facts about the effects of your actions on your health enables you to make informed choices. Using behavioral self-management enables you to make important lifestyle changes.

This chapter briefly addresses some other skills that are important for a lifetime of wellness: developing and maintaining meaningful interpersonal relationships, meeting the challenges of aging, using the health care system intelligently, and understanding environmental health.

DEVELOPING SUCCESSFUL INTERPERSONAL RELATIONSHIPS

People need social relationships; we cannot thrive as solitary creatures. Many research studies have shown that social isolation is a strain for human beings. For example, one study found that people who have had a heart attack and who live alone have a higher chance of having a second heart attack than do those not living alone. Another study found that women with few or no social contacts were twice as likely to die of cancer. These and other studies make it clear that social and emotional connections to others are a crucial element in physical and mental health.

Forming Relationships

Intimate relationships satisfy many human needs, including the need for approval and affirmation, for companionship, for a sense of belonging, and for sexual expression. Many of society's needs are also fulfilled by relationships, particularly the need to nurture and socialize children within that society.

Self-Image and Self-Esteem Relationships begin with individuals. To have successful relationships, people first have to accept and feel good about themselves. A positive self-image and reasonably high self-esteem help people love and respect others. The roots of a positive sense of self are found in childhood. People are likely, as adults, to have the sense that they are basically lovable, worthwhile people if, as children, they felt loved, valued, and respected; if their parents or other important adults responded to their needs in appropriate ways; and if they were given the freedom to explore and develop a sense of being separate individuals.

Even if people's earliest experiences and relationships were less than ideal, however, they can still establish satisfying relationships in adulthood. Humans are resilient and flexible; we have the ability to change our ideas and patterns of behavior. We can learn ways to enhance our self-esteem and become more trusting and appreciative of others. We also have the ability to acquire the communication and conflict resolution skills needed to maintain successful relationships.

Friendship, Love, and Intimacy The first relationships people form outside the family are friendships—reciprocal relationships between equals, held together with ties of respect, affection, trust, tolerance, and loyalty. Whether with members of the same or the other sex, friendships give us the opportunity to share ourselves and discover others. Like love relationships, friendships bind society together, providing people with emotional support and buffering them from stress.

Intimate love relationships are among the most profound human experiences. They may not give people perfect happiness, but they do tend to give life much of its meaning. For most adults, love, sex, and commitment are closely linked ideals in intimate relationships. Love reflects the positive factors that draw people together and sustain them in a relationship—trust, caring, respect, loyalty, interest in the other, and concern for the other's well-being. Sex brings excitement and passion to the relationship, adding fascination and pleasure. Commitment, the determination to continue, reflects the stable factors that help maintain the relationship—responsibility, reliability, and faithfulness. Although love, sex, and commitment are related, they are not necessarily connected. One can exist without the others. Despite the various permutations of the three, most people long for a special relationship that contains them all.

When two people fall in love, their relationship at first is likely to be characterized by high levels of passion and rapidly increasing intimacy. In time, passion decreases as the partners become familiar with each other. The disappearance of passionate love is often experienced as a crisis in a relationship. If a quieter, more lasting love fails to emerge, the relationship will likely break up, and each person will search for another who will once again ignite his or her passion.

But love does not necessarily have to be passionate. When intensity diminishes, partners often discover a more enduring love. They can now move from absorption in each other to a relationship that includes external goals and projects, friends, and family. In this kind of more secure love, satisfaction comes not just from the relationship but also from achieving other creative objectives, such as work or child rearing. The key to successful relationships isn't in intensity but in transforming passion into an intimate love, based on closeness, caring, and the promise of a shared future.

Choosing a Partner Although the pool of potential partners for a relationship may appear huge, most people pair with someone who lives in the same geographical area and who is similar in racial, ethnic, and socioeconomic background, educational level, lifestyle, physical appearance, and other traits. In simple terms, people select partners like themselves.

When choosing intimate companions, perhaps the most important question two people can ask is, "How much do we have in common?" Although differences add interest to a relationship, similarities increase the chances of a relationship's success. If there are major differences, partners should ask, first, "How accepting of differences are we?" and second, "How well do we communicate?" Acceptance and communication skills go a long way toward making a relationship work, no matter how different the partners.

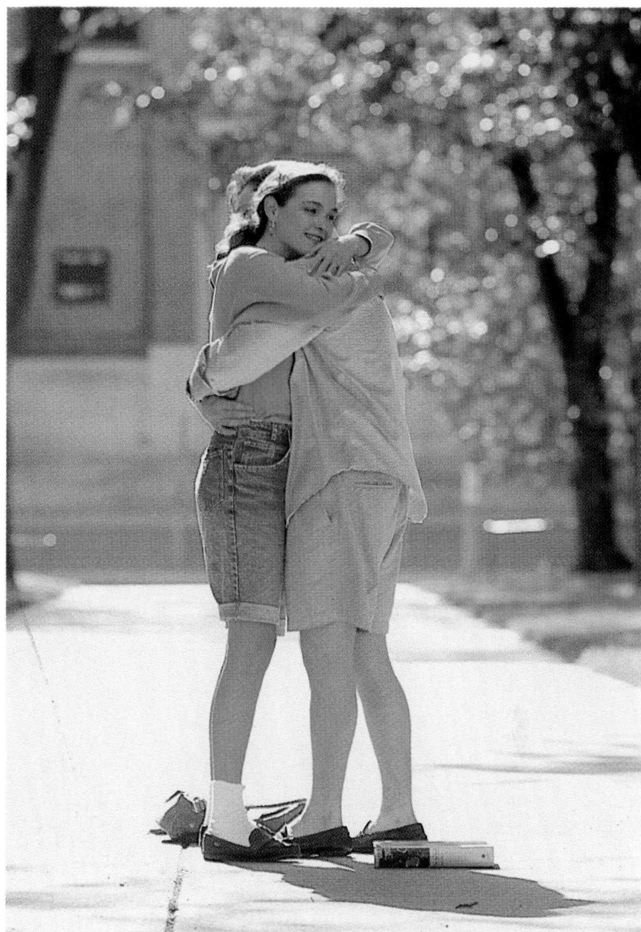

Although the selection process may seem haphazard and random, most people choose their romantic partners carefully and through a fairly predictable process. Like many couples, this young man and woman are similar in racial, ethnic, and socioeconomic background and probably have important values and interests in common.

Marriage

Although half of all marriages in our society now end in divorce, the popularity of getting married hasn't diminished. The primary functions and benefits of marriage are those of any intimate adult relationship, including affection, personal affirmation, companionship, sexual fulfillment, and emotional growth. But marriage also provides a setting in which to raise children, and it affords some provision for the future. By committing themselves to their relationship by getting married, people provide themselves with lifelong companions.

Although most people would like to believe otherwise, love is not enough to make a successful marriage. Couples have to have strengths; they have to be successful in their relationship before marriage. Problems in relationships are magnified rather than solved by marriage. The following relationship characteristics appear to be the best predictors of a happy marriage:

- The partners have realistic expectations about their relationship.
- Each feels good about the personality of the other.
- They communicate well.
- They have effective ways of resolving conflicts.
- They agree on religious/ethical values.
- They have an egalitarian role relationship.
- They have a good balance of individual versus joint interests and leisure activities.

Coping with the challenges of marriage requires couples to be committed to remaining married through the inevitable ups and downs of the relationship. They need to be tolerant of each other's imperfections, keep their sense of perspective and their sense of humor, and be willing and able to put energy into providing and sustaining mutually sufficient levels of intimacy, sexual satisfaction, and commitment. The most important skills they bring to these challenges are their communication and conflict resolution skills.

Communication Skills The key to developing and maintaining an intimate relationship is good communication. Most of the time, we don't think about communicating; we simply talk and act in natural ways. But when problems arise—when we feel others don't understand us or when someone accuses us of not listening, for example—we become aware of our limitations or, more commonly, what we think are other people's limitations. Miscommunication creates frustration and distances us from our friends and partners.

As much as 65% of face-to-face communication is nonverbal. Even when we're silent, we're communicating. We send messages when we look at someone or look away, lean forward or sit back, smile or frown. The ability

TACTICS AND TIPS
Resolving Conflict

Although there are many theories about and approaches to conflict resolution, some basic strategies are generally useful in successfully negotiating with a partner:

- *Clarify the issue.* Take responsibility for thinking through your feelings and discovering what is really bothering you. Agree that one person will speak first and have the chance to speak fully while the other listens. Then reverse the roles. Try to understand the other's position fully by repeating what you've heard and asking questions to clarify or elicit more information. Agree to talk only about the topic at hand and not get distracted by other issues. Sum up what the other person has said.
- *Find out what each person wants.* Ask the other person to express his or her desires. Don't assume you know what the other wants and speak for him or her.
- *Identify various alternatives.* There may be alternative approaches that will help each person get what he or she wants. Practice brainstorming to generate a variety of options.
- *Decide how to negotiate.* Work out some agreements or plans for change, such as agreeing that if one person will do one task, the other will do another task, or that one person will do a task in exchange for being able to do something else he or she wants.
- *Solidify the agreements.* Go over the plan verbally, and write it down if necessary, to ensure that you both understand and agree to it.
- *Review and renegotiate.* Decide on a time frame for trying out the new plan, and set a time to discuss how it's working. Make adjustments as needed.

to interpret nonverbal messages correctly is important to the success of relationships. It's also important, when sending messages, to make sure body language agrees with spoken words. When verbal and nonverbal messages are incongruent with each other, the message is confusing.

Three keys to good communication in relationships are:

1. *Self-disclosure:* Revealing personal information that ordinarily wouldn't be revealed because of the riskiness involved. It usually increases feelings of closeness and allows the relationship to move to a deeper level of intimacy.
2. *Listening:* Good listening skills require that we spend more time and energy trying to fully understand another person's "story" and less time judging, evaluating, blaming, advising, analyzing, or trying to control. To connect with other people and develop real emotional intimacy, good listening is essential.
3. *Feedback:* A constructive response to another's self-disclosure. Giving positive feedback means acknowledging that the friend's or partner's feelings are valid, no matter how upsetting or troubling, and offering self-disclosures in response. Feedback opens up the possibility for change where silence, anger, or indifference do not.

For tips on effective communication, refer to the box "Clear Communication" in Chapter 10.

Conflict and Conflict Resolution Conflict is natural in intimate relationships. In fact, as the relationship gets closer, more differences will be discovered and more opportunities for conflict will arise. Conflict itself isn't dangerous to intimate relationships; it may simply indicate that the relationship is growing. But if conflict isn't handled in a constructive way, it will damage—or even destroy—the relationship. See the box "Resolving Conflict" for tips on handling conflict effectively.

Conflict is often accompanied by anger, a natural enough emotion but one that can be difficult to handle. The best way to manage anger in a relationship is to recognize it as a symptom of something that requires attention and needs to be changed. When partners are angry, they should wait until they calm down, then come back to the issue later and try to deal with it rationally. Negotiation helps dissipate anger so that the conflict can be resolved.

To resolve conflicts, partners in a relationship have to feel safe in voicing their disagreements. Both have to trust that the discussion won't get out of control, that they won't be abandoned by the other, and that their partner won't take advantage of their own vulnerability. Partners should follow some basic ground rules when they argue, including the following:

- Don't give ultimatums.
- Don't resort to the silent treatment.
- Don't "hit below the belt."
- Don't use sex to smooth over differences.

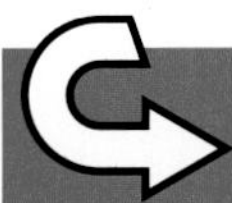

TACTICS AND TIPS

Building Healthy Relationships

- Take the time every day to talk to others. Be willing to invest time, energy, and effort in your relationships.
- Share your thoughts and feelings with friends and loved ones.
- Listen carefully to what people say to you. Don't interrupt.
- Express yourself directly and honestly, but respect the feelings and opinions of others.
- Express your appreciation of people around you. Compliment them on their strengths and special qualities.
- Give and seek emotional support when it is needed.
- When you're angry with a friend, family member, or partner, discuss the problem with him or her, but wait until you can do it calmly and fairly.
- Accept responsibility for your feelings, thoughts, and actions and for your own happiness.
- Allow your friends or partner the freedom to grow and change.
- Be realistic and accepting of your friends, family members, and partner. No one is perfect; everyone is occasionally a source of disappointment to others. Don't let human flaws keep you from loving and respecting the significant people in your life.

- Don't generalize or accuse: "You always . . ."
- Don't bring up old issues.
- Use humor; try to laugh at yourself.

Successful Relationships, Successful Families

Some people view relationships as mysterious connections between people that develop naturally and require no effort to maintain, but this is far from true. Without time spent together and energy invested in maintaining intimacy, people drift apart and relationships die. Because of the importance of healthy, satisfying relationships, people should take the time to develop and nurture this aspect of their lives. For tips on staying connected with others, see the box "Building Healthy Relationships."

Family relationships are another important part of a healthy life. A strong family isn't a family without problems; it's a family that copes successfully with stress and crisis. Researchers have proposed that six major qualities or themes appear in strong families:

1. *Commitment.* The family is very important to its members; sexual fidelity between partners is included in commitment.
2. *Appreciation.* People care about one another and express that caring. The home is a positive place to be.
3. *Communication.* People spend time listening to one another and enjoying one another's company. They talk about disagreements and attempt to solve problems.
4. *Time together.* People do things together, often simple activities that don't cost money.
5. *Spiritual wellness.* The family promotes sharing, love, and compassion for other human beings.
6. *Coping with stress and crisis.* When faced with illness, death, marital conflict, or other crises, family members pull together, seek help, and use other coping strategies to meet the challenge.

It may surprise some people that partners in committed relationships and members of strong families often go to counseling centers. They know that the smartest thing to do in some situations is to get help. Many resources are available for individuals and families seeking counseling, including marriage and family counselors, clergy, psychologists, and other trained professionals in the community. (To rate your own family's strengths, see Lab 15-1.)

MEETING THE CHALLENGES OF AGING

Aging is a normal process of development that occurs over the entire life span. It happens to everyone, but at different rates for different people. Although youth is not entirely a state of mind, your attitude toward life and your attention to your health significantly influence the satisfaction you will derive from life, especially when new physical and mental challenges occur in later years. If you take charge of your health during young adulthood, you can exert great control over the physical and mental aspects of aging, and you can respond better to events that might be out of your control. With foresight and energy, you can shape a creative, graceful, and even triumphant old age (see the box "Words of Wisdom: Attitudes Toward Aging Among Native Americans and Hispanic Americans").

DIMENSIONS OF DIVERSITY

Words of Wisdom: Attitudes Toward Aging Among Native Americans and Hispanic Americans

The following is excerpted from an article written by Dr. Robert Coles, a professor of psychiatry and medical humanities at Harvard Medical School.

Why are so many Americans afraid of growing old? This question occurred to me often during the three years my wife and I lived in New Mexico and Arizona. Not a day went by when we weren't reminded of how much Native American and Hispanic families value old age. These are cultures that grant dignity and authority to their elders.

One young Hispanic woman described to us her relationship with her parents, both in their seventies, in this way: "When I am wondering what to do about a problem, I turn to my mother or my father. Even if they are not here, I still turn to them. I picture them in my mind and I hear them saying words that make good sense." One day, this woman's father made a show of his humorous and practical good sense before his young grandson. "You know what my son said to me that night when he was going to bed?" the woman asked. "He told me he wished he could be old like his grandpapa!"

To be old is to "last" oneself—to go through ups and downs, to survive bad luck and avoid successfully all sorts of hazards. To be old, then, is to be blessed by fate, by chance and circumstance. Pueblo Indians know that. One Hopi child drew me a picture of an old woman shaking hands with the moon. Then she explained, "When you're old, you're a full moon; you make the night a little less dark." For Hopi children, an older person is a source of encouragement, instruction, inspiration, a part of nature's awesome presence.

For many young people living in other parts of America, old age is regarded not as a major achievement but rather as a last, sad, brief way station. One boy in Boston commented, "It's no fun to be old; it's the worst thing in the world, except to die." To many of us, old age means abandonment, rejection, loneliness, a loss of respect from others, and subsequently a loss of self-respect. This is not the case, though, in Hispanic and Native American cultures. The elders we met in New Mexico and Arizona showed a great deal of self-confidence, and in general they seemed contented with their lives. In their contentment and harmony with nature lies a lesson for all of us.

Source: Coles, R. 1989. Full-moon wisdom. *New Choices for the Best Years,* September.

What Happens as You Age?

Aging results from biochemical processes that we don't yet fully understand. Physiological changes are caused by a combination of gradual aging and injury from disease. Because most organ systems have an excess capacity for performing their functions, the body's ability to function is not affected until damage is fairly extensive. Studies of healthy people indicate that general functioning remains essentially constant until after age 70.

Some of the physical changes that accompany aging are these:

- Skin becomes looser, drier, and less elastic.
- The ability to hear high-pitched and certain other sounds declines in most people.
- Presbyopia, the inability of the eyes to focus sharply on nearby objects, occurs gradually in most people beginning in their forties. The eyes require more time to adapt to dark conditions, and depth perception may become distorted.
- The sensations of taste and smell diminish somewhat.
- Cells at the base of hair follicles produce progressively less pigment and eventually die. (Hair is thickest at age 20; individual hair shafts shrink after that.)
- Bone mass is lost and muscles become weaker, although both of these changes can be minimized significantly through regular exercise, a proper diet, and other measures.
- The heart pumps less blood with each beat, and maximum heart rate drops. Most of the other changes in the cardiovascular system that are associated with aging can be largely controlled through lifestyle.
- Sexual response slows, but an active and satisfying sex life can continue for both men and women throughout life.

Life-Enhancing Measures

Many of the characteristics associated with aging aren't due to aging at all. They are the result of neglect and abuse of our bodies and minds. These assaults lay the foundation for later mental problems and chronic conditions like arthritis, heart disease, diabetes, hearing loss, and high blood pressure. We sacrifice our optimal health by smoking, eating a poor diet and overeating, abusing alcohol and drugs, bombarding our ears with excessive noise, and exposing our bodies to too much ultraviolet radiation from the sun. We also jeopardize our bodies through inactivity, encouraging our muscles and even our bones to wither and deteriorate.

You can prevent, delay, lessen, or even reverse some of the changes associated with aging through good health habits. A few simple things you can do every day will make a vast difference to your health, your appearance, and your energy and vitality. The following suggestions have been mentioned throughout this text, but because they are profoundly related to health in later life, they are highlighted here.

- *Challenge your mind.* Creativity and intelligence remain stable in healthy individuals. Staying involved in learning as a lifelong process can help you stay sharp and retain all your mental abilities.
- *Plan for social changes.* Social roles change over time and require a period of adjustment. Retirement and an "empty nest" confer the advantage of increased leisure time, but many people do not know how to enjoy it. Throughout life, cultivate interests and hobbies you enjoy, both alone and with others, so that you can continue to live an active and rewarding life in your later years. Try new activities, take classes, and meet new people. Volunteering in your community can enhance self-esteem and allow you to be a contributing member of society. (See the box "Help Yourself by Helping Others" on p. 354 for more on the wellness benefits of volunteering.)
- *Develop physical fitness.* Exercise enhances both mental and physical health. Enough cannot be said for the positive effects of appropriate exercise throughout your life, particularly when weighed against the physical and mental deterioration of older people who have not stayed fit. Exercise significantly improves both the quantity and the quality of your life by keeping your body functioning at peak levels and by protecting you from chronic diseases and injuries, even as you age.
- *Eat wisely.* Health at every age is helped by a varied diet with special attention to a lower intake of fat and calories. Eat meals low in fat and high in complex carbohydrates. Concentrate on fresh fruits and vegetables, whole grains, no-fat or low-fat dairy products, and lean portions of fish and poultry.
- *Maintain a healthy body composition.* Obesity is not physically healthy, and it leads to premature aging. Sensible eating habits and an active lifestyle can help you maintain a healthy body composition throughout your life.
- *Control drinking and overdependence on medications.* Alcohol abuse ranks with depression as a common hidden mental health problem, affecting 20% of the elderly population. The problem is often not identified because the effects of alcohol or drug addiction can mimic disease, such as Alzheimer's disease. Don't use alcohol to relieve anxiety or emotional pain; don't take medications when safer forms of treatment are available.
- *Don't smoke.* The average pack-a-day smoker can expect to live about 12 years less than a nonsmoker and to be susceptible to disabilities that affect the quality of life. Premature balding and skin wrinkling are also associated with smoking.
- *Recognize and reduce stress.* Don't wear yourself out through a lack of sleep, the misuse or abuse of drugs, or overworking. Practice relaxation and stress management, using the techniques described in Chapter 10.

Other strategies for successful aging include the following:

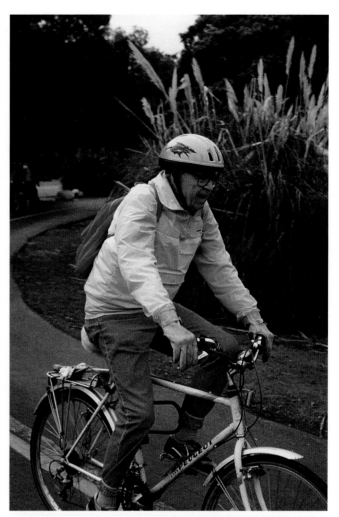

Regular exercise throughout life is an important key to graceful aging. By keeping fit, this man has retained a high level of physical functioning. Regular exercise also helps prevent depression, boredom, and losses in intelligence typically associated with aging.

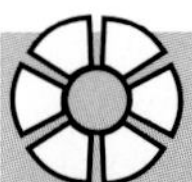

WELLNESS CONNECTION
Help Yourself by Helping Others

Choosing to help others—whether as a volunteer for a community organization or through spontaneous acts of kindness—can enhance emotional, social, spiritual, and physical wellness. Surveys and studies indicate that the sense of purpose and service, and the feelings of generosity and kindness, that go with helping others may be as important a consideration for wellness as good nutrition and regular exercise. For example, in a study of nearly 3000 male residents of Michigan, those who volunteered for community organizations were two-and-a-half times less likely to die than their nonhelping peers.

In a national survey of volunteers from all fields, helpers reported the following benefits:

- "Helper's high"—physical and emotional sensations such as sudden warmth, a surge of energy, and a feeling of euphoria that occur immediately after helping
- Feelings of increased self-worth, calm, and relaxation
- A perception of greater physical health
- Fewer colds and headaches, improved eating and sleeping habits, and some relief from the pain of chronic diseases such as asthma and arthritis

Just how might helping benefit the health of the helper? By helping others, we may relieve our own distress and guilt over their problems. We focus on things other than our own problems, and we get a special kind of attention from the people we help. Helping others can be effective at banishing a bad mood or a case of the blues. Helping may block physical pain because most of us can only pay attention to a limited number of things at a given time. Helping others can also expand our perspective and enhance our appreciation for our own lives. Helping may benefit physical health by providing a temporary boost to the immune system and by combatting stress and hostile feelings linked to the development of chronic diseases.

Helping others doesn't require a huge time commitment or a change of career. To get the most out of helping, keep the following guidelines in mind:

- *Make contact.* Choose an activity that involves personal contact.
- *Help as often as possible.* If your schedule allows, volunteer at least once a week. However, as with many parts of a wellness lifestyle, any amount of time spent helping is better than none.
- *Make helping voluntary.* Voluntary helping has positive results, whereas obligatory helping situations can actually increase stress.
- *Volunteer with others.* Working with a group enables you to form bonds with other helpers who can support your interests and efforts.
- *Focus on the process, not the outcome.* We can't always measure or know the results of our actions.
- *Practice random acts of kindness.* Smile, let people go ahead of you in line, pick up litter, and so on.
- *Adopt a pet.* Several studies suggest that pet owners enjoy better health, perhaps by feeling needed or by having a source of unconditional love and affection.
- *Avoid burnout.* Recognize your own limits, pace yourself, and try not to feel guilty or discouraged. Take pride in being a volunteer or caregiver, and give yourself frequent pats on the back.

You can experience the "helper's high" and the other personal rewards of volunteerism as soon as you begin helping others. In addition to the benefits for you, volunteering has the added bonus of having a positive impact on the health and wellness of others. It fosters a sense of community and can provide some practical help for many of the problems facing our society today.

Source: Adapted from Sobel, D. S. 1993. Rx: Helping others. *Mental Medicine Update,* Winter.

- Get regular physical examinations to detect treatable diseases (see the discussion about health care in the next section).
- Protect your skin from the sun by using hats, gloves, sunglasses, and sunscreen.
- Avoid extremely loud noises, such as from stereo earphones or loud machines, that can contribute to hearing loss.

The health behaviors you practice now, in your early adulthood, weigh more heavily in determining how long and how well you will live than your behaviors at a later age. By taking care of yourself now, you're buying some insurance for the future.

USING THE HEALTH CARE SYSTEM INTELLIGENTLY

Just as people can prevent many illnesses through healthy lifestyle choices, they can also avoid many visits to the medical clinic by managing their own health care—by gathering information, soliciting advice, making their own decisions, and taking responsibility for following through. People who manage their own health care are informed partners in medical care; they also practice safe, effective self-care.

How can you develop this self-care attitude and take a more active role in your own health care? First, you have to learn to identify and manage medical problems. Second, you have to learn how to make the health care system work for you. This section will help you become more competent in both these areas.

Managing Medical Problems

The first step in managing medical problems is observing your body and assessing your symptoms. Symptoms—pain, fever, coughing, diarrhea, and so on—are signals that something isn't working right. In most cases, and with sufficient time and rest, the body heals itself. The decision to seek professional assistance for a symptom is generally guided by the nature of the symptom and by your own previous history of medical problems. If you're unsure about a symptom, call your physician. You may be able to obtain medical advice over the telephone. About 15% of all outpatient medical advice and 30% of all pediatric advice is now given by telephone.

Professional assistance is appropriate for any symptom that is severe, unusual, persistent, or recurrent. Medical emergencies requiring a trip to the nearest hospital emergency room include broken bones, severe burns, deep wounds, uncontrollable bleeding, chest pain, loss of consciousness, poisoning or drug overdose, and difficulty breathing.

Self-treatment with over-the-counter (nonprescription) drugs is an important part of our health care system. These drugs include antihistamines for allergies; expectorants and cough suppressants for coughs; decongestants for nasal congestion; laxatives for constipation; binding agents for diarrhea; aspirin, acetaminophen, ibuprofen, and naproxen sodium for fever or pain; antacids for heartburn and indigestion; syrup of ipecac for poisoning; hydrocortisone cream for skin rashes; lozenges for sore throats; ice packs, heating pads, and elastic bandages for sprains; and bandages and antibacterial creams for minor wounds.

In many cases, however, symptoms and conditions can be handled without drugs, using such treatments as massages, ice packs, neck exercises, relaxation exercises, and other stress-management techniques (refer to Chapter 10). Relying on drugs can be a waste of money and, more importantly, can divert attention from better ways of coping with symptoms.

If you do decide to medicate yourself, be sure to use drugs responsibly:

- Read drug labels, and follow the instructions carefully.
- Do not exceed the recommended dosage or length of treatment.
- Never take a drug from an unlabeled container.
- Use caution with aspirin. Because of an apparent connection between aspirin and a rare but serious problem known as Reye's syndrome, aspirin should not be given to children or adolescents with symptoms of flu or chicken pox.
- Consult your physician if you are taking other medications, if you are pregnant or nursing, or if you have a chronic illness.
- Dispose of any expired medications.

If people were to seek professional care for even a small percentage of the problems they usually manage themselves—colds, backaches, headaches, stomach upset, and so on—the professional health care system would be overwhelmed. Individuals play a key role in our health care system, not just as consumers but also as providers of their own health care. With increased knowledge of when and how to self-treat, people can become even more competent in self-care.

Getting the Most Out of Medical Care

Although many health problems can be self-treated, many others require treatment by trained professionals. The key to using the health care system effectively is good communication between patient and physician. In interacting with health care providers, people need to be assertive in a firm (but not aggressive) manner; they should ask questions, express their concerns, and be persistent. The box "Getting the Most from Your Medical Visit" provides tips for good communication with a health care provider.

Another important part of preventive health care is regular screening for various conditions and diseases. The guidelines shown in Table 15-1 (p. 357) represent the minimum testing recommended for people without symptoms. People who have symptoms or who are at risk for a particular disease should discuss their individual needs with their physician.

Knowing how and where to get information on health topics is another key skill of informed health care consumers. Use the resources in your community, including the library and health care facilities, to obtain information about health issues, locate health information centers, and find self-help and mutual aid groups. Refer to Chapter 1 for a listing of health-related newsletters and magazines, and to the For More Information section at the end of this chapter for helpful books and other publications.

Paying for health care is another critical concern. Health insurance enables people to budget in advance for health care costs that may otherwise be unpredictable and ruinously high. Having insurance makes an individual more likely to use health services and receive adequate care. Most people are insured through a group policy obtained through their place of employment, or through their parents' or spouse's employer. (Group policies generally offer more coverage and cost less than individual policies.) Others are covered by government programs

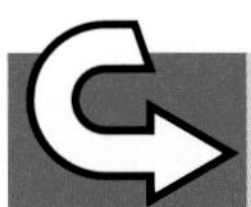

TACTICS AND TIPS
Getting the Most from Your Medical Visit

Preparing for the Visit

- Make a written list of your questions and concerns; include notes about your symptoms.
- Bring a list of all medications (prescription and nonprescription) you are taking, or bring them with you to the office.

During the Visit

- Take notes during the visit, or bring someone else along to help you understand and remember what is said.
- Try to be as open as you can in sharing your thoughts, feelings, and fears.
- Don't be afraid to ask questions.
- If you're not sure you remember or understand something your physician says, ask to go over it again. If appropriate, ask your physician to write down his or her instructions or recommend reading material for more information.
- In your own words, briefly repeat back what you understood the physician to say about your problem and what you are supposed to do.

After the Visit

- Give your physician feedback about the way you're treated by your health care team, and how the treatment he or she recommended worked for you.
- Make sure you understand what the next steps are: return for another visit, phone for test results, obtain a prescription drug, and so on.
- Keep track of your medical history by making notes in a section of your health journal about your medical status.

such as Medicare and Medicaid. For more information on choosing a policy that is appropriate for you, see the box "Choosing Health Insurance" (p. 358).

ENVIRONMENTAL HEALTH

Because of the close relationship between human beings and the environment, even the healthiest lifestyle can't protect a person from the effects of polluted air, contaminated water, or a nuclear power plant mishap. Environmental health encompasses all the interactions between humans and the environment and the health consequences of these interactions (see the box "The Sense of Wonder," p. 359).

While environmental health still focuses on such longstanding concerns as clean air and clean water, food inspection, and waste disposal, in recent years its focus has expanded and become more complex. Many of the health challenges of the next century will involve protecting the environment from the by-products of human activity. Technological advances and rapid population growth have increased the ability of humans to affect and damage the environment. Water supplies are being depleted; landfills are filling up with paper trash, disposable diapers, and plastic packaging; and toxic wastes threaten to contaminate both soil and water. But today there is a growing recognition that we hold the world in trust for future generations and for other forms of life. Our responsibility is to pass on an environment no worse—and preferably better—than the one we enjoy today.

Population Growth

The rapid expansion of the human population, particularly during the last 50 years, is generally believed to be responsible for most of the stress humans put on the environment. At the beginning of the first century A.D., there were about 200 million people alive. By the seventeenth century, world population had gradually increased to 500 million. But then it started to rise exponentially, increasing to 1 billion by about 1830, to 2 billion by 1930, to 4 billion by 1975, to 5 billion by 1987, and to 5.6 billion by 1994. Experts predict that world population will reach 10 billion by the year 2050 and level off at about 11.6 billion in about 2150. With so many people consuming and competing for the Earth's resources, it is difficult for societies to provide such basics as clean air and water and to work toward a better environment.

Although population trends are difficult to influence, many countries recognize the importance of population management. A key goal of population management is to improve the conditions of people's lives so they feel less pressure to have large families. Research indicates that improved health, better education, and increased opportunities for women work together with family planning to cut fertility rates and uncontrolled population growth.

TABLE 15-1 Recommended Medical Tests for Healthy People

Screening Test	Frequency
Medical and family history	Periodically
Total blood cholesterol level	Every 5 years
Blood pressure	Every 2 years
Weight	Periodically
Sigmoidoscopy (visual examination of the lower colon to detect colon and rectal cancer)	Every 5–10 years for anyone over age 50. Anyone at higher risk due to personal or family history should discuss appropriate screening with a physician.
Fecal occult blood test (test for hidden blood in the stool to detect colon cancer)	Every 1–2 years. Anyone at increased risk due to personal or family history should discuss appropriate screening with a physician. (This test is of uncertain benefit for average-risk people age 50 and over.)
Skin examination	Periodically for anyone with a history of excessive sun exposure or severe sunburns, skin cancer or precancerous skin conditions, or a family history of malignant melanoma.
Blood glucose (sugar) level (blood test for diabetes)	Periodically for anyone more than 50 pounds overweight, with a family history of diabetes or a history of diabetes during pregnancy, or of Native American heritage.
Clinical breast exam (physical examination by a health professional for breast cancer detection)	Every 1–2 years for all women over age 40; women at higher risk due to a history of previous breast cancer or family history of breast cancer should have an exam every year beginning at age 35.
Breast self-exam (self-examination for breast cancer detection)	Every month for all women over age 20.
Mammogram (x-ray examination for breast cancer detection)	Every 1–2 years for women 50–75 who are of average risk (the test has less certain benefit for age 40–50 and over age 75). Every year beginning at age 35 for women at higher risk due to personal or family history.
Pap test (examination of the cells of the cervix to detect cervical cancer)	Every 1–3 years for women 18–65 (less certain benefit after age 65 if previous tests were normal).
Rubella antibodies (blood test for immunity to German measles)	Once for women of childbearing years who are fertile and do not know from previous blood tests whether they are immune.
STD tests (gonorrhea, chlamydia, and syphilis)	Periodically for anyone with multiple sex partners or a history of other recent sexually transmissible diseases.
HIV testing (test for AIDS virus antibodies)	Periodically for anyone at risk.
Tuberculin skin test (to detect infection with tuberculosis)	Periodically for anyone with close contact in the last 2 years with someone known to have tuberculosis or anyone who recently moved to the United States from Asia, Africa, Central America, South America, or the Pacific Islands, where TB is more common.
Testicular self-exam (self-examination for testicular cancer)	Every month for men age 18–45.

Source: Adapted from U.S. Task Force Staff. 1989. *Guide to Clinical and Preventive Services: Report of the U.S. Preventive Services Task Force.* Baltimore: Williams & Wilkins.

CRITICAL CONSUMER
Choosing Health Insurance

Because of the many types of insurance plans and contracts currently available, choosing health insurance can be complicated. It's important that you evaluate the services provided by different plans, and choose the one that's best for you.

If you work for a large company, you may be given a choice of several types of plans, some with a traditional framework and some offering "managed care." In a traditional plan, you pay a premium up front, a fixed deductible, and a percentage of expenses thereafter. In a managed care plan, you (or your employer) pay just the premium and usually a small per-visit fee. When services are used, the fixed fees remain the same, regardless of the amount or level of services that are provided. Managed care plans tend to cost consumers less money, but they have restrictions governing which physicians, facilities, tests, and treatments are available to patients.

When you are choosing between several plans, obtain a copy of each policy that sounds suitable, read it carefully, and be sure you understand what it says. The following questions are designed to help you choose the most appropriate insurance for you:

- What services are covered? Different policies may cover any of the following:
  - Physicians' office visits
  - X-ray examinations
  - Outpatient diagnostic tests
  - Medications
  - Inpatient hospital costs
  - Surgical costs, including anesthesia
  - Inpatient medical services
  - Physical therapy
  - Maternity fees
  - Vision care
  - Emergency room care
  - Mental health services
  - Skilled nursing home care
  - Alcohol and drug dependence treatment
- Which of these services am I most likely to need?
- Are there exclusions for any preexisting conditions or chronic problems?
- What preventive health services are covered?
- How do the various policies compare in cost?
- Are the deductible and copayments (coinsurance provisions) suitable?
- Are the maximum limits high enough?
- Will I be able to see the physicians I prefer?
- Does my present physician participate?

Pollution

Many modern environmental problems are problems of pollution—contaminants in the environment that may pose a health risk. Air pollution is not a human invention—it can be caused by a forest fire, a dust storm, a pollen bloom, or the eruption of a volcano—but it is magnified by human activities, particularly the burning of fossil fuels like coal and gasoline. Air pollution can cause illness and death if pollutants become concentrated for a period of several days or weeks. Increased amounts of carbon monoxide and acids and decreased amounts of oxygen in the air put extra strain on people suffering from heart or respiratory illnesses.

Three atmospheric problems have surfaced in recent years that may have long-range effects on human health.

1. *The greenhouse effect, or global warming.* This is a gradual raising of the temperature of the lower atmosphere of the Earth. Warming occurs as a result of the burning of fossil fuels, which releases "greenhouse gases." Experts predict that temperatures on Earth will increase by 3–4°C by the end of the next century, a change that could melt polar ice caps, raise the level of the sea, and change weather patterns. The health implications of such an increase are unknown.
2. *Depletion of the ozone layer.* Ozone depletion in the Earth's atmosphere is occurring primarily as a result of the release of chlorofluorocarbons (CFCs), industrial chemicals used in coolants, propellants, solvents, and foaming agents. The ozone layer absorbs ultraviolet (UV) radiation from the sun. If this layer becomes too thin or disappears in spots, increased exposure to UV light may cause more cases of skin cancer, increase the incidence of cataracts and blindness, and impair immune system functioning.
3. *Acid precipitation.* When atmospheric pollutants, most of which are produced by coal-burning electric power plants, combine with moisture in the air, they fall to Earth as highly acidic rain or snow. Acid precipitation has damaged trees and aquatic life in many parts of the world, including the northeastern United States, Canada, and northern Europe.

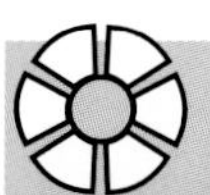

WELLNESS CONNECTION

The Sense of Wonder

In this excerpt from her book, *The Sense of Wonder,* noted scientist and author Rachel Carson affirms the nurturing power of the natural world and urges us to appreciate the deep relationship between nature and the human spirit.

> What is the value of preserving and strengthening this sense of awe and wonder, this recognition of something beyond the boundaries of human existence? Is the exploration of the natural world just a pleasant way to pass the golden hours of childhood or is there something deeper?
>
> I am sure there is something much deeper, something lasting and significant. Those who dwell, as scientists or laymen, among the beauties and mysteries of the earth are never alone or weary of life. Whatever the vexations or concerns of their personal lives, their thoughts can find paths that lead to inner contentment and to renewed excitement in living. Those who contemplate the beauty of the earth find reserves of strength that will endure as long as life lasts. There is symbolic as well as actual beauty in the migration of the birds, the ebb and flow of the tides, the folded bud ready for spring. There is something infinitely healing in the repeated refrains of nature—the assurance that dawn comes after night, and spring after the winter.

Source: Carson, R. 1956. *The Sense of Wonder.* New York: Harper & Row.

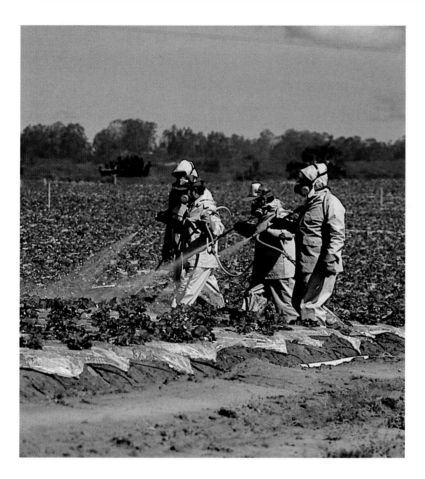

Some pesticide residue may remain on fruits and vegetables when they reach consumers, but the greatest health risks from toxic chemicals occur for agricultural workers. Special clothing and equipment help protect these workers as they spray strawberries.

Other forms of pollution pose problems as well. Chemical substances, including lead, asbestos, pesticides, herbicides, solvents, flame retardants, and hundreds of other products, can cause illness and death. Radiation, whether from the sun, x-rays, nuclear power plants, or other sources, can cause cancer, chromosome damage, sterility, and other health problems. Even noise pollution—loud or persistent noise in the environment—can cause hearing loss and stress.

What Can You Do?

Faced with an array of complex and confusing environmental issues, you may feel overwhelmed and conclude

TACTICS AND TIPS
What You Can Do for the Environment

- Ride your bike, walk, use public transportation, or carpool in a fuel-efficient vehicle instead of driving.
- Keep your car tuned up and well maintained.
- Make sure your home is well insulated.
- Use compact fluorescent light bulbs instead of incandescent bulbs to save energy.
- Buy energy-efficient appliances, and use them only when necessary.
- Run the washing machine or dishwasher only when they have full loads.
- Don't buy products containing CFCs or halon fire extinguishers.
- Buy products with the least amount of packaging you can, or buy products in bulk. Avoid disposable products. Buy recycled or recyclable products.
- Recycle newspapers, glass, cans, paper, and other recyclable items.
- Snip plastic six-pack rings (when they end up in the environment, birds and animals can strangle in them).
- Store food in glass jars and reusable plastic containers rather than plastic wrap.
- Take your own bag along when you go shopping.
- Dispose of household hazardous wastes according to instructions.
- Take showers rather than baths to save water.
- Install sink faucet aerators and water-efficient showerheads.
- Don't let the water run when you're brushing your teeth, shaving, or hand-washing clothes.
- Don't leave anything behind when you're hiking or camping.
- Buy products and services from environmentally responsible corporations. Don't buy products made from endangered species.
- Join or support organizations working on environmental causes.
- Vote for political candidates who support environmentally sound practices. Communicate with your elected representatives about environmental issues.

that there isn't anything you can do. This isn't true. People can take many actions to limit their negative impact on the environment and to promote environmentally sound practices in the social and political arenas. If everyone made individual changes in his or her life, the impact would be tremendous. Refer to the box "What You Can Do for the Environment" for a sampling of actions you can take.

Assuming responsibility for your actions in relation to the environment isn't very different from assuming responsibility for your own health behaviors. It involves knowledge, awareness, insight, motivation, and commitment. The same strategies that work to change personal health behaviors can be used to change environment-related behaviors.

FIT AND WELL FOR LIFE

Adopting a wellness lifestyle is the most important thing you can do to ensure a high quality of life for yourself, now and in the future. The first chapter of this book described a behavioral self-management program that can be used to change problem behaviors and move toward wellness. Subsequent chapters have provided information on important areas of health and wellness—physical fitness, nutrition, weight management, stress management, cardiovascular health, cancer, substance use and abuse, and sexually transmissible diseases. As you learned about these aspects of health and assessed your own health status in relation to each of them, you probably identified personal behaviors that fell short of the ideal. Take the opportunity now (if you haven't already) to consider which of these behaviors you can begin to change. As you do so, let's review the basics of behavioral self-management:

- Choose one behavior to change at a time. Begin with something simple.
- Make sure your motivation and commitment are sufficient to carry you through to success. If they're not, review the health consequences of *not* changing this behavior.
- Follow the six-step program outlined in Chapter 1: (1) monitor your behavior and gather data; (2) analyze the data and identify patterns; (3) set specific goals; (4) make a personal contract; (5) devise a strategy and put it into action; (6) keep track of progress and revise the plan if necessary. Lab 15-2 contains a blank contract and program plan, which you can adapt to fit most behavior change programs.

- Build rewards into the plan.
- Make sure the new behavior is enjoyable and fits into your routine.
- Get support from family and friends.
- Forgive yourself when you slip. Don't blame yourself or others or undermine yourself by feeling guilty.
- Expect to succeed. Use positive self-talk to create a new self-image—one that includes your new behavior.

You live in a world in which your own choices and actions have a tremendous impact on your health. Statistics show that Americans have become healthier in recent years because of lifestyle changes, the kind of changes described in this book. Don't let the broad scope of wellness be an excuse for apathy; instead, let it be a call to action. The time to start making changes in *your* lifestyle—to start becoming fit and well—is right now!

SUMMARY

- A lifestyle of wellness includes healthy interpersonal relationships, an ability to meet the challenges of aging, knowledge of the health care system, and an understanding of environmental issues—as well as an understanding of fitness and specific health problems.
- Individual and social needs are fulfilled by interpersonal relationships. Self-esteem, trust, and communication skills are the essential elements for building and maintaining good relationships.
- Intimate love relationships must be built on the same qualities found in friendship—respect, trust, tolerance, and loyalty—if they are to survive, but they also encompass passion and long-term commitment. Passion normally decreases with time and is replaced by closeness, caring, shared goals, and family activities.
- Similarities between partners increase the chance of having a successful relationship.
- Conflict resolution and communication skills are especially important to a successful marriage.
- Strong families are characterized by commitment, appreciation, communication, time spent together, spiritual wellness, and the ability to cope with stress and crisis.
- Many of the changes associated with aging are the result of an unhealthy lifestyle. There are many things that people can do to prevent, delay, lessen, or reverse them.
- Managing one's own health care involves identifying and managing medical problems and making the best use of the existing health care system.
- Self-care means knowing which symptoms need professional attention, understanding how to use over-the-counter and prescription drugs responsibly, and finding nondrug treatments whenever possible.
- The best use of the health care system requires good communication with physicians, getting regular medical screenings, and knowing where to get information.
- Today's environmental health challenges include protecting the environment from the by-products of human activity. Overpopulation contributes to environmental problems, as do the greenhouse effect, depletion of the ozone layer, and acid precipitation—all results of human activities such as the burning of fossil fuels and using CFCs. Continued individual attempts to minimize negative environmental effects can have a tremendous impact.

BEHAVIOR CHANGE ACTIVITY

Maintaining Your Program

If you maintain your new behavior for at least 6 months, your chances of lifetime success are greatly increased. However, you may find yourself sliding back into old habits at some point. If this happens, there are some things you can do to help maintain your new behavior.

- Remind yourself of the goals of your program (list them here).

____

____

____

(continued)

- Pay attention to how your new pattern of behavior has improved your wellness status. List the major benefits of changing your behavior, both now and in the future.

____

____

____

- Consider the things you enjoy most about your new pattern of behavior. List your favorite aspects.

____

____

____

- Think of yourself as a problem solver. If something begins to interfere with your program, devise strategies for dealing with it. Take time out now to list things that have the potential to derail your program, and develop possible coping mechanisms.

Problem	Solution

- Remember the basics of behavior change. If your program runs into trouble, go back to keeping records of your behavior to pinpoint problem areas. Make adjustments in your program to deal with new disruptions. And don't feel defeated if you lapse. The best thing you can do is to renew your commitment and continue with your program.

FOR MORE INFORMATION

Refer to Chapter 1 for resource materials on general wellness. The books listed below provide additional information about the wellness topics introduced in this chapter.

The Bennett Information Group. 1990. *The Green Pages: Your Everyday Shopping Guide to Environmentally Safe Products.* New York: Random House. *A practical guide covering over 900 items by brand name, including detergents, cleansers, shampoo, paper towels, flea collars, and many more.*

Benson, H., and E. M. Stuart. 1992. *The Wellness Book: The Comprehensive Guide to Maintaining Health and Treating Stress-Related Illness.* New York: Birch Lane Press. *Combines relaxation response techniques with other behavioral medicine approaches, such as stress management, exercise, and nutrition, to provide the best practical guide to mind-body health now available.*

Birkedahl, N. 1991. *Older and Wiser: A Workbook for Coping with Aging.* Oakland, Calif.: New Harbinger Publications. *Exercises and activities for self-reflection about money, diet, exercise, family, stress, and health.*

Buscaglia, L. F. 1984. *Loving Each Other: The Challenge of Human Relationships.* Thorofare, N.J.: Charles B. Slack. *A university professor and popular public speaker, Buscaglia is witty and energetic on his favorite topic, the nature of love.*

Carson, R. 1962. *Silent Spring.* Boston: Houghton Mifflin. *The classic that awakened people to the dangers of wide-scale insecticide spraying.*

Clayman, C. B., ed. 1994. *The American Medical Association Family Medicine Guide,* 3d ed. New York: Random House. *A comprehensive volume discussing more than 650 diseases, containing question-and-answer charts to help evaluate common medical symptoms and decide when to see a physician.*

The Earth Works Group. 1989. *50 Simple Things You Can Do to Save the Earth.* Berkeley, Calif.: Earthworks Press. *An indispensable guide to improving the environment.*

Ehrlich, P. R. 1990. *The Population Explosion.* New York: Ballantine Books. *An update of Ehrlich's landmark 1971 book calling attention to the problems associated with population growth.*

Gaylin, W., and E. Person. 1988. *Passionate Attachments: Thinking About Love.* New York: The Free Press. *A fresh and compelling collection of essays in which humanists and scientists explore the nature and complexities of love, relating it to sexual behaviors, personality development, mythology, mental health, and the essence of humanity.*

Greenwood, S., B. Hasselbring, and M. Castleman. 1987. *The Medical Self-Care Book of Women's Health.* New York: Doubleday. *A self-help consumer's guide to women's health issues.*

Griffith, H. W. 1994. *Complete Guide to Prescription and Nonprescription Drugs, 1995 edition.* New York: Putnam. *A comprehensive guide to side effects, warnings, and precautions for the safe use of over 4000 brand-name and generic drugs.*

Madara, E. J., and A. Meese. 1992. *The Self-Help Sourcebook: Finding and Forming Mutual Aid Self-Help Groups.* Denville, N.J.: American Self-Help Clearinghouse (St. Claire's–Riverside Hospital, Pocono Road, Denville, NJ 07834). *Provides a national listing of self-help groups and guidelines for anyone interested in forming a self-help group.*

Myers, N., ed. 1993. *Gaia: An Atlas of Planet Management,* rev. ed. New York: Anchor Books. *A beautifully illustrated and informative guide to environmental problems and possible solutions.*

Rees, A. M., ed. 1994. *Consumer Health Information Source Book,* 4th ed. Phoenix, Ariz.: Oryx Press. *An annotated bibliography of popular books and pamphlets on a wide variety of health topics, as well as a listing of health-related clearinghouses, hot lines, and resource organizations.*

Sobel, D., and R. Ornstein. 1995. *Minding Your Own Health.* New York: HarperCollins. *A self-help guide to mind-body medicine using prescriptions for the internal pharmacy of the brain.*

Stutz, D. R., and F. Feder. 1991. *The Savvy Patient.* New York: Consumer Reports Books. *Describes how patients can communicate effectively with their physicians and be active participants in their medical care.*

Tannen, D. 1990. *You Just Don't Understand: Women and Men in Conversation.* New York: Morrow. *A discussion of gender differences in language showing how men and women use language differently; also provides many helpful ideas about how to improve communication in relationships.*

Vickery, D. M., and J. F. Fries. 1992. *Take Care of Yourself: The Consumer's Guide to Medical Care,* 5th ed. Reading, Mass.: Addison-Wesley. *An excellent self-care guide containing over 100 easy-to-follow decision charts outlining when to see a physician and how to apply safe and effective home treatments.*

There are many national and international organizations working on environmental health problems. For information about these organizations, call their local chapter or national headquarters, or consult the *Conservation Directory,* published annually by the National Wildlife Federation. A few of the largest and best-known environmental organizations are listed below.

Greenpeace, USA, Inc.
1436 U Street NW
Washington, DC 20009
202-462-1177

National Wildlife Federation
1400 16th Street NW
Washington, DC 20036
202-797-6800

National Audubon Society
700 Broadway
New York, NY 10003
212-979-3000

The Nature Conservancy
1815 North Lynn Street
Arlington, VA 22209
703-841-5300

Sierra Club
730 Polk Street
San Francisco, CA 94109
415-776-2211

SELECTED BIBLIOGRAPHY

Aging successfully: How to succeed at the business of growing older. 1992. *Mayo Clinic Health Letter,* November.

Crosby, J. 1991. *Illusion and Disillusion.* Belmont, Calif.: Wadsworth.

Ehrlich, P. R., and A. H. Ehrlich. 1991. *Healing the Planet: Strategies for Solving the Environmental Crisis.* Reading, Mass.: Addison-Wesley.

Fehr, B. 1988. Prototype analysis of the concepts of love and commitment. *Journal of Personality and Social Psychology* 55(4): 557–579.

Fries, J. F., et al. 1993. Reducing health care costs by reducing the need and demand for medical services. *New England Journal of Medicine* 329:321–325.

Guide to Clinical Preventive Services: Report of the U.S. Preventive Services Task Force. 1989. Baltimore, Md.: Williams & Wilkins.

Johnson, O., ed. 1994. *1995 Information Please® Almanac.* Boston: Houghton Mifflin.

Lips, H. 1992. *Sex and Gender,* 2d ed. Mountain View, Calif.: Mayfield.

Lemonick, M. D. 1992. The ozone vanishes. *Time,* 17 February.

Myers, N., ed. 1993. *Gaia: An Atlas of Planet Management,* rev. ed. New York: Anchor Books.

Naar, J. 1990. *Design for a Livable Planet: How You Can Help Clean Up the Environment.* New York: Harper & Row.

Olson, D., and J. DeFrain. 1997. *Marriage and the Family: Diversity and Strengths,* 2d ed. Mountain View, Calif.: Mayfield.

Olson, D., H. McCubbin, H. Barnes, A. Larsen, A. Muxem, and M. Wilson. 1983. *Families: What Makes Them Work?* Beverly Hills, Calif.: Sage.

The ozone hole: Is it really there? 1994. *Consumer Reports,* August.

Pifer, A., and L. Bronte. 1986. *Our Aging Society.* New York: Norton.

Porter, S. 1991. *Planning Your Retirement.* New York: Prentice-Hall.

Porterfield, J. D., and R. St. Pierre. 1992. *Healthful Aging.* New York: Dushkin.

Rice, F. P. 1996. *Intimate Relationships, Marriages, and Families,* 3d ed. Mountain View, Calif.: Mayfield.

Sadik, N. 1991. Healthy people—in numbers the world can support. *World Health Forum* 12:347–355.

Shaver, P., et al. 1988. Love as attachment: The integration of three behavioral systems. In *The Psychology of Love,* ed. R. Sternberg and M. Barnes. New Haven: Yale University Press.

Shephard, R. J., T. Kavanagh, D. J. Mertens, S. Qureshi, and M. Clark. 1995. Personal health benefits of Masters athletics competition. *British Journal of Sports Medicine* 29:35–40.

Sherman, C. 1992. The aging process: How to cope with growing older. *San Francisco Chronicle,* 20 October.

Sternberg, R., and M. Barnes, eds. 1988. *The Psychology of Love.* New Haven: Yale University Press.

Stevens, W. K. 1992. Humanity confronts its handiwork: An altered planet. *New York Times,* 5 May.

Stinnett, N., and J. DeFrain. 1986. *Secrets of Strong Families.* Boston: Little, Brown.

Strong, B., and C. DeVault. 1992. *The Marriage and Family Experience.* St. Paul, Minn.: West.

Strong, B., and C. DeVault. 1996. *Core Concepts in Human Sexuality.* Mountain View, Calif.: Mayfield.

Stuart, R. B. 1983. *Improving Communication.* Champaign, Ill.: Research Press.

U.S. Bureau of the Census. 1991. Marital and living arrangements: March 1990. *Current Population Reports.* Series P-2. Washington, D.C.: U.S. Government Printing Office.
U.S. Bureau of the Census. 1991. *Statistical Abstract of the United States.* 111th ed. Washington, D.C.: U.S. Government Printing Office.
Vickery, D. M., and D. Iverson. 1993. Medical self-care and the use of the medical care system. In *Health Promotion in the Workplace,* 2d ed., ed. M. O'Donnell and J. Harris. Albany, N.Y.: Delmar.
Vickery, D. M., H. Kalmer, D. Lowry, M. Constantine, E. Wright, and W. Loren. 1983. Effect of a self-care education program on medical visits. *Journal of the American Medical Association* 250:2952–2956.

Name ______________________ Section ______________ Date ______________

LAB 15-1 *Rating Your Family's Strengths*

This Family Strengths Inventory was developed by researchers who studied the strengths of over 3000 families. To assess your family (either the family you grew up in or the family you have formed as an adult), circle the number that best reflects how your family rates on each strength.

	Low				High
1. Spending time together and doing things with each other	1	2	3	4	5
2. Commitment to each other	1	2	3	4	5
3. Good communication (talking with one another often, listening well, sharing feelings with one another)	1	2	3	4	5
4. Dealing with crises in a positive manner	1	2	3	4	5
5. Expressing appreciation to each other	1	2	3	4	5
6. Spiritual wellness	1	2	3	4	5
7. Closeness of relationship between spouses	1	2	3	4	5
8. Closeness of relationship between parents and children	1	2	3	4	5
9. Happiness of relationship between spouses	1	2	3	4	5
10. Happiness of relationship between parents and children	1	2	3	4	5
11. Extent to which spouses make each other feel good about themselves (self-confident, worthy, competent, and happy)	1	2	3	4	5
12. Extent to which parents help children feel good about themselves	1	2	3	4	5

Scoring Add the numbers you have circled. **Score:** __________

A score below 39 indicates below-average family strengths. Scores between 39 and 52 are in the average range. Scores above 53 indicate a strong family. Low scores on individual items identify areas that families can profitably spend time on. High scores are worthy of celebration but shouldn't lead to complacency. Like gardens, families need loving care to remain strong.

LABORATORY ACTIVITIES

Name ____________________ Section ____________ Date ____________

LAB 15-2 *Monitoring Your Progress*

As you completed the 10 labs listed below, you entered the results in the Preprogram Assessment column of this lab. Now that you have been involved in a fitness and wellness program for some time, do the labs again and enter your new results in the Postprogram Assessment column. You will probably notice improvement in several areas. Congratulations! If you are not satisfied with your progress thus far, refer to the tips for successful behavior change in Chapter 1 and throughout this book. Remember—fitness and wellness are forever. The time you invest now in developing a comprehensive, individualized program will pay off in a richer, more vital life in the years to come.

	Preprogram Assessment	*Postprogram Assessment*
LAB 2-1 Activity Index	Activity index: _______ Classification: _______	Activity index: _______ Classification: _______
LAB 3-1 Cardiorespiratory Endurance		
1-mile walk test	$\dot{V}O_{2max}$: ____ Rating: ____	$\dot{V}O_{2max}$: ____ Rating: ____
3-minute step test	$\dot{V}O_{2max}$: ____ Rating: ____	$\dot{V}O_{2max}$: ____ Rating: ____
1.5-mile run-walk test	$\dot{V}O_{2max}$: ____ Rating: ____	$\dot{V}O_{2max}$: ____ Rating: ____
Åstrand-Rhyming test	$\dot{V}O_{2max}$: ____ Rating: ____	$\dot{V}O_{2max}$: ____ Rating: ____
LAB 4-1 Muscular Strength		
Maximum bench press test	Weight: ____ lb Rating: ____	Weight: ____ lb Rating: ____
Maximum leg press test	Weight: ____ lb Rating: ____	Weight: ____ lb Rating: ____
Hand grip strength test	Weight: ____ kg Rating: ____	Weight: ____ kg Rating: ____
LAB 4-2 Muscular Endurance		
60-second sit-up test	Number: ____ Rating: ____	Number: ____ Rating: ____
Curl-up test	Number: ____ Rating: ____	Number: ____ Rating: ____
Push-up test	Number: ____ Rating: ____	Number: ____ Rating: ____
LAB 5-1 Flexibility		
Sit-and-reach test	Score: _________ in. Rating: _________	Score: _________ in. Rating: _________

LABORATORY ACTIVITIES

	Preprogram Assessment	*Postprogram Assessment*
LAB 6-1 Body Composition		
Body mass index	BMI: ________ kg/m^2	BMI: ________ kg/m^2
	Desirable range (yes/no): ____	Desirable range (yes/no): ____
	Relative risk rating: ____	Relative risk rating: ____
Skinfold measurements	Sum of 3 skinfolds: ____ mm	Sum of 3 skinfolds: ____ mm
	Percent body fat: ____%	Percent body fat: ____%
	Rating: ______	Rating: ______
Waist-to-hip-circumference ratio	Ratio: _______	Ratio: _______
	Relative risk: _______	Relative risk: _______
LAB 8-2 Dietary Analysis		
Percentage of calories	From protein: ____%	From protein: ____%
Percentage of calories	From fat: ____%	From fat: ____%
Percentage of calories	From saturated fat: ____%	From saturated fat: ____%
Percentage of calories	From carbohydrate: ____%	From carbohydrate: ____%
LAB 9-1 Daily Energy Balance	Approximate daily energy expenditure: _____ cal/day	Approximate daily energy expenditure: _____ cal/day
LAB 10-1 Identifying Stressors	Total weekly stress score: ______	Total weekly stress score: _____
LAB 11-1 Risk Factors for CVD	Score: ______	Score: ______
	Estimated Risk: ______	Estimated risk: ______

Injury Prevention and Personal Safety

Injuries are the fourth leading cause of death among Americans. Injuries affect all segments of the population, but they are particularly common among minorities and people with low income, primarily due to social, environmental, and economic factors. The economic cost of injuries in the United States last year alone was over $400 billion.

Injuries are generally classified into four different categories, depending on the situation in which they occur: motor vehicle injuries, home injuries, work injuries, and public injuries. The greatest number of deaths occurs in motor vehicle crashes, but the greatest number of disabling injuries occurs in the home.

CAUSES OF INJURIES

Injuries may be caused by human factors, by environmental factors, or by a combination of both (multiple causation).

Human factors include:

- Physical conditions (hunger, illness, fatigue)
- Natural physical limitations (in strength, endurance, sensory abilities, skill)
- Physical impairments caused by drugs or alcohol
- Psychological factors (amount of knowledge or information, awareness of risk, beliefs and attitudes toward safety, emotional states)

Environmental factors include:

- Natural conditions (weather conditions, earthquakes)
- Societal conditions (stop-and-go traffic, drunk drivers)
- Work-related conditions (faulty equipment)
- Home-related conditions (throw rugs)
- Any other dangerous conditions

When unsafe states (human factors) and unsafe conditions (environmental factors) interact, an injury often results. At a critical moment, the individual must make a decision that influences the outcome of the situation. If the decision is a good one, the injury may be avoided. If the decision is not as good, or if the incident is unavoidable at this point, someone may be injured or killed.

MOTOR VEHICLE INJURIES

Incidents involving motor vehicles are the most common cause of death for people under age 45, the most common cause of paralysis due to spinal injury, and the leading cause of severe brain injury.

Nearly two-thirds of all motor vehicle injuries are caused by bad driving, especially speeding. As speed increases, momentum and force of impact increase and the time allowed for the driver to react (reaction time) decreases. Speed limits are posted to establish the safest *maximum* speed limit for a given area under *ideal* conditions.

A second factor contributing to injury and death in motor vehicle collisions is failure to wear a safety belt. A person who doesn't wear a safety belt is twice as likely to be injured in a crash as a person who does wear a safety belt. Safety belts not only prevent the individual from being thrown from the car at the time of the crash but also provide protection from the "second collision," which occurs when the occupant of the car hits something inside the car, such as the steering column, dashboard, or windshield. The safety belt also spreads the stopping force of the collision over the body.

Although air bags provide some supplemental protection in the event of a collision, they are useful only in head-on collisions. They also deflate immediately after inflating and therefore do not provide protection in collisions involving multiple impacts. They should be used in conjunction with safety belts.

A third common factor in motor vehicle injuries is alcohol; it is involved in about half of all fatal crashes. Alcohol-impaired driving, defined by blood alcohol concentration (BAC), is illegal in all states. The legal BAC limit varies from 0.08 to 0.10, but people are impaired at much lower BACs. All psychoactive drugs have the potential to impair driving ability.

About 75% of all motor vehicle collisions occur within 25 miles of home and at speeds lower than 40 miles per hour. These crashes often occur because the driver believes safety measures are not necessary for short trips.

A

Clearly, the statistics prove otherwise.

To prevent motor vehicle injuries:

- Obey the speed limit. If you have to speed to get there on time, you're not allowing enough time. Try leaving 10–15 minutes earlier.
- Always wear a safety belt. Strap infants and toddlers into government-approved car seats (consult the product specifications before purchasing). Never hold a child in your lap while a car is moving.
- Never drive under the influence of alcohol or other drugs. Never ride with a driver who has been drinking or using drugs.
- Keep your car in good working order. Regularly inspect tires, oil and fluid levels, windshield wipers, spare tire, and so on.
- Always allow enough following distance. Follow the "3-second rule": When the vehicle ahead passes a reference point, count out 3 seconds. If you pass the reference point before you finish counting, drop back and allow more following distance.
- Always increase following distance and slow down if weather or road conditions are poor.
- Choose interstate highways rather than rural roads. Highways are much safer because of better visibility, wider lanes, fewer surprises, and other factors.
- Always signal when turning or changing lanes.
- Stop completely at stop signs. Follow all traffic laws.
- Take special care at intersections. Always look left, right, and then left again. Make sure you have plenty of time to complete your maneuver in the intersection.
- Don't pass on two-lane roads unless you're in a designated passing area and have a clear view ahead.

Motorcycle and Moped Injuries

About one out of every ten traffic fatalities among people age 15–34 involves someone riding a motorcycle. Most motorcycle collisions occur because the other driver did not see the motorcyclist. Injuries from motorcycle collisions are more severe than those from automobile crashes. Because head injuries are the major cause of death, the use of a helmet is critical for rider safety.

To prevent injuries when riding a motorcycle:

- Maximize your visibility by wearing light-colored clothing, driving with your headlights on, and correctly positioning yourself in traffic.
- Develop the skills necessary to operate the motorcycle. Lack of skill, especially when evasive action is needed to avoid a collision, is a major factor in motorcycle injuries. Skidding from improper braking is the most common cause of loss of control.
- Wear a helmet. Helmets should conform to safety standards established by the U.S. Department of Transportation, the American National Standards Institute, or the Snell Memorial Foundation.
- Wear eye protection in the form of goggles, a face shield, or a windshield.

To prevent injuries when riding a moped:

- Follow the guidelines for motorcyclists, but remember that mopeds have a maximum speed of 30–35 miles per hour and have less power for maneuverability, especially in an emergency situation.
- Develop appropriate skills. Mopeds move fast enough to result in injury in the event of a crash, so be sure you know how to handle the moped in traffic.

Pedestrian and Bicycle Injuries

Injuries to pedestrians and bicyclists are considered motor-vehicle-related because they are usually caused by motor vehicles. About one-fifth of all motor vehicle deaths each year involve pedestrians; over 100,000 pedestrians are injured each year. In most injuries, poor decision making is the crucial factor, not the traffic situation itself.

To prevent injuries when walking or jogging:

- Walk or jog in daylight.
- Maximize your visibility by wearing light-colored, reflective clothing.
- Face traffic when walking or jogging along a roadway, and follow traffic laws.
- Avoid busy roads or roads with poor visibility.
- Cross only at marked crosswalks and intersections.
- Don't listen to a radio or tape on headphones while walking.
- Don't hitchhike; it places you in a potentially dangerous situation.

Bicycle injuries result primarily from not knowing or understanding the rules of the road, failing to follow traffic laws, and not having sufficient skill or experience to handle traffic conditions. *Bicycles are considered vehicles; bicycle riders must obey all traffic laws that apply to automobile drivers, including stopping at traffic lights and stop signs.*

To prevent injuries when riding a bike:

- Maximize your visibility by wearing light-colored, reflective clothing. Make sure your bicycle is equipped with reflectors. Use lights, especially at night or when riding in wooded or other dark areas.

- Ride with the flow of traffic, not against it, and follow traffic laws. Use bike paths when they are available.
- Ride defensively; never assume that drivers have seen you.
- Know and use hand signals. Look around and signal before turning.
- Be especially careful when turning or crossing at corners and intersections. Watch for cars turning right.
- Stop at all traffic lights and stop signs.
- Continue pedaling at all times to help keep the bike stable and to maintain your balance.
- Properly maintain the working condition of your bike.
- Secure your pants with clips, and secure your shoelaces so they don't get tangled in the chain.
- Wear a helmet. Three out of four cyclists killed in crashes die as a result of head injuries. The brain is very sensitive to any impact, even at low speeds.
- Wear other safety equipment, including eye protection, proper footwear, and gloves.

HOME INJURIES

Contrary to popular belief, home is one of the most dangerous places to be. The most common fatal home injuries are caused by falls, fires, poisoning, and incidents involving firearms.

Falls

Falls are second only to motor vehicle injuries in terms of causing deaths. They are the fifth leading cause of unintentional death for people under age 25. Nearly two-thirds of the deaths occurring from falls are from falls at floor level (tripping, slipping, and so on) rather than from a height.

To prevent injuries from falls:

- Place skidproof backing on rugs and carpets.
- Install handrails and nonslip applications in the shower and bathtub.
- Keep floors clear of objects or conditions that could cause slipping or tripping, such as heavy wax coating, electrical cords, and toys.
- Outside the house, clear dangerous surfaces created by ice, snow, fallen leaves, or rough ground.
- Install handrails on stairs. Keep stairs well lit and clear of objects.
- When climbing a ladder, use both hands. Never stand higher than the third step from the top. When using a stepladder, make sure the spreader brace is in the locked position.
- If there are small children in the home, place gates at the top and bottom of stairs. Never leave a baby unattended on a bed or table.

Fires

Each year about 80% of fire deaths and 65% of fire injuries occur in the home. Most home fires begin in the kitchen, living room, or bedroom. Many are caused by careless actions such as smoking in bed or leaving a cigarette burning in an ashtray.

To prevent fires:

- Dispose of all cigarettes in ashtrays. Never smoke in bed.
- Do not overload electrical outlets.
- Do not place extension cords under rugs or where people walk. Replace worn or frayed extension cords.
- Place a wire screen in front of fireplaces and wood stoves. Remove ashes carefully and store them in airtight metal containers, not paper bags.
- Properly maintain electrical appliances, kerosene heaters, and furnaces, and clean flues and chimneys annually.
- Keep portable heaters at least 3 feet away from curtains, bedding, towels, or anything that might catch fire. Never leave heaters on when you're out of the room or sleeping.

To be prepared for a fire:

- Plan at least two escape routes out of each room. Designate a location outside the home as a meeting place.
- Install a smoke-detection device on every level of your home. Clean the detectors and test batteries once a month, and replace the batteries at least once a year.
- Keep a fire extinguisher in your home, and know how to use it. Most fire extinguishers are operated by breaking the seal and pulling the pin on the handle, aiming the discharge at the base of the flames, and using a sweeping motion to cover the burning area.

To prevent injuries from fire:

- Get out as quickly as possible and go to the designated meeting place. Don't stop for a keepsake or a pet. Never hide in a closet or under a bed. Once outside, count heads to see if everyone is out. If you think someone is still inside the burning building, tell the firefighters. Never go back inside a burning building.
- If you're trapped in a room, feel the door. If it is hot, or if smoke is coming in through the cracks, don't

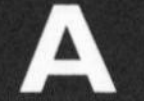

open it; use the alternative escape route. If you can't get out of a room, go to the window and shout or wave for help.

- Smoke inhalation is the largest cause of death and injury in fires. To avoid inhaling smoke, crawl along the floor away from the heat and smoke. Cover your mouth and nose, ideally with a wet cloth, and take short, shallow breaths.
- If your clothes catch fire, don't run. Drop to the ground, cover your face, and roll back and forth to smother the flames. Remember: stop-drop-roll.

Poisoning

Over 2 million poisonings occur every year, a majority of them among children under age 5.

To prevent poisoning:

- Store all medicines out of reach of children. Use medicines only as directed on the label or by a physician.
- Use cleaners, pesticides, and other dangerous substances only in areas with proper ventilation. Store them out of the reach of children.
- To prevent poisoning by gases, never operate a vehicle in an enclosed space, have your furnace inspected yearly, and use caution with any substance that produces potentially toxic fumes, such as kerosene.
- Many common house and garden plants are poisonous if ingested, including azalea, oleander, poinsettia, rhododendron, wild mushrooms, daffodil bulbs, hyacinth bulbs, mistletoe berries, apple seeds, morning glory seeds, larkspur seeds, wisteria seeds, and the leaves and stems of potato, rhubarb, and tomato plants. Keep these plants out of the reach of young children.

To be prepared in case of poisoning:

- Keep the number of the nearest Poison Control Center (or emergency room) in an accessible location.
- Keep a bottle of syrup of ipecac (which induces vomiting) on hand.

In case of poisoning, take the following emergency steps, and then call the Poison Control Center:

- For swallowed poison, don't follow the emergency instructions on labels of containers (they may be old or incorrect). Give water immediately *except* in these important cases: (1) the person is unconscious, having convulsions, or cannot swallow; (2) you don't know what the person swallowed; (3) the person swallowed a strong acid or alkali (toilet bowl cleaner, rust remover, chlorine bleach, dishwasher detergent, etc.) or a petroleum product (kerosene, gasoline, furniture polish, lighter fluid, paint thinner, etc.).
- For inhaled poison, get the person to fresh air immediately, and open doors and windows.
- For poison on the skin, remove contaminated clothing and flood the skin with water for 10 minutes. Wash the skin gently with soap and water, and rinse thoroughly.
- For poison in the eye, gently hold the eye open and flood it with lukewarm water poured from a glass held 2–3 inches from the eye. Continue for 15 minutes.
- When you call the Poison Control Center, be prepared to provide (1) the age and weight of the victim, (2) the name of the product or poison, (3) how much was taken, and (4) when it was taken. Have syrup of ipecac handy in case you are instructed to induce vomiting.

Unintentional Injury from Firearms

Firearms pose a significant threat, especially to people between ages 15 and 24, with most fatalities involving males who are cleaning or handling guns they thought were unloaded.

To prevent firearm injuries:

- Never point a loaded gun at something you do not intend to shoot.
- Store unloaded firearms under lock and key and separately from ammunition.
- Inspect firearms carefully before handling them.
- Follow the safety procedures advocated in firearms safety courses.

Other Home Injuries

Burns, choking, suffocation, and electrocution are other dangers in the home, particularly for small children. Burns are the third leading cause of death in young children (following motor vehicle collisions and drowning). House fires cause the most deaths, but hot water causes the most nonfatal burns. When a burn occurs, cold water should be poured on it immediately to cool the tissue and prevent the burn from going deeper.

To prevent burns in children:

- Place barriers around stoves and radiators, and keep children out of the kitchen where they might be burned by spills.
- Set your hot water heater no higher than 120°F.
- Always test the contents of a baby bottle on the wrist before feeding the baby. When bottles are heated in

microwave ovens, the liquid can become scalding before the outside of the bottle gets very hot.

- Unplug and store extension cords when not in use.
- Apply sunscreen to children's skin when they are out in the sun.

To prevent other home injuries:

- Keep small objects out of the reach of children under age 3, and don't give them raw carrots, nuts, popcorn, or hard candy. Inspect toys for small parts that could be put in the mouth. Balloons also pose a serious choking hazard for young children.
- Keep infants away from plastic bags, which can suffocate them, and don't put infants to bed wearing jackets with drawstring hoods, which can strangle them.
- Keep electrical appliances away from a filled tub or sink. Use plastic covers over electrical outlets.

PUBLIC INJURIES

Public injuries are defined as those that occur in public places but do not involve a motor vehicle. Most public injuries involve recreational activities, such as swimming and boating, playground activities, the use of all-terrain vehicles, and sports.

Drowning

Drowning is a special danger for children and for adults who are using alcohol. Children under age 5 and people between ages 15 and 24 have the highest rates of death from drowning. Many drownings of children occur in residential pools, often when there is inadequate supervision. Many drownings also occur when people on boats fall overboard. Between one-third and two-thirds of these drownings involve alcohol.

To prevent drowning:

- Develop adequate swimming skill, and make sure children learn to swim.
- Make sure residential pools are fenced.
- Use caution when swimming in unfamiliar surroundings (such as the ocean) or for an unusual length of time.
- Avoid being chilled by water colder than 70°F.
- Don't swim under the influence of alcohol or other drugs.
- Don't swim alone.
- When on a boat, use a personal flotation device. The U.S. Coast Guard recommends six different types, keyed to particular water conditions.

Playground Injuries

Over 200,000 injuries occur on school, park, and residential playground equipment every year. Most injuries are the result of falls from equipment to the ground; deaths are usually the result of head injuries.

To prevent playground injuries:

- Make sure equipment and surfaces under equipment comply with safety standards.
- Teach children to use equipment properly.

All-Terrain Vehicle Injuries

Most of the injuries associated with all-terrain vehicles (ATVs) are head injuries, which account for about 70% of the deaths.

To prevent ATV injuries:

- Develop the skills needed to operate the vehicle safely.
- Use safety equipment, especially helmets.
- Don't drink and drive.

In-line Skating Injuries

In-line skating, or rollerblading, has become a very popular recreational activity among people of all ages. Most injuries occur because users are not familiar with the equipment and do not wear appropriate safety gear. Injuries to the wrist and head are the most common. To reduce your risk of being injured while rollerblading, wear a helmet, elbow and knee pads, a long-sleeved shirt, and long pants.

Sports Injuries

An increase in the number of people exercising to improve their health has brought with it an increase in sports-related injuries.

To prevent sports injuries:

- Develop the skills required for the activity.
- Recognize and guard against the hazards associated with the activity.
- Include appropriate exercises for warming up and cooling down.
- Make sure facilities are safe.
- Follow the rules, and practice good sportsmanship.
- Use proper safety equipment, including, where appropriate, helmets; eye protection; knee, elbow, and wrist pads; and correct footwear.
- When it is excessively hot and humid, avoid heat stress by following the guidelines given in the box "Exercising in Hot Weather" in Chapter 3.

A

WORK INJURIES

Many aspects of workplace safety are monitored by the Occupational Safety and Health Administration (OSHA), a federal agency. The highest rate of work-related injuries occurs among laborers, whose jobs usually involve extensive manual labor and lifting—two areas not addressed by OSHA safety standards. Back injuries are the most common work injury.

To protect your back when lifting:

- Don't try to lift beyond your strength. If you need it, get help.
- Get a firm footing, with your feet shoulder width apart. Get a firm grip on the object.
- Keep your torso in a relatively upright position and crouch down, bending at the knees and hips. Avoid bending at the waist. To lift, stand up or push up with your leg muscles. Lift gradually, keeping your arms straight. Keep the object close to your body.
- Don't twist. If you have to turn with an object, change the position of your feet.
- Plan ahead. Make sure your pathway is clear before you pick up the object.
- Put the object down gently, reversing the rules for lifting.

A new type of work-related injury involves damage to the musculoskeletal system caused by repeated strain on the hand, arm, wrist, or other part of the body. Such injuries and disorders are referred to as cumulative trauma disorders, repetitive stress injuries, or repetitive motion disorders. Carpal tunnel syndrome is one type. It is characterized by pain and swelling in the tendons of the wrists and sometimes numbness and weakness. Its growing incidence is associated with the use of computers.

To prevent carpal tunnel syndrome:

- Maintain good posture at the computer. Use a chair that provides back support, and place the feet flat on the floor or on a foot rest.
- Position the screen at eye level and the keyboard so the hands and wrists are straight.
- Take breaks periodically to lessen the cumulative effects of stress.

VIOLENCE AND INTENTIONAL INJURIES

Violence is emerging as a major public health concern. The United States ranks first among developed nations in the rate of violent deaths; the number of such deaths exceeds the combined total of violent deaths in the next 17 nations. Violence includes assault, homicide (murder), sexual assault, domestic violence, suicide, and various forms of abuse. About 2.2 million Americans are victims of violent injury every year.

Assault

Assault is the use of physical force to inflict injury or death on another person. Most assaults occur during arguments or in connection with another crime, such as robbery. Poverty, urban settings, and the use of alcohol and drugs are associated with higher rates of assault.

Homicide is the tenth leading cause of death in the United States. Homicide victims are most likely to be male, between ages 19 and 24, and members of minority groups. Most homicides are committed with a firearm; the murderer and the victim usually know each other.

To protect yourself at home:

- Secure your home with good lighting and effective locks, preferably deadbolts.
- Make sure that all doors and windows are securely locked. Always lock windows and doors, including sliding glass doors, whenever you go out.
- Get a dog, or post "Beware of Dog" signs.
- Ensure that the landscaping around your home doesn't provide opportunities for concealment.
- Don't hide keys in obvious places. Don't give anyone the chance to duplicate your keys; for example, don't give your entire set of keys to a parking attendant, only the car key.
- Install a peephole in your front door. Don't open your door to people you don't know.
- Don't let strangers into your home or yard. When repair or delivery people or utility workers come to the door, ask to see identification, or call the company to verify that they've sent someone out.
- If you or a family member owns a weapon, store it securely. Store guns and ammunition in separate locations.
- If you are a woman living alone, use your initials rather than your full name in the phone directory. Don't use a greeting on your answering machine that implies you live alone or are not home.
- Teach everyone in the household how to obtain emergency assistance.
- Know your neighbors. Work out a system for alerting each other in case of an emergency.
- Establish a neighborhood watch program.

To protect yourself on the street:

- Avoid walking alone, especially at night. Stay where people can see and hear you.

- Dress sensibly, in clothing that allows you freedom of movement.
- Walk purposefully. Act alert and confident.
- Walk on the outside of the sidewalk, facing traffic.
- Know where you are going. Appearing to be lost increases your vulnerability.
- Don't hitchhike.
- Carry valuables in a fanny pack, pants pocket, or shoulder bag strapped diagonally across the chest. Conceal small purses inside a tote or shopping bag. Keep at least one hand free.
- Always have your keys ready as you approach your vehicle or home.
- Carry enough change so that you can make a telephone call or take public transportation. Carry a whistle to blow if you are attacked or harassed.
- Be aware of suspicious behavior. Listen to your own inner warning signals.
- If possible, allow at least two arm lengths between yourself and a stranger.
- If you feel threatened, run and/or yell. Go into a store or knock on the door of a home. If someone grabs you, yell "Help!" or "Fire!"

To protect yourself in your car:

- Keep your car in good working condition, carry emergency supplies, and keep the gas tank at least half full.
- When driving, keep doors locked and windows rolled up at least three-quarters of the way.
- Park your car in well-lighted areas or parking garages, preferably those with an attendant or security guard.
- Lock your car when you leave it, and check the interior before opening the door when you return.
- Don't pick up strangers. Don't stop for vehicles in distress; drive on and call for help.
- Note the location of emergency call boxes along highways and in public facilities. If you travel alone frequently, consider investing in a cellular phone.
- If your car breaks down, raise the hood and tie a white cloth to the aerial or door handle. Wait in the car with the doors locked and windows rolled up. If someone approaches to offer help, open a window only a crack and ask the person to call the police or a towing service.
- When you stop at a light or stop sign, leave enough room to maneuver out if you need an escape route.
- If you are involved in a minor automobile crash and you think you have been bumped intentionally, don't leave your car. Motion to the other driver to follow you to the nearest police station. If confronted by a person with a weapon, give up your car.
- Don't get into disputes or arguments with drivers of other vehicles.

To protect yourself on public transportation:

- While waiting, stand in a populated, well-lighted area.
- Sit near the driver or conductor in a single seat or an outside seat.
- If traveling to an unfamiliar location, call the transit agency for the correct route and time. Make sure that the bus, subway, or train is bound for your destination before you board it.
- If you flag down a taxi, ensure that it's from a legitimate service. When you reach your destination, ask the driver to wait until you are safely inside the building.

To protect yourself on campus:

- Ensure that door and window locks are secure and that halls and stairwells have adequate lighting.
- Don't give dorm or residence keys to anybody.
- Don't leave your door unlocked or allow strangers into your room.
- Avoid solitary late-night trips to the library or laundry room. Take advantage of on-campus escort services.
- Don't jog or exercise outside alone at night. Don't take shortcuts across campus that are unfamiliar or seem unsafe.
- If security guards patrol the campus, know the areas they cover, and stay where they can see or hear you.

Sexual Assault, or Rape

Sexual assault, or rape, is sexual coercion that relies on the threat and use of physical force or takes advantage of circumstances that render a person incapable of giving consent (such as when drunk). If the victim is younger than the legally defined age of consent, the act constitutes statutory rape, regardless of whether consent is given. Coerced sexual activity in which the victim knows the rapist is often referred to as acquaintance rape or date rape. At least 3.5 million females are raped annually in the United States, and perhaps 10,000 males are raped each year by other males.

Rape victims suffer both physical and psychological injury. For most, the physical wounds are not severe, but the psychological pain can be substantial and long-lasting. Many victims experience shock, anxiety, depression, shame, and psychosomatic symptoms. These psychological reactions are called rape trauma syndrome; other symptoms include fear, nightmares, fatigue, crying spells, and digestive upset. Self-blame is common, a reaction reinforced by our society's tendency to blame the victim. Fortunately, this tendency is giving way to a more realistic view of the violent nature of rape.

A

To protect yourself against rape:

- Follow the guidelines listed above for protecting yourself against assault.
- Think out in advance what you would do if you were threatened with rape. However, no one knows what he or she will do when scared to death. Trust that you will make the best decision at the time—whether to scream, run, fight, or give in to avoid being injured or killed.

If you are raped:

- Tell what happened to the first friendly person you meet.
- Call the police. Tell them you were raped, and give your location.
- Try to remember everything you can about your attacker, and write it down.
- Don't wash or douche before the medical exam. Don't change your clothes, but bring a new set with you if you can.
- At the hospital you will have a complete exam. Show the physician any bruises or scratches.
- Tell the police exactly what happened. Be honest, and stick to your story.
- If you do not want to report the rape to the police, see a physician as soon as possible. Be sure you are checked for pregnancy and STDs.
- Contact an organization with skilled counselors so you can talk about the experience. Look in the telephone directory under "Rape" or "Rape Crisis Center" for a hotline number.

Acquaintance Rape

Most women are in much less danger of being raped by a stranger than of being sexually assaulted by a man they know or date. Surveys suggest that as many as one woman in four has had sex forced on her by a man she knew or was dating. Victims of acquaintance rape tend to shoulder much of the responsibility for the incident, questioning their own judgment rather than blaming the aggressor.

One factor in acquaintance rape appears to be the double standard about appropriate sexual behavior for men and women. It is still a cultural belief in our society that "nice" women don't say yes to sex, even when they want to, and that "real" men don't take no for an answer. There are also widespread differences between men and women in how romantic signals are perceived. Researchers in one study found that men tend to interpret women's actions on dates, such as smiling or talking in a low voice, as indicating an interest in having sex, while the women interpreted the same actions as being "friendly." Men who rape their dates also tend to have certain characteristics, including hostility toward women and an acceptance of sexual violence. Both men and women must take responsibility for reducing the incidence of rape.

To protect yourself from acquaintance rape:

- Believe in your right to control what you do. Set limits, and communicate them clearly, firmly, and early. Be assertive.
- Remember that some men think flirtatious behavior or sexy clothing indicates an interest in having sex.
- Use the statement that has proven most effective in stopping acquaintance rape: "This is rape and I'm calling the cops!"

Guidelines for men:

- Be aware of social pressure. It's OK not to "score."
- Understand that "No" means "No." Stop making advances when your date says to stop.
- Don't assume that flirtatious behavior or sexy clothing means a woman is interested in having sex, that previous permission for sex applies to the current situation, or that your date's relationships with other men constitute sexual permission for you.
- Remember that alcohol and drug use interferes with judgment, perception, and communication about sex.

PROVIDING EMERGENCY CARE

You can improve someone else's chances of surviving if you are prepared to provide emergency help. A course in first aid, offered by the American Red Cross and on many college campuses, can teach you to respond appropriately when someone needs help.

Emergency rescue techniques can save the lives of people who have stopped breathing, are choking, or whose hearts have stopped beating. Pulmonary resuscitation (also known as rescue breathing, artificial respiration, or mouth-to-mouth resuscitation) is used when a person is not breathing (Figure A-1). Cardiopulmonary resuscitation (CPR) is used when a pulse can't be found. Training is required before a person can perform CPR. Courses are offered by the American Red Cross and the American Heart Association.

Many choking victims can be saved with the Heimlich maneuver (also called abdominal thrusts). For instructions on performing this maneuver, see Figure A-1. Blows to the upper back in conjunction with chest thrusts are an acceptable way to dislodge an object from an infant's throat.

When you have to provide emergency care:

- Remain calm, and act sensibly.
- Make sure the scene is safe for both you and the injured person. Don't put yourself in danger; if you

American Red Cross

TO SAVE A LIFE

RESCUE BREATHING

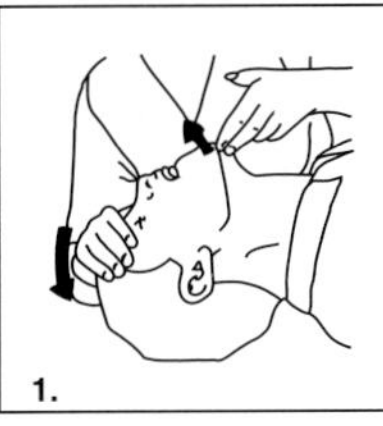

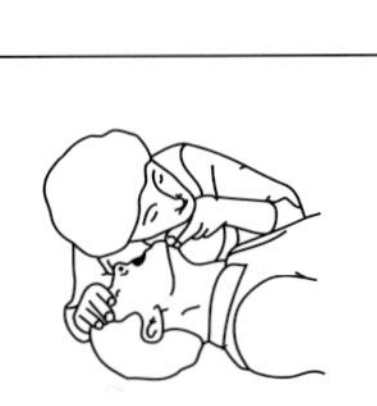

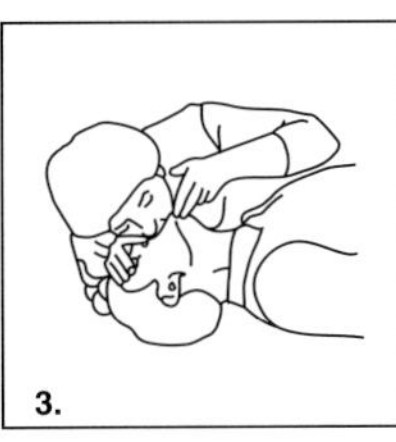

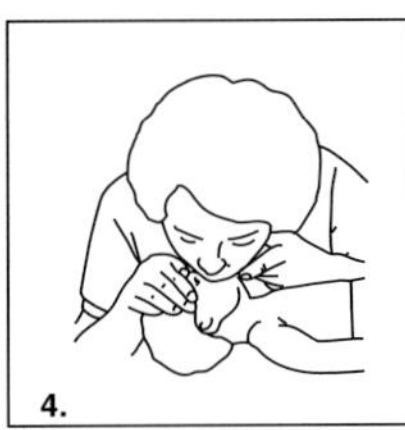

IF VICTIM APPEARS TO BE UNCONSCIOUS, TAP VICTIM ON THE SHOULDER AND SHOUT "ARE YOU OKAY?"

1. Apply the major force with the hand on the forehead.

- Place fingertips under the bony part of the jaw.
- Support and lift the jaw with your fingertips. Avoid closing the mouth.
- Do not push the soft tissues of the throat; it may block the airway.

If necessary, pull the lower lip down slightly, with your open thumb to keep the mouth open.

2. Look, listen and feel for breathing for 3-5 seconds.

3.
- If the person is not breathing, pinch nose closed.
- Place your mouth tightly around victim's mouth and blow into his mouth.
- Give two full breaths

Stop blowing when victim's chest has expanded.

- Turn head and listen for exhalation.
- Give 1 breath every 5 seconds.

4. INFANTS AND SMALL CHILDREN

- Tilt head slightly.
- Cover & seal nose with your mouth.
- Blow shallow breaths.
- Give 1 breath every 3 seconds.

FIRST AID FOR CHOKING

1. ASK:
"ARE YOU CHOKING?"

If victim cannot breathe, cough, or speak...

GIVE THE HEIMLICH MANEUVER.

Stand behind the victim.

Wrap your arms around the victim's waist.

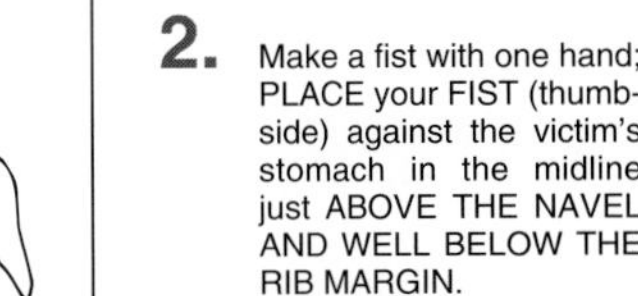

2. Make a fist with one hand; PLACE your FIST (thumb-side) against the victim's stomach in the midline just ABOVE THE NAVEL AND WELL BELOW THE RIB MARGIN.

Grasp your fist with your other hand.

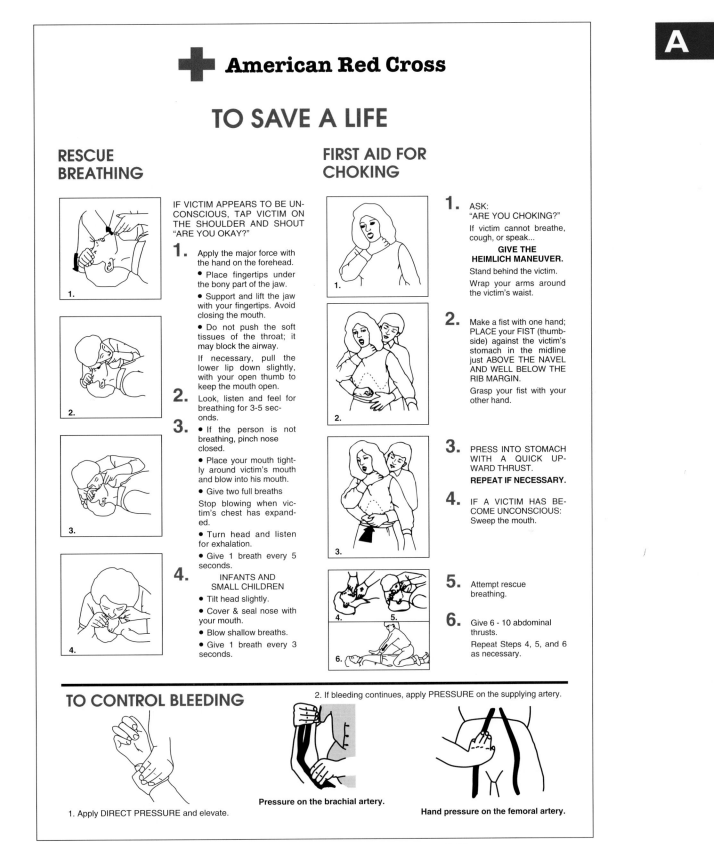

3. PRESS INTO STOMACH WITH A QUICK UPWARD THRUST.

REPEAT IF NECESSARY.

4. IF A VICTIM HAS BECOME UNCONSCIOUS: Sweep the mouth.

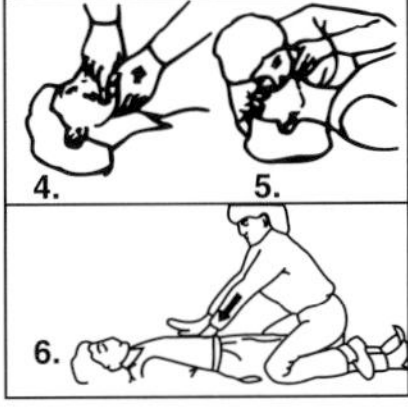

5. Attempt rescue breathing.

6. Give 6 - 10 abdominal thrusts.

Repeat Steps 4, 5, and 6 as necessary.

TO CONTROL BLEEDING

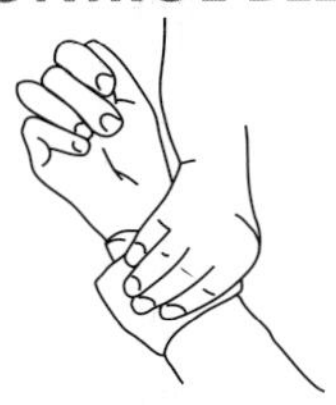

1. Apply DIRECT PRESSURE and elevate.

2. If bleeding continues, apply PRESSURE on the supplying artery.

Pressure on the brachial artery.

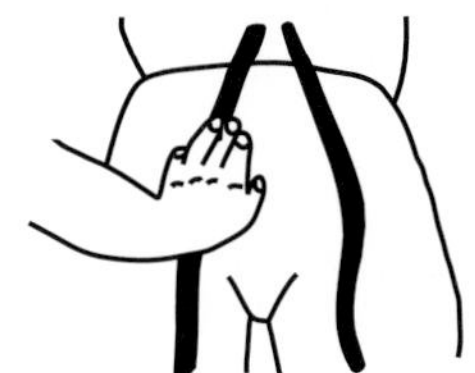

Hand pressure on the femoral artery.

Figure A-1 *Rescue breathing and first aid for choking, procedures recommended by the American Red Cross.*

A

get hurt too, you will be of little help to the injured person.

- Identify yourself to the victim, say you are there to help, and ask what happened. This information will help you give appropriate first aid and is crucial for medical personnel when they arrive or are contacted.
- Conduct a quick head-to-toe examination. Assess the victim's signs and symptoms, such as level of responsiveness, pulse, breathing, size of pupils, and the color, texture, and temperature of the skin. Look for bleeding and any indications of broken bones or paralysis.
- If the situation requires immediate action (no pulse, shock, etc.), provide first aid if you are trained to do so. If you are alone, provide assistance first, and then seek help. If several people are available, one should go for help while the rest give first aid.

SUMMARY

Like other behaviors, acting in a safe way involves choices you make every day.

To improve your chances of avoiding and preventing injuries:

- Increase your knowledge and level of awareness.
- Examine your attitudes to see if they are realistic.
- Know your capacities and limitations.
- Adjust your behavior when environmental hazards exist.
- Take responsibility for your actions.

SELECTED BIBLIOGRAPHY

American Red Cross. 1993. *Community First Aid and Safety.* St. Louis: Mosby Year Book.

Bever, D. L. 1992. *Safety: A Personal Focus,* 3d ed. St. Louis: Mosby Year Book.

DiMona, L., and C. Herndon, eds. 1994. *The 1995 Information Please® Women's Sourcebook.* Boston: Houghton Mifflin.

Fike, R. A. 1994. *Staying Alive! Your Crime Prevention Guide.* Washington, D.C.: Acropolis Books.

National Safety Council. 1994. *Accident Facts, 1994 Edition.* Itasca, Ill.: National Safety Council.

Out of harm's way. 1994. *Harvard Women's Health Watch,* April.

Reducing your risk of becoming a carjacking victim. 1993. *Healthline,* August.

Rosenberg, M. L., and M. A. Fenley. 1991. *Violence in America.* New York: Oxford University Press.

U.S. Department of Health and Human Services. 1990. *Healthy People 2000.* Washington, D.C.: U.S. Government Printing Office, DHHS Publication No. (PHS) 91-50212.

B

Nutritional Content of Common Foods

This food composition table has been prepared for Mayfield Publishing Company and is copyrighted by DINE Systems, Inc., the developer and publisher of the DINE System family of nutrition software for personal computers. The values in this food composition table were derived from the USDA Nutrient Data Base for Standard Reference Release 10 and nutrient composition information from over 300 food companies. Nutrient values used for each food were determined by collapsing similar foods into one food, using the median nutrient values. In the food composition table, foods are listed within the following eight groups: fruits, vegetables, beverages, alcoholic beverages, grains, dairy, fats/sweets/other, and protein foods. Further information can be obtained from:

DINE Systems, Inc.
586 N. French Road
Amherst, NY 14228
716-688-2492
716-688-2505 fax

Order of fields: Name, Amount/Unit, Calories, Protein, Total Fat, Saturated Fat, Carbohydrates (minus added sugar), Added Sugar, Fiber, Cholesterol, Sodium, Calcium, Iron.

FRUITS

Name	Amount/Unit	Cal	Pro. g	TFat g	SFat g	Carb. g	Sug. g	Fbr. g	Chol. mg	Sod. mg	Calc. mg	Iron mg
Apples, sweetened	½ cup	68	0	0.11	0	12.5	3.25	2	0	4	4	0.3
Apples, unsweetened	½ frt, ½ cup	41	0.25	0	0	9.5	0	2.1	0	0	4	0.2
Applesauce, sweetened	½ cup	97	0.25	0	0	12	11	1.8	0	4	4	0.4
Applesauce, unsweetened	½ cup	53	0.25	0	0	12.5	0	2.5	0	2	4	0.2
Apricots, sweetened	3 hlv, ¼ cup	65	0.5	0	0	3.75	10.75	1.1	0	3	8	0.4
Apricots, unsweetened	3 halves	27	0.5	0	0	5.5	0	1.1	0	3	8	0.3
Banana	1 fruit	105	1	0.33	0.22	24	0	2.3	0	1	7	0.4
Blueberries, sweetened	½ cup	103	0.5	0.11	0	8.5	16.25	2.3	0	3	7	0.4
Blueberries, unsweetened	½ cup	41	0.5	0.22	0	9	0	1.7	0	2	5	0.2
Cherries, sweetened	½ cup	106	0.75	0	0	12.25	13	0.9	0	4	13	0.4
Cherries, unsweetened	10 frt, ½ cup	44	0.75	0	0	10	0	0.9	0	2	12	0.4
Dates	5 frt, ¼ cup	118	0.75	0.22	0.11	28.5	0	3.7	0	1	14	0.5
Dried fruit	¼ cup	92	1	0	0	21.75	0	2.4	0	9	11	0.7
Figs, sweetened	2 fruit	45	0.25	0	0	7	3.75	1.3	0	1	15	0.2
Figs, unsweetened	2 frt, ¼ cup	74	0.75	0.33	0.11	17.5	0	4.2	0	3	39	0.6
Fruit cocktail, sweetened	½ cup	83	0.5	0	0	8.75	11	1.4	0	8	8	0.3
Fruit cocktail, unswtnd	½ cup	50	0.5	0	0	11.5	0	1.4	0	4	6	0.3
Grapefruit, sweetened	½ cup	76	0.5	0	0	10	8	0.5	0	2	18	0.5
Grapefruit, unsweetened	½ frt, ½ cup	39	0.5	0	0	9	0	0.7	0	0	14	0.2
Grapes, sweetened	½ cup	94	0.5	0	0	10.5	12	0.5	0	7	12	1.2
Grapes, unsweetened	20 frt, ½ cup	48	0.5	0	0	11.5	0	0.5	0	2	8	0.2
Guava	1 fruit	45	0.5	0.33	0.11	9.5	0	5	0	2	18	0.3
Juice, unsweetened	¾ cup	90	0.5	0	0	22.5	0	0.2	0	8	16	0.5
Kiwi fruit	1 fruit	46	0.75	0.33	0.11	10	0	2.1	0	4	20	0.3
Mango	½ frt, ½ cup	61	0.5	0.11	0	14.25	0	1.8	0	2	9	0.2
Melon	½ cup	30	0.5	0	0	7	0	0.7	0	9	8	0.2
Nectarines	1 fruit	68	1	0.56	0	14.5	0	3.3	0	0	6	0.2
Orange	1 frt, ¾ cup	63	1	0	0	14	0	3.9	0	1	53	0.2
Papaya	½ frt, ½ cup	56	0.75	0	0	12.75	0	1.8	0	4	35	0.2
Peaches, sweetened	½ cup	94	0.5	0	0	5.25	17	1.2	0	8	3	0.4
Peaches, unsweetened	1 frt, ½ cup	44	0.5	0	0	10.75	0	1.3	0	3	5	0.1
Pears, sweetened	2 halves	103	0.5	0	0	6	18.5	3.2	0	8	8	0.4
Pears, unsweetened	2 hlvs, ½ cup	60	0.5	0	0	15	0	3	0	4	10	0.2
Pineapple, sweetened	2 slices, ½ cup	93	0.5	0	0	7.5	15	0.9	0	2	15	0.4
Pineapple, unsweetened	2 slices, ½ cup	70	0.25	0	0	17.5	0	0.9	0	2	6	0.4
Plums, sweetened	2 plums	67	0.5	0.11	0	8	7.75	0.7	0	17	9	0.7
Plums, unsweetened	1 raw, 2 canned	37	0.5	0	0	8.25	0	0.9	0	1	5	0.2
Prunes, cooked	½ cup	136	1.25	0.33	0	32	0	4.9	0	3	29	1.4
Prunes, dried	½ cup	209	2	0.44	0	49.25	0	6.8	0	4	45	2.1
Pumpkin, canned	½ cup	41	0.75	0.11	0.11	8.75	0	3.5	0	6	32	1.7
Raisins	¼ cup	109	1	0	0	26	0	2.5	0	5	19	0.8
Raspberries, sweetened	½ cup	117	0.75	0.11	0	12	18.25	4.2	0	0	19	0.5
Raspberries, unsweetened	½ cup	30	0.5	0.22	0	6.5	0	3	0	0	14	0.3
Strawberries, sweetened	½ cup	100	0.5	0.11	0	9	15	2	0	4	14	0.6
Strawberries, unsweetened	½ cup	24	0.5	0.22	0	5.5	0	1.6	0	2	11	0.5
Tangerines, sweetened	½ cup	76	0.5	0	0	10	8.5	0.9	0	8	9	0.4
Tangerines, unsweetened	1 frt, ½ cup	43	0.5	0	0	9.75	0	0.9	0	2	14	0.1
Watermelon	½ cup	25	0.5	0.22	0.22	5	0	0.3	0	2	6	0.2

VEGETABLES

Name	Amount/Unit	Cal	Pro. g	TFat g	SFat g	Carb. g	Sug. g	Fbr. g	Chol. mg	Sod. mg	Calc. mg	Iron mg
Asparagus	6 spears, ½ cup	24	1.75	0.33	0.11	3.75	0	1.5	0	4	22	0.6
Asparagus, canned	½ cup	21	1.5	0.33	0.11	2.75	0	1.9	0	425	17	1.5
Avocados	½ frt, ½ cup	166	2	14.22	2.56	7.25	0	2.7	0	10	12	1
Bamboo shoots	¼ cup	4	0.25	0	0	0.5	0	0.3	0	1	4	0.1
Bamboo shoots, canned	¼ cup	6	0.5	0.11	0	1	0	0.6	0	2	1	0.1
Bean sprouts	½ cup	16	1.25	0	0	2.75	0	2.2	0	3	7	0.5
Bean sprouts, canned	½ cup	8	0.75	0	0	1.25	0	2.3	0	149	9	0.3
Beets, canned	½ cup	36	0.75	0	0	8	0	2.9	0	324	17	0.8
Beets, pickled	½ cup	82	0.75	0	0	8.5	11.25	2.8	0	250	13	0.5
Beets, raw, cooked	½ cup	31	0.75	0	0	6.75	0	2.5	0	49	11	0.6
Bok choy, chinese cabbage	½ cup	5	0.25	0	0	0.75	0	0.6	0	23	37	0.3
Broccoli, cooked	½ cup	24	1.75	0.11	0	4.25	0	2.5	0	15	68	0.8
Broccoli, raw	½ cup	12	0.75	0.11	0	2	0	1.5	0	12	21	0.4
Brussels sprouts	½ cup	32	1.5	0.33	0.11	5.75	0	2.4	0	18	24	0.8
Cabbage, raw or cooked	½c rw, ¼c ck	9	0.25	0	0	1.75	0	1	0	7	13	0.2
Carrots, canned	½ cup	17	0.25	0.11	0	3.75	0	2.7	0	176	19	0.5
Carrots, raw or cooked	½ cup	26	0.5	0	0	5.75	0	2.2	0	43	21	0.4
Cauliflower, raw or cooked	½ cup	15	0.75	0.11	0	2.5	0	1.3	0	7	15	0.3
Celery, raw or cooked	½ cup	10	0.25	0	0	2.25	0	1.4	0	51	25	0.2
Coleslaw	½ cup	154	0.5	14.44	2.67	4.25	1	1.5	7	287	32	0.4
Corn	½ cup	80	1.75	0.33	0	17.5	0	4.6	0	4	2	0.5
Corn, canned	½ cup	83	1.5	0.44	0.11	13	5.5	4.7	0	324	5	0.4
Cucumber	½ cup	7	0.25	0	0	1.5	0	0.7	0	1	7	0.1
Eggplant	½ cup	13	0.25	0	0	3	0	1	0	2	3	0.2
French fries	½ cup	174	1.75	7.33	3.22	19	0	2.6	0	37	6	0.6
Fried vegetables/onions	½ cup, 6 rings	180	2	10.78	2.67	15.5	0	1	0	150	12	0.7
Green beans, canned	½ cup	13	0.75	0	0	2.5	0	1.5	0	170	18	0.6
Green beans, raw or cooked	½ cup	20	1	0	0	4	0	1.8	0	3	30	0.7
Greens, mustard, turnip, ckd	½ cup	15	1	0.11	0	2.5	0	1.4	0	16	87	0.7
Greens, mustard, turnip, raw	½ cup	7	0.5	0	0	1.5	0	0.9	0	9	41	0.4
Greens, turnip, canned	½ cup	17	1	0.22	0.11	2.5	0	2.2	0	325	138	1.8
Kale, raw or cooked	½ cup	20	0.75	0.11	0	3	0	1.7	0	15	47	0.6
Lettuce, endive	½ cup	4	0.25	0	0	0.75	0	0.7	0	6	13	0.2
Lettuce, iceberg	1 leaf	3	0	0	0	0.5	0	0.3	0	2	4	0.1
Miso	½ cup	284	14.25	7.33	1.11	39.25	0	7.4	0	5032	92	3.8
Mixed vegetables, canned	½ cup	39	1.25	0.11	0	8	0	3.5	0	122	22	0.9
Mixed vegetables, frozen	½ cup	22	0.75	0	0	4.5	0	2	0	22	27	0.6
Mushrooms, canned	½ cup	19	1	0.11	0	3.25	0	1.1	0	178	1	0.6
Mushrooms, fresh, cooked	½ cup	25	1.75	0.11	0	4.25	0	1.5	0	1	7	1.7
Mushrooms, raw	½ cup	9	0.5	0	0	1.5	0	0.6	0	1	2	0.4
Okra	½ cup	26	1	0.11	0	5.5	0	2.1	0	5	55	0.5
Onions	½ cup	29	0.5	0.11	0	6.25	0	1.4	0	8	20	0.3
Parsnips	½ cup	64	0.75	0.11	0	14.75	0	3.2	0	8	30	0.5
Peas, green	½ cup	63	3.75	0.11	0	11.5	0	3.5	0	70	19	1.2
Peas, green, canned	½ cup	59	3.25	0.11	0	8	2.75	5.3	0	186	17	0.8
Peas, snowpeas	½ cup	35	2.25	0.11	0	5.75	0	3.4	0	4	37	1.6
Peppers, hot	2 tablespoons	8	0.25	0	0	1.5	0	0.2	0	1	3	0.2
Peppers, sweet, green	½ cup	12	0.25	0.11	0	2.25	0	0.6	0	2	3	0.6
Peppers, sweet, red	½ cup	12	0.25	0.11	0	2.25	0	0.8	0	2	3	0.6
Potato skins, cheese, bacon	2 halves	302	11	15.89	7.44	27.5	0	1.4	34	267	225	4.5

continued

Vegetables, continued

Name	Amount/Unit	Cal	Pro. g	TFat g	SFat g	Carb. g	Sug. g	Fbr. g	Chol. mg	Sod. mg	Calc. mg	Iron mg
Potato, baked/boiled	½ bkd/1 bld	113	1.5	0	0	26.5	0	2.6	0	7	9	0.4
Potatoes, mashed	½ cup	118	1.5	4.56	1.44	17	0	1.8	4	340	40	0.3
Rutabaga	½ cup	35	0.75	0.11	0	7.5	0	2.1	0	19	43	0.5
Salad, potato	½ cup	153	3	7.78	1.89	15	1.5	1.9	47	512	19	0.5
Salad, three bean	½ cup	80	2	0	0	16.25	1.75	5	0	540	20	3.6
Sauerkraut	½ cup	22	0.75	0.11	0	4.5	0	4.1	0	780	36	1.7
Soup, vegetable	1 cup	81	2	1.56	0.44	11.25	2.25	0.5	2	892	16	1
Spaghetti sauce	½ cup	118	2	5	0.89	12.75	1.5	3.3	0	589	20	1.1
Spaghetti sauce with meat	½ cup	80	2	3.11	0.67	12.5	2	3.3	2	630	20	1.1
Spinach, canned	½ cup	25	1.75	0.33	0.11	3.25	0	3.9	0	29	135	2.5
Spinach, fresh, cooked	½ cup	24	1.75	0.11	0	3.75	0	3	0	73	131	1.7
Spinach, raw	½ cup	6	0.5	0	0	0.75	0	1.1	0	22	28	0.8
Squash, summer	½ cup	18	0.5	0.11	0	3.75	0	1.5	0	3	22	0.4
Squash, winter	½ cup	41	0.75	0.11	0	9.5	0	3	0	4	23	0.6
Squash, zucchini, fresh, ckd	1c rw, ½c ck	18	0.75	0	0	3.5	0	1.4	0	2	19	0.5
Sweet potato	½ cup	98	1.25	0	0	23	0	4	0	11	30	0.5
Sweet potato, candied	½ cup	190	1	0	0	26.5	20	4.4	0	60	20	0.7
Tomatoes, canned or stewed	½ cup	34	0.75	0.11	0	6.5	0.25	2.4	0	305	33	0.7
Tomatoes, raw	½ cup	17	0.5	0.11	0	3.5	0	1.3	0	8	6	0.5
Waterchestnuts, canned	½ cup	34	0.25	0	0	8.25	0	1.5	0	3	3	0.3
Waterchestnuts, raw	½ cup	66	0.75	0	0	15.75	0	1.4	0	9	7	0.4
Watercress, raw	½ cup	2	0.25	0	0	0.25	0	0.2	0	7	20	0

BEVERAGES

Name	Amount/Unit	Cal	Pro. g	TFat g	SFat g	Carb. g	Sug. g	Fbr. g	Chol. mg	Sod. mg	Calc. mg	Iron mg
Beer, non-alcoholic	12 fluid ounces	55	0.75	0	0	11	0	0	0	19	25	0.1
Wine, non-alcoholic	5 fluid ounces	42	0.5	0	0	9.75	0	0	0	7	12	0.6
Cola	12 fluid ounces	150	0	0	0	0	37	0	0	70	0	0
Cola, diet	12 fluid ounces	2	0.25	0	0	0.25	0	0	0	70	0	0
Cola, diet, no caffeine	12 fluid ounces	2	0	0	0	0	0	0	0	70	0	0
Cola, no caffeine	12 fluid ounces	155	0	0	0	0	38.75	0	0	73	0	0
MellowYellow, MountainDew	12 fluid ounces	177	0	0	0	0	44	0	0	30	0	0
Noncola, diet, no caffeine	12 fluid ounces	4	0	0	0	0.5	0	0	0	42	0	0
Noncola, no caffeine	12 fluid ounces	157	0	0	0	0	37.75	0	0	46	2	0.1
Juice drink	¾ cup/1 box	106	0	0	0	6.5	19.5	0	0	7	1	1
Coffee	1 cup	5	0.25	0	0	1	0	0	0	7	6	0.6
Coffee, decaffeinated	1 cup	3	0.25	0	0	0.75	0	0	0	8	8	0.1
Postum	1 teaspoon	12	0	0	0	3	0	1.3	0	0	0	0
Tea, herbal, no caffeine	1 cup	4	0	0	0	0.75	0	0	0	3	5	0.2
Tea, plain	1 cup	3	0	0	0	0.5	0	0	0	0	0	0

B

ALCOHOLIC BEVERAGES

Name	Amount/Unit	Cal	Pro. g	TFat g	SFat g	Carb. g	Sug. g	Fbr. g	Chol. mg	Sod. mg	Calc. mg	Iron mg
Beer	12 fluid ounces	145	1	0	0	13.25	0	0	0	8	12	0
Beer, light	12 fluid ounces	110	1	0	0	7	0	0	0	8	15	0
Chianti	5 fluid ounces	106	0.25	0	0	2.5	0	0	0	8	12	0.6
Cocktail, mixed drink	1 cocktail	139	0	0	0	1	1.5	0	0	6	4	0.1
Liqueur	1 glass, 1½ oz	167	0	0.11	0	8.5	9.5	0	0	4	1	0
Liquor	1 jigger	110	0	0	0	0	0	0	0	0	0	0
Vermouth	5 fluid ounces	100	0.25	0	0	1	0	0	0	8	12	0.4
Wine cooler	12 fluid ounces	173	0.75	0	0	7.75	9.75	0	0	25	32	1.4
Wine	5 fluid ounces	104	0.25	0	0	2.5	0	0	0	12	12	0.4
Wine, light	5 fluid ounces	73	0.5	0	0	1	0	0	0	10	13	0.6

GRAINS

Name	Amount/Unit	Cal	Pro. g	TFat g	SFat g	Carb. g	Sug. g	Fbr. g	Chol. mg	Sod. mg	Calc. mg	Iron mg
Cereal, bran, fiber	⅓ cup	62	2	0.78	0.22	7.75	2.75	3.8	0	113	13	3
Cereal, frosted	1 cup	147	1.75	0.11	0	18.75	14.75	0.5	0	93	4	2.4
Cereal, fruit flavored	1 cup	110	1.75	0.22	0.11	12	13	0.5	0	168	5	4.5
Cereal, granola	¼ cup	130	3	4.89	0.89	13.5	4.5	1.7	0	55	19	0.9
Cereal, oat flakes	1 cup	182	5	1.78	0.44	24.75	4.5	3.2	0	115	32	5.8
Cereal, other, cold	1 cup	110	2	0.22	0.11	19.5	3	0.6	0	226	4	1.8
Cereal, other, hot	⅔ cup	100	3	0	0	22	0	0.7	0	54	18	1.1
Cereal, whole grain	¾ cup	105	3	0.78	0.22	19	0	2.3	0	160	8	1.4
Granola, fat free	¼ cup	90	2	0	0	21	0.25	2.5	0	20	0	0.4
Oatmeal, flavored	1 packet	140	4	2.22	0.44	18	8.25	2.4	0	181	100	4.5
Oatmeal, plain	⅔ cup cooked	109	4	1.78	0.33	18.25	0	3.3	0	1	15	1.9
Pancakes, waffles	2 pnck/2 wfl	173	4.75	4	1.11	26	3.5	1	44	503	100	1.5
Bagel	1 bagel	175	7	1.22	0.22	32.5	2.25	1.5	0	325	20	1.8
Biscuit	1 biscuit	100	2	3.78	1.22	13.5	0	0.5	2	262	47	0.7
Bread or roll, wheat	1 slice, 1 roll	65	2	0.89	0.22	10	2	1.4	0	106	20	0.7
Bread or roll, white	1 slice, 1 roll	70	2.75	1.11	0.33	11	2	0.5	0	132	20	0.7
Bread, mixed grain	1 slice	65	2	0.89	0.22	9.75	2.25	1.4	0	106	27	0.8
Bread, oatmeal	1 slice	90	4	1.78	0.33	10.5	4	1.5	0	140	40	1.1
Bread, pita, wheat	1 pita (6″ diam)	145	5.5	0.89	0.22	28.5	0.5	4.1	0	360	50	1.4
Bread, pita, white	1 pita (6″ diam)	160	6	1	0.22	30	1	1.1	0	300	80	0.7
Bread, raisin	1 slice	70	2	1	0.33	8.25	3	0.9	0	85	20	0.7
Bread, rye, pumpernickel	1 slice	80	2.75	0.89	0.11	13	1	1.1	0	185	22	1.1
Bread, wheat, diet	1 slice	40	2.5	0.56	0.11	4.25	2	2	0	120	40	0.7
Bread, white, diet	1 slice	40	3	0	0	6	1	2	0	110	40	0.7
Bread, whole wheat	1 slice, 1 roll	70	2.75	1.11	0.22	10	1.25	1.9	0	160	20	1
Breadsticks	⅓ lrg, 2 sm	36	1.25	0.78	0.22	6	0.5	0.6	0	72	0	0.2
Cornbread, hushpuppies	2.5″ sq, 3 hpup	166	3	5.33	1.78	25.75	0	1.6	42	421	87	0.8

continued

Grains, continued

Name	Amount/Unit	Cal	Pro. g	TFat g	SFat g	Carb. g	Sug. g	Fbr. g	Chol. mg	Sod. mg	Calc. mg	Iron mg
Croissants	1 croissant	310	7	19	11.22	27	6	2	0	240	38	1.8
Danish, nonfat	1 piece	90	2	0	0	20	9.75	0.2	0	85	20	0
English muffin	1 muffin	130	5	0.89	0.33	25	1.5	1.6	0	280	96	1.7
Muffin	1 muffin	140	3	4.67	1.56	11.75	8	1.2	21	198	42	1.1
Muffins, fat free	1 muffin	155	3	0.11	0	35	11.5	0.9	0	140	50	0.5
Roll, hmbrgr, hotdog, wheat	1 roll	114	4	1.11	0.22	21.25	0.75	2.5	0	242	46	1
Roll, hmbrgr, hotdog, white	1 roll	138	3.25	2.44	0.67	22.5	2	1.4	0	271	67	1.3
Roll, hoagie, sub	½ roll	200	5.5	3.56	0.89	34.25	2	0.9	0	342	50	1.9
Stuffing	½ cup	210	4.5	12.67	3	17.5	2.5	0.5	22	578	40	1.1
Cake, nonfat	1 piece/slice	70	1.5	0	0	16	7.75	0.6	0	85	0	0
Cookies, nonfat	2 cookies	75	1	0	0	17.5	6.5	0.6	0	115	0	0.2
Cracker sandwiches	2 lrg, 5 sm	70	1.75	3.11	1.11	7.75	0.75	0.2	1	135	20	0.4
Crackers, butter type	5 lrg, 10 sm	70	1	3.56	1.11	8	0.25	0.2	1	193	4	0.4
Crackers, crispbread	1 lrg, 2 sm	40	1	0.89	0.33	8.5	0	1.6	0	112	0	0.5
Crackers, lowfat	2 lrg, 5 sm	60	2.25	2.33	0.33	10	0	0.6	0	100	0	0.4
Crackers, wheat	4 crackers	70	1	2.22	0.44	8	0.5	1.5	0	75	0	0.4
Matzo or melba toast	½ matzo, 5 melba	72	2.75	0.67	0.22	14	1.5	0.6	0	189	2	1
Barley, cooked	½ cup	84	2.25	0.11	0	18.5	0	2.5	0	3	11	0.5
Bulgur	½ cup	113	4.25	0.22	0	23.5	0	3	0	3	13	3.7
Couscous	⅔ cup	120	4	0	0	26	0	4.3	0	5	0	0.7
Grits	½ cup	73	1.5	0.11	0	16	0	0.3	0	136	0	0.8
Lasagna, meat	1 serving	350	27.5	23.11	6	31	1.5	2.6	73	1040	275	2.1
Lasagna, vegetable	1 serving	315	22	12	5.89	27	0.5	4.6	40	970	350	2.3
Macaroni and cheese	½ cup	191	6	8.56	2.67	22.75	0	1.4	18	434	71	1.2
Macaroni, whole wheat	1 cup	202	8	1.11	0.22	39	0	7.4	0	10	20	4.5
Noodles, chow mein	½ cup	130	3	6.44	1.11	14.5	0	0.5	2	228	4	0.8
Noodles, egg, macaroni	1 cup	190	7	0.56	0.11	37	0	1.1	0	30	14	2.1
Pasta w/parmesan cheese	½ cup	252	6.5	14.67	6.33	22.5	0	1.1	38	479	78	1.5
Salad, pasta	½ cup	250	4	16	3.33	20.75	0	0.7	28	410	40	0.7
Spaghetti	1 cup	200	7.5	1	0.22	40.5	0	1.1	0	19	14	2
Spaghetti w/meatballs	1 cup	307	12	10.56	3.89	37	0	2.7	34	1220	53	3.3
Spaghetti, whole wheat	1 cup	200	9	1.11	0.22	39.5	0	5.8	0	10	20	2.7
Rice cake	1 large cake	35	0.75	0	0	7.5	0	0.3	0	13	0	0
Rice, brown	½ cup	115	2.5	0.67	0.22	25	0	1.8	0	2	12	0.5
Rice, long grain/wild, mix	½ cup	137	3	2	0.56	23	2	0.9	0	579	11	1.1
Rice, seasoned	½ cup	150	3.5	3.78	1.67	23	1	1	5	700	13	1.2
Rice, white	½ cup	92	2	0	0	20.5	0	0.5	0	225	10	0.7
Tabouli	½ cup	170	3	8.67	1.33	20	0	1.6	0	290	0	0.7
Taco shell	1 shell	50	0	2	1.11	8	0	0.2	0	5	0	0
Tortilla	1 tortilla	65	2	1	0.11	12	0	0.9	0	1	42	0.6

DAIRY

Name	Amount/Unit	Cal	Pro. g	TFat g	SFat g	Carb. g	Sug. g	Fbr. g	Chol. mg	Sod. mg	Calc. mg	Iron mg
Buttermilk	1 cup	99	8.75	2	1.33	11.25	0	0	9	257	285	0.1
Hot cocoa prepared w/milk	1 cup	218	8	9	5.67	13.5	11.25	3	33	123	298	0.8
Meal replacement drinks	1 cup	200	14	1	0.44	36	17	4	5	230	500	6.3
Milk, chocolate	1 cup	179	8.5	4.67	3	10.5	14.5	1.1	17	150	284	0.6
Milk, lowfat	1 cup	112	8.75	3.56	2.22	11.25	0	0	14	123	299	0.1
Milk, skim	1 cup	86	9	0.44	0.33	11.5	0	0	4	126	302	0.1
Milk, whole	1 cup	150	8.5	7.67	5	11	0	0	33	120	291	0.1
Cheese spread	2 tablespoons	81	3.5	6.56	4.33	2	0	1	89	293	95	1
Cheese, American	1 ounce, 1 slice	106	6.75	8.22	5.44	0.5	0	0	27	406	174	0.1
Cheese, cheddar	1 ounce, 1 slice	113	7.5	8.67	5.89	0.5	0	0	30	177	203	0.2
Cheese, cottage	½ cup	113	14.5	4.78	3.11	3	0	0	17	440	65	0.2
Cheese, cottage, nonfat	½ cup	90	14	0	0	7	0	0	10	400	60	0
Cheese, cottage, lowfat	½ cup	96	15	1.22	0.78	4	0	0	5	440	74	0.2
Cheese, mozzarella	1 ounce, 1 slice	80	6	5.67	3.67	0.5	0	0	22	106	147	0.1
Cheese, mozzarella, light	1 ounce	72	7.25	4.11	2.78	0.75	0	0	16	150	183	0.1
Cheese, parmesan	1 tablespoon	23	2.25	1.44	0.89	0.25	0	0	4	93	69	0.1
Cheese, provolone	1 ounce, 1 slice	100	7.75	7	4.78	0.5	0	0	20	248	214	0.2
Cheese, reduced fat	1 ounce	80	8	5	3	1	0	0	20	220	350	0
Cheese, ricotta	½ cup	216	15	14.89	10	3.75	0	0	63	104	257	0.5
Cheese, ricotta, part skim	½ cup	166	14.5	8.67	5.67	6.25	0	0	37	143	369	0.3
Cheese, Swiss	1 ounce	101	8	6.89	4.67	0.75	0	0	25	231	246	0.1
Ice cream	½ cup	148	2.5	7.44	4.67	4.5	11.75	0.2	30	58	88	0.3
Ice milk	½ cup	110	3	2.78	1.89	10	8	0.3	8	75	100	1
Tofutti	½ cup	150	2.5	6.67	1.11	9	11	1.5	0	105	1	0.6
Yogurt, frozen	½ cup	100	3	1.78	1.11	8	10.25	0.1	7	59	100	1
Yogurt, lowfat w/fruit	1 container	240	9	3	2	27	16	0.3	10	120	330	1
Yogurt, nonfat w/fruit	1 container	95	3.5	0	0	8	12	0	0	70	150	1
Yogurt, plain, lowfat	1 container	142	11.25	3.67	2.44	15.75	0	0	15	160	422	0.6
Yogurt, plain, nonfat	1 container	110	11	0.22	0.22	16	0	0	4	160	430	1
Yogurt, plain, whole milk	1 container	145	8.75	6.89	4.56	11.5	0	0	32	123	312	0.6
Yogurt, w/frt, art. swtner	1 container	90	7	0.67	0.44	14	0	0.5	5	110	250	1

FATS/SWEETS/OTHER

Name	Amount/Unit	Cal	Pro. g	TFat g	SFat g	Carb. g	Sug. g	Fbr. g	Chol. mg	Sod. mg	Calc. mg	Iron mg
Bacon	1 slice	36	5.25	1.78	0.67	0	0	0	12	360	2	0.2
Bacon bits	1 tablespoon	21	2.5	1.11	0.33	0	0	0	6	181	1	0.1
Butter	1 tablespoon	104	0	11.44	7.22	0	0	0	32	119	2	1
Gravy	¼ cup	30	1	1.44	0.56	2.25	0.5	0.1	1	260	3	0.4
Lard	1 tablespoon	115	0	12.22	5	0	0	0	12	0	0	0
Margarine, stick	1 tablespoon	101	0	10.56	2	0	0	0	0	133	4	0
Margarine, stick, light	1 tablespoon	60	0	6.67	1	0	0	0	0	110	1	1
Margarine, tub	1 tablespoon	101	0	8.89	2	0	0	0	0	152	4	0
Margarine, tub, light	1 tablespoon	50	0	5.89	1	0	0	0	0	110	1	1
Mayonnaise	1 tablespoon	100	0.25	11	1.89	0.25	0.25	0	8	74	1	1
Mayonnaise, light	1 tablespoon	48	0.25	4.56	1	0.75	1	0	5	95	1	1
Mayonnaise, nonfat	1 tablespoon	12	0	0	0	3	3	0	0	190	0	0
Miracle Whip	1 tablespoon	64	0	5.89	0.89	2.5	0.5	0	5	95	2	1
Miracle Whip, nonfat	1 tablespoon	20	0	0	0	5	5	0	0	210	0	0
Oil	1 tablespoon	120	0	12.78	1.89	0	0	0	0	0	0	0.1
Salad dressing	1 tablespoon	80	0	8.22	1.33	0.25	0.25	1	0	146	2	1
Salad dressing, light	1 tablespoon	16	0.25	0.33	0.11	0.75	0.5	0.3	0	137	1	1
Salad dressing, no oil	1 tablespoon	12	0	0	0	2.5	0	0.7	0	0	1	1
Salad dressing, nonfat	1 tablespoon	16	0	0	0	3	3	0	0	143	0	0
Brownie	1¾″ square	150	2	6.22	1.67	6.5	15	0.9	10	105	1	0.7
Cake	1 piece/slice	280	4	11.33	3	15.25	22.25	0.5	56	285	57	1
Candy, choc/peanut butter	1 pkg, 1½ oz	237	6	13.78	5.89	4	22	2.5	3	90	34	0.7
Candy, chocolate	1 ounce piece	150	2	8.22	4.78	2.25	15	0.8	6	24	50	0.3
Candy, chocolate covered	1 ounce	132	1.25	5.56	2.11	3	13.25	1.5	3	43	33	0.4
Candy, fudge	1″ cube	88	0.75	3	0.78	1.25	13.25	0.3	2	40	20	0.2
Candy, hard	5 pieces	110	0	0	0	0	27.5	0	0	7	1	0.1
Cookies, fig bars	2 fig bars	100	1	1.78	0.44	10.5	10.5	1.2	1	90	20	0.7
Cookies, oatmeal raisin	3 cookies	195	2.25	8.11	1.89	13.5	13.5	1.4	1	150	0	0.8
Cookies, other	3 cookies	180	1.5	8.11	2.89	10	15	0.3	3	131	1	0.7
Danish	1 roll	252	4.5	11.67	3.67	10.25	19	0.7	14	249	36	1.1
Diet bar	1 bar	120	2	4	1.44	19	9.5	3	1	30	150	2.7
Doughnut or sweet roll	1 serving	201	3	8.11	2.89	12.5	13.25	0.6	19	145	21	0.8
Frozen desserts, nonfat	½ cup	100	2	0.22	0.11	23.5	9.5	0.4	1	48	100	0
Frzn yogurt cone, lowfat	1 serving	105	4	1	0.56	22	13	0.1	3	80	112	0.2
Frzn yogurt sundae, lowfat	1 serving	240	6	3	2.33	50.5	43	0.8	6	170	190	0.1
Gelatin	½ cup	105	2	1	1	23	22	0	0	57	0	0
Gelatin, sugar free	½ cup	8	1.5	0	0	0	0	0	0	31	0	0
Granola bars	1 bar	133	2	6	2	18.25	13	0.6	0	70	20	0.5
Pie, custard or cream	⅙ of 9″ pie	346	6.75	13.11	6.22	20.75	25.75	1	125	375	122	0.8
Pie, fruit	⅙ of 9″ pie	405	4	16.22	5.33	34.75	25.25	4	6	423	17	1.6
Pie, pecan	⅙ of 9″ pie	575	7	29.67	5.67	33	37.25	2.2	100	305	65	4.6
Pudding	½ cup	150	4.5	2.22	1.44	10	18	0	9	443	152	0
Pudding, diet	½ cup	90	4	2.44	1.56	13	0	0.4	9	423	152	0.1
Cream, whipped	1 tablespoon	15	0.25	1.33	1.11	0.25	0.25	0	2	4	3	1

continued

Fats, Sweets, Other, continued

Name	Amount/Unit	Cal	Pro. g	TFat g	SFat g	Carb. g	Sug. g	Fbr. g	Chol. mg	Sod. mg	Calc. mg	Iron mg
Dessert topping, no sugar	1 tablespoon	5	0	0.56	0.44	0	0	1	4	5	2	1
Jam or jelly	2 teaspoons	35	0	0	0	1	7.5	0.1	0	1	1	1
Cream, coffee, half&half	1 tablespoon	25	0.5	2.22	1.44	0.5	0	0	8	6	15	0
Nutrasweet, Equal	1 packet	4	0.5	0	0	0	0.5	0	0	0	0	0
Saccharin	1 packet	2	0	0	0	0	0	0	0	2	0	0
Salt	4 shakes	0	0	0	0	0	0	0	0	64	0	0
Sugar	1 teaspoon	15	0	0	0	0	3.75	0	0	0	0	0
Syrup, pancake, table	2 tablespoons	110	0	0	0	0	27.5	0	0	21	1	1
Coffee whitener	1 tablespoon	22	0	2.11	1.33	0	1	0	0	12	1	1
Cream cheese	2 tablespoons	106	2.5	10.22	6.67	1	0	0	34	90	24	0.4
Cream cheese, light	2 tablespoons	80	3	7	4	1	0	0	25	115	20	1
Sour cream	1 tablespoon	26	0.25	2.56	1.56	0.5	0	0	5	17	14	0
Sour cream, imitation	1 tablespoon	25	0.75	2.33	2	0.75	0	0	1	10	7	0
Sour cream, nonfat	1 tablespoon	8	1	0	0	1	0	0	0	10	20	0
Catsup	1 tablespoon	17	0	0	0	2.75	1.5	0.2	0	168	3	0.1
Cheese sauce	¼ cup	71	3.5	3.56	1.89	6.5	0	0	10	412	139	0.1
Chili sauce	1 tablespoon	17	0.25	0	0	2.75	1.25	0.9	0	196	2	0.1
Hollandaise sauce	¼ cup	230	2.25	23.22	8.44	2.5	0	0	140	316	50	1
Mustard	1 teaspoon	6	0.25	0.33	0	0.25	0	0	0	60	0	0
Olives	3 olives	15	0.25	1.56	0.22	0.25	0	0.3	0	234	8	0.2
Pickles, dill	2 spears	7	0	0.11	0	1	0.75	0.9	0	584	9	0.4
Pickles, sweet	1 pickle, 3 sl.	18	0	0	0	0.5	4	0.3	0	107	2	0.2
Soy sauce	1 tablespoon	10	1.25	0	0	1.25	0	0	0	1015	3	0.4
Steak,Worcestershire sce	1 tablespoon	11	0	0	0	1	1.75	0	0	143	0	0
White sauce	¼ cup	99	2.5	5.67	2.22	6	0	0.1	8	222	73	0.2
Soup, beef or chicken	1 cup	74	4.25	2.22	0.67	8.5	0	1	7	910	17	0.9
Soup, bouillon, broth	1 cube/packet	9	0.75	0.22	0.11	0.25	1	0	1	965	1	0.1
Soup, broth based, no salt	1 cup	135	5.75	3.89	0.78	16.5	0	2.8	0	115	47	1.8
Soup, cream, chowder	1 cup	140	5.5	6.11	2.89	14	0	0.9	22	1010	150	0.6
Soup, low salt	1 cup	110	4	3	1	12	0	0.5	2	100	17	1.3
Soup, miso	1 cup	152	4.5	6.44	0.89	19	0	3	0	490	20	1.3
Breakfast milk powder	1 packet	130	6	0	0	0	26.25	0.4	0	185	80	4.5
Hot chocolate mix	1 envelope	110	1.5	2.78	1.56	3.5	16	1.1	2	165	40	0.7
Meal replacement bar	1 serving	270	11	14	5	24	22.5	0	0	330	250	4.5
Milkshake	10 oz, 1¼ cup	368	10	12.78	8.22	26.5	19.25	0.5	54	243	375	0.5
Milkshake, lowfat	1 serving	320	10.75	1.33	0.56	66	44.75	0	10	170	327	0.1
Popcorn	1 cup	32	0.75	1.44	0.44	5.5	0	0.8	0	68	0	0.2
Potato chips, corn chips	1 cup	152	2	9.44	1.78	15	0	1.4	0	229	15	0.4
Pretzels	⅔ cup	110	2.75	0.89	0.22	21.75	1	0.9	0	610	9	1.4
Tortilla chips	1 cup	95	1.25	4.67	1.33	12	0	0.9	0	123	23	0.3

B

PROTEIN FOODS

Name	Amount/Unit	Cal	Pro. g	TFat g	SFat g	Carb. g	Sug. g	Fbr. g	Chol. mg	Sod. mg	Calc. mg	Iron mg
Biscuit w/egg, meat, cheese	1 biscuit	489	18.75	31.22	9.67	29	4	0.8	347	1240	151	2.9
Egg salad	½ cup	267	11	22.89	5.78	1	3	0.3	418	513	43	1.8
Egg, boiled, poached	1 egg	79	6.5	5.56	2.11	0.5	0	0	274	69	28	1
Egg, fried, scrambled	1 egg	89	6.25	6.78	3	1	0	0	281	150	37	0.9
Egg, omelet	1 omelet	342	23.25	25.44	12.56	4	0	0	861	553	243	2.8
Egg, substitute	¼ cup	43	5.5	1.56	0.22	1.5	0	0	0	115	30	0.8
Chicken breast sandwich	1 sandwich	509	26	26.89	4.78	34.75	1.75	1.2	83	1082	80	2.7
Chicken salad	½ cup	179	14.75	12.22	2.89	0.75	0.75	0.3	118	329	21	0.9
Chicken wings	10 wings	1282	90	91.11	35.78	11.5	5	0.2	326	1750	62	4
Chicken, turkey, no skin	4 ounces	137	27.25	3.33	1.11	0	0	0	77	58	12	1.3
Chicken, turkey, w/skin	4 ounces	145	19.75	7.22	2.44	0	0	0	57	49	10	0.9
Chicken, fried, no skin	4 ounces	107	19.25	4.22	1.33	0.25	0	0	50	46	9	0.8
Chicken, fried, w/skin	4 ounces	206	21	11.22	3.22	6.25	0	0.2	69	199	14	1.1
Chicken, mixed dish	1 cup	365	15.25	17.78	5.56	13.5	0	1	103	600	30	2.2
Beef stew	1 cup	207	15.25	9	4.22	16.5	0.5	2.5	53	616	29	2.6
Beef, corned	4 ounces	242	24.25	16.11	7	0	0.25	0	87	1024	15	2
Beef, grnd, hmbrgr, not fried	4 ounces	200	21.25	13.67	6.11	0	0	0	70	60	8	1.9
Beef, grnd, hmbrgr, fried	4 ounces	207	21.25	13.56	5.89	0	0	0	68	62	8	1.9
Beef, mixed dish	1 cup	310	19.25	13.56	5.89	23.5	1.25	2.1	68	840	52	3.5
Beef, roast beef	4 ounces	198	21.25	11.11	4.89	0	0	0	59	47	6	2.1
Cheeseburger (large) w/roll	1 sandwich	711	32	43.33	16.78	33	4	1	113	1164	295	5
Cheeseburger (lowfat) w/roll	1 sandwich	370	24	14	5	35	3.5	1.6	75	890	200	3.6
Cheeseburger (small) w/roll	1 sandwich	461	29	27.56	13.67	25.25	3	0.8	95	906	245	3.3
Hamburger (large) w/roll	1 sandwich	594	27.5	33	12.67	33.25	2	0.9	101	688	87	4.8
Hamburger (lowfat) w/roll	1 sandwich	320	22	10	4	35	3.5	1.6	60	670	150	3.6
Hamburger (small) w/roll	1 sandwich	355	22	19.33	8.22	22.25	3	1.7	95	556	71	3.2
Liver	4 ounces	169	23.5	6	2.67	3.25	0	0	344	69	10	7.7
Pate	1 tablespoon	41	2	3.67	1.44	0	0	0	51	91	9	0.7
Roast beef sandwich	1 sandwich	353	27.25	14.89	7.33	30.25	2.25	0.7	49	766	87	4.1
Tripe	4 ounces	61	12.5	1.11	0.67	0	0	0	58	44	77	0.3
Veal	4 ounces	177	21.75	9.78	4.78	0	0	0	78	52	9	2.7
Veal, mixed dish	1 serving	327	28.25	17.78	9.78	9.5	0.75	1.7	137	634	138	3.7
Bacon substitute	1 strip	52	3	4.11	1.56	0	0	0	13	207	1	0.2
Ham	4 ounces	165	21	8.67	3.11	0	0	0	54	1419	8	1
Hot dog	1 hot dog	144	5.75	12.89	5.22	0.25	1.25	0	30	547	20	0.7
Hot dog and roll	1 sandwich	298	9.25	17.56	6.67	20	2.5	0.7	29	880	60	2.2
Pork feet	8 ounces	138	14.5	8.78	3.22	0	0	0	71	597	32	1.1
Pork rinds	4 ounces	610	69	34.67	13.33	0	0	0	106	3033	25	0.7
Pork spareribs	4 ounces	176	13.75	13.11	5.22	0	0	0	54	41	21	0.8
Pork, fresh, fried	4 ounces	192	14.5	14.89	5.67	0	0	0	55	33	5	0.5
Pork, fresh, roasted	4 ounces	164	15.75	10.22	3.89	0	0	0	54	37	4	0.6
Sausage	1 ounce	88	4	7.44	2.89	0	0.5	0	14	258	4	0.4
Lamb	4 ounces	225	26.25	14.78	7.11	0	0	0	91	65	10	2
Caviar	1 tablespoon	40	4.25	2.11	0.78	0.5	0	0	94	240	44	1.8
Clams, oysters, shrimp, fried	4 pieces	103	5.25	6.11	1.11	6	0	0.1	23	183	20	0.6
Clams, oysters, shrimp	½ cup	71	12.25	1.22	0.33	2.5	0	0	62	108	41	6
Crabmeat	3 ounces	86	12.5	1	0.22	4.5	0	0	26	713	25	0.4
Fish casserole	1 cup	407	18.5	23.78	7.56	26.25	0.75	1.8	70	1314	182	2.3
Fish sandwich	1 sandwich	488	19	26.56	5.89	39.25	3.75	1.5	70	928	46	2
Fish, fried	4 ounces	279	11.5	15.33	3.56	21.5	1.5	0.9	52	467	0	0.7

continued

Protein Foods, continued

Name	Amount/Unit	Cal	Pro. g	TFat g	SFat g	Carb. g	Sug. g	Fbr. g	Chol. mg	Sod. mg	Calc. mg	Iron mg
Fish, not fried	4 ounces	108	22.75	1.33	0.44	10	0	0	60	76	17	0.5
Fish, smoked, pickled	1 ounce	56	6.25	2.33	0.67	0	0	0	14	235	5	0.3
Seafood or fish salad	½ cup	160	13.5	9.78	2.33	1.75	0.25	0.4	142	250	31	0.9
Tuna in oil	½ cup	142	22	5.44	1.11	0	0	0	18	275	7	0.8
Tuna in water	½ cup	90	19.25	1.44	0.44	0	0	0	28	400	0	0.7
Chili con carne	1 cup	286	15.75	12.44	5.78	28.5	0	6.5	43	964	86	3
Chili, vegetarian	1 cup	240	18	12	1.78	13	2	16.4	0	860	6	3.2
Luncheon meat, beef, pork	1 ounce slice	76	4.25	6.11	2.56	0	0.5	0	18	348	3	0.4
Luncheon meat, chkn, trky	1 ounce slice	32	5.75	0.67	0.22	0	0	0	12	358	3	0.3
Pepperoni	1 slice	27	1.25	2.33	0.89	0.25	0	0	5	112	1	0.1
Pizza, cheese topping	2 slices	352	21.75	13.44	7.33	36.25	0.75	3	33	890	474	2.3
Pizza, French bread	1 slice	410	17.5	19.22	8	39	2	2	35	1030	200	2.7
Pizza, meat topping	2 slices	445	25	17	8	50	0.5	4.3	31	906	263	3
Pizza, vegetable topping	2 slices	419	24.75	10.33	5.56	64.25	1	10	19	685	285	5
Chop suey	1 cup	300	26	16	4.33	13	0	1.5	68	1053	60	4.8
Chow mein, beef or chicken	¾ cup	65	6.5	1.44	0.56	5.25	0.75	1.4	26	845	80	1.3
Eggroll	1 eggroll	173	6.75	4.56	0.89	25	3	0.8	7	471	20	1.1
Sweet & sour chicken, pork	1 cup	426	17.5	13.89	3.33	23.5	31.75	1.3	83	1209	27	1.9
Burrito	2 burritos	426	16	14.33	7.11	57.75	0	6.4	65	1116	105	4.5
Chimichanga	1 chimichanga	425	18.5	17.11	8.33	41.25	0	5.2	30	933	145	4
Enchilada	1 enchilada	322	10.5	16.89	9.67	30	0	5.8	42	1052	276	2.2
Taco	1 small	370	21	18.44	11.11	26.5	0	3.4	57	802	221	2.4
Taco salad	1½ cup	279	13.5	13.33	6.67	24	0	4.3	44	763	192	2.3
Tostada	1 tostada	325	13.75	13.89	9.67	28	0	7.5	40	834	214	2.2
Beans, baked	½ cup	140	6	1.67	0.67	15	7.5	6	8	423	60	2.1
Beans, black	½ cup	113	6.5	0.33	0.11	20.75	0	4.4	0	1	24	1.8
Beans, kidney, pinto	½ cup	115	6.5	0.33	0.11	22.25	0	4.5	0	2	33	2.4
Beans, kidney, pinto, canned	½ cup	104	5.75	0.22	0	19.5	0	6.1	0	445	35	1.6
Beans, lima	½ cup	94	5.5	0.22	0.11	17.5	0	4.6	0	26	25	1.8
Beans, lima, canned	½ cup	93	4.75	0.22	0.11	17.5	0	5.8	0	309	35	2
Beans, navy, chickpeas	½ cup	132	6.75	1	0.22	23.75	0	4.8	0	4	52	2.4
Beans, navy, chickpeas, cnd	½ cup	146	7	0.78	0.11	27.5	0	5	0	473	51	2
Beans, white, canned	½ cup	153	8.25	0.22	0.11	29.25	0	5	0	7	96	3.9
Beans, white, split peas	½ cup	125	7	0.22	0.11	23	0	5.3	0	2	66	2.6
Broadbeans, fava	½ cup	93	5.5	0.22	0	17	0	4.4	0	4	31	1.3
Broadbeans, fava, canned	½ cup	91	6	0.11	0	16.25	0	4.5	0	580	34	1.3
Chickpeas	½ cup	138	6.5	1.67	0.11	24.75	0	4.8	0	183	39	2
Lentils	½ cup	115	7.75	0.22	0	20.25	0	2.8	0	2	19	3.3
Peas, black eyed	½ cup	100	5.75	0.33	0.11	18.25	0	8.3	0	3	21	2.2
Peas, black eyed, canned	½ cup	92	5	0.33	0.11	16.5	0	8.2	0	359	24	1.2
Soybeans, roasted	¼ cup	205	14.25	10.22	1.56	13.5	0	1.9	0	1	89	2
Tahini	1 tablespoon	92	2.5	7.33	1.11	3.75	0	1.5	0	10	109	2.2
Nuts, mixed	3 tablespoons	170	4.25	13.56	2.22	6.25	0	1.6	0	170	20	1.1
Peanut butter	2 tablespoons	190	9	14.56	2.78	4.5	2	2.4	0	150	11	0.6
Peanuts	3 tablespoons	164	6.25	12.33	1.78	5.25	0	2.5	0	110	7	0.5

C Nutritional Content of Popular Items from Fast-Food Restaurants

Arby's

	Serving size	Calories	Protein	Total fat	Saturated fat	Total carbohydrate	Sugars	Fiber	Cholesterol	Sodium	Vitamin A	Vitamin C	Calcium	Iron	% calories from fat
	g		g	g	g	g	g	g	mg	mg	% Daily Value				
Regular roast beef	155	383	22	18	7	35	N/A	N/A	43	936	*	*	6	27	42
Super roast beef	254	552	24	28	8	54	N/A	N/A	43	1174	3	15	9	36	46
Light roast beef deluxe	182	294	18	10	4	33	N/A	N/A	42	826	4	13	13	25	31
Roast chicken club	238	503	31	27	7	37	N/A	N/A	46	1143	*	13	18	16	48
Turkey sub	277	486	33	19	5	47	N/A	N/A	51	2033	10	22	40	26	35
Light roast turkey deluxe	195	260	20	6	2	33	N/A	N/A	33	1262	4	20	13	19	21
Italian sub	297	671	34	39	13	47	N/A	N/A	69	2062	10	19	41	24	52
Potato cakes	85	204	2	12	2	20	N/A	N/A	0	397	*	15	*	8	53
Cheddar fries	142	399	6	22	9	46	N/A	N/A	9	443	*	*	8	8	50
Roast chicken salad (no dressing)	400	204	24	7	3	12	N/A	N/A	43	508	97	85	17	11	31
Thousand island dressing	62	298	1	29	4	10	N/A	N/A	24	493	2	2	*	4	88
Jamocha shake	326	368	9	11	3	59	N/A	N/A	35	262	6	*	25	*	27
Ham/cheese croissant	119	345	16	21	12	29	N/A	N/A	90	939	*	*	15	15	55

N/A: not available.
*Contains less than 2% of the Daily Value of these nutrients.

Burger King

	Serving size	Calories	Protein	Total fat	Saturated fat	Total carbohydrate	Sugars	Fiber	Cholesterol	Sodium	Vitamin A	Vitamin C	Calcium	Iron	% calories from fat
	g		g	g	g	g	g	g	mg	mg	% Daily Value				
Whopper®	270	640	27	39	11	45	8	3	90	870	10	15	8	25	55
Whopper Jr.®	168	420	21	24	8	29	5	2	60	570	4	8	6	20	51
Double Whopper® with cheese	375	960	52	63	24	46	8	3	195	1360	15	15	25	40	59
BK Big Fish sandwich	255	720	25	43	8	59	4	2	60	1090	2	2	6	20	54
BK Broiler® chicken sandwich	248	540	30	29	6	41	3	2	80	480	4	10	4	30	48
Chicken Tenders®	88	250	16	12	3	14	0	2	35	530	*	*	*	4	43
Broiled chicken salad (no dressing)	302	200	21	10	5	7	4	3	60	110	100	25	15	20	45
Garden salad (no dressing)	215	90	6	5	3	7	0	3	15	110	110	50	15	6	50
Bleu cheese salad dressing	30	160	2	16	4	1	0	<1	30	260	*	*	*	*	90
French fries (medium)	116	400	5	20	5	43	0	3	0	240	*	4	*	6	45
Onion rings	124	310	4	14	2	41	6	5	0	810	*	*	*	*	41
Chocolate shake (medium)	284	310	9	7	4	54	48	3	20	230	6	*	20	10	20
Croissan'wich® w/bacon, egg, and cheese	118	350	15	24	8	18	2	<1	225	790	8	*	15	10	62
French toast sticks	141	500	4	27	7	60	11	1	0	490	*	*	6	15	49
Dutch apple pie	113	310	3	15	3	39	22	2	0	230	*	10	*	8	44

*Contains less than 2% of the Daily Value of these nutrients.

Domino's Pizza

(1 serving = 2 slices for hand-tossed and deep-dish pizzas, ⅓ of pizza for thin-crust pizzas)

	Serving size	Calories	Protein	Total fat	Saturated fat	Total carbohydrate	Sugars	Fiber	Cholesterol	Sodium	Vitamin A	Vitamin C	Calcium	Iron	% calories from fat
	g		g	g	g	g	g	g	mg	mg	% Daily Value				
Hand-tossed—cheese	147	344	15	10	4	50	1	2	19	981	9	4	28	22	26
pepperoni	159	406	18	15	7	50	1	3	32	1179	9	5	28	24	33
extra cheese & pepperoni	175	455	21	19	9	51	1	3	42	1304	12	5	41	25	38
ham	161	362	17	10	5	50	1	2	26	1143	9	5	28	23	25
Ital. sausage & mushroom	176	403	18	14	6	52	1	3	31	1151	10	5	29	25	31
veggie	176	360	15	10	5	52	1	3	19	1028	10	21	29	18	25
Thin crust—cheese	141	364	16	16	6	40	2	2	26	1012	11	6	42	8	40
pepperoni	157	447	20	23	9	40	2	2	43	1277	12	6	43	10	46
extra cheese & pepperoni	178	512	24	28	12	41	2	2	56	1443	15	6	60	12	49
ham	159	388	19	17	7	41	3	2	35	1229	11	6	42	9	39
Ital. sausage & mushroom	179	442	20	21	9	43	3	3	41	1240	12	7	43	12	43
veggie	179	386	17	17	7	43	3	3	26	1076	12	28	43	11	40
Deep dish—cheese	205	560	24	24	9	63	4	3	32	1184	15	5	45	27	39
pepperoni	218	621	26	29	11	63	4	3	45	1383	16	5	46	28	42
extra cheese & pepperoni	235	671	30	33	13	64	4	3	54	1508	18	5	59	29	44
ham	220	577	26	25	9	64	5	3	38	1347	15	5	45	27	40
Ital. sausage & mushroom	236	618	26	28	11	66	5	4	43	1356	16	6	46	29	41
veggie	236	576	24	25	9	65	5	4	32	1233	16	22	46	28	39

Jack in the Box

	Serving size	Calories	Protein	Total fat	Saturated fat	Total carbohydrate	Sugars	Fiber	Cholesterol	Sodium	Vitamin A	Vitamin C	Calcium	Iron	% calories from fat
	g		g	g	g	g	g	g	mg	mg	% Daily Value				
Breakfast Jack®	121	300	18	12	5	30	5	0	185	890	8	15	20	15	36
Supreme croissant	172	570	21	36	15	39	4	2	245	1240	15	20	10	20	57
Hamburger	97	280	13	11	4	31	5	0	25	470	2	2	10	15	35
Jumbo Jack®	229	560	26	32	10	41	6	0	65	740	4	10	10	25	51
Grilled sourdough burger	223	670	32	43	16	39	4	0	110	1180	15	10	20	25	58
Chicken fajita pita	189	290	24	8	3	29	<1	3	35	700	10	10	25	15	25
Grilled chicken fillet	211	430	29	19	5	36	7	0	65	1070	6	10	15	35	40
Chicken supreme	245	620	25	36	11	48	5	0	75	1520	10	4	20	15	52
Monterey roask beef sandwich	238	540	30	30	9	40	4	3	75	1270	8	8	30	20	50
Garden chicken salad	253	200	23	9	4	8	4	3	65	420	70	20	20	4	41
Blue cheese dressing	57	210	1	18	4	11	3	0	15	750	0	0	0	0	77
Chicken teriyaki bowl	440	580	28	2	<1	115	20	6	30	1220	110	15	10	10	3
Super taco	126	280	12	17	6	22	1	3	30	720	0	4	15	10	55
Egg rolls (3 pieces)	165	440	3	24	7	54	6	4	30	960	0	6	8	15	49
Chicken strips (6 pieces)	177	450	39	20	5	28	<1	0	80	1100	0	0	0	6	40
Stuffed jalapeños (7 pieces)	136	420	15	27	12	29	3	3	55	1620	15	15	35	4	58
Barbeque dipping sauce	28	45	1	0	0	11	7	0	0	300	0	0	0	0	0
Seasoned curly fries	109	360	5	20	5	39	0	4	0	1070	0	8	2	8	50
Onion rings	103	380	5	23	6	38	4	0	0	450	0	4	2	10	54
Chocolate milkshake	322	390	9	6	4	74	66	<1	25	210	*	*	30	4	14

*Contains less than 2% of the Daily Value of these nutrients.

KFC

	Serving size	Calories	Protein	Total fat	Saturated fat	Total carbohydrate	Sugars	Fiber	Cholesterol	Sodium	Vitamin A	Vitamin C	Calcium	Iron	% calories from fat
	g		g	g	g	g	g	g	mg	mg	% Daily Value				
Original Recipe®: breast	137	360	33	20	5	12	0	1	115	870	*	*	6	6	50
thigh	92	260	19	17	5	9	0	1	110	570	*	*	4	6	59
Extra Tasty Crispy™: breast	168	470	31	28	7	25	0	1	80	930	*	*	4	6	54
thigh	118	370	19	25	6	18	0	2	70	540	*	*	2	6	61
Hot & Spicy: breast	180	530	32	35	8	23	0	2	110	1110	*	*	4	6	59
thigh	107	370	18	27	7	13	0	1	90	570	*	*	*	6	66
Tender Roast™: breast (as served)	139	251	37	11	3	1	<1	0	151	830	*	*	*	*	39
breast (skin removed)	118	169	32	4	1	1	0	0	112	797	*	*	*	*	23
thigh (as served)	90	207	18	12	4	<2	<1	0	120	504	*	*	*	*	52
thigh (skin removed)	59	106	13	6	2	<1	<1	0	84	312	*	*	*	*	46
Hot Wings™ Pieces	135	471	27	33	8	18	N/A	N/A	150	1230	*	*	4	8	63
Crispy Strips™ (3)	92	261	20	16	4	10	0	3	40	658	*	*	*	3	25
Pot pie	368	770	29	42	13	69	8	5	70	2160	80	2	10	10	49
Corn on the cob	151	222	4	12	2	27	4	8	0	76	4	3	0	2	49
Mashed potatoes w/gravy	120	109	1	5	<1	16	0	2	<1	386	*	*	*	*	41
Mean Greens™	111	52	3	2	1	8	1	3	6	477	43	8	14	9	35
BBQ baked beans	110	132	5	2	1	24	9	4	3	535	5	0	4	8	14
Garden rice	107	75	2	1	0	15	1	1	0	576	7	9	1	1	12
Cole slaw	90	114	1	6	1	13	N/A	N/A	<5	177	*	45	3	2	47
Biscuit (1)	56	200	3	12	3	20	2	1	2	564	*	*	4	6	54

N/A: not available.

*Contains less than 2% of the Daily Value of these nutrients.

McDonald's

	Serving size	Calories	Protein	Total fat	Saturated fat	Total carbohydrate	Sugars	Fiber	Cholesterol	Sodium	Vitamin A	Vitamin C	Calcium	Iron	% calories from fat
	g		g	g	g	g	g	g	mg	mg	% Daily Value				
Hamburger	105	270	12	10	4	34	6	2	30	520	2	4	15	15	33
Cheeseburger	120	320	15	14	6	35	6	2	45	750	6	4	15	15	39
Quarter-Pounder®	172	420	23	21	8	37	7	2	70	690	4	4	15	25	45
Quarter-Pounder® w/cheese	200	530	28	30	13	38	8	2	95	1160	10	4	15	25	51
Big Mac®	216	530	25	28	10	47	8	3	80	960	6	4	20	25	48
Filet-O-Fish®	143	360	14	16	4	40	6	2	35	690	2	*	10	10	40
McGrilled Chicken Classic®	189	260	24	4	1	33	6	2	45	500	4	8	10	10	14
French fries (large)	147	450	6	22	4	57	0	5	0	290	*	30	2	6	44
Chicken McNuggets® (6 pc)	109	300	19	18	4	16	0	0	65	530	*	*	2	6	54
Barbeque sauce	28	45	0	0	0	10	10	0	0	250	*	6	*	*	0
Garden salad (no dressing)	234	80	6	4	1	7	5	2	140	60	60	35	6	8	45
Fajita chicken salad (no dressing)	285	160	20	6	2	9	6	3	65	400	160	50	4	10	34
Bleu cheese dressing	60	190	2	17	3	8	3	0	30	650	2	*	6	2	81
Lite vinaigrette dressing	62	50	0	2	0	9	6	0	0	240	6	6	*	*	36
Egg McMuffin®	137	290	17	13	5	27	3	1	235	730	10	2	15	15	40
Bacon, egg, cheese biscuit	152	450	17	27	9	33	3	1	240	1340	10	*	10	15	54
Hash browns	53	130	1	8	2	14	0	1	0	330	*	4	*	2	55
Hotcakes w/margarine & syrup	222	580	9	16	3	100	42	2	15	760	8	*	10	15	25
Chocolate shake, small	N/A	340	12	5	3	64	57	1	25	300	4	6	45	4	13
Apple pie	77	260	3	13	4	34	13	<1	0	200	*	40	2	6	45

*Contains less than 2% of the Daily Value of these nutrients.

Taco Bell

	Serving size	Calories	Protein	Total fat	Saturated fat	Total carbohydrate	Sugars	Fiber	Cholesterol	Sodium	Vitamin A	Vitamin C	Calcium	Iron	% calories from fat
	g		g	g	g	g	g	g	mg	mg	% Daily Value				
Taco	78	180	10	11	5	11	N/A	N/A	30	276	7	2	8	6	55
Light taco	78	140	11	5	2	11	N/A	N/A	20	290	6	0	8	0	36
Soft taco	99	220	12	11	5	19	N/A	N/A	30	554	4	2	12	13	45
Light soft taco	99	180	13	5	3	19	N/A	N/A	25	550	4	0	4	6	28
Taco supreme®	106	230	11	15	8	12	N/A	N/A	45	276	11	5	11	6	59
Light taco supreme®	106	160	13	5	2	14	N/A	N/A	20	340	10	4	8	0	31
Light soft taco supreme®	128	200	14	5	3	23	N/A	N/A	25	610	10	4	4	6	25
Tostada w/red sauce	156	243	9	11	4	27	N/A	N/A	16	596	13	75	18	9	41
Chicken soft taco	107	213	14	10	4	19	N/A	N/A	52	615	4	4	8	35	42
Bean burrito w/red sauce	206	357	15	14	4	63	N/A	N/A	9	1148	7	88	19	21	35
Burrito supreme® w/red sauce	255	503	20	22	8	55	N/A	N/A	33	1181	18	43	19	22	39
Fiesta bean burrito	114	226	8	9	3	29	N/A	N/A	9	652	5	57	15	15	35
Nachos Bell Grande®	287	649	22	35	12	61	N/A	N/A	36	997	23	96	30	19	48
Chicken Mexi Melt®	107	257	14	15	7	19	N/A	N/A	48	779	10	4	22	20	53
Mexican pizza	223	575	21	37	11	40	N/A	N/A	52	1031	20	51	26	21	58
Taco salad	535	860	32	55	19	64	N/A	N/A	80	910	33	125	32	33	58
Light taco salad	535	680	35	25	N/A	81	N/A	N/A	50	N/A	N/A	N/A	N/A	N/A	33

N/A: not available.

Wendy's

	Serving size	Calories	Protein	Total fat	Saturated fat	Total carbohydrate	Sugars	Fiber	Cholesterol	Sodium	Vitamin A	Vitamin C	Calcium	Iron	% calories from fat
	g		g	g	g	g	g	g	mg	mg	% Daily Value				
Single w/everything	219	420	26	20	7	37	9	3	70	810	6	10	10	30	43
Big Bacon Classic	287	610	36	33	13	45	11	3	105	1510	15	25	25	35	49
Jr. hamburger	117	270	15	10	3	34	7	2	30	560	2	2	10	20	33
Jr. bacon cheeseburger	170	410	22	21	8	34	7	2	60	910	8	15	15	20	46
Grilled chicken sandwich	177	290	24	7	2	35	8	2	55	720	4	10	10	15	22
Caesar side salad (no dressing)	89	110	8	5	2	8	0	2	10	660	35	25	4	6	41
Grilled chicken salad (no dressing)	338	200	25	8	2	10	5	4	50	690	110	60	20	10	36
Taco salad (no dressing)	510	590	29	30	11	53	8	10	65	1230	35	40	40	25	46
Blue cheese dressing (2T)	28	170	1	19	3	0	0	0	15	190	0	0	2	0	100
Ranch dressing, reduced fat (2T)	28	60	0	5	1	2	1	0	10	240	0	0	2	0	75
Soft breadstick	44	130	4	3	1	24	N/A	1	5	250	0	0	4	8	21
French fries, medium	130	380	5	19	4	47	0	5	0	120	0	10	2	6	45
Baked potato w/broccoli & cheese	411	470	9	14	3	80	6	9	5	470	35	120	20	25	27
Baked potato w/chili & cheese	439	620	20	24	9	83	7	9	40	780	20	60	35	30	35
Chili, small, plain	227	210	15	7	3	21	5	5	30	800	8	6	8	15	30
Chili, large w/cheese & crackers	363	405	27	17	7	37	8	7	60	1380	14	10	20	27	38
Chicken nuggets (6)	94	280	14	20	5	12	N/A	0	50	600	0	0	2	4	64
Barbeque sauce	28	50	1	0	0	11	N/A	N/A	0	100	6	0	0	4	0
Frosty dairy dessert, medium	324	460	12	13	7	76	63	4	55	260	10	0	40	6	25
Chicken club sandwich	220	500	32	23	5	44	7	2	70	1090	4	15	10	20	41

N/A: not available.

Index

Boldface numbers indicate pages on which glossary definitions appear. "*t*" indicates that the information is in a table.